AUGMENTATIVE AND ALTERNATIVE COMMUNICATION

AUGMENTATIVE AND ALTERNATIVE COMMUNICATION

A HANDBOOK OF PRINCIPLES AND PRACTICES

LYLE L. LLOYD

Purdue University

DONALD R. FULLER

University of Arkansas at Little Rock

HELEN H. ARVIDSON

Purdue University

ALLYN AND BACON

Boston • London • Toronto • Sydney • Tokyo • Singapore

Senior Vice President and Editor-in-Chief, Education: Nancy Forsyth
Executive Editor: Stephen D. Dragin
Editorial Assistant: Elizabeth McGuire
Cover Administrator: Jenny Hart
Composition Buyer: Linda Cox
Manufacturing Buyer: Suzanne Lareau
Production Coordinator: Deborah Brown
Editorial-Production Service: Anne Rebecca Starr

Copyright © 1997 by Allyn and Bacon
A Viacom Company
160 Gould Street
Needham Heights, Massachusetts 02194

Internet: www.abacon.com
America Online: Keyword: college online

Library of Congress Cataloging-in-Publication Data

Augmentative and alternative communication : a handbook of principles
   and practices / [edited by] Lyle L. Lloyd, Donald R. Fuller, Helen
   H. Arvidson.
      p.   cm.
   Includes bibliographical references and indexes.
   ISBN 0-205-19884-8
   1. Communicative disorders—Patients—Rehabilitation.
   2. Communication devices for the disabled.   I. Lloyd, Lyle L.
   II. Fuller, Donald R.   III. Arvidson, Helen H.
   RC423.A927   1997
   616.85′503—dc21   97-26195
                                             CIP

Printed in the United States of America
10 9 8 7 6 5 4 3 2 1   02 01 00 99 98 97

Dedicated to our spouses—Myrna, Michele, and John—for their tolerance and support throughout the development of this text and our other professional activities.

CONTENTS

PART 2   SYMBOLS

CHAPTER 9   LOW TECHNOLOGY   127

Charlotte A. Wasson, Helen H. Arvidson, and Lyle L. Lloyd

CHAPTER 10   HIGH TECHNOLOGY   137

Raymond W. Quist and Lyle L. Lloyd

PART 4   AAC ASSESSMENT

PART 5   AAC INTERVENTION

CHAPTER 18   INTERVENTION FOR PERSONS WITH DEVELOPMENTAL DISABILITIES   299

Doreen M. Blischak, Filip Loncke, and Amy Waller

CHAPTER 19   INTERVENTION FOR PERSONS WITH ACQUIRED DISORDERS   340

Rajinder Koul, Helen H. Arvidson, and G. S. Pennington

PART 6   CURRENT ISSUES AND TRENDS

PREFACE

Augmentative and alternative communication (AAC) has emerged in recent years as one of the significant advances in special education, speech-language pathology, and other areas that serve individuals with disabilities. AAC is the supplementation and/or replacement of natural speech and/or writing using aided and/or unaided symbols (e.g., Blissymbols, fingerspelling, gestures, ideographs, logographs, manual signs, pictographs) and the related means of selection and transmission of such symbols. The term is also used to refer to the transdisciplinary clinical/educational practice related to the AAC process.

In the 1950s, when I completed the academic and practicum requirements for an Illinois teaching license and for ASHA certification in both audiology and speech-language pathology, none of the university programs offered AAC coursework. That made sense then, because during my first two positions—first at a public school and then as a university aural rehabilitation supervisor—we did not see any students requiring AAC. But times have changed. Schools, university clinics, and other service providers are serving an increasing number of individuals with little or no functional speech. Back then, the common view was that if individuals with little or no functional speech were taught to use manual signs or other alternatives to speaking, it would prevent them from learning to speak. Now we know better. Although personnel preparation programs in special education and speech-language pathology did not teach AAC, many programs emphasized the importance of understanding the scientific bases of clinical/educational practice and the literature and practices of other professionals. We were also taught to question. It was this questioning that ultimately led to the uses of AAC in the 1950s and 1960s.

AAC has come a long way in the last four decades, but it still has a long way to go. AAC evolved primarily from clinical and educational practices with only a limited research base that was extrapolated from other fields. During the last two decades, research directly relevant to AAC clinical/educational practice has emerged. This evolution was reflected by the inclusion of scattered articles in various refereed journals and became more prominent with the initiation of the journal *Augmentative and Alternative Communication* in 1985. The first three AAC courses were offered during the 1977–1978 academic year at Marquette University, Purdue University, and the University of Wisconsin. This led to the publication of the first AAC texts in the early 1980s, the ASHA text in 1986, and subsequent other texts. So why did we write this text? There are several reasons. In two decades of teaching AAC, I have diligently searched for a book with a strong theoretical and research base for professional practice that reflected the transdisciplinary nature of AAC—I wanted a book that could serve as a text for preservice professional preparation and inservice or continuing education, as well as serve as a resource for practicing professionals.

This text is the first to provide an AAC model and taxonomy that can serve as a basis for both application and further development of the field. It is organized into major units, providing basic or fundamental information that leads to practical applications. The practical application chapters provide a systematic and integrated approach to AAC, combining the educational perspective of special education and the clinical perspective of speech-language pathology in a broad transdisciplinary context. Chapter 1 makes a clear distinction between AAC as a process and assistive technology (AT) as the tools. Later chapters focus on AAC symbols as a fundamental element of both aided and unaided AAC. Because these symbols help distinguish AAC from other areas of special education and speech-language pathology, it is important for clinicians/educators to understand why such wide variety is needed and to understand the symbols so they can design optimal AAC systems for each individual. Other chapters focus on the technology that provides the means for some of the symbols to be communicated.

The evolution of AAC as a transdisciplinary field has resulted in confusion in the use of terminology. This text is the first to provide a chapter—Chapter 4—that discusses basic terminology issues. It is also one of the first texts to provide an extensive glossary. Within the chapters, terms representing critical aspects or concepts have been boldfaced; the glossary includes all of these terms as well as additional relevant terms.

This text includes areas that have received little or no attention in most texts—funding based on the legal issues of AAC, due process and expert testimony, and ethics, which is emerging as a critical area in AAC. It also includes full chapters (with additional material integrated throughout the text) on multicultural issues; literacy; communication alternatives to problem behaviors; and seating, other positioning, and motor control.

To orient students to research and literature that support our clinical/educational practice, this text has the most extensive referencing of any published text. These references will also serve as valuable resources for practicing professionals. The appendices further enhance this book's value as a complete resource in the field.

The material in this text is organized so that instructors can customize their courses by selecting the chapters they choose to emphasize depending on their orientation and preference. However, we do recommend that instructors start with the introduction. At Purdue we teach a broad three-credit overview course, a requirement for all students seeking certification as speech-language pathologists or teachers of students with severe disabilities. We also offer elective, advanced AAC courses for one to three credits each, depending on topics and requirements. When we taught the basic three-credit course, we used earlier drafts of Chapters 1 and 3 through 19 as required reading. Chapters 2, 20, and 21 were recommended and discussed briefly. We referred to the materials from Chapters 22 though 25, but did not require or recommend

them. However, several of these chapters were required in our advanced courses.

To facilitate the book's use as a resource or reference, there is a detailed table of contents, a subject index, and an author index.

A text this extensive is the result of the efforts of many individuals. When I began the text, I selected Donald R. Fuller (a former doctoral student) and Helen H. Arvidson (a current doctoral student) to work extensively as my co-editors. We then collaborated in selecting individuals who could author the chapters. This way, we were able to obtain more in-depth coverage of each topic. Most of the contributing authors have done either advanced graduate study or postdoctoral work at Purdue. Although Heleen Bos and Martine Smith (two of the international contributors), Kevin C. McDowell (a lawyer with the Indiana Department of Education), and Orlando Taylor (Howard University) are not part of the Purdue AAC Group, they were selected for their particular expertise. Other members of the AAC Group—particularly Kate Kellum, Lisa Pufpaff, and Amy Waller—have contributed by compiling guides or various resource materials.

The text reflects much that we have learned from our students since we taught our first AAC course 20 years ago. We have learned from both their research and practical questions and their innovative procedures and writing. Therefore, we extend appreciation not only to the contributors but to the many students who have taken AAC courses. Likewise, our colleagues over the past 40 years—especially those who have been active in AAC—have contributed greatly to this text.

I would also like to thank many of my own professors who introduced me to the professions of special education and speech-language pathology. Some contributed to my clinical inquiry and showed me the importance of knowing the *why* and not just the *how* of assessment and intervention. Others contributed to my appreciation and knowledge of the scientific approach to both basic and applied questions. Many contributed to my professional development and my lifelong learning approach. These professors at Eastern Illinois University, University of Illinois, and the University of

Iowa, plus the many others who served as mentors during my various administrative, research, teaching, and service-delivery positions, as well as those in various professional organizations, are too numerous to mention, but I would like to thank two in particular. Wayne L. Thurman, at Eastern Illinois University, was my first professor and mentor and Joseph E. Spradlin, at the Parsons (Kansas) Research Center, was my first colleague mentor. They contributed in many ways, but were probably the greatest influence on my publication efforts, including my approach to this text.

Appreciation goes to the following reviewers for their comments on the manuscript: John M. Costello, Children's Hospital—Boston; Carolyn W. Watkins, Watkins and Associates; Thomas W. King, University of Wisconsin/Eau Claire; Joan Miller, Mount Saint Mary College; Joe Reichle, University of Minnesota; Shirley McNaughton, Ontario Institute for Studies in Education—Toronto; and Linda I. House, SUNY/Geneseo.

Also, we wish to thank our families for their indulgence and support through not only the writing of this text, but in many of our other writing and related professional activities over the years.

We are extremely indebted to those AAC users and their family members who have taught us so much. They not only challenge us to question our strategies and techniques; they provide insights and answers as well.

L.L.L.

List of Contributors

Helen H. Arvidson, Editor
AAC Program, Special Education
Purdue University
West Lafayette, IN 47907

Doreen M. Blischak
Department of Speech Pathology and Audiology
Ball State University
Muncie, IN 47306

Heleen Bos
Institute of General Linguistics
University of Amsterdam
Spuistraat 210
1012 VT Amsterdam
The Netherlands

Donald R. Fuller, Editor
Department of Audiology and Speech Pathology
University of Arkansas at Little Rock
2801 South University Avenue
Little Rock, AR 72204

Mary Blake Huer
Department of Speech Communication
California State University—Fullerton
Fullerton, CA 92634

Kathleen A. Kangas
Department of Speech Pathology and Audiology
Idaho State University
Campus Box 8116
Pocatello, ID 83209

Rajinder Koul
Department of Communication Disorders
Texas Tech Health Sciences Center
Texas Tech University
Lubbock, TX 79409

Filip Loncke
Research Department
Royal Institute
Jules De Streelaan 67
9050 Gentbrugge
Belgium

Lyle L. Lloyd, Editor
Special Education, Audiology, and Speech
    Sciences
Purdue University
West Lafayette, IN 47907

Kevin C. McDowell
Indiana Department of Education
Room 229 State House
Indianapolis, IN 46204

Irene R. McEwen
Department of Physical Therapy
University of Oklahoma
P.O. Box 26901
Oklahoma City, OK 73190

G. S. Pennington
Speech-Language Pathology
Indiana Veterans Home
3851 North River Road
West Lafayette, IN 47906

Raymond W. Quist
Department of Communication Disorders and
    Special Education
Indiana State University
SOE 410
8th and Sycamore Streets
Terre Haute, IN 47809

Ralf W. Schlosser
Bloorview MacMillan Centre
350 Rumsey Road
Toronto, Ontario M4G 1R8
Canada

Martine M. Smith
School of Clinical Speech and Language Studies
Trinity College
184 Pearse Street
Dublin 2
Ireland

Gloria Soto
Department of Special Education
San Francisco State University
San Francisco, CA 94132

Michele M. Stratton
Speech-Language Pathologist
Conway Human Development Center
150 Siebenmorgan Road
Conway, AR 72032

Orlando Taylor
The Graduate School
Howard University
2400 6th Street NW
Washington, DC 20058

Amy Waller
Speech-Language Pathologist
2541 De Soto Road
Sarasota, FL 34234

Charlotte A. Wasson
Total Rehab Services
1206 South 5th Street
Effingham, IL 62041

Carole Zangari
LaBonte Institute for Hearing, Speech,
    and Language
Nova Southeastern University
3375 SW 75th Avenue
Fort Lauderdale, FL 33314

CHAPTER 1

INTRODUCTION AND OVERVIEW

LYLE L. LLOYD, DONALD R. FULLER, AND HELEN H. ARVIDSON

> *. . . If all of my possessions were taken from me with one exception, I would choose the power of communication, for by it I would regain all the rest.*
>
> —Daniel Webster

It has been said many times in many ways that communication is the essence of life. One can see it when an individual glances or gestures to share feelings with a family member or uses a microphone to lecture to a large audience. These two major purposes of communication—socialization and information transfer—can be accomplished by individuals with a wide range of abilities and disabilities not only through natural speech and writing, but also through **augmentative and alternative communication (AAC)**. In recent years AAC, which is the supplementation or replacement of natural speech and/or writing, has allowed many individuals with disabilities to more fully realize their potential and enjoy the essence of life.

AAC is described in this text as being a process. The term is also used, however, to refer to the transdisciplinary field that uses a variety of symbols, strategies, and techniques to assist people who are unable to meet their communication needs through natural speech and/or writing. A wide variety of these are introduced in this text. The defining characteristics that place all these symbols, strategies, and techniques under the category of AAC are that they are either not used or not relied on by most individuals to meet the communication needs of daily life.

In general, AAC symbols and techniques may be divided into two broad categories—**aided** and **unaided** (Lloyd & Fuller, 1986). **Aided communication** involves use of some external device or equipment, which may range from very simple handmade materials, such as a picture board or wallet, to highly complex electronic devices that produce computer-synthesized speech. **Unaided communication** requires no additional pieces of equipment, using only the individual's own body as the mode of communication. One of the most common examples of unaided AAC is manual signing. Gesturing, miming, pointing, and eye gazing are also unaided communication means.

PERSPECTIVES

AAC may be viewed from many perspectives, including those of AAC users as well as etiological, historic, theoretical and fundamental, basic human communication model, assistive technology, assessment, intervention, transdisciplinary and integrated, legal and ethical, and visionary or futuristic. These perspectives are not mutually exclusive, but rather interconnected and interrelated. This chapter provides a brief overview of each of these perspectives, which are discussed in detail in the chapters that follow. Because of its overriding importance, the perspective of the user not only is discussed first in this chapter, but is woven throughout the text.

AAC Users and Etiological Perspectives

> *As long as . . . people considered my brain useless and my facial expressions and*

sounds meaningless, I was doomed to remain "voiceless."

—Ruth Sienkiewicz-Mercer

All the nurses aides were really afraid of me because I was the only person who could not talk.

—Diana Creer-Berti

A growing body of literature provides access to the viewpoints of individuals who use AAC techniques and those who have been recipients of professional services (e.g., Creech, 1992; Sienkiewicz-Mercer & Kaplan, 1989). These reports have important, although sometimes painful, messages regarding communication. Huer and Lloyd (1990) found that frustration was a particularly common theme expressed by AAC users. The frustration seems to be very common among individuals with severe communication disabilities.

> I can remember those silent years when my mind was overflowing with questions that were not being answered: remembering the want to verbalize my thoughts, dreams, and hopes, and desiring to share and grow in my world. Life began turning into a room with many windows and a door without a key. (Marshall, 1990, p. 5)

According to Huer and Lloyd (1990), concerns expressed about professional services included lack of knowledge about severe disabilities and lack of concern or respect for the client as an individual. Concerns included the practices of educational, medical, and speech-language pathology professionals. Most of the users who commented on their devices reported that the devices themselves were valuable, but they continued to believe that communication, not the use of the device, is the key.

> I had a few speech teachers. Every speech teacher had their own way of doing things. I was confused. One would say do it this way and another would say do it another way. The last speech teacher I had in elementary school said "O.K. it's time for a Canon" but the one I had before she came said "Use speech." . . .
>
> [T]he speech teacher did ask me if I liked it [the Canon] and I said "no" but she said, "Hang in there; it's not going to be overnight." Most of the time nobody asked. And, if they did, it didn't seem

to make them change anything. (Dawn, in Smith-Lewis & Ford, 1987, pp. 15–16)

AAC interventions offer valuable options for persons with severe disabilities when individual strengths and needs are carefully assessed and appropriate goals are established. Understanding the etiology of communication disorders is basic to the provision of AAC services. Significant differences exist, for example, between goals developed for children whose communication disorders result from congenital conditions and goals developed for adults who have acquired communication disorders. These differences relate to a variety of aspects, such as the relationship of caregivers to AAC users. Parents often take the major role in directly providing or arranging care and services for their children with congenital conditions, whereas spouses and/or adult children often take the major role in providing or arranging care and services for individuals with acquired disorders. Service providers must be sensitive to the impact that these different relationships can have on the intervention process and use different approaches, as appropriate, with the different caregivers who will be facilitating the communication of the AAC users.

Whether a condition is congenital or acquired may affect a user's level of acceptance or resistance to AAC intervention. Providing functional and motivational intervention is enough to engage some individuals in interactions that will quite naturally lead to improved communication, but may not engage others. Individuals with acquired, progressive disorders, for example, may be dealing with psychological and emotional factors that challenge intervention. Individuals with progressive diseases such as multiple sclerosis or Parkinson's disease may not realize the need to develop AAC skills until the disease has progressed to the point that learning new ways to communicate requires more energy and effort than they can expend. Providing services for individuals with acquired, nonprogressive conditions, such as traumatic brain injury (TBI), that affect language and memory skills, poses still different challenges and underscores the importance of knowing and respecting individual needs and desires.

Individuals with little or no functional speech

usually have related impairments in language, memory, cognition, hearing, vision, and/or motor skills, which must be carefully assessed and addressed. Intervention must be approached with a clear understanding of individual strengths and needs. Individuals do not, however, live in a vacuum. Needs will be influenced by the environments in which individuals live and the people with whom they interact. These influences must be considered carefully if intervention is to be effective.

The perspective of AAC users is of paramount importance in the provision of AAC services. Their needs and desires regarding the direction of the intervention process should be respected. Their rights should be protected. In November 1991, the **American Speech-Language-Hearing Association (ASHA)** approved guidelines developed by the National Joint Committee for the Communication Needs of Persons with Severe Disabilities (1992), which included a Communication Bill of Rights. Following are the 12 specific rights designed to enhance the ability of individuals to affect conditions of their own existence through communication.

1. The right to request desired objects, actions, events, and persons, and to express personal preferences, or feelings.
2. The right to be offered choices and alternatives.
3. The right to reject or refuse undesired objects, events, or actions, including the right to decline or reject all proffered choices.
4. The right to request, and be given, attention from and interaction with another person.
5. The right to request feedback or information about a state, an object, a person, or an event of interest.
6. The right to active treatment and intervention efforts to enable people with severe disabilities to communicate messages in whatever modes and as effectively and efficiently as their specific abilities will allow.
7. The right to have communication acts acknowledged and responded to, even when the intent of these acts cannot be fulfilled by the responder.
8. The right to have access at all times to any needed augmentative and alternative communication devices and other assistive devices, and to have those devices in good working order.
9. The right to environmental contexts, interactions, and opportunities that expect and encourage persons with disabilities to participate as full communicative partners with other people, including peers.
10. The right to be informed about the people, things, and events in one's immediate environment.
11. The right to be communicated with in a manner that recognizes and acknowledges the inherent dignity of the person being addressed, including the right to be part of communication exchanges about individuals that are conducted in his or her presence.
12. The right to be communicated with in ways that are meaningful, understandable, and culturally and linguistically appropriate. (pp. 2–3)

Historic Perspective

History gives us a kind of chart, and we dare not surrender even a small rushlight in the darkness. The hasty reformer who does not remember the past will find himself condemned to repeat it.

—John Buchan

The next best thing to knowing something is knowing where to find it.

—Samuel Johnson

The importance for researchers and clinicians/educators to have a solid historic perspective of their field should not be underestimated. AAC is a relatively young transdisciplinary field with roots in a number of different scientific and technical fields, but it is a professional and scholarly field that has emerged with its own research, **models**, and **taxonomies**. During the last two decades, it has established its own body of literature.

The senior editor of this text, who is currently active in AAC, was also active in the early development of the field, and has had a long-standing interest in the historic perspective. He and others have contributed to the literature on the historic perspective (Galyas, Fant, & Hunnicutt, 1993; Lloyd, 1986, 1993; Lloyd & Karlan, 1984; McNaughton, 1990; Vanderheiden & Yoder, 1986; Zangari, Lloyd, & Vicker, 1994). Chapter 2 discusses the historic perspective in more detail.

Theoretical and Fundamental Perspective

I start where the last man left off.

—Thomas A. Edison

AAC emerged from clinical/educational practice (with little or no research base) out of the need to provide services for individuals who had not benefited from traditional speech therapy. In the 1970s, after anecdotal reports of success with AAC strategies and techniques began to appear, interest in understanding why AAC was successful when more traditional approaches failed became more widespread. Fristoe and Lloyd (1979a) hypothesized 16 factors and characteristics that could account for the facilitative effects reported in the literature. These factors, identified more from clinical/educational observation than research, are based on consideration of AAC as both a stimulus mode and a response medium. Lloyd and Karlan (1984) modified and arranged these factors and characteristics into six groups with general descriptors added for conceptual clarity. With minor rewording (to update terminology), Lloyd and Kangas (1994) summarized the underlying factors and characteristics of AAC as follows.

I. **General simplification of input.** The information presented to the individual, when presented in an AAC form, is simplified in both context and manner of presentation. This simplification, which would presumably facilitate processing and hence understanding of the communicative messages, is accomplished in two ways:
   A. **Verbiage (noise) is reduced.** When speech and AAC symbols are simultaneously presented, irrelevant or parenthetical comments are eliminated from the clinician's speech.
   B. **Rate is adjustable.** When AAC symbols such as manual signs or graphic symbols are presented simultaneously with speech, the rate of presentation is slowed, allowing more processing time. Even the most experienced users of manual sign, for example, slow their rate when signing and speaking, so it can be expected that trainers who are less experienced with AAC symbol use would slow their presentation rate even more.

II. **Response production advantages.** Four advantages have been identified that relate to the training of expressive language responding and actual production. The training of expressive language responding is facilitated, and production becomes easier for the AAC symbol user when contrasted with natural speech production in the following ways:

A. **Pressure for speech is removed.** It is apparent with some autistic and some mentally retarded individuals, especially those capable of some limited, though often barely intelligible speech production, that parents or others exert great pressure on them to speak. Because expected performance may exceed capacity or readiness to produce speech, the pressure may become detrimental to further speech and language development. AAC symbols provide alternative modes by which messages can be sent, thus relieving the pressure on speech production, which, in some cases, subsequently improves.

B. **Physical demands are decreased.** The motor acts necessary to produce a response with AAC are far less complex than those required for spoken responding. With unaided symbols, the motor coordination required for manual sign or gestural production, while seemingly complex, is still far simpler than that required for phonation and articulation. Aided symbols, because they are typically graphic and not produced at the time of the response, require only a means to select (i.e., it is an indicating response, not a producing response).

C. **Physical manipulation of the response is possible.** Just as the difficulty of the response production is decreased when AAC symbols are employed, so too is the difficulty of actual physical manipulation by the trainer. Although it is possible to physically guide the individual in producing an oral response, it is quite arduous. The far greater ability of the trainer to physically guide either the formation of manual or gestural responses or the indication of graphic symbols undoubtedly adds greatly to the more rapid acquisition of AAC.

D. **Clinician's observation of shaping is facilitated.** The visual modality in which AAC symbols (with the exception of digitized and synthetic speech) occur, facilitates the trainer's judgment of how close attempts at response production are coming to the criterial response. Analysis of the characteristics and topography of approximations to the desired production requires far less training and technical background than such an analysis of oral responses.

III. **Advantages for individuals with severe cognitive impairment.** For those individuals exhibiting severe cognitive deficits, use of AAC symbols has some particular features or consequences which would contribute to the acquisition of AAC. Two of these follow:

    A. Vocabulary is limited and functional. The vocabulary has been kept small, often as a consequence of training trainers and parents to use and understand the symbol forms. The lexical items selected for representation with AAC symbols have been more broadly functional to the user, such as *drink*, *play*, *no*, *more*. In this fashion, conceptual rather than syntactic learning is emphasized.

    B. Individual's attention is easier to maintain. With visually presented and produced symbols (e.g., manual signs), evaluation and hence maintenance of attention can be done through assessment of eye contact or direction of gaze. Visible evaluation of attention to auditory/oral symbols cannot be done.

IV. Receptive language/auditory processing advantages. The employment of AAC symbols has direct advantageous effects on the comprehension of language and auditory processing, which in turn affects the comprehension of communicative messages. The two apparent causes for these effects reflect different levels of comprehension and include the following:

    A. Structure of language input is simplified. When AAC symbols are presented simultaneously with spoken symbols, the full syntactic structure of the spoken message is often not represented by the AAC symbols. The AAC symbols often represent only the semantically relevant or meaningful information in the message, thus highlighting what is critical to comprehend.

    B. Auditory short-term memory and/or auditory processing problems are minimized. Because of their visual modality, AAC symbols bypass the auditory channel and thus eliminate any particularly pronounced auditory processing deficits that may exist.

V. Stimulus processing/stimulus association advantages. Again, because it occurs primarily in a visual modality, AAC symbols in communication have certain advantages for the processing of the visual symbol stimuli or for the development of associations between visual symbols and their referents. These are the following:

    A. Figure-ground differential is enhanced. The visual mode of the symbols may help to differentiate the figure from the ground with respect to the communicative message from the visual background. Auditory symbols may not be as easy to differentiate from the ambient background of noise.

    B. Stimulus consistency is optimized. Visual symbols appear to have greater consistency in representation and production than do auditory/oral symbols. With manual signs or gestures, especially at slow rates, contextual or co-production influences are minimal compared with speech where contextual and co-articulatory influences may greatly affect what the listener perceives as the same or different phonemes or words. Certainly, aided symbols have an even greater consistency, because they are selected rather than formed (with the exception of handwritten symbols) on each occasion.

    C. Temporal duration is greater. The temporal duration of the presentation of most AAC symbols is greater than that occurring for natural speech symbols, with the exception of AAC symbols such as digitized or synthesized speech and vibral tactile analogs of speech. This duration can be adjusted to be even longer without altering what the individual perceives to be the form of the stimulus. This is a special advantage for individuals who require greater orientation, perception, and processing time for stimulus presentations. The presentation of AAC symbols can easily be adjusted without loss of relevance or information value. Graphic symbols have the advantage of permanency.

    D. Modality consistency is facilitated. A unimodal rather than cross-modal relationship exists between most AAC symbols and visual referents. AAC symbols, being visual in modality, are more easily associated with visual referents than are speech symbols, which exist in a separate modality. Learning that a symbol represents a referent is easier when both exist in the same stimulus mode (i.e., the object and the symbol for that object are both visual). In addition, the temporal characteristics of the stimulus and referent can be more easily matched when the relationship is unimodal.

VI. Symbolic representational advantages. Another aspect of symbols that can help to explain the facilitative effects on communication development of the use of AAC symbols is the amount and type of information conveyed within the symbol itself and the use to which it is put. Two possibilities follow:

   A. **Supplemental representation is possible.** When used simultaneously with speech, AAC symbols supplement the representational input of the speech symbols. This supplementation has led, with some individuals, to accelerated development of both speech comprehension and production. The success of this supplementation is possibly the result of a type of representation found within certain AAC symbols themselves.

   B. **Visual representation is possible.** AAC symbols such as pictures, rebuses, certain manual signs, and Blissymbols among others, contain within the symbols themselves visual representations of the referents. This representational characteristic has been referred to as *iconicity*; the iconicity of symbols varies, but where greater iconicity exists, meaning, memory, and/or concept visualization can be facilitated. (pp. 630–634)

Clinicians/educators should consider factors such as these in selecting AAC assessment and intervention strategies and evaluating outcomes, remembering that (a) the preceding factors are based primarily on clinical/educational observation with limited research, (b) none of the hypothesized factors is applicable to each AAC user, and (c) more applied and basic research to test these hypothesized factors (i.e., careful empirical investigation) is needed to establish the role and relative contribution of each factor. Although more is known now than when Fristoe and Lloyd (1979a) hypothesized these factors, especially about iconicity, establishing the relative contributions of the factors and the relationships among them would greatly clarify the directions that could be taken in developing facilitative AAC strategies and techniques.

The theoretical and fundamental perspective evolves from an understanding of the human communication model. The decision that Sanders's (1976, 1982) model is robust enough to serve as a framework for AAC with only minor modifications (see Chapter 3) provides support for what aspects of communication are critical in organizing theory. For example, the AAC processes and in-

terface modifications proposed by Lloyd, Quist, and Windsor (1990) are based on a taxonomy using aided and unaided communication as the superordinate structure. This structure is applicable to the **means to represent**, the **means to select**, and the **means to transmit**, which, in turn, has implications for the interaction process and the important transmission and communication environments in the AAC process. Clinicians/educators, as well as researchers/academics, can use the aided/unaided aspect of the taxonomy as a way of viewing their clinical/educational assessment and intervention issues and aiding in the development of basic as well as applied research questions. The aided/unaided taxonomy has been further developed by Fuller, Lloyd, and Schlosser (1992) with subordinate classification dimensions of static versus dynamic, iconic versus opaque, and set versus system aspects of AAC symbols as the means to represent (see Chapter 3), but to date there have been no published reports of developing subordinate levels of the taxonomy for the means to select or the means to transmit.

Basic Human Communication Model

The thinking man or woman or the man or woman of feeling . . . can experience no greater affront to their humanity than denial of freedom of expression.

—Archibald Cox

Communication Model. This text is based on a broad view of human communication. It is organized around the basic human communication model of a sender and a receiver, both of whom bring to the process experience and physical, psychological, social, cognitive, and linguistic abilities. Communication involves the transmission of a message by a sender to a receiver who may or may not respond. It is also generally considered to be an interactive process between at least two communicators, with the sender and receiver reversing roles. The initial receiver becomes the sender, and the initial sender becomes the receiver. Figure 1.1 provides a simplified illustration of the human communication model.

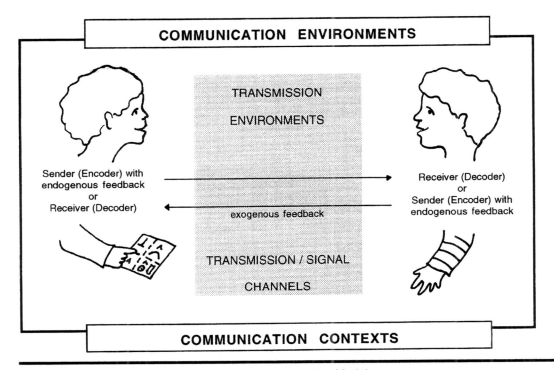

COMMUNICATION ENVIRONMENTS

TRANSMISSION

ENVIRONMENTS

Sender (Encoder) with
endogenous feedback
or
Receiver (Decoder)

exogenous feedback

Receiver (Decoder)
or
Sender (Encoder) with
endogenous feedback

TRANSMISSION / SIGNAL

CHANNELS

COMMUNICATION CONTEXTS

FIGURE 1.1   Basic Elements of the Human Communication Model

AAC may be viewed as a broad or robust communication model including (a) a sender who has the intention of communicating (e.g., a message); (b) a receiver who is engaged in an interaction with the sender; (c) a set/system of symbols to represent messages (e.g., feelings, requests, information); (d) a channel through which one sends a message (e.g., acoustic, optic, vibratory); (e) the broader contexts or environments in which the communication act is taking place; and (f) complex feedback systems within (endogenous) and between (exogenous) individuals (Lloyd, Quist, & Windsor, 1990). The success of communication depends on many factors, including the degree to which the sender and receiver share common linguistic and nonlinguistic symbols, their cultural background, and their experience and skill for combining the symbols. Communication involves linguistic (verbal) symbols, which are typically spoken or written, and nonlinguistic (nonverbal) symbols such as gestures, facial expressions, and hand movements. Individuals with functional natural speech frequently augment their spoken communication with nonlinguistic (nonverbal) com-

munication. Likewise, AAC users tend to use a variety of both linguistic and nonlinguistic forms of communication (Basil & Ruiz, 1985; Liberoff, 1992; Lloyd & Fuller, 1986; Lloyd et al., 1990; van Balkom & Welle Donker-Gimbrere, 1985; Vanderheiden & Lloyd, 1986).

Lloyd et al. (1990) proposed that the AAC model should be based on a robust human communication model and not be considered categorically different. In essence, the only differences involve the AAC processes and interfaces, means to represent the message (symbols), means to select, and means to transmit. This proposed model is presented by Fuller and Lloyd in Chapter 3. Some individuals suggest that AAC requires a different model. The position espoused in this text, however, is that the AAC model is not different; rather it is the applications, standards, and expectations that may be different. In other words, the differences between individuals with no apparent communication disorders and individuals with little or no functional speech are not categorical differences, but differences in expectations, emphasis, and repair strategies, to name a few.

AAC may be viewed as a process composed of three aspects: (a) means to represent an idea, (b) means to select the representation of the idea, and (c) means to transmit the representation of the idea (Lloyd et al., 1990). Each of these three aspects may be aided or unaided (Lloyd & Fuller, 1986; Lloyd et al., 1990). Although the three aspects are discussed sequentially, they do not necessarily occur in this order. They are typically interactive and frequently occur concurrently. They are discussed in more detail in Chapter 3.

A robust communication model involves two types of environments: **transmission environments** (often referred to as **transmission/signal channels**) and **communication environments** (often referred to as **communication contexts**). These multiple environments must be considered in applying the human communication model to individuals with little or no functional speech. The application of the human communication model to AAC is an important aspect of the theoretical and fundamental perspective previously discussed.

Communication typically involves a dyad (i.e., two individuals interacting). In a group situation, however, the particular individuals engaged in a communication dyad at any one time typically change as conversation shifts. In an even more robust communication model, more than two people are involved in the interaction.

A significant part of communication involves language that includes both the symbols or tokens (e.g., printed words, manual signs, spoken words) to represent a message and the rules or logic for combining the symbols (e.g., grammar, syntax). Human communication also includes nonlinguistic (e.g., pictures, gestures) and paralinguistic (e.g., prosody) forms.

Purposes of Communication. Light (1988) outlined four purposes that can be accomplished during communicative interactions: (1) communication of needs/wants, (2) information transfer, (3) social closeness, and (4) social etiquette. Communicating needs/wants involves regulation of a partner's behavior to the extent that the sender of the message can obtain something or cause something to happen. In information transfer, the emphasis is on the content of the message. In communication

for social closeness, the emphasis is not on the content of the message, but rather the establishment, maintenance, and/or development of an interpersonal relationship. Social etiquette can be accomplished through the use of polite social conventions such as "Nice to see you" and "Thank you very much."

More generally, communication may be used for information transfer, socialization, or a combination thereof. In addition to face-to-face communication, however, one should consider aspects of communication such as those that relate to on-line or real-time interaction and recorded or stored messages. The success of communication is strongly related to the match of the sender and receiver, especially their means to represent their messages (symbols or tokens).

Multimodal Communication. Human communication is **multimodal**. Most frequently it involves the auditory and visual channels, but it may also involve the tactile channel. Most people use **multimodal communication** (Vanderheiden & Lloyd, 1986). People speak to convey thoughts, but even when speaking, senders typically use not only the speech mechanism, but also the face, hands, arms, and other body parts to convey messages. Additional meaning is conveyed by facial expressions, gestures (e.g., pointing to the coffee mug one wants), tone of voice, and even posture. A typical speaker uses not only speech but also gestures, writing, typing, and tape recordings (e.g., as on a telephone answering machine). In the span of a single hour, a teacher might speak, write on a chalkboard, show pictures or diagrams on an overhead projector, and point to a map or wall chart. Receivers typically use eyes, ears, and touch receptors to receive messages, but may also use olfactory cells and taste buds.

There are numerous examples of multimodal communication. People switch easily from one mode to another and combine modes within a single situation. They select the modes of communication that will be most effective and efficient in a given situation for a given listener. For example, one might write a note to a spouse that ends with the words "I love you," but draw a heart to express the same idea to a 4-year-old child. People also select the mode that will best set the tone to achieve specific goals. One might be content to rely only on speech when having a casual chat with an employer, but when discussing a specific idea to improve business, one might choose to put an idea in writing so that an employer will attend to it as a serious proposal.

Users of AAC systems should be viewed as multimodal communicators. Their communication systems should include both aided and unaided modes and strategies. They should include both the communication modes they have developed naturally without formal intervention and those modes, strategies, and techniques that can be facilitated or taught by clinicians/educators. A variety of techniques may be needed to address a varied audience. For example, a person who uses manual sign with familiar listeners would need some other approach to communicate with store clerks or bank tellers who have no knowledge of signing. In addition, an individual who uses an electronic device must also have a backup system available for times when the device is broken or the battery needs charging.

Viewing an AAC user as a multimodal communicator implies that whatever communication mode the individual chooses should be respected and accepted. Clinicians/educators, in their enthusiasm to teach what they view as more effective communication modes, sometimes refuse to accept simpler, more effective modes. For example, they might put "yes" and "no" on an individual's communication device. When the student attempts to answer a question by nodding or shaking the head, the clinician/educator might respond with "Use your device to tell me." This is unnecessary, because the clinician/educator probably understand the gesture. Users report incidents such as this to be very frustrating (Huer & Lloyd, 1988a, 1988b) and they may have the inadvertent, negative effect of causing students to become discouraged about even trying to communicate.

Communicative Competence. **Communicative competence** is an important concept of the human communication perspective. Competence should be considered within the framework of communication. According to Light (1989), four distinct competencies contribute to overall com-

municative competence. These are **linguistic competence**, **operational competence**, **social competence**, and **strategic competence**. These four were recently summarized by Lloyd and Kangas (1994) as follows:

Linguistic competence refers to knowledge of the language, or linguistic code. According to Chomsky (1965), linguistic competence refers to the internal abilities of the individual. It includes everything the person knows about the language and how the units can be combined. Light (1989) points out that for the AAC user, linguistic competence may include knowledge of both the native language used in the environment (e.g., English or Spanish) and special AAC symbols (e.g., Blissymbolics).

Operational competence is a unique concern of AAC, especially for aided communication. Operational competence refers to the user's ability to manage the specific devices or techniques that are used in the communication process. This might include the ability to turn a device on or off, adjust the volume, operate a scanning system, and so on. This is, perhaps, the competence that most people focus on first when communicating with an AAC user, mainly because it represents an aspect of AAC that is different from typical spoken communication.

Social competence refers to the broad communication skills addressed by sociolinguistics (Hymes, 1971). This includes discourse strategies, interaction functions, and pragmatic adjustments to context. Examples of abilities that relate to social competence include maintaining a topic, using transitions to change topic, adjusting the type of language used to the ability of the listener, gaining someone's attention before giving information, and giving appropriate indications of maintaining interest and/or understanding the communication partner. Social competence may be a serious issue that is easily overlooked for an AAC user. It is not unusual for AAC approaches to be introduced to an individual who has had extremely limited communication abilities for many years. Social competence abilities that are developed quite naturally for typically developing children may be problematic for AAC users, simply because AAC users have not experienced successful communication to facilitate these abilities.

Strategic competence (defined by Canale, 1983) refers to adapted strategies that are called into play when there is some breakdown in the communication process. Examples include asking for additional information, recognizing when the listener has not understood, and repeating or changing a message to clarify the error. As pointed out by Light (1989), this is especially important for AAC users. AAC approaches remain imperfect replacements for the ability to use speech easily and effectively. There are probably a greater number of difficulties and barriers to achieving efficient communication when AAC strategies are being used. The ability to adjust and respond to these problems will be critical to the overall success of an AAC user. (pp. 635-636)

Assistive Technology Perspective

My communication aid is fantastic, but without me, it does not do anything. I could not function in society without a communication system. However, the communication system is just the key that unlocks the door to the candy shop. I'm the candy.

—Rick Creech

The technology perspective is extremely important in AAC. Unfortunately, it is related to a common misconception in the field. Many administrators and clinicians/educators think that AAC and **assistive technology (AT)** are synonymous. Additionally, confusions and concerns related to similarities and differences between AAC and AT often arise. To clarify this relationship, one should remember that AAC is a process, while on the other hand, AT refers to the tools used to assist individuals with functions and activities. There is an overlap of the AAC process and the AT tools, but they are not synonymous. AAC frequently involves the use of AT, but there is much more to AAC than simply AT. Conversely, there is more to AT than just communication devices. AAC should not, however, be considered a subset or a specialty of AT. An assistive communication device is one of the more critical tools in aided communication. However, an AAC system should include both aided and unaided means to represent, means to select, and means to transmit. In other words, the use of AT may be only a small part of an overall AAC system.

In fact, surveys about the use of technology suggest that communication by AAC users is predominantly unaided (e.g., gestures, speech, or even vocalizations of limited intelligibility) (Burd, Hammes, Bornhoeft, & Fisher, 1988; Matas, Mathy-Laikko, Beukelman, & Legresley, 1985).

Figure 1.2 illustrates the overlapping relationship of the AAC process and the AT tools. The left oval shows that AAC consists of both aided and unaided approaches. The right oval provides a small sample of different types of AT. Aided AAC approaches that use prostheses overlap with AT. The figure shows that visual and hearing prostheses are related to AAC, but not typically thought of as AAC. Likewise, some aspects of job accommodation (e.g., computer access for communication) would overlap with AAC, but many other devices and structure modifications would not be considered part of AAC. Other types of AT, such as mobility orthoses/prostheses, are not part of AAC per se. However, in some cases, wheelchairs, walkers, and crutches may be used to transport or hold assistive communication devices and, therefore, may indirectly be considered a part of AAC.

A related misconception about AAC and AT is that providing an assistive communicative device solves the communication problem. Without appropriate training and backup support, most assistive devices are of little or no value. Lack of training and support often result in expensive devices not being used and ultimately ending up on shelves. It is as if nothing has been learned from colleagues in audiology about another type of assistive device, the hearing aid. Just as one cannot give a hearing aid to an individual and expect to solve a hearing problem, one cannot give an assistive communication device to an individual and expect to solve an expressive communication problem.

Making wise use of the technology which is now available is also absolutely essential for a person like me to be able to continue on through high school in a regular class setting. Electric wheelchair, laptop computer, voice synthesizer, ultralight computers are some examples of the modern technology I have been using in recent years. . . . Once the decision about my education was made by myself and my parents, plans for how to mange that

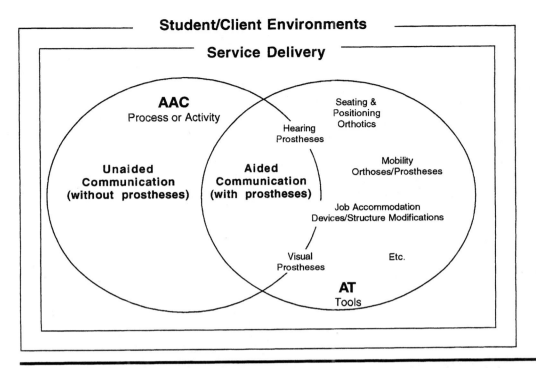

Student/Client Environments

Service Delivery

AAC
Process or Activity

Hearing
Prostheses

Seating &
Positioning
Orthotics

**Unaided
Communication
(without prostheses)**

**Aided
Communication
(with prostheses)**

Mobility
Orthoses/Prostheses

Job Accommodation
Devices/Structure Modifications

Visual
Prostheses

Etc.

AT
Tools

FIGURE 1.2   Relationship of Augmentative and Alternative Communication (AAC) to Assistive Technology (AT)

education were soon underway, and still are today as I complete high school and head for college. We have a formula; as problems present themselves, solutions are sought, and at times, we have learned that you never give up, just keep on trying. (Valentic, 1991, p. 9)

Assessment Perspective

You can observe a lot by watching.

—Yogi Berra

To be able to ask a question clearly is two-thirds of the way to getting it answered.

—John Ruskins

Everything should be made as simple as possible, but not one bit simpler.

—Albert Einstein

Assessment and evaluation are critical to developing an appropriate intervention plan. Knowing what questions to ask, why they should be asked, how to ask them, whom to ask, when to ask, and where to ask are the essence of assessment. Know-

ing how to interpret and use the answers to the questions are the essence of evaluation. AAC assessment should be field-based (involving assessment in natural environments), extensive (including multiple natural environments and communication partners), transdisciplinary (involving role release and collaboration across disciplines), and ongoing (involving as many assessment sessions as appropriate and also follow-up). Assessment of the existing communication abilities and the abilities of the related cognitive, motor, and sensory domains are important, as is the understanding of the etiology of the communication disabilities. Especially critical are assessment and evaluation of auditory, visual, and motor abilities because they are the means to represent (symbols), select, and transmit messages in AAC approaches. Also, AAC users have a high probability of having sensory and/or motor impairments. A combination of the primary impairment (e.g., aphasia, cerebral palsy, or mental retardation) and concomitant sensory and/or motor impairments results in a disability that is greater than one would expect from the sum of these impairments. In addition to discussion of the critical roles of these impairments in the Assessment unit of this text, sensory impairments are discussed in Chapter 16, and motor impairments are discussed in Chapter 17.

Team Approach.   One of the most basic premises of AAC assessment is that it must involve a team approach. The diversity and complexity of issues involved in AAC require knowledge and skill from many individuals and disciplines. The specific services required by any particular individual with little or no functional speech will vary, but individuals who might typically be on an assessment team for a school child are the child, occupational therapist, paraprofessional, parents, teacher, special educator, and speech-language pathologist. Depending on the specific needs of the child, such individuals as an audiologist, personal aide, physical therapist, psychologist, rehabilitation engineer, social worker, or vision specialist may also be included on the assessment team.

Field-Based Assessment.   To provide a true picture of the strengths and needs of AAC users, assessment must be conducted in natural environments. What an individual can do in a testing situation in an isolated, unfamiliar location may not give an accurate indication of communication strengths and needs. Direct observation, videotapes, and interviews in familiar environments with familiar communication partners provide important information about an individual's functional communication abilities.

Standardized and Norm-Referenced Tests.   Standardized and norm-referenced tests are sometimes used during the assessment process, but use of these tests is a critical issue in AAC in several ways. The responses required in the assessment of cognitive as well as both receptive and expressive language abilities may need to be adapted for AAC users. Similarly, stimulus material may need to be presented in nonstandard ways, which can affect the processing and/or response assessment of the test. AAC users may also express different fatigue factors than typical individuals of the normative group. The norms provided for standardized and norm-referenced tests will not be valid if modifi-

cations have to be made. Test results may give some index of performance level, but they should not be reported as normed scores. A description of any modifications made for the administration of a test must be included in the reporting of results and caution must be used in the interpretation of scores. Standardized and norm-referenced tests, however, need not be completely discarded because of these limitations. They can provide important information. Criterion-referenced tests, however, are often preferred.

Criteria-Based Assessment.   Some areas take considerable time to assess because of the extent of information that must be gathered to begin a particular intervention. It is not always necessary, however, to gather the most extensive information. Criteria-based assessment, which includes criterion-referenced tests, may be more appropriate. In criteria-based assessment, the clinician does not attempt to determine an individual's ability to use specific symbol sets/systems, specific switches or other technology, and levels of functioning, but rather attempts only to discover whether the skills are sufficient to support a particular AAC strategy. That is, the clinician/educator might not need to complete assessment of fine motor skills to determine whether they are sufficient to make use of manual signing. Although many initial speech and language assessments can be completed within 3 to 6 hours, the initial AAC assessment rarely can be completed within one day.

Criteria-based assessment is more appropriate than norm-referenced assessment for clients who may be expected to show changes as various communication interventions are implemented. Individuals with congenital impairments may never have been successful in most communication interactions, and the introduction of a strategy that provides success may have a rather dramatic impact on the further development of language and communication skills. Many clients with acquired disabilities can also be expected to show changes over time. As previously discussed, some individuals may show patterns of improvement; that is, the level of disability may actually diminish over time. Individuals with progressive disabilities, on the other hand, may develop more severe disabilities. Criteria-based assessment may be more sensitive to these changes and may lead more quickly to decisions to vary or change the AAC intervention strategies.

Capability Profile. For most areas of speech and language assessment, the clinician is interested in obtaining maximal assessment; that is, to determine a capability profile that accurately details a person's level of functioning in various important domains. In AAC, however, it is often more effective to operate from a criteria-based approach (Beukelman & Mirenda, 1992; Yorkston & Karlan, 1986). The abilities of many AAC users are extremely difficult to assess, but time must be taken to assess them properly. Assessment may require a long time because the diagnostic procedures might be extremely tiring for the individual, who may need to take many breaks. Reducing the assessment for those aspects that will determine possible intervention strategies can both benefit the AAC user and make the clinician/educator more efficient. Assessment and intervention are very much intertwined and usually continue simultaneously. Thus, one could expect that the more extensive maximal assessment type of information would be gathered over a longer time during intervention.

Feature Matching. Once strengths and needs have been assessed and goals have been developed, **feature matching** should be employed to select components for an appropriate AAC system. Needs and goals that are determined by assessing abilities in natural environments with a variety of communication partners should be outlined and prioritized. Specific aided and unaided approaches should then be evaluated. For example, if an individual with cognitive impairment has good motor control, manual sign might be considered. If an individual has high cognitive abilities but limited motor control, a computer with switch access might be considered. AAC systems and communication approaches are different from those used by typical speakers and must be well matched to the real communication needs of individuals and their environments. Feature matching is critical in the assessment process presented in this text (see Chapters 8, 14, and Appendix A).

Follow-Up. Regardless of the assessment model employed, follow-up is an important component of the assessment process. Abilities and disabilities as well as communication needs of individuals change over time. As individuals become successful with one communication approach, new or additional approaches should be considered. Ongoing assessment and reassessment of AAC systems and intervention plans will be needed.

Intervention Perspective

The primary question is not what you know, but how you know it.

—Aristotle

Whatever is worth doing at all, is worth doing well.

—Lord Chesterfield

AAC intervention often begins with the development of goals to expand a repertoire of communication behaviors, develop intentional and symbolic abilities, and/or increase participation in daily routines (Kangas & Lloyd, 1988). Some authors have suggested that AAC intervention should not be initiated until certain levels of cognitive functioning, social skills, and receptive language have been reached (Owens & House, 1984) or until a gap between receptive and expressive language has been demonstrated (Chapman & Miller, 1980). Evidence to support this prerequisite approach, however, has been based mainly on observations of typically developing children and not on research with children with disabilities. More recently, authors have challenged this approach, suggesting that intervention can be effective for individuals exhibiting a wide range of skill levels related to both congenital and acquired disabilities.

Several models of service delivery are described in the literature. The **unidisciplinary model** typically includes one professional who is primarily responsible for providing services to improve communication skills. Although this model has been effective with individuals with poor articulation, stuttering, or language delays, one service provider is unlikely to be effective in meeting the many needs of individuals with little or no functional speech. Individuals with sensory, motor, cognitive, and language impairments typically require services from specialists in many fields.

The **multidisciplinary team model** involves the provision of services from many disciplines including, for example, audiology, career counseling, computer science, medicine, occupational therapy, ophthalmology, physical therapy, general and special education, social work, and speech-language pathology. Specialists may provide the specific expertise and strategies to meet an individual's needs; however, intervention may become disjointed and fragmented rather than coherent and holistic (Beukelman & Mirenda, 1992). When individuals with severe communication disabilities are removed from their natural environments to obtain services in the environments of each specialist, the danger of fragmentation is very real.

The **interdisciplinary team model** involves more disciplines and provides for a greater exchange and sharing of information. Specialists may meet on a regular basis to determine goals and discuss intervention strategies. In this model, specialists have access to a variety of perspectives, which allows them to better understand the implications of the impairments and disabilities that affect communication. Planning intervention includes consultation and collaboration.

AAC services typically require more than sharing, collaborating, and implementing, however. The success of AAC intervention depends on the coordination and offering of services not just between disciplines, but across disciplines. The **transdisciplinary team model** involves individuals and professionals from different disciplines sharing knowledge and ideas as they work together to provide services through cotreatment that focus not on the specific disabilities of an individual, but on an individual as a whole. The hallmark characteristic of the transdisciplinary team is role release, the sharing of information and function across disciplines. Divisions between disciplines become less distinct. A more thorough discussion of AAC service delivery models appears in Chapter 21.

Intervention is based on the development and prioritization of long-range goals and objectives. Exactly what these goals will be, however, depend on an individual's specific needs and expectations.

AAC needs may not be readily apparent in individuals with neurogenic progressive diseases such as amyotrophic lateral sclerosis (ALS), multiple sclerosis (MS), or Parkinson's disease (Beukelman & Garrett, 1988). Intervention for these individuals will focus on changing needs that can be expected to increase. Intervention for individuals with short-term neurogenic diseases such as Guillain-Barré syndrome, on the other hand, will focus on immediate needs that can be expected to diminish.

Intervention typically focuses on developing skills that will enhance participation and independence in the environments in which individuals are expected to function. Specific intervention strategies are discussed in Chapters 18 and 19. An individual with a congenital condition such as cerebral palsy or an acquired condition such as TBI, for example, may be expected to begin or return to active participation in society. Goals for such integration will come from several sources (e.g., individuals with disabilities, communication partners, and professionals) and will vary widely with respect to individual needs and different environments. Intervention for an individual who is always with caregivers in a familiar setting will certainly differ from the program designed for an individual who is learning to function more independently in home, school, work, and community environments. The transdisciplinary model can be effective in meeting these goals of integration.

Transdisciplinary and Integrated Perspective

. . . [G]rant me the serenity to accept the things I cannot change, courage to change the things I can, and wisdom to know the difference.

—St. Francis of Assisi

Many ideas grow better when transplanted into another mind than in the one where they sprang up.

—Oliver Wendell Holmes

The transdisciplinary team approach, which incorporates collaboration and promotes role release, is basic to AAC assessment and intervention. It allows professionals with knowledge and expertise in a variety of disciplines to work together to share information that is known and to develop new ideas and strategies to improve the communication skills of individuals with little or no functional speech. Although improvement in functional communication often appears as a goal, this goal should not be interpreted as being an end but rather as being the means to an end. Individual AAC users have their own ideas as to what ends or outcomes are important to them. For many, the desired end or outcome is acceptance.

> We people with disabilities have historically been separated from the rest of society. This practice of segregation has often been justified as the best to serve our special needs. But the practice has had a very serious consequence. It has taught people in the community that people with disabilities are not part of the community. It has caused them to believe that the exclusion of people with disabilities is the natural order of things, which obviously works against us, as we struggle to be accepted. . . .
>
> The best way to build acceptance is to deemphasize the idea that our disabilities are the most important difference between us and other individuals. People should be treated equally, regardless of their level of ability. All children should go to school with their age mates from their neighborhood. (Sienkiewicz-Mercer, 1995)

Inclusion into general education classrooms is one way in which individuals can gain acceptance into a group of their peers. If the inclusion is only physical, however, it may do little or nothing to facilitate real acceptance. Unless academic participation and integration is carefully planned, AAC users can feel excluded even in the presence of physical inclusion. Like assessment and intervention, inclusion must be carefully designed to meet individual needs and should be encouraged to the optimal extent that is beneficial.

> Acceptance is not something that can happen overnight. Negative attitudes can be overcome, but we have to be patient, and we have to work together. (Sienkiewicz-Mercer, 1995)

The ability to effectively communicate is critical to achieving integration and inclusion for individuals with severe disabilities. Like typically speaking individuals, AAC users often want to enjoy a sense of community with others. This is

difficult to achieve without effective communication. Improving the communication skills of AAC users is often the focus when working toward integration and inclusion, but this should not be the only focus. Improving the communication skills of communication partners is also important and should not be overlooked.

> Many people seem to be interested in helping people with disabilities in all sorts of ways. Their ability to communicate with us is the key. They must talk to us, and they must listen to us. (Sienkiewicz-Mercer, 1995)

Legal and Ethical Perspective

There are no whole truths; all truths are half truths. It is trying to treat them as whole truths that plays the devil.
—Alfred North Whitehead

Legal and ethical issues arise in the field of AAC, as they do in any field of service delivery. These issues can be particularly complicated, however, when they involve individuals with little or no functional speech whose messages are typically not sent as completely or received as accurately as messages of typically speaking individuals. Administrators and researchers, as well as clinicians/educators and others who work with AAC users, must understand and be able to appropriately deal with the legal and ethical issues that affect the lives of AAC users.

The 1992 Communication Bill of Rights outlines a number of rights designed to facilitate an AAC user's impact on the environment. These rights reflect a social mandate to improve communication and increase participation in social, educational, and vocational settings. AAC users have more than just social mandates behind them, however. Early broad-based civil rights legislation that laid the groundwork to protect the rights of all individuals has special implications for individuals with severe disabilities. The Americans with Disabilities Act (ADA; PL 101-336, 1990) assigns responsibility and outlines more specifics related to providing services for individuals with disabilities. A comprehensive review of relevant legislation appears in Chapter 20.

Legislation provides a solid base on which to develop programs to meet the needs of individuals with little or no functional speech. Different interpretations contribute to variation in the particulars of providing a free, appropriate public education (FAPE), but the mandate is clear. Administrators and service providers must be secure in the knowledge of their responsibilities in carrying out such legal mandates. They must also, however, be secure in handling the many ethical issues that may arise as they work to implement legislation. Professional organizations provide codes of ethics, but these are typically general guidelines. Administrators and service providers must be prepared to follow not only these general guidelines, but also know how to deal with specific ethical issues.

One ethical issue that has received considerable attention involves the interpretation of messages conveyed by AAC users. Because of the nature of AAC, service providers are often called on to interpret messages whether through repeating more intelligibly what they believe the AAC user has said or by saying the symbols to which the AAC user appears to be gazing. Interpreters must be vigilant in guarding against injecting subjective thoughts that would bias an AAC user's message in any way.

A second ethical issue involves confidentiality. Professionals who work with AAC users must be above reproach. Information that is obtained from AAC users can only be shared when permission is granted. This information may be spoken communication, written documents, and/or videotapes.

A third ethical issue concerns the dissemination of written messages. AAC users send spoken messages through voice output communication aids (VOCAs), but they may also send a considerable number of messages through computers and printers. Service providers must be sensitive to the wishes of AAC users regarding the distribution of these written messages which endure. AAC users should be secure in knowing that their messages are not indiscriminately distributed to individuals for whom they were not intended. A more thorough discussion of ethical issues appears in Chapter 20.

Visionary or Futuristic Perspective

If you have built castles in the air, your work need not be lost; that is where they should be. Now put the foundations under them.
—Henry David Thoreau

If I have seen further, it is by standing on the shoulders of giants.
—Sir Isaac Newton

The important thing is not to stop questioning.
—Albert Einstein

AAC has many dimensions that must be viewed from many perspectives. New challenges emerge as more and more individuals become involved as both users and providers of AAC services. Progress has been made in the brief history of the field by the provision of means of communication that were not previously available. Individuals have always had the means to use unaided communication modes such as gesturing and signing, but these modes are limited by the number of communication partners who can interpret the messages. Advancements in technology have affected the manufacture and distribution of a variety of communication devices that are smaller, lighter, more functional, and more user friendly in terms of improved storage and retrieval systems, memory, and voice output. Advances in ergonomics and the development of sophisticated switches and software have done much to facilitate operational competence. Relatively little improvement, however, has been made in improving social competence. AAC users can store and retrieve large amounts of text and graphics for oral presentation and written documents, but efficiency in on-line, real-time interactive communication is lacking. Communication partners are often reluctant to engage in true interactive communication with AAC users because of the time it takes to generate spontaneous messages.

As in most areas of endeavor, funding has been—and will most likely continue to be—a factor that influences the future directions of AAC. Funding for the research that forms the very foundation of the field is necessary. Additionally, funding for personnel preparation, training programs for service providers and individual AAC users who need systems, and educational support must not be forgotten, especially as managed care becomes more prevalent.

Funding alone, however, cannot meet the challenge of achieving communicative competence. Human factors must also be in place. Communication is complex. Achieving competence requires the cooperation, collaboration, and creativity of AAC users and other members of their transdisciplinary teams. Providing AAC users with opportunities to become functional, spontaneous communicators as they move toward becoming independent, participating individuals is a challenge that will carry the field into the future.

SUMMARY

The ability to communicate with others is one of the most important human assets. AAC provides options that may replace or support conventional means of communication for individuals who experience severe communication disabilities. The two broad categories of AAC are aided and unaided. Aided strategies involve some external device or equipment, whereas unaided communication is done with the individual's own body. The many aided and unaided strategies and techniques differ from conventional communication because they often use different means to represent, select, and transmit messages. Selection of appropriate AAC strategies requires careful assessment of an individual's abilities and environmental communication needs, and this is best accomplished with a team approach. The goals of AAC intervention should be to enhance the individual's communicative competence in the context of current and future home, school, work, and community settings. When AAC interventions are carried out with the needs and the perspective of the AAC user as a central focus, basic human rights are respected and new opportunities and life choices are made possible.

CHAPTER 2

HISTORY OF AAC

HELEN H. ARVIDSON AND LYLE L. LLOYD

Augmentative and alternative communication (AAC), as a recognized field involved in providing services to improve the communication skills of individuals with little or no functional speech, is relatively young. Although AAC was being used by some clinicians/educators in the 1950s, it was not until the next decade that it gained recognition, and not until the 1970s that it became recognized as a field of its own (Zangari, Lloyd, & Vicker, 1994). Communicating through augmentative and alternative means, however, is not new. Ancient history suggests that early humans used symbols (e.g., drawings and paintings) to communicate. Reference to the use of manual signs by individuals who were deaf dates back to the works of Plato (Levinson, 1967). Additional documentation of the use of manual sign alphabets and sign systems appeared during the Middle Ages (Bebian, 1825, cited in Stokoe, 1960; Bulwer, 1644; Dixon, 1620/1890; Savage, Evans, & Savage, 1981). The use of manual signs extended beyond individuals who were deaf, however. Benedictine monks who had taken vows of silence communicated through manual signs (Chaves & Solar, 1974). Manual signs were used with individuals with cognitive impairments during the 1800s (Bonvillian & Miller, 1995). Gestural communication was used among individuals from different cultures to facilitate communication across languages (Skelly, 1979).

Several reports have been written chronicling the history of AAC (Galyas, Fant, & Hunnicut, 1993; Lloyd, 1980, 1986, 1993; Lloyd & Karlan, 1984; McNaughton, 1990; Vanderheiden & Yoder, 1986). To date, however, the most extensive account of the development of AAC is the historic perspective paper by Zangari et al. (1994) written as part of the observance of the tenth anniversary celebration of the **International Society for Augmentative and Alternative Communication (ISAAC)**.

This chapter introduces readers to background information on the development and growth of AAC as a recognized field, beginning with a brief description of antecedents and concluding with a short discussion of controversial issues. The field of AAC, with its own research, theories, models, and taxonomies, investigates, collaborates, develops technology, and delivers services to individuals who, for a variety of reasons, do not communicate through natural speech and/or writing. Looking forward in an attempt to discover how the field will progress is inviting; it stimulates ideas that lead to future growth and development. One must not only look forward, however. One should also look backward. Looking backward allows one to know and understand the history of AAC. Gaining knowledge of the past is critical, because it improves the chances of avoiding mistakes of the past, aids in understanding the present, and promotes a promise of progress toward a productive future.

ANTECEDENTS

Several scientific, technologic, and social antecedents spurred the development of AAC. Although the impact and importance of each of these antecedents varied over the decades, they all played a role in shaping AAC into the field it is today.

Scientific Antecedents

AAC grew out of the need to provide methods and materials to meet the communication needs of individuals with little or no functional speech. Traditional speech therapy, which focused on improving the intelligibility and articulation of natural speech, was found to be generally ineffective for individuals with severe communication disabilities. Innovative clinicians/educators were prompted to develop and use new intervention strategies that focused not on natural speech, but rather on augmentative and alternative methods of communication, including manual signs and graphic symbols. Early uses of AAC were based on the knowledge and skill of individual service providers, however, not on science. The scientific base developed when special education and rehabilitation programs began to apply the principles of operant technology in their teaching programs. Single subject research design and the use of the stimulus equivalence paradigm (Sidman, 1971; Sidman & Cresson, 1973; Spradlin, Karlan, & Wetherby, 1976) influenced the educational aspects of AAC. Remington (1994) described a partnership between behavior analysis and the teaching of pragmatics, semantics, and syntax related to AAC.

Basic research on the ability of chimpanzees to communicate with manual signs and symbols (Gardner & Gardner, 1969, 1979; Premack, 1971a; Premack & Premack, 1974; Rumbaugh, 1977; Rumbaugh, Gill, & von Glasserfield, 1973) laid the foundation for investigating the use of manual signs and graphic symbols to improve the communication skills of individuals with cognitive impairments (Carrier, 1974; Deich & Hodges, 1977). The investigation of using manual signs and graphic symbols was not, however, restricted to controlled environments. The use of AAC began to be studied in more meaningful contexts and natural environments, as well (Lorrett, 1969). Kopchick and Lloyd (1976), for example, developed a 24-hour **total communication** program to promote the functional use of manual signs in the residential living environments of individuals with cognitive and hearing impairments. They incorporated a variety of communication modes, including gestures, postures, manual signs, and natural speech in their total communication approach. The emphasis of their approach to total communication, however, was not on the different modes being used, but rather on the fact that the modes were being used 24 hours a day throughout the environment.

A project based at the University Hospital School in Iowa during the 1960s was one of the first projects to use empirical data to justify AAC services for individuals with cerebral palsy (Vicker, 1974). Researchers who investigated the impact of neurologic impairment of the articulatory system began to develop clinical AAC programs for individuals whom they considered unlikely to develop natural speech (Kladde, 1974). AAC strategies were also introduced to unintelligible adults who had demyelinating conditions such as amyotrophic lateral sclerosis (ALS) (Adams, 1966) and neurological impairments such as aphasia (Chen, 1968).

By the late 1970s and early 1980s, a research base began to develop. Before that time, however, little empirical data on AAC assessment and intervention were available. Reports in the literature were largely anecdotal, consisting of surveys, pilot projects, and success stories (Lloyd, 1986). By the 1980s, however, research began to catch up with service delivery, and AAC began to grow into a field of its own, responding to the needs of individuals with severe communication disabilities.

Technologic Antecedents

As early as the 1920s, 1930s, and 1940s, Bell Telephone Labs and others began work on speech intelligibility, **speech synthesis** (Egan, 1948; Fletcher, 1929; French & Steinberg, 1947; Licklider & Miller, 1951), and the transistor (Schure, 1961), thus laying the foundation for developing the technology that affected the field of AAC. Technical developments in bioengineering and computers in the 1940s and 1950s also paved the way. The development of control devices during the 1960s offered opportunities for communication to individuals with severe physical and communication disabilities (Perron, 1965). Two significant technological developments were the Patient Operated Selector Mechanism, commonly called POSM or POSSUM, and the Patient Initiated Light Operated Telecontrol, known as PILOT. POSSUM, a special typewriter control involving scanning and selection through the activation of a switch, was considered to be an enormous advancement in the technology that improved the communication skills of individuals with severe physical and communication disabilities (Zangari et al., 1994). PILOT, an indicator controlled by movements of the head, provided access opportunities for individuals who could not make selections with other parts of their bodies (Collins, 1974; Copeland, 1974). Switches used in conjunction with the **Morse code** provided AAC systems for individuals with physical disabilities (Clement, 1961). The development of the microprocessor in the late 1960s (Rosch, 1989) had a major impact on AAC because of the use of personal computers in communication and the development of dedicated AAC devices (Lloyd, 1993).

Social Antecedents

Historical events and medical advances created an increasing need to provide AAC services. Because of the introduction of antibiotics and other medical advances, many injured World War II veterans were among the growing number of individuals with physical and cognitive impairments affecting communication. Antibiotics and improved medical health care were also responsible for an increasing number of infant survivors who began to exhibit developmental delays and communication disabilities (Begab, 1977; Gorga, 1989). The number of individuals surviving injuries also increased; many individuals who might previously have died from accidents, falls, and gunshot wounds were now surviving with head injuries that left them with physical and cognitive impairments and little or no functional speech. The number of individuals surviving strokes and neurological diseases also increased.

Because of these increases in the number of individuals with physical and cognitive impairments, the general public became more aware of the need to provide services. Public opinion moved away from the previously held idea that individuals with disabilities needed custodial care and toward the notion that education and opportunities to develop more independence were important (Scheerenberger, 1987). This notion prompted advocacy for the rights of individuals with disabilities and the passage of legislation that mandated services and educational opportunities.

NEEDS OF INDIVIDUALS

Demographics

The growing number of individuals who needed AAC exhibited a variety of specific communication needs. Some individuals needed AAC because they did not have the physical structures such as the tongue or larynx to produce natural speech. These individuals often used writing or an **electrolarynx** to communicate (Zangari et al., 1994). Other individuals needed AAC systems because of sensory impairments. Individuals who were deaf or had dual sensory impairments needed visual and/or tactile cues to communicate. Still other individuals needed AAC because of motor impairments that precluded their ability to produce natural, intelligible speech. These individuals were able to formulate ideas and encode messages, but unable to produce them because of conditions such as apraxia or dysarthria. Motor impairment was sometimes so severe that individuals could not gesture, use manual signs, or direct select graphic symbols on communication boards or devices. Still other individuals demonstrated communication needs because of congenital or acquired cognitive impairments. Many individuals exhibited a combination of physical, sensory, motor, and cognitive impairments.

Awareness

Public awareness of the needs of individuals with disabilities grew as information was disseminated through the media. Individuals with disabilities shared information and stories about themselves with the general population through newspaper and magazine articles, radio interviews, and television broadcasts. Public awareness and support gained impetus when prominent figures such as John Kennedy and Hubert Humphrey revealed that they had relatives with cognitive impairments. The Panel on Mental Retardation, developed by President Kennedy in 1961, became a powerful resource for the distribution of information and prompted public support for programs designed to improve services for individuals with disabilities (Zangari et al., 1994).

Legislation, Advocacy, and Social Policy

Public awareness of individuals with disabilities led to government involvement and legislation. In 1971, the United Nations issued a Declaration of the General and Specific Rights of the Mentally Handicapped (United Nations, 1971). Federal legislation, including Section 504 of the Vocational Rehabilitation Act (PL 93-112, 1973), Education for All Handicapped Children Act (PL 94-142, 1975), Education of the Handicapped Act (EHA) Amendments of 1986 (PL 99-457, 1986), Technology-Related Assistance for Individuals with Disabilities Act (Tech Act) (PL 100-407, 1988), Americans with Disabilities Act (ADA) (PL 101-336, 1990), Individuals with Disabilities Education Act (IDEA) (PL 101-476, 1990) were passed to prevent discrimination of individuals solely on the basis of disabilities and to provide equal opportunities. Legislation affecting individuals with disabilities and the field of AAC is discussed in Chapter 20.

Advocacy for individuals with disabilities had begun some time before federal legislation passed in the United States, however. Scandinavian countries were instrumental in promoting the concept of normalization. They advocated that individuals with disabilities should have access to educational opportunities that would help them develop skills that would allow them to live more independently in a manner more similar to their peers (Scheerenberger, 1987). Parent groups that shared information and resources were formed in several countries. In the United States, for example, the **Association for Retarded Children (ARC)** (later called Association for Retarded Citizens, now known as **the Arc**) was founded in 1950. This organization identified individuals with cognitive impairments who could benefit from AAC services. It was instrumental in securing educational opportunities and paving the way for the provision of special services in the public schools (Zangari et al., 1994).

Professionals took a role in advocating for the rights of individuals with disabilities in general and with communication disabilities in particular. **Speech-language pathologists** in the health field, for example, recognized the potential benefits that AAC could have for individuals with diseased or damaged speech mechanisms and individuals who were dependent on ventilators (Zangari et al., 1994). **Special educators** began to engineer environments and adapt curricula to meet student needs. Professionals who provided services for individuals with cerebral palsy advocated that communication was a fundamental right.

Advocacy to provide educational and communication opportunities for individuals with hearing impairments increased during the 1960s. The shift from the oralist approach to a total communication approach expanded the use of **American Sign Language (ASL)** for communication (Denton, 1970; Evans, 1982; Garretson, 1976; Vernon, 1972). Americans who were deaf advocated for the right to be educated in their own natural language. ASL began to be studied by linguists and gained serious attention (Stokoe, 1960). At the same time, other manual sign and gesture sets/systems were developed and taught in the public schools to individuals with cognitive impairments. By the early 1970s, the use of manual signs became an unaided form of AAC used with individuals with both hearing and cognitive impairments (Burrows & Lloyd, 1972; Hall & Conn, 1972; Hall & Talkington, 1970; Hoffmeister & Farmer, 1972). New interest in pragmatics and communicative intent also influenced the increased use of manual signs and other AAC strategies (Zangari et al., 1994). The use of graphic symbols was promoted (McNaughton & Kates, 1974).

Public figures, family, and professionals all advocated for AAC users, but AAC users also advocated for themselves. AAC users published printed material and made presentations at conferences and conventions in an effort to improve their position. Although social policy often changes slowly, the mandates of federal legislation and continued advocacy have aided in the movement toward recognizing and making accommodations to meet the needs of individuals with disabilities. The provision of closed-captioned television programming, the use of telephone devices for the deaf (TDDs), state relay systems, the increasing availability of AAC devices, and special educational programming are just a few visible illustrations of this movement.

AAC MODES AND METHODS

A variety of modes and methods were used to provide AAC for individuals long before AAC evolved as a field of its own. Individuals who could not speak, for example, intuitively used gestures, made drawings, or wrote messages. They sometimes developed an augmentative or alternative system of communication of their own (Brown, 1954).

In the beginning, health care providers, speech-language pathologists, and educators often experimented to find viable modes and methods of communication, because there was no research base to guide them. However, as more and more individuals who needed AAC were identified and served, different modes and methods developed.

The use of manual signs appeared early as a legitimate AAC strategy for improving the communication skills of individuals with hearing impairments. Manual signs were subsequently used as a method of AAC for individuals with cognitive impairments (Kiernan, Reid, & Jones, 1982; Kopchick & Lloyd, 1976) and individuals with both hearing and cognitive impairments (Burrows & Lloyd, 1972; Furth, 1961; James, 1963; Leshin, 1961; Mangan, 1963). Although the teaching of signs often evolved out of a general need to produce signs in specific situations according to the capability of the signer, more structured plans for the presentation of signs based on motor abilities and iconicity evolved to guide the teaching. Sign languages and systems are discussed in Chapter 7.

The early use of aided AAC modes was documented by a few service providers and AAC users. **Communication boards** and charts were used with individuals with aphasia (Goldstein & Cameron, 1952; Sklar & Bennett, 1956) and physical disabilities (Feallock, 1958; Goldberg & Fenton, 1960). Roe (1948), an individual with cerebral palsy, described the evolution of his communication board. He and his teachers first tore off the back cover of an old book and had large alphabet letters printed on it. Later, he used a black lucite board with white letters. Much of the early work done with communication boards, however, was undocumented. Data providing information regarding optimal size, type, and layout of symbols were not routinely collected. Yet, symbol communication boards appeared in the educational programming and daily living environments of individuals with little or no functional speech. They included a variety of symbol types such as photographs, line drawings, and **traditional orthography (TO)**. **Blissymbolics**, first developed for international communication, was introduced as a system that allowed symbols to be combined into linguistic codes (Bliss, 1949, 1965; McNaughton, 1976, 1985). Fuller, Lloyd, and Stratton discuss symbols and aided communication in Chapter 6.

In the early days of AAC service provision, modes and methods were borrowed from other disciplines. Methods that were effective for teaching skills to typically developing children, for example, were used with children with disabilities. Sensitive and innovative service providers, however, recognized special needs and adapted resources and methods of teaching. Meaningful, optimally accessible, and appropriately sized symbols were created by service providers sensitive to cognitive, motor, and visual impairments. Aided language stimulation and prompt hierarchies were used to enhance the teaching of language. Some service providers collected data to determine what worked best for particular AAC users, but in the beginning, most service providers worked from their own knowledge bases, and methods varied widely. Stories of successes generated enthusiasm and optimism, but there were also doubts about the value and promise of AAC, because there was no research.

AAC RESEARCH

As more individuals began receiving services and more questions related to efficacy and best practices arose, more research was initiated. Investigators began to look at how to assess and provide intervention that would optimally benefit AAC users in achieving functional communication skills. They looked at physical and cognitive issues of AAC users and physical and technical issues of AAC devices. Improved understanding of symbol use and language acquisition; innovations in educational practices; increased knowledge of physical, medical, and cognitive conditions; and developments in technology brought together the expertise of many disciplines that contributed to the emergence of AAC as a recognized, transdisciplinary field. Service providers collaborated with professionals from many disciplines such as medicine, occupational therapy, physical therapy, psychology, special education, speech-language pathology, rehabilitation engineering, and technology.

The need for AAC grew and service delivery expanded, but it was not until research provided a knowledge base and theories were developed that AAC became recognized as a field of its own. Leaders in the field began to conceptualize information (e.g., Light, 1988), develop taxonomies (e.g., Lloyd & Fuller, 1986), and create models (e.g., Lloyd, Quist, & Windsor, 1990; Sanders, 1971, 1976, 1982). Fuller and Lloyd present and discuss communication models in Chapter 3.

ASSISTIVE COMMUNICATION DEVICES

Advancements in technology were responsible for some of the most visible contributions to AAC during the 1970s (Lloyd, 1986). Personal computers developed for the public at large were adapted for use by individuals with special needs. Additionally, devices developed specifically as assistive communication devices were being manufactured and became commercially available. Devices that accepted a variety of input methods and produced a variety of output products were developed. Early AAC devices that produced visual output included the Talking Brooch, developed in the United Kingdom. Input came from a miniature keyboard and output appeared on a light-emitting diode (LED) display that could be worn on the clothing (Newell, 1974). Another innovative AAC device was the Auto-Com™, developed at the Trace Research and Development Center for the Severely Handicapped (Vanderheiden & Harris-Vanderheiden, 1976), which a user could take to different environments. The Auto-Com had the capability to display words input by the user on an LED display and also to print them out on a strip of paper. An important feature of the Auto-Com was that an AAC user could program and correct messages.

The introduction of voice output was a major advancement in the development of communication devices. With voice output, AAC users did not have to rely on the proximity and visual attention of communication partners. They had more power to initiate and engage someone in a communication exchange, because they could attract attention auditorily.

Despite advancements in technology and assistive communication devices, however, the process of communicating has often been fatiguing and slow for individuals with severe disabilities. The amount of energy and time required to send messages have been reduced through word prediction, abbreviation expansion, and a variety of coding techniques, but the problem of achieving efficient communication remains. AAC users are often unable to complete messages, because they became too fatigued or because their communication partners do not allow time.

Improvements in the speed, durability, dependability, and affordability of communication aids have contributed to the increase in options available for AAC users. The 1980s brought a notable increase in the involvement of manufacturers and vendors of communication aids who have supported the field directly through the publication of newsletters, awarding of scholarships, and the organization of the **Communication Aid Manufacturers Association (CAMA)**, which hosts seminars featuring the latest in communication aids. Communication aids are discussed in detail in Chapters 9 and 10.

INSTITUTIONALIZATION

Dissemination

The field of AAC grew as professionals began to share their experiences. Anecdotal accounts of successes and research findings were recorded and disseminated through the print media. Articles about AAC began to appear in refereed journals. Professionals in one part of the world began reading what was happening in another. One comprehensive report that came to be regarded as an influential international addition to the knowledge base of AAC was put out by the Swedish Institute for the Handicapped in the 1970s. "Technical Aids for the Speech-Impaired: An International Survey on Research and Development Projects" provided a comprehensive compilation of information on the research and development of AAC in different parts of the world up to that time (Lundman, 1978). This report led to further cooperation, collaboration, and dissemination of information related to professional and technological developments in AAC through the International Project on Communication Aids for the Speech Impaired (IPCAS) (Zangari et al., 1994). The circulation of newsletters describing the use of AAC strategies also contributed to the spread of information about AAC, as did the publication of books and book chapters.

Professional Preparation

Although information became available to a large number of practicing professionals through the print media, it became available to students through coursework at colleges and universities. During the academic year 1977–78, the first coursework in AAC became available at the university level (Zangari et al., 1994). In 1983, government grants began to support graduate work in AAC for students at a few institutions of higher learning. Academic programs included coursework and research opportunities that provided students with the knowledge and skills necessary to design and implement appropriate AAC intervention programs. By the end of the 1980s and the beginning of the 1990s, more than 100 colleges and universities in the United States offered at least one course in AAC (Koul & Lloyd, 1994b).

Organizations

The field of AAC grew in the 1980s with the expansion of research, developments in technology, dissemination of information, and increased opportunities to take coursework in AAC. During this decade, however, another important dimension was added. In 1980 and 1982, the Blissymbolics Communication Institute and the Ontario Institute for Studies in Education at the University of Toronto organized and sponsored the International Conferences on Nonspeech Communication to share information and discuss issues. These conferences paved the way for the organization of ISAAC, an organization devoted exclusively to the field of AAC (Zangari et al., 1994).

ISAAC has been a major force in the development of the field since it was organized in 1983 and held its first biennial conference in 1984. Its membership, which includes more than 2,000 individuals from more than 40 different countries, works to encourage scholarship, promote research, and improve service delivery. ISAAC has organized national chapters, with the first being ISAAC-UK (United Kingdom) in 1986, followed by ISAAC-Sverige (Sweden) in 1987, and USSAAC (United States) in 1988. There are now over 10 chapters. ISAAC brings together the expertise of researchers, service delivery providers, and AAC users from many nations at biennial conferences where they make formal and informal presentations about their work in the field. Research symposia are often held in conjunction with the conferences.

In addition to sharing information at conferences, ISAAC sponsors two periodicals devoted exclusively to AAC. *Augmentative and Alternative Communication*, the official journal of ISAAC, publishes clinical, educational, and research papers with an international perspective. Manuscripts, which typically include descriptive papers, research studies, and position papers, are submitted and put through a review process to ensure selection of high-quality work for publication. *The ISAAC Bulletin* is the quarterly newsletter.

Other organizations that developed an AAC focus as a part of their broader professional missions include ASHA (American Speech-Language-Hearing Association) and RESNA (Rehabilitation Engineering Society of North America, subsequently renamed the Rehabilitation Engineering and Assistive Technology Society of North America). The RESNA AAC Special Interest Group, organized in 1988, focuses on assistive technology (AT) and aided AAC approaches. In 1992, ASHA formed its AAC Special Interest Division, which has a broader focus than just AT (that is, it includes both aided and unaided AAC approaches). The ASHA AAC Division's quarterly newsletter has emerged as a major source of practical information.

During the 1980s, AAC users began to take

more initiative in improving the availability and quality of AAC services, forming self-advocacy organizations such as Hear Our Voices. More recently, AAC users have used the computer to network by subscribing to list servers such as ACOLUG (Augmented Communicators On-Line Users' Group). Information about AAC-relevant list servers (e.g., ACOLUG) and organizations (e.g., ASHA, ISAAC, RESNA) is provided in Appendix B.

Research

AAC services grew out of the need to improve the communication skills of individuals with little or no functional speech. Service providers responded by adapting materials and teaching methods to improve communication skills even before their efficacy was researched. Now, however, research guides and supports the provision of AAC services. Research continues to be of paramount importance in broadening the knowledge base of the field, as reflected by the organization of conferences such as ISAAC's biennial research symposium; an increase in the number of research presentations at conferences sponsored by ASHA, ISAAC, and other professional organizations; and an increase in the number of research articles published in professional journals such as *Augmentative and Alternative Communication.*

Theories, Models, and Taxonomies

The expansion of research and the collection of empirical data have led to the development of theories, models, and taxonomies that make the field what it is today. Clinicians/educators must no longer rely on their own knowledge base and innovative ideas. They can look to the theories that have been developed on the basis of research and apply principles of assessment and intervention in their service delivery. They can use the models and taxonomies that provide structure and organization to aid in understanding AAC as a process.

CONTROVERSIAL ISSUES

Theories, models, and taxonomies create structure for the field. Different interpretations and imple-

mentations, however, occasionally cause controversy. One such issue involved the move away from providing traditional pull-out services in isolated environments to providing services in the natural environments of the home, classroom, and job site. A related issue involved the move toward full inclusion of children with severe disabilities into general education classrooms. Information related to best practices was published to assist educators in integrating AAC users (Calculator & Jorgenson, 1991), but, in many cases, personnel were not adequately prepared. There was a lack of empirical data to guide the implementation of the legislative mandate, which provided for a free, appropriate public education (FAPE) for everyone, prohibiting discrimination on the basis of disabilities.

A second controversial issue revolved around facilitated communication, an intervention strategy in which a facilitator provides emotional and physical support to help users access keyboards to type messages. Although the intervention was thought to be a major breakthrough by some, others remained skeptical in the absence of empirical data to verify authorship of the messages (Shane, 1993).

A third issue involved the allocation of resources for AAC users. AAC services require the expertise of not just one professional, but a team of many, and this can be expensive. The rental or purchase of a communication aid can also be expensive, depending on how much high technology is involved. AAC users can look to a variety of funding sources, described in Chapter 21, but there has often been disagreement over who is responsible for providing an AAC system and services. The determination of who should provide funding for the necessary training and ongoing education that allows AAC users to develop skills to use their AAC systems effectively has also been a controversial issue.

SUMMARY

Despite these controversial issues, the field of AAC has developed to the point that individuals with a variety of communication disabilities are benefiting from AAC services more than ever before. Today, AAC services are offered by members of transdisciplinary teams at home, at school, in the workplace, in medical settings, and in extended care facilities. The development of improved educational strategies, increasing availability of assistive communication devices, increasing opportunities for academic and professional preparation service providers, and increasing educational opportunities for individuals with communication disabilities have all played roles in bringing the field of AAC to where it is today.

Service delivery is no longer driven by the needs of AAC users and the knowledge of individual service providers. It grows in concert with what research finds to be effective. Research serves as the foundation for the development and implementation of AAC programs so that individuals with severe communication disabilities have optimal opportunities to reach their full potential in becoming effective communicators. Clinicians/educators must review the research as they continue to provide services.

CHAPTER 3

AAC MODEL AND TAXONOMY

DONALD R. FULLER AND LYLE L. LLOYD

Webster's Third International Dictionary (1976) defines a **model** as ". . . a theoretical projection in detail of a possible system of human relationships . . ." (p. 1451). The operative words in this definition are *theoretical* and *human relationships*. A model is typically a construction based on one's current understanding of how a particular phenomenon operates; that is, a model is simply a representation of theory. Human relationships can include economics, psychology, or any other system in which humans are an integral part including **communication**. Communication is an extremely complex phenomenon that is not fully understood to this day. As such, the best one can do is offer a theory for how communication within the human species takes place. To assist in conceptualizing all the various aspects that make up communication, a model can be employed based on current knowledge of the process. Lloyd, Quist, and Windsor (1990) identified several benefits of constructing a model for **augmentative and alternative communication (AAC)**. A model allows for the formulation of questions and hypotheses about the individual aspects of AAC and how the individual aspects interrelate. From this, systematic quantitative and qualitative research can be designed to address the questions and hypotheses. In the short term, research affords the opportunity to adjust the model, if necessary, to reflect new knowledge. In turn, the expansion of the knowledge base through research ultimately allows for the development of effective assessment and intervention strategies. Another benefit of a model is that it provides structure to the knowledge base. At the same time, the relationships between and among various fields can be better conceptualized through the use of a model. This is especially important for AAC, which can be described as a field of fields that includes occupational therapy, physical therapy, social work, special education, speech-language pathology, rehabilitation engineering, and other professions.

With the vast amount of information that exists in the field of AAC, it is not only beneficial, but also necessary, to conceptualize the AAC process by developing a model based on current theory. This model will serve as the basis for organizing and presenting the information concerning AAC for the remainder of this textbook. Before presenting the model, however, the reader may be in a better position to understand the complex process of AAC if a brief background discussion on the evolution of communication models in general is provided. Therefore, the following section examines a representative number of models that have come from information processing, speech production, and communication. From this discussion, the reader should be able to see a direct relationship between these fields and AAC.

COMMUNICATION MODELS IN GENERAL

The process of human communication has been conceptualized by several individuals over the past four decades (Berko, Wolvin, & Wolvin, 1977; Fairbanks, 1954; Sanders, 1971, 1976, 1982; Shannon & Weaver, 1949). Each model presented in this section is based on a different orientation or school of thought, but they all share similar aspects. The model proposed by Shannon and Weaver (1949) was developed to illustrate general information processing and not necessarily communication per se, although human communication could be considered a form of information processing. The key aspects or elements of their model include a *source, message, transmitter, sig-*

nal channel, receiver, and *destination.* In human speech communication, the source represents the individual's brain, where the message (the idea to be transmitted) is formulated. The message is sent through the transmitter (the speech mechanism) as an acoustic signal. This signal channel may or may not include noise. Eventually, the signal is perceived by the receiver (the listener's ear) and then interpreted at the destination (the listener's brain). This model does not consider the reciprocality of communication, but simply describes a single **message** being conveyed from **sender** to **receiver**.

Fairbanks (1954) presented a model to describe speech production, which for most individuals is the primary mode of communication. As such, his model is not concerned with communication but instead with how speech is produced. This does not lessen the impact of his model, because it provides a rather detailed account of at least one half of the communication process (the sender). A unique feature of Fairbanks's model is that it is a closed-loop or servosystem, meaning that ongoing **feedback** is an integral part of the model. In essence, the signal (i.e., the message that is to be conveyed by speech) is stored in a controller unit, then sent through an effector unit (the speech mechanism), where it is finally sent out as an acoustic signal. The unique feature of this model is the sensor unit, which is responsible for comparing the signal that went out to the message that was intended. According to this model, the hearing mechanism is the chief anatomical structure responsible for receiving feedback, with the output acoustic signal being fed back to the hearing mechanism through air and bone conduction. Other sensors are also responsible for the feedback mechanism (e.g., tactile and kinesthetic receptors of the individual speech organs). Feedback has direct implications for AAC, as iterated by Lloyd et al. (1990):

> Speech, or any communication output, is self-corrective in most senders. This is possible because the sender is able to constantly monitor the output via various forms of feedback (auditory, visual, and tactile) and adjust such output according to a preconceived standard based on previous experience. If the sender lacks the experience or receives distorted sensory feedback, there may be a serious deterioration in communication effectiveness. In

AAC, message distortions may be related to the nature of the input or output system used (e.g., poor visual acuity and hearing impairment). Furthermore, such sensory distortions may alter perception of the environment and result in inappropriate understanding and interaction with that environment. This may have serious implications for the individual's cognitive and social development. In AAC, distortions in sensory feedback may result because of the significant variations in the form and/or latency of the feedback. For example, synthesized speech provides no proprioceptive or kinesthetic feedback and may be substantially delayed as compared with the instantaneous feedback of the output of the vocal mechanism. (p. 182)

Clearly, an AAC model should include some form of feedback mechanism.

The model proposed by Berko, Wolvin, and Wolvin (1977) attempts to describe how such variables as attitudes, experiences, and physical states, enter into the process of communication. According to their model, two communicators (a source and a receiver) convey information and ideas to one another through a communication environment that may or may not be superimposed by a noise component (either internally or externally generated). In this sense, their model is similar to the model proposed by Shannon and Weaver (1949). The uniqueness of the part that intangible variables play in communication sets this model apart from the others. The source communicator's (i.e., the sender's) attention is first aroused by an idea or a need to communicate. The sender then chooses to communicate a message by using language symbols. Memory and past experiences are used to govern the selection of language symbols for encoding the message. The sender's message is then tempered by the sender's attitudes, physical state, and expectations. The message is sent through a channel within the communication environment and is received by the receiver communicator. This person's attention is aroused by aural stimuli or the need to communicate. The message is received in distorted form (due to the introduction of the noise component). The receiver communicator must then rely on memory and past experiences to decode the message. The information is then stored and the receiver communicator offers feedback to the source communicator.

Sanders's (1971, 1976, 1982) model includes aspects from the models of Fairbanks (1954) and Berko et al. (1977). It addresses the complexity of interaction between a sender and receiver within a communication environment and also addresses the issue of feedback. It is, however, a much more widely expanded model of communication, because it describes in greater detail the sender and receiver. The message **encoding** and **decoding** processes are also explained in more detail. A key component of Sanders's model is the multimodal description of message sending and receiving. Irrespective of disability, most individuals do not rely solely on speech as a means of communication. Some may rely on facial expressions, gestures, and posture and movement, in addition to speech. The use of pictures is also a possibility when speech or gestures fail to get the message across (e.g., when two persons of differing languages attempt to communicate). As such, communication tends to be a multimodal phenomenon. This is especially important for AAC, because any and all modalities (e.g., gesture, pointing, speech, writing) must be manipulated to maximize the probability of successful communication. An AAC model should therefore include a multimodal component.

The reader who is interested in a more thorough discussion of these models is encouraged to locate the original papers (Berko et al., 1977; Fairbanks, 1954; Sanders, 1971, 1976, 1982; Shannon & Weaver, 1949). In addition, compendium of these models can be found in the article by Lloyd et al. (1990).

AAC MODEL

The preceding discussion indicates that these models share several aspects of general communication and information processing. These include the sender, message, receiver, feedback, and communication environment (Lloyd et al., 1990). Successful communication must have at least two individuals—a sender of an idea and a receiver of that idea. In addition, communication implies that a message is being transmitted. This message is transmitted and the communicators exchange ideas within a communication environment, which may have noise components (internally and/or externally generated). Finally, feedback—both internal (e.g., auditory and kinesthetic) and external (e.g., linguistic and nonlinguistic indicators that the message has been understood)—is a crucial component of the communication process. Communication is a multimodal process. Speech is not the only mode by which ideas are transmitted. Facial expression, gestures, pointing, and writing are also legitimate means of conveying information. Typically, several of these tend to be transmitted in parallel. For persons with disabilities, a multimodal approach to communication is essential, and an AAC model should contain all these aspects.

Lloyd et al. (1990) proposed an AAC model, illustrated in Figure 3.1, that takes into consideration all these aspects. This model is an expansion of Sanders's (1971, 1976, 1982) model of general communication, with modifications made to reflect what occurs during the AAC process. Lloyd et al. (1990) argued that an AAC model could be subsumed under a general communication model instead of being designed as a categorically different entity for three reasons. First, AAC is typically an intentional, symbol-based, and rule-governed form of communication, consisting of a message being transmitted from a sender to a receiver within a communication environment with appropriate feedback being given. Second, a model based on general communication lends itself to direct observation and comparison between AAC and other forms of communication (e.g., animal communication, spoken communication, and other forms of human communication between individuals with and without disabilities). Finally, AAC is an interactive process between communicators, one of whom may not have communication disabilities. In other words, communication often takes place between an AAC user and a person without disabilities. An AAC model must consider these facts.

In Figure 3.1, the key elements of a general communication model are the sender, message, transmitter, communication environment, receiver, and feedback (both endogenous and exogenous). Lloyd et al. (1990) added to Sanders's model the

communication environment. The communication process is influenced by different communication environments. Recognition of this is critical for effective AAC intervention. Therefore, clinicians/educators must consider communication environment as a critical part of the AAC model. With this addition, what Sanders referred to as the environment was retitled the **transmission environment** or **transmission/signal channels** for the AAC model (see Figure 3.1). Whereas the communication environment includes the people, places, and contexts in which communication is taking place, the transmission environment is the actual propagating medium or signal environment. The transmission environment is typically air for conducting light and/or sound waves, but it could

be some other medium such as water. In other words, there are two different types of environments, and each has multiple possibilities.

Another addition was the AAC **transmission processes** and AAC **interface** component, which will be explained in more detail later. For purposes of discussion, the process of AAC will be described in terms of the sender being an AAC user. Keep in mind, however, that in the natural environment either the sender or receiver, or both, may be using AAC.

The upper half of Figure 3.1 shows a typical scenario between two communicators in which the sender is using AAC: Person A (the sender) forms an idea to be communicated. Coded neural impulses are generated via the sender's cognitive and

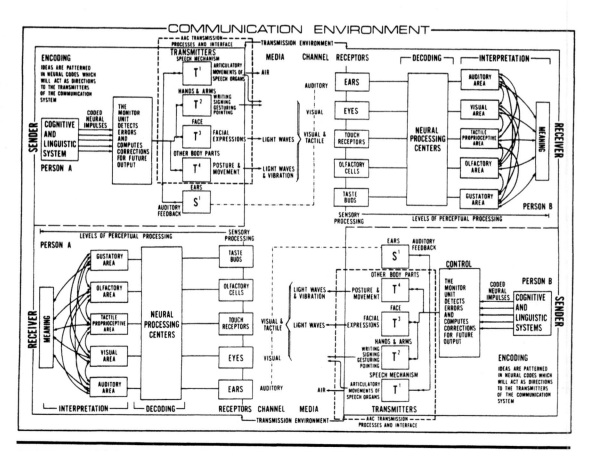

FIGURE 3.1 AAC Communication Model
From Lloyd, Quist & Windsor, 1990, pp. 172–183. Used by permission.

linguistic systems. These impulses pass through a monitor unit that detects errors and makes corrections for future output (a form of endogenous feedback). Coded impulses then drive any one or number of the transmitters (speech mechanism, hands and arms, face, and other body parts) to encode the message. If the speech mechanism is driven, the output will be speech via the articulatory movements of the speech organs. If the hands and arms are driven, the output could be pointing, gesturing, manual signing, or writing. Facial expressions will be generated if the face is driven. Finally, other body parts (e.g., shoulders, legs) when driven will assist in generating communication through posture and movement. Any one or all of these modes of communication may be in operation at a given time. The output message then passes through the transmission environment (e.g., speech as an acoustic signal or sound/vibration waves and manual signs as a visual signal or light waves) to Person B's receptors (ears, eyes, touch receptors, etc.) where sensory processing takes place. (Simultaneous with this process, Person A's ears may be receiving auditory feedback, either endogenously from within self or exogenously from Person B or some other source in the communication environment.) The sensory organs of Person B transduce the incoming signal(s) where the information is decoded at neural processing centers. The message is interpreted in the various somatic areas of the brain (auditory, visual, tactile, proprioceptive, etc.), and meaning is finally achieved. The lower half of Figure 3.1 is simply a reversal of the upper half. That is, the two communicators have changed places so that Person B is now the sender and Person A is the receiver of a message. The process of *general* communication is thereby described. Keep in mind that this is only a superficial discussion that does not adequately describe the true complexity of AAC.

Housed within the AAC transmission processes are three important components: the **means to represent** (symbol), the **means to select** a symbol, and the **means to transmit** a symbol. Although these processes can equally describe how persons without disabilities transmit information via different modes, the main focus of this part of the model is to describe how persons with severe communication disabilities may form, select, and transmit messages. Because speech is typically not sufficient to meet these individuals' daily communication needs, they may have to rely on other forms of communication such as graphic (printed) symbols or words, gestures, manual signs, or other types of symbols.

Symbols used for AAC are typically categorized as either **aided symbols** or **unaided symbols**. In keeping with the definitions proposed by Lloyd and Fuller (1986), aided symbols require some type of external assistance, aid, or device (e.g., communication board, electronic aid, or paper and pencil) to produce a message. On the other hand, unaided symbols require nothing external to the user's body to produce a message. The aided/unaided dichotomy can also be used to describe the selection and transmission of symbols.

At this point, the AAC transmission process will be described more fully. First, the user must formulate a message and then choose symbols to represent it. As already stated, symbols can be classified as either aided or unaided. This is not to imply that a typical AAC user will be using symbols from only one of the two domains. To the contrary, an effective AAC communicator will in all likelihood be communicating using symbols from both.

Second, once the symbols are chosen to represent the various concepts to be communicated, they must be selected from the pool of all symbols available to the AAC user. If the AAC user chooses to use unaided symbols, the means to select will also be unaided. For example, if the user is communicating with Amer-Ind gestures, the selection of the symbols will be by hand and arm movements. On the other hand, if the AAC user is communicating with aided symbols, the means to select those symbols can be either aided or unaided. Consider the individual who communicates with Blissymbols. In an unaided selection, the user has the motor ability to point to the symbols on a communication board. Because the user is selecting the symbols with body parts (in this case, the finger of one hand), the means to select is unaided. Suppose, however, that the user does not possess adequate motor control to use a finger or any other body part. The only consistent motor control the user possesses is adequate head movement. Obviously this user will not be able to select the Blissymbols directly through body parts. However, if the user is fitted with a head stick or light pointer, the ability to point to the symbols on the communication board can be achieved. Because a device is being used to select symbols, the means to select in this case is aided.

Once the symbols are chosen and selected, the message is transmitted through some means. Once again, if the AAC user communicates with unaided symbols, both the means to select and the means to transmit will be unaided. In this case, the individual is considered to be directly transmitting the message through the movements of body parts. Direct transmission is classified as an unaided means to transmit.

When a person uses aided AAC symbols, those symbols must be displayed on some type of aid or device. This can include anything from simple communication boards to wallets, booklets, and sophisticated electronic devices. Aided symbols are different from unaided symbols, because they are typically graphic (printed) or three-dimensional (e.g., objects) and therefore cannot be simply committed to memory, as unaided symbols can. Because some type of external aid or device is required to display aided symbols, the means to transmit is always aided if the symbols are aided, regardless of whether the means to select is aided or unaided. Therefore, for the two examples mentioned above, the means to transmit is aided even though the individual may have had the ability to directly select symbol choices.

The Lloyd et al. (1990) AAC model, based primarily on Sanders' (1971, 1976, 1986) communication model, is a broad multimodal model that accounts for the major aspects of AAC. The degree of communication and miscommunication is directly related to the match or mismatch of the sender and receiver. In general, communication is more effective and efficient when the sender and receiver are more closely matched on cognitive ability, culture and experience, linguistic competence, motivation and interest, and perceptual skills and abilities. This model can be used as a framework to aid in understanding which communication modes will be selected. External factors

that influence communication and the interactive nature of communication are key aspects of the model. The formulation of a message and the selection of modes are influenced by the way communication partners perceive each other's abilities. In the communication process, the communicative intent or function is more important than the form. Communicators are driven by seeking relevance in the message (Sperber & Wilson, 1986). Relevance has been considered crucial in recent discussions of AAC models (von Tetzchner et al., 1996). While the model is robust in its multimodality and consideration of environmental and external factors, it does not elaborate on the internal cognitive and linguistic systems nor does it explain how neuroprocessing centers encode and decode messages. More recently, psycholinguists have proposed models, such as Levelt's blueprint for the speaker, that account for underlying communication processes (Levelt, 1993). Levelt's model, however, focuses only on spoken language and does not account for the multimodal nature of AAC. Loncke, Vander Beken and Lloyd (1997) have extended Levelt's model to account for both linguistic and nonlinguistic communication in various modes. An AAC model considers more than just spoken language.

With an AAC model in place, it is now time to focus more fully on describing an AAC taxonomy for symbols, selection techniques, and transmission modes.

AAC TAXONOMY

By definition, **taxonomy** is the science of classification. Humans tend to categorize and group things in their environment to enhance memory, storage, and retrieval. In AAC, a system of classification not only provides for the organization of various symbols, selection techniques, and modes of transmission, but also provides insight into how these phenomena interact. A taxonomy affords the opportunity to make direct comparisons between and among symbols, selection techniques, and modes of transmission.

In the discussion of the AAC model, the communication environment was described. Housed within this environment are the AAC transmission processes and interface. The AAC transmission processes include the means to represent, the means to select that representation, and the means to transmit the message. Recall that in each case, the *aided/unaided* dichotomy was used to classify the phenomena associated with it. In essence, a simple taxonomy has already been described for the means to represent, select, and transmit. More specifically, a superordinate level (aided versus unaided) has been described for each of the three AAC transmission processes.

Table 3.1 provides examples of the means to represent, select, and transmit according to the aided/unaided dichotomy. For the means to select and means to transmit, the aided/unaided classification as proposed by Lloyd et al. (1990) is an excellent *superordinate* level of a taxonomy. In fact, at present, *subordinate* levels (i.e., levels of subclassification) may not even need to be described for the means to select and the means to transmit. Aided means to select include mechanical pointers (e.g., head pointers, mouthsticks), switches, and other mechanical or electronic devices that use direct selection or scanning techniques. Unaided means to select include various body movements (e.g., blinking, eye gaze, gesturing). Aided means to transmit include communication boards, electronic devices, and other items external to the user's body. Finally, unaided means to transmit involve direct transmission through the user's own body parts. Illustrative examples of these are provided later.

Of the three AAC transmission processes, the means to represent has received the most attention (Fuller, Lloyd, & Schlosser, 1992; Lloyd & Fuller, 1986; Lloyd et al., 1990). Examples of the various AAC symbols as classified under the aided/unaided dichotomy show the original superordinate taxonomic level as proposed by Lloyd and Fuller (1986). However, for the means to represent, Fuller et al. (1992) proposed further subordinate levels. These levels, along with the original superordinate level of aided/unaided, are illustrated in Figure 3.2. These subordinate taxonomic levels include *static/dynamic*, *iconic/opaque*, and *set/system*.

Vanderheiden and Lloyd (1986) defined **static** symbols as being permanent and enduring. These symbols do not require any movement or

change to express meaning. Conversely, **dynamic** symbols are not permanent and enduring, and do require movement or change to convey meaning. This level is immediately subordinate to the aided/unaided superordinate level. However, the static/dynamic classification scheme is not a true dichotomy because within some AAC symbol sets/systems, there may actually be a combination of static and dynamic symbols. An example of this is the American manual alphabet, in which all of the letters are static except for *j* and *z*. These two letters require movement to be understood, and therefore they are dynamic. (The determination as to whether a symbol is static or dynamic is made if the symbol itself does or does not require movement; the natural movement from one letter to another or from one manual sign to another does not influence the determination of static or dynamic.) Because the static/dynamic classification is not truly dichotic, symbol sets and systems can only be described in terms of whether the symbols in that set/system are *predominantly* static or dynamic (i.e., the larger proportion of symbols in any given set/system are either static or dynamic).

This situation also exists for the second subordinate level of the symbol taxonomy—**iconic** versus **opaque**. Any given symbol set/system will in all likelihood include a number of symbols that are iconic (i.e., the symbols visually resemble the referents they represent) and a number of symbols that are opaque (i.e., the symbols have no discernible relationship to the referents they represent). Only a very few examples exist in which all symbols in a set/system are either iconic or opaque. Objects, if used to represent themselves (e.g., an apple used to represent the referent *apple*), are totally iconic. Lexigrams and Premack symbols are examples of totally opaque symbol sets. For the most part, AAC symbol sets and systems can only be described as *predominantly* iconic or opaque. In other words, for a given set/system the larger proportion of symbols are either iconic or opaque.

The final subordinate taxonomic level for the means to represent is the set/system classification. **Symbol sets** are simply collections of symbols in which each symbol has one or more specified meanings. Although sets can be expanded to some

TABLE 3.1   Aided and Unaided Means to Represent an Idea, Means to Select the Representation of the Idea, and Means to Transmit the Representation of the Idea

AIDED	UNAIDED
Means to Represent	
Objects	Gestures (e.g., pointing, yes/no head shakes, mime, Amer-Ind, generally understood gestures, esoteric signs/gestures)
Pictures (e.g., photographs, Picture Communication Symbols or PCS)	
Pictogram Ideogram Communication (PIC)	Natural sign languages (e.g., ASL, BSL, PSL, SSL; American, British, Portuguese, and Swedish Sign Language, respectively)
PICSYMS	
Blissymbols	Gestuno
Graphic representation of manual signs and/or gestures (e.g., Sigsymbols)	Manually coded English (MCE) (e.g., Signed English, Paget-Gorman Sign System or PGSS, Seeing Essential English or SEE-I, Signing Exact English or SEE-II, or the manual or gestural coding of other spoken languages)
Synthetic or animated manual signs and/or gestures	
Expanded (complex) rebus	
Other logographs with referent relationships	Fingerspelling or manual alphabets
Modified orthography and other symbols	Eye blink, gestural, and/or vocal alphabet codes (e.g., Morse code)
Arbitrary logographs (e.g., Yerkish lexigrams) and shapes (e.g., Premack symbols)	
Traditional orthography (TO)	Eye blink, gestural, and/or vocal word and/or message codes
Graphic representations of fingerspelling	Tadoma and other vibrotactile codes
Synthetic fingerspelling	
Braille and other static-tactile codes	Hand-cued speech (e.g., Cued Speech and Danish Mouth Hand)
Electronic-cued speech	
Digitized speech	Natural speech
Synthetic speech	
Electrolarynx-generated speech	
Means to Select	
Mechanical pointers	Blinking
Switches	Body movements
Other mechanical or electronic indicating prostheses/devices that may use either direct selection or scanning	Eye gaze
	Gesturing
	Pointing with a body part
	Speech
	Vocalization
	Writing
Means to Transmit	
Communication boards, charts, cards, books	Direct transmission using various body parts (e.g., arms, face, hands, vocal tract)
Microprocessors that can be either adapted or dedicated as AAC aids	
Paper and pen	

Adapted from Lloyd and Kangas, 1994, pp. 607–657. Used by permission.

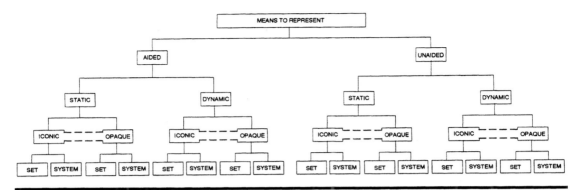

FIGURE 3.2 AAC Symbol Taxonomy for the Means to Represent. The iconic/opaque level is represented as a continuum rather than a dichotomy because of the limited research base.

From Fuller, Lloyd, & Schlosser, 1992, pp. 67–74. Used by permission.

small degree, they have no specified rules for expansion. Examples of aided symbol sets include iconic sets such as Picture Communication Symbols (PCS) (Johnson, 1981, 1985, 1992) and opaque sets such as Yerkish lexigrams (Romski, Sevcik, Pate, & Rumbaugh, 1985; Rumbaugh, 1977). Unaided symbols such as common gestures or the more formalized gestures from Amer-Ind (Skelly, 1979) are also sets. While some may argue that Amer-Ind is a system because of its capacity for agglutination (combining symbols to form new concepts), it is technically classified as a set because there are no formal rules or internal logic to govern the creation of new symbols. **Symbol systems**, on the other hand, do have formal rules and internal logic for the creation of new symbols. Examples of aided symbol systems are Blissymbolics (Bliss, 1965; McNaughton, 1976, 1985; Wood, Storr, & Reich, 1992) and Sigsymbols (Cregan, 1982; Cregan & Lloyd, 1990). American Sign Language (ASL) and British Sign Language (BSL) are examples of unaided systems that have their own syntactic and morphological structures. Signed English and the Paget-Gorman Sign System (PGSS) do not have their own syntactic structures, but are still considered systems because they mimic the syntax of English (that is, subject-verb-object).

Typically symbol sets represent concrete referents better than abstract referents while symbol systems represent both equally well, thus providing greater **representational range**. The set/system classification is a true dichotomy, clearly subdividing AAC symbols into mutually exclusive groups. Aided symbols are discussed in greater detail in Chapter 6, and unaided symbols are more thoroughly discussed in Chapter 7. Also, Appendix A-1 provides a Symbol Set and System Guide to assist in the analysis of the four taxonomic levels and other aspects of symbol sets/ systems.

Table 3.2 lists the various AAC symbols according to the full symbol taxonomy. Symbols are classified according to the successive levels of the taxonomy, in the order in which the successive levels appear (i.e., aided/unaided, followed by static/dynamic, iconic/opaque, and set/system). All symbols used for AAC can be classified according to this taxonomy. For example, Blissymbols can be classified as an aided-static-iconic system. That is, all symbols in Blissymbolics require an external device or aid to be displayed and are permanent and enduring. The larger proportion either strongly or somewhat resemble their referents. Finally, Blissymbolics is a system in that rules and a logic exist for the expansion of vocabulary beyond the original collection. It is very powerful in that it can allow the user to convey virtually any idea, no matter how abstract or complex. As a second example, fingerspelling is classified as an unaided-static-opaque system. Nothing foreign to the user's body parts is used to display the sym-

TABLE 3.2   Listing of Symbol Sets and Systems According to the AAC Symbol Taxonomy

AIDED	UNAIDED

Aided-static-iconic set
  Basic (simple) rebus
  Objects
  PCS
  PIC
  Pictures
  Tangible symbols
	Unaided-static-iconic set
	  (None)

Aided-static-iconic system
  Blissymbols
  Expanded (complex) rebus
  Picsyms
  Sigsymbols
	Unaided-static-iconic system
	  (None)

Aided-dynamic-iconic set
  Animated gestures
  Animated manual signs
	Unaided-dynamic-iconic set
	  Amer-Ind
	  Gestuno
	  Gestures
	  Mime

Aided-dynamic-iconic system
  (None)
	Unaided-dynamic-iconic system
	  Manually coded languages
	  Natural sign languages

Aided-static-opaque set
  Premack symbols
  Yerkish lexigrams
	Unaided-static-opaque set
	  (None)

Aided-static-opaque system
  Animated fingerspelling
  Braille
  Graphic Morse code
  Traditional orthography (TO)
	Unaided-static-opaque system
	  Fingerspelling

Aided-dynamic-opaque set
  (None)
	Unaided-dynamic-opaque set
	  (None)

Aided-dynamic-opaque system
  Digitized speech
  Synthesized speech
	Unaided-dynamic-opaque system
	  Cued speech
	  Gestural Morse code
	  Natural speech
	  Tadoma

Adapted from Fuller, Lloyd, & Schlosser, 1992, pp. 67–74. Used by permission.

bols; therefore, fingerspelling is unaided. Twenty-four of the 26 letters do not require movement or change to convey meaning (only *j* and *z* do), so fingerspelling is predominantly static. Alphabets are rather arbitrary inventions that have little visual relationship to their referents and are therefore opaque. Finally, because fingerspelling from the American alphabet mimics the English language, it is classified as a system. With this symbol taxonomy in place, symbols can be grouped into meaningful categories. Furthermore, the similarities and differences between and among the various AAC symbols can be determined by using this taxonomy.

Examples of an Integrated Taxonomy

A taxonomy has been described for the AAC transmission processes. Two examples are provided in this section to illustrate how the taxonomy operates. The first AAC user is an individual in the Deaf community who communicates in American Sign Language (ASL). The first transmission process is the means to represent, or simply the symbols this person uses to communicate his thoughts. He uses the manual signs from ASL. These symbols are classified as an unaided-dynamic-iconic system. The user conveys meaning by using his body parts to generate the symbols; therefore, the symbols are unaided. Most symbols require movement to be understood (movement is one of the primary parameters of natural sign languages). Therefore, ASL is predominantly dynamic. Manual signs from ASL are predominantly iconic as well; there is some visual relationship between most manual signs and their referents, although this relationship may not be readily apparent. Finally, as with all languages, ASL is a system because it has its own syntactic, morphological, and pragmatic rules. The second transmission process is the means to select the representation. This individual is selecting the manual signs from ASL by various body movements; therefore, the means to select is unaided. The final transmission process is the means to transmit. In this case, transmission is direct through body movements and therefore is also unaided. Remember from the discussion of the AAC transmission processes that if the symbols are unaided, the means to select and the means to transmit will also always be unaided.

The second AAC user communicates with an electronic voice output communication aid (VOCA). To assist this individual in encoding messages, PCS are pasted to the keys of the device. She has the ability to activate the keys by depressing them with the index finger of her right hand. The first AAC transmission process is the means to represent. PCS are used for this purpose. The symbol taxonomy describes PCS as an aided-static-iconic set. These symbols require a device external to this user's body for display, but are permanent and enduring. Therefore, PCS are aided and static. Most PCS visually represent their referents (i.e., they are predominantly iconic). Finally, PCS are a commercially available collection of symbols that do not have a rule base for further development of symbols beyond the original collection. Therefore, PCS are a set. The second transmission process is the means to select. In this case, the user selects her choices by depressing keys on the electronic device. Therefore, the means to select is unaided (had she used a headstick or other device to access the keys, the means to select would have been aided). Finally, remember that if the means to represent is aided, the means to transmit will also be aided, regardless of whether the means to select is aided or unaided. Because PCS are aided, the means to transmit is aided because the symbols are being displayed on the electronic device, which is external to this user's body.

SUMMARY

Any AAC situation can be described in rather striking detail, as can be seen from the preceding examples. With the AAC model in place, the overall process of communication and the symbols, selection techniques, and modes of transmission can be thoroughly described to allow the clinician/educator to gain insight into the complexity of AAC. The symbol taxonomy provides the structure for the systematic classification of symbols so important to the process of symbol selection. The model and taxonomy presented in this chapter will serve as the framework for the remainder of this text. The reader's attention is now turned toward the use of terminology in AAC—the topic of the next chapter.

CHAPTER 4

TERMINOLOGY ISSUES

DOREEN M. BLISCHAK, LYLE L. LLOYD, AND DONALD R. FULLER

Use of consistent terminology in a rapidly growing, international, transdisciplinary field such as **augmentative and alternative communication (AAC)** is of critical importance. Because individuals involved in the provision of AAC services and AAC users themselves come from a broad variety of clinical, educational, medical, and vocational backgrounds, varying terms are often used to designate the same concept. Terms may also be used somewhat differently across various cultures and disciplines. Consistency in terminology is important not only among individuals within the AAC community, but also among individuals outside the field of AAC. This chapter describes and defines terms that are often ambiguously or incorrectly used in AAC to provide consistency across chapters in this text and across disciplines in the field.

GENERAL TERMINOLOGY

Of primary importance is the term *augmentative and alternative communication (AAC)* itself. Although work has been done to provide communication alternatives to individuals with severe **speech impairments** since the 1950s, it was not until the 1980s that the term came into accepted usage (see Chapter 2 for an historic perspective). Some continue to use the terms *alternative communication, aug com, augmentative communication,* or *nonoral, nonspeech, nonverbal,* or *nonvocal communication.* In this text, the broader term *augmentative and alternative communication* is used to describe the use of special strategies, methods, and techniques to *augment* and/or serve as an *alternative* to natural speech and/or writing, in keeping with the name of the journal of the International Society for Augmentative and Alternative Communication (ISAAC). Use of the term *AAC* implies that some individuals may (in some circumstances) use alternatives to natural speech and/or writing and in other situations may augment their speech and/or writing. Other individuals may use strictly alternative, or conversely, augmentative methods. Thus, the broader term *AAC* covers a continuum of communication use.

AAC symbols and approaches may be described along various dimensions. In this text, the superordinate classification is aided (Chapter 6) or unaided (Chapter 7), according to the taxonomy and AAC model discussed in Chapter 3 (Fuller, Lloyd, & Schlosser, 1992; Lloyd & Fuller, 1986; Lloyd, Quist, & Windsor, 1990). Other ways to classify AAC symbols and approaches include static or dynamic, iconic or opaque, and set or system (see Chapter 3).

Aided communication involves the use of any aid that is external to the body, such as graphic symbols, mechanical pointers, switches, and microcomputers. **Aided symbols** are discussed in Chapters 5 and 6. Technology for using aided symbols is discussed in Chapters 8, 9, and 10. **Unaided communication**, on the other hand, involves use of the body only and includes vocalization, natural speech, blinking, gestures, and manual signs (Fuller et al., 1992; Lloyd & Fuller, 1986; Lloyd et al., 1990). **Unaided symbols** are discussed in Chapters 5 and 7. Most individuals use a combination of aided and unaided AAC methods, which is referred to as **multimodal communication**.

Various terms have also been used to describe individuals who use AAC, such as *augmented communicators, consumers, nonspeakers, nonspeaking individuals* (Lloyd & Blischak, 1992) or nonoral, nonverbal, or nonvocal, which have largely fallen out of common usage (Vanderheiden & Yoder, 1986). Although it is most accurate to describe individuals who use AAC as *individuals with little or no functional speech and/or writing*, such wording can be cumbersome. In general, this text will use the term *AAC user* to include both potential and current users of AAC, with the assumption that even before formal AAC intervention, many individuals may naturally use techniques such as eye gaze or other body postures and movement as an augmentation or alternative to natural speech (see Chapter 1 for a discussion of other AAC methods).

Additional terms used to describe individuals who use or may use AAC are *severely speech-impaired individuals*, *individuals with severe speech and physical impairments* (SSPI), or *individuals with severe communication disabilities*. Use of these terms is in keeping with those adopted by the World Health Organization (WHO), which delineates the differences between the terms ***impairment***, ***disability***, and ***handicap*** (see Lloyd & Blischak, 1992).

Impairment: The absence or deficiency of a specific structure or physiological function, such as speech impairment, hearing impairment, or cognitive impairment.

Disability: The limitation to engage in activities or perform skills due to an impairment. For example, an individual with a severe speech impairment may experience a communication disability. With appropriate AAC intervention, however, an individual may function adequately and independently, thereby reducing or eliminating the disabling effects of the speech impairment. In a similar vein, individuals with profound degrees of hearing impairments are not necessarily disabled, because they may function without difficulty in the Deaf community.

Handicap: The negative impact of a disability on an individual's ability to participate in society, which can be viewed as a disadvantage. A *handicap* is not the inevitable result of a *disability*, but may occur as adaptations for participation in mainstream society are limited by a variety of physical and attitudinal barriers.

As described in Chapter 22, the extent to which an individual experiences a disability or handicap as a consequence of having an impairment (or multiple impairments) is largely culturally determined. In this text, the terms *impairment* and *disability* are used predominantly, except in cases where *handicap* is appropriate.

Because of the lack of consistency in the use of terms common in the field of AAC, (e.g., sign language), definitions for terms as used in this text are provided. For additional discussion, see Lloyd and Blischak (1992).

Communication: The transmission of meaning from one individual to another, via gestural, signed, spoken, and/or written means. Communication is generally considered to be intentional and involve social interaction.

Speech: The human or electronic production of spoken language. Speech is considered to be *vocal*, although not all vocalizations are speech (see Table 4.1).

Symbol: Something used to represent another thing or concept. Although some use this term to describe only linguistic symbols involved in the reception and production of spoken and/or written language (e.g., Siegel-Causey & Guess, 1989), in this text, *symbol* is used to denote any representation of a referent (object, idea, action, relationship, etc.), including use of body movements such as gesture, pantomime, and facial expression, which are more appropriately referred to as *nonlinguistic*.

Language: A conventional set of arbitrary symbols (spoken or written) and a set of rules for combining them to represent ideas about the world for the purpose of communication.

Verbal: An ambiguous term related to speech and language. Although the term *verbal* has been used to mean spoken or speech, as in "The child follows verbal instructions," it is also used to refer to the use of *language* in the broader sense of linguistic symbols. For this reason, use of the term *verbal* is generally avoided in this text; instead, the less ambiguous terms *spoken*, *written*, and *gestural* are used as appropriate.

Nonverbal: Another ambiguous term which technically means without language. It is generally used to describe types of evaluation tools that, utilizing spatial and motor tasks with gestural instructions, purport to measure the nonverbal intelligence of individuals who have difficulty comprehending or producing the spoken language of their present

TABLE 4.1 Verbal/Nonverbal and Vocal/Nonvocal Communication

	VERBAL	NONVERBAL
VOCAL	Human speech Synthetic speech	Cries Moans Sighs
NONVOCAL	Writing Sign language Blissymbolics	Drawing Gestures Pictures

Adapted from Vanderheiden & Lloyd, 1986, p. 73.

community (e.g., individuals with hearing impairments, individuals with brain damage, non-native speakers) (e.g., Leiter, 1959). In the field of AAC, it is occasionally used to describe individuals with little or no functional speech, as in "The child was nonverbal." In this text, the term *nonverbal* will only be used in the former case to describe communication or tasks that are truly nonverbal and will not be used to describe individuals.

Vocal: Voice or oral production of sounds that may or may not be speech sounds (e.g., cries, moans, sighs).

Nonvocal/Nonoral: Literally, without voice or oral production, once used to describe AAC methods that were produced without vocal output.

Table 4.1, adapted from Vanderheiden and Lloyd (1986), provides a delineation of verbal/nonverbal and vocal/nonvocal communication.

SYMBOL TERMINOLOGY

In describing symbols, particularly graphic symbols, terms borrowed from the fields of linguistics and psychology have been used to describe the degree to which a symbol resembles its referent (Fuller & Stratton, 1991; Lloyd & Blischak, 1992). Descriptions of graphic symbols in Chapters 5 and 6 include discussion of iconicity and related terms applied to various graphic symbol sets and systems:

Symbol set: ". . . (a) set of symbols that is closed in nature; it could be clinician-produced or it could consist of purchased symbol books, stamps, and/or cards containing a limited number of symbols. A symbol set can be expanded, but it does not have clearly defined rules for expansion" (Vanderheiden & Lloyd, 1986, p. 71).

Symbol system: ". . . (a) set of symbols specifically designed to work together to allow for maximum communication. Symbol systems include rules or a logic for the development of symbols not already represented in the system. These rules may be internal to the symbol system . . . or may be a part of the language coded by the symbol system" (Vanderheiden & Lloyd, 1986, p. 71).

Iconicity: A general term referring to the visual relationship between a symbol and its referent (the entity represented by a symbol).

Transparency: A more specific term than iconicity. Transparency is used to describe the *guessability* of a symbol in the absence of the referent. For example, in transparency studies, individuals may be shown manual signs such as MILK or BOOK, which are relatively transparent, and be asked to guess their meanings.

Translucency: A term similar in meaning to the term *representativeness* (Fuller & Lloyd, 1991; Fuller & Stratton, 1991). Translucency refers to the degree to which individuals perceive a relationship between a symbol and its referent when the referent is known. In translucency studies, individuals may be shown, for example, the Blissymbol for "house" and be asked to rate it on a 5- or 7-point scale according to the extent to which the symbol looks like a house.

Iconic: An adjective that describes a symbol that readily depicts a referent or some easily identifiable aspect of a referent.

Opaque: An adjective that describes a symbol that has very little or no visual relationship to its referent.

Arbitrary: An adjective that describes a symbol, similar in meaning to the term *opaque* used to describe a symbol that is rated as having very little to no visual relationship to its referent. For example, the traditional orthography (TO) of most written languages is highly arbitrary; there is no perceived relationship between the symbol (letter, word) and the referent (speech sound, object).

Concrete/Abstract: Terms that refer to the tangible or intangible nature of the referent and the ease with which a stimulus evokes an image. In general, tangibles such as people, places, and objects tend to be concrete; intangibles such as beliefs, emotions, concepts, and ideas tend to be more abstract. These terms should be used only to describe the *referent* and not the *symbol*.

Other terms that have been problematic in the field of AAC are those related to the use of manual signs (see Chapter 7). Two of these terms are *sign language* and *total communication*, both of which have been borrowed from the literature related to the education of individuals with hearing impairments. Both relate to AAC methods that incorporate the use of manual signs. These terms have been adopted according to what is appropriate in that body of literature.

Manual signs: A general term that may refer to a natural sign language (e.g., American Sign Language [ASL]) or to the use of manual signs as a code for a spoken language. In the latter case, production of manual signs is often paired with speech production, by signing each spoken word or each key word (see simultaneous communication).

Sign language: A term that refers only to the use of a natural sign language (e.g., ASL) and not to the use of manual signs as a code for a spoken language.

American Sign Language (ASL): The natural sign language used by the Deaf community in the United States and some provinces of Canada. Comparable sign languages in other countries are also often referred to with similar acronyms, such as BSL (British Sign Language) and SSL (Swedish Sign Language).

Simultaneous communication: The simultaneous use of two modes of communication, often manual signing and speaking. Simultaneous communication is multimodal.

Total communication: A philosophy in the education of individuals with hearing impairments that refers to the use of whatever means are appropriate to establish communication, which may include speech, written words or other graphic symbols, manual signs, fingerspelling, and/or gestures. In this way, the term is similar to the term *AAC*, and as such represents the concurrent development of similar approaches to communication intervention in different fields.

Gestures: The use of the body to represent objects, ideas, actions, or relationships without the linguistic constraints of manual signs. Most gestures are culturally determined.

TECHNOLOGY TERMINOLOGY

The advent of high technology in everyday life has created an enormous new collection of terms and acronyms, which many individuals have incorporated into their working vocabulary with relatively little effort (e.g., software, mainframe, ATM or automated teller machine). Much of the technology terminology used in AAC has been taken from such familiar terms, along with less frequently used terms that are specific to AAC, and are discussed in Chapters 8, 9, and 10 and the glossary. A few terms, however, require explanation to differentiate their use in this text.

AAC system: "[An] integrated network of symbols, techniques, aids, strategies, and skills that an individual uses to communicate" (Vanderheiden & Yoder, 1986, p. 13). This term may be considered synonymous with the term *communication system* in that they both describe the integrated use of many components for communication. An assistive communication device is considered to be one component of an AAC system.

Assistive communication device: "Any electronic or nonelectronic aid or device that provides external assistance for communication" (Lloyd & Blischak, 1992, p. 106).

Dedicated communication device: An assistive communication device that has been specifically designed for communication, as opposed to the type of assistive device that comprises specially developed adaptations (e.g., software, switch interface) used in conjunction with commonly available personal computers.

Voice output communication aid (VOCA): An assistive communication device that features electronically produced voice/speech.

SUMMARY

AAC services are being provided for individuals with severe communication disabilities throughout the world by persons engaged in a wide variety of occupations, including education, engineering, medicine, occupational and physical therapy, psychology, and speech-language pathology. As such, common, widely accepted terminology must be adopted and used. Development of consistent terminology is critical in building any scientific or professional area; thus, recognition of a common set of terms is a critical step in the establishment of AAC as a viable discipline.

Additional key terms are included in a comprehensive glossary in this text. These terms are those most commonly used and accepted by AAC service providers and users as noted in AAC texts (Beukelman & Mirenda, 1992; Blackstone, 1986)

and as delineated in the quarterly journal of the field, *Augmentative and Alternative Communication* (see Lloyd & Blischak, 1992). For some terms, alternate definitions which do not have direct application to AAC have been excluded. Although some glossary subdefinitions are numbered, the numbers are not meant to reflect order of preference.

CHAPTER 5

INTRODUCTION TO AAC SYMBOLS

LYLE L. LLOYD, DONALD R. FULLER, FILIP LONCKE, AND HELEEN BOS

Human communication consists of an intricate complex of language use and all kinds of other communicative behaviors, such as eye gaze and eye contact, facial expression (changes in), body posture, pointing, and hand movements. This complex of communicative behaviors is often referred to as **total communication** (TC), the simultaneous or alternate use of various human communication modes. For example, most individuals may use hand gestures to emphasize a particular point during a conversation. Facial expression can also be used to enhance spoken communication. Multiple modes of communication are common in everyday social interaction between humans without cognitive and/or physical disabilities.

A close look at the characteristics of human communication and language in general will provide a better understanding of the characteristics of **symbols** that can be used within AAC. Everyone involved in the use of AAC should be aware of what AAC is and is not, as seen from a linguistic perspective. Decades of linguistic research in various areas of communication has shown quite convincingly that the characteristics of genuine human communication and language are to some extent universal and form part of each individual's biological endowment. Hence, one could argue that the organization of AAC—and the communication modes within it—should as much as possible follow these general principles of human communication and language. Although the linguistic and communication capacities of AAC users may be restricted in some ways, there is no reason to assume that they consist of substantially different components than those that exist for communicators without disabilities. Therefore,

before discussing some basic characteristics of AAC symbols, this chapter focuses on some of the most basic features of natural languages and human communication.

NATURAL LANGUAGES AND AAC SYMBOLS

A natural human language is a conventional system of arbitrary symbols and grammatical rules to combine these symbols into larger units (e.g., phrases, clauses, sentences) in order to convey meaning. A *natural* language is one that has evolved from social interaction between human beings—that is, it has not been expressly invented. It is typically acquired by children as their first language. Spoken languages are natural languages. Sign languages used by persons with profound hearing impairment are also the result of natural development. These individuals are often hindered in their communication through spoken language, but the adaptational powers of the human being have resulted in the evolution of sign languages, well suited for the physical condition of deafness, as an alternative means of communication. Sign languages are languages in a different modality: they are not spoken and heard like spoken languages, but instead used in the manual-visual channel, produced mainly with the hands and perceived by vision. Deaf children acquire a sign language as their first language, and the course and pace of this acquisition are much the same as for the acquisition of a spoken language (Newport & Meier, 1985; Siple & Fischer, 1991). Sign languages are nonvocal but not nonverbal forms of communication. The notion *verbal* should be equated with *linguistic*, not with *speech* per se. Sign languages are *linguistic* systems. In human social interaction, natural languages transmitted through the spoken modality are the benchmark by which all other forms of communication are compared. For persons with cognitive and/or physical impairments, modes other than spoken communication may have to be used. These modes are often judged by listeners in comparison with spoken communication. An AAC system designed for an individual with a severe communication disability should approximate spoken, natural language as closely as possible in terms of symbols used, **representational range**, and rate of message transmission.

Chapter 3 described AAC as a process composed of three aspects: (1) means to represent, (2) means to select, and (3) means to transmit. Each of these three aspects may be aided or unaided. Although these three aspects are usually discussed sequentially, they do not necessarily occur in this order. They are typically interactive and frequently occur concurrently. Of primary importance to this chapter is the **means to represent**, including the aided and/or unaided symbols that are used to convey messages by persons with severe communication disabilities.

AAC SYMBOLS: THE MEANS TO REPRESENT

In typical communication by individuals without disabilities, meanings are represented by symbols, usually spoken or printed words. In AAC, meanings must also be represented by symbols, but often these symbols are designed specifically for this type of communication. Symbols may be described as belonging to **sets** or **systems**. Table 5.1 provides examples of the many aided and unaided communication symbols for consideration in AAC. It also includes symbols typically used by individuals without disabilities who communicate through natural speech and writing (traditional orthography [TO]). To understand how different types of symbols can facilitate communication and information processing for individuals with disabilities, the concept of multiple modes is important. One of the breakthroughs for the development of AAC has been the realization that systems for organizing meaning are internal cognitive structures not necessarily linked or tied to any one mode of expres-

sion. A language such as English, for example, is typically expressed unimodally through speech or writing. However, it can also be expressed multimodally as, for example, through speech and manual signs or speech and photographic symbols. The selection of appropriate modalities typically results in improved communication for individuals with disabilities (e.g., many individuals with cognitive impairments may have stronger skills in processing visual modalities).

The aided and unaided AAC symbol sets and systems in Table 5.1 are listed in relative order according to several criteria: (1) the concreteness or abstractness of the referents being represented by the symbols, (2) the cognitive and physical demands the symbols place on the user, (3) the iconicity of the symbols, and (4) the degree to which the symbols correspond to the oral and/or written language of the general community. Only *relative* comparisons can be made between symbol sets and systems according to these criteria. To illustrate, any given aided or unaided set/system typically has a number of symbols that may be highly iconic, some that may be somewhat iconic, and still yet a small number that may be so arbitrary that the symbols are opaque. As such, symbol sets and systems are usually classified according to how their symbols *generally* meet the criteria mentioned above. The arrangement of the symbol sets and systems in Table 5.1 allows the clinician/educator to make general comparisons between and among the various aided and unaided symbols.

Typically, symbol sets in which the symbols tend to be limited to representing concrete referents are listed at the top of each column, whereas symbol systems that have symbols representing both concrete and abstract concepts are listed toward the bottom. Symbols that tend to be less taxing from a cognitive and/or physical standpoint appear toward the top. Symbols that require more cognitive and/or physical demands on the user tend to be toward the bottom of each column. Relatively more iconic symbols are found within the symbol sets appearing at the top of each column, whereas more opaque symbols are found within the sets and systems at the bottom. Finally, as one proceeds down each column, the symbols generally correspond more readily to the community

TABLE 5.1   AAC Symbol Sets and Systems

AIDED	UNAIDED
Objects	Gestures (e.g., pointing, yes/no head shakes, mime, Amer-Ind, generally understood gestures, esoteric signs/gestures)
Pictures (e.g., photographs and drawings including basic [simple] rebus, PCS* and Sigsymbol pictures)	
	Natural sign languages (e.g., ASL, BSL, CSL, FSL, JSL, KSL, SSL, and TSL†)
PIC*	
Picsyms	Gestuno
Blissymbols	Manually coded English (MCE) (e.g., Signed English, PGSS, SEE-I, and SEE-II‡) or manual coding for other spoken languages (e.g., manually coded Swedish)
Graphic representations of manual signs and/or gestures (e.g., HANDS, pictures of signs, Sign Writer, Sigsymbols, and Worldsign)	
Synthetic or animated manual signs and/or gestures	Fingerspelling or manual alphabet
	Eye blink, gestural, and/or vocal alphabet codes (e.g., Morse code)
Expanded (complex) rebus	
Other logographs with referent relationships	Tadoma and other vibrotactile codes
Modified orthography and other symbols	Hand-cued speech (e.g., Cued Speech and Danish Mouth Hand)
Arbitrary logographs (e.g., Yerkish lexigrams) and shapes (e.g., Premack symbols)	
	Natural speech
Traditional orthography (TO)	
Graphic representation of fingerspelling	
Synthetic fingerspelling	
Braille and other static-tactile codes	
Electronic vibrotactile codes	
Electronic-cued speech	
Linear printing	
Digitized speech	
Electrolarynx-generated speech	
Synthesized speech	

Modified from Lloyd & Fuller, 1986, and Lloyd & Kangas, 1994. These are formal, or conventionalized, symbol sets and systems; informal nonverbal behaviors or ritualized behaviors have not been included. Used by permission.

*PCS, Picture Communication Symbols; PIC, Pictogram Ideogram Communication

†ASL, American Sign Language; BSL, British Sign Language; CSL, Chinese Sign Language; FSL, French Sign Language; JSL, Japanese Sign Language; KSL, Korean Sign Language; SSL, Swedish Sign Language; TSL, Taiwanese Sign language

‡PGSS, Paget-Gorman Systematic Sign; SEE-I, Seeing Essential English; SEE-II, Signing Exact English

language. With these dimensions in mind, the clinician/educator can make simple comparisons between symbols when trying to determine which would be more effective for use with a potential user. From a clinical/educational standpoint, however, there are other variables to consider in choosing specific symbols. These are mentioned briefly in the next section and will be discussed more thoroughly in other chapters.

ISSUES RELEVANT TO AIDED AND UNAIDED SYMBOLS

There is a growing body of research on the characteristics of symbols that are used in AAC. For aided symbols, these characteristics include **iconicity, complexity, perceptual distinctness, size, degree of ambiguity**, and number of messages that can be encoded by an individual with a set/system. These characteristics affect symbol production, reception, and/or cognitive processing. *Iconicity* refers to the degree to which a symbol resembles its **referent** or some aspect of its referent. *Complexity* involves the sophistication of a graphic symbol; the more information contained within a graphic symbol, the greater the complexity of that symbol. *Perceptual distinctness* refers to the degree to which a symbol seems obviously different and distinct from other symbols. *Size* refers to the physical, measurable dimensions of a symbol, an important variable for persons with visual impairments. *Degree of ambiguity* describes the number of concepts a single symbol can represent. Symbols with more ambiguity represent a larger number of distinct concepts than symbols with less ambiguity. Finally, the *number of messages that can be encoded* is determined by the size of the symbol set/system and the presence (or absence) of rules for generating symbols beyond the original set. These variables are discussed in greater depth in Chapter 6.

For unaided symbols, characteristics include iconicity, touch vs. nontouch, symmetrical vs. asymmetrical, one-handed vs. two-handed, complexity of handshape and/or movement, topical similarity vs. dissimilarity, visible vs. invisible, and one movement vs. repetitive movements. *Iconicity* has been shown to be a powerful variable in the acquisition of unaided as well as aided AAC

symbols. *Touch vs. nontouch* refers to whether there is physical contact between the hands, or between the hands and body during the production of the symbol. *Symmetry* is determined according to what the two hands are doing during production. If both hands are making the same handshape and/or movement, the symbol is considered symmetrical. How many hands are used to produce an unaided symbol determines if it is *one-handed vs. two-handed*. *Complexity of handshape and/or movement* refers to the physical intricacy and difficulty in producing a particular handshape or movement. *Topical similarity vs. dissimilarity* is determined by the number of features that make symbols similar or dissimilar. *Visibility* is determined according to whether any part or aspect of the symbol is obscured or hidden by another. For example, in some manual signs, one hand may be partially blocking the full view of the other hand. Such manual signs would be considered *invisible*. Finally, the number of times a particular movement is generated during the production of an unaided symbol determines whether the symbol consists of *one movement vs. repetitive movements*. These characteristics are discussed more thoroughly in Chapter 7.

In addition to considering the characteristics of aided and unaided symbols, the selection of symbol sets and/or systems must be a careful process based on many considerations, including, but not limited to, acceptability, accessibility, assertability, cognitive demands, correspondence to community language, cost, intelligibility, logic, perceptual and memory demands, portability, representational range, sensory and motor demands, and training demands (Beukelman & Mirenda, 1992; Fuller, Lloyd, & Schlosser, 1992; Lloyd & Karlan, 1983, 1984). These variables are referred to as symbol selection considerations and are discussed more thoroughly in Chapter 13.

SUMMARY

This chapter provides a broad overview of the wide variety of aided and unaided AAC symbol sets and systems. Following a brief discussion on symbol use in natural languages, specialized symbols for AAC were introduced, and the characteristics of iconicity, complexity, perceptual distinctness, size, degree of ambiguity, and number of messages that can be encoded by an individual using a specific set/system were defined. Table 5.1 provides a listing of aided and unaided symbols, ordered according to several criteria, to aid clinicians/educators in understanding the basic characteristics of symbols. It is imperative that clinicians/ educators have a clear understanding of symbol characteristics so they can select symbols to meet the specific needs of AAC users. The chapter serves primarily as an introduction, or preorganizer, for Chapter 6 on aided symbols and Chapter 7 on unaided symbols.

AIDED AAC SYMBOLS

DONALD R. FULLER, LYLE L. LLOYD, AND MICHELE M. STRATTON

Chapter 3 described a model of **augmentative and alternative communication (AAC)**. An integral component of that model was the AAC transmission processes, which include the **means to represent**, **means to select**, and **means to transmit**. These three processes were further defined according to an **aided/unaided** dichotomy. The aided/unaided dichotomy subsequently was used as the superordinate level of the AAC symbol taxonomy. By definition, aided symbols require some type of device or aid that is external to the user's body in order for a message to be transmitted. Unaided symbols, on the other hand, require nothing other than the user's body parts to convey a message (these symbols will be the topic of Chapter 7).

This chapter discusses aided AAC symbols as the means to represent. In addition to the aided/unaided classification, the taxonomy discussed in Chapter 3 further differentiates symbols according to several subordinate levels including **static/dynamic**, **iconic/opaque**, and **set/system**. The aided AAC symbols known today can be categorized into one of eight groups (see Figure 3.2). This taxonomy allows the grouping of aided AAC symbols according to shared characteristics. For example, objects, pictures, simple line drawings such as basic (simple) rebus symbols, Picture Communication Symbols (PCS), and Pictogram Ideogram Communication (PIC) symbols are very similar because each is classified as an aided-static-iconic set. Similarly, PICSYMS, Blissymbols, Sigsymbols, and expanded (complex) rebus symbols are aided-static-iconic systems. Logically, one can then deduce that the major difference between the former and latter groups of symbols is that the latter are more powerful because they are systems,

whereas the former are only finite sets without an internal logic or rules for expansion.

Chapter 5 introduced a wide array of aided and unaided symbol sets and systems currently available, arranged according to several criteria, including relative concreteness/abstractness of referents represented, cognitive and physical demands placed on the user, degree of iconicity, and degree to which the symbols correspond to the spoken and written language of the community (see Table 5.1). Although the aided AAC symbols in this chapter are discussed in the same general order as they are listed in Table 5.1, they are grouped according to characteristics and implications for clinical/educational use.

Table 6.1 categorizes several aided AAC symbol sets and systems as (1) object-based symbols; (2) primarily picture-based symbols without linguistic characteristics; (3) partially picture-based symbols with linguistic characteristics; (4) primarily picture-based symbols dedicated to voice output communication aid (VOCA) use; (5) aided representations of manual signs and gestures; (6) alphabet-based symbols; (7) phonemic- or phonic-based symbols; (8) arbitrary logographs and shapes; or (9) electronically-produced vibratory/acoustic symbols. In the next section, a number of the most commonly known or used aided AAC symbol sets and systems are discussed.

AIDED AAC SYMBOL DESCRIPTIONS

Object-Based Symbols

Object-based symbols include real **objects**, miniature objects, and **tangible** and **textured symbols**. According to the symbol taxonomy in Chapter 3, all three types of symbols are classified as aided-

TABLE 6.1   Categorization of Aided Symbols According to Their Functional Similarities

OBJECT-BASED SYMBOLS

Real objects	Tangible and textured symbols
Miniature objects	

PRIMARILY PICTURE-BASED SYMBOLS WITHOUT LINGUISTIC CHARACTERISTICS

Photographs	Brady-Dobson Alternative Communication (B-DAC)
Simple line drawings (e.g., basic (simple) rebus)	Pictogram Ideogram Communication (PIC)
Core Picture Vocabulary	Mosman Sounds and Symbols
Picture Communication Symbols (PCS)	Other commercially available symbols (e.g., Touch 'n Talk)
Oakland Picture Dictionary	

PARTIALLY PICTURE-BASED SYMBOLS WITH LINGUISTIC CHARACTERISTICS

PICSYMS	CyberGlyphs (formerly Jet Era Glyphs)
Blissymbolics	Sigsymbols

PRIMARILY PICTURE-BASED SYMBOLS OF DEDICATED VOCAs

DynaSyms	Lingraphica Concept-Images

AIDED REPRESENTATIONS OF MANUAL SIGNS AND GESTURES

Sigsymbols (sign-linked symbols)	HANDS
Pictures or illustrations of signs and gestures	Sign Writing
Worldsign	Synthetic or animated manual signs and gestures
Makaton symbols	

ALPHABET-BASED SYMBOLS

Traditional orthography (TO)	Morse code
Modified orthography	Aided representations of fingerspelling
Braille	

PHONEMIC- OR PHONIC-BASED SYMBOLS

Expanded (complex) rebus	Phonetic alphabets (e.g., IPA, ITA)
Visual Phonics	NU-VUE-CUE

ARBITRARY LOGOGRAPHS AND SHAPES

Yerkish lexigrams	Premack Symbols

ELECTRONICALLY PRODUCED VIBRATORY/ACOUSTIC SYMBOLS

Vibrotactile codes	Electronically produced speech
Electronic-cued speech	

static-iconic sets. Real objects can be used in several ways. At the simplest level, an exact duplicate of an object can be used to represent its real counterpart, for example, a comb of the same size, shape, and color as the one an individual actually uses. At a slightly more complex level, a similar or miniature object may be used to represent the real object. In this case, a comb of a slightly different size, shape, and/or color, or a miniature, can be used to represent the individual's real comb. An even more complex level involves the use of an object (either real or miniature) to represent a concept associated with that object. A miniature comb, for example, may be used to represent the concept of morning and/or evening grooming (e.g., brushing teeth, taking bath, combing hair). Finally, using a part of an object to represent the real object or a concept associated with the object may be the most complex level of representation with objects. For example, a shoelace may be used to represent a shoe or the process of going for a daily walk in the park. Objects are typically displayed through the use of communication vests (Goossens' & Crain, 1986), object boxes (Porter et al., 1985), or other displays conducive to holding or storing objects (Musselwhite, 1986).

Real Objects.
Real objects can be an effective choice for individuals who are beginning to communicate as well as for persons with cognitive, physical, and sensory impairments (Beukelman & Mirenda, 1992; Musselwhite & St. Louis, 1988; Rowland & Schweigert, 1989a, 1989b, 1990). For persons with cognitive impairments, the similarity of object symbols to their concrete referents makes them a powerful means of communication. The additional three-dimensional nature of objects allows them to be easily manipulated by persons with visual impairments. The major drawback for real objects is their size. For some concepts (e.g., chair, bed), the use of real objects would be practically impossible. The size of objects limits the number that can be displayed at a given time. Because of this, miniature objects may be a more viable means of representation.

Miniature Objects.
One should be cautious in the selection of miniature objects, because they might not be as representative of the real object or concept for a particular individual as one might expect (Vanderheiden & Lloyd, 1986). Mirenda and Locke (1989) noted that for some persons with cognitive impairments, two-dimensional representations may be more easily recognizable than miniature objects. A second caution concerns tactile discrimination. Some individuals with visual impairments may experience difficulty understanding that the miniature of a particular real object represents that object, because the two in all likelihood will not feel the same (Beukelman & Mirenda, 1992). On the whole, however, miniature objects have been found to be a viable means of representation for persons having cognitive (Mirenda & Locke, 1989), physical (Landman & Schaeffler, 1986), and sensory impairments (Rowland & Schweigert, 1989a, 1989b, 1990), including dual impairments. The clinician/educator should keep in mind that miniature objects (and parts of objects) must be carefully matched to the potential user.

Tangible and Textured Symbols.
Rowland and Schweigert (1989a, 1989b) described the use of what they referred to as tangible symbols with persons having sensory impairments. Tangible symbols can be either two- or three-dimensional and must be permanent, easily discriminated tactilely, highly iconic, and easy to manipulate. Shape and texture are important properties of tangible symbols. Symbols that use textures to represent referents are known as textured symbols. Symbols can either be purposefully or arbitrarily associated with their referents. In the former case, a square of sandpaper could be used to represent "woodwork shop" for an individual who is employed in a work shelter that makes wooden furniture. In the latter case, a swatch of cotton fabric could be used by an individual to represent his favorite Rush compact disc. Tangible symbols also include raised line drawings that can be felt by persons with visual impairments (Edman, 1991; Garrett, 1986). Case studies by Locke and Mirenda (1988), Mathy-Laikko, et al. (1989), and Murray-Branch, Udavari-Solner, and Bailey (1991) have shown that tangible symbols can be used effectively with persons having sensory (in-

cluding multiple) as well as severe cognitive impairments.

Should a symbol user be capable of moving from objects to a higher level of representation, a pairing process may be used to help that individual generalize from objects to pictures (Van Tatenhove, 1979). Objects are typically matched with symbols that have a higher level of representation (e.g., line drawings or PCS) and then are gradually faded so that the line drawings remain. Goossens' and Crain (1986) also suggested another strategy involving the use of "object pictures" to provide a transition from objects to a higher level of representation. In this strategy, a cross-section of the object is mounted on a surface, resulting in a three-dimensional "picture." This picture then evolves into raised pictures, where the height of the raised picture is gradually decreased. Eventually, a flat surface (i.e., two-dimensional picture) is used.

Primarily Picture-Based Symbols without Linguistic Characteristics

Symbols in this category are classified as aided-static-iconic sets and may include (but are not limited to) photographs, simple line drawings (e.g., basic [simple] rebus symbols, hand drawings), Core Picture Vocabulary™, PCS, Oakland Picture Dictionary, Brady-Dobson Alternative Communication (B-DAC), PIC, Mosman Sounds and Symbols, and other commercially available symbols (e.g., Self-Talk, Talking Pictures, Touch 'n Talk). These tend to be collections of line drawings and/or pictures that have no logic base for the expansion of symbols beyond the original finite vocabulary. The initial vocabulary size varies greatly from set to set. All are generically referred to as pictures. Illustrations of some of these symbols can be found in Figures 6.1 and 6.2.

Mirenda (1985) suggested that pictures can be classified into one of two categories: (1) constructed pictures, which include color and black-and-white photographs and drawings either produced by camera or hand, or taken from various sources such as magazines, picture books, or catalogs; and (2) commercially available pictures, which are prepackaged sets. (All the symbols

listed above are commercially available except photographs and simple line drawings.) Musselwhite and St. Louis (1988) suggest that the use of simple pictures and line drawings (especially those that are highly iconic) ". . . may provide an intermediate step between real objects, events, and people, and more abstract aided symbols such as PICSYMS, rebuses, or Blissymbols" (p. 195). However, Vanderheiden and Lloyd (1986) emphasize that the clinician/educator must ensure that the pictures are clearly representational for the potential user, and not just for the persons who work with that individual.

Photographs.   Good quality photographs can be either made by the clinician/educator with a camera or obtained from any number of sources such as magazines, catalogs, children's picture dictionaries, travel aids, picture books, and other printed media (Mirenda, 1985). Photographs can be either color or black-and-white and are typically used to represent people, objects, places, easily depicted verbs, and other activities (Beukelman & Mirenda, 1992). Few AAC systems are composed of photographs exclusively; typically, photographs are used as more realistic representations of important entities in the user's life (e.g., specific people with whom the user comes into daily contact or specific possessions that the user requests frequently). Reichle, York, and Sigafoos (1991) suggest that the addition of contextual information is very important in the production of a photograph. Whatever contextual information is required to allow the user to understand the photograph should be included in the photograph.

A number of studies have been conducted using photographs. Dixon (1981) reported that persons with severe disabilities had less difficulty in associating color photographs with their referents if the figure was cut out, as opposed to remaining intact. Mirenda and Locke (1989) determined that for their sample of persons with intellectual impairments, color photographs were matched with somewhat better accuracy to their referents than black-and-white photos of the same referents. Finally, Sevcik and Romski (1986) found that their subjects with mental retardation were able to more accurately match black-and-

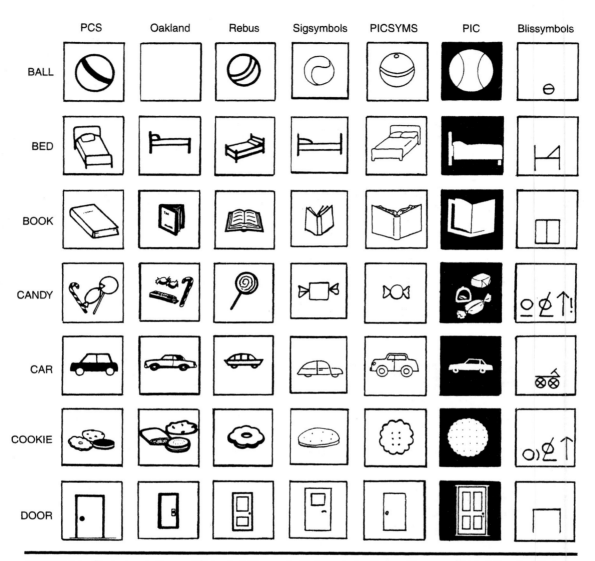

FIGURE 6.1 Representations of Selected Concrete Referents by Seven Common Aided Symbol Sets and Systems
From Vanderheiden, G. C., & Lloyd, L. L., 1986. Reprinted by permission.

white photographs to their referents than line drawings. The findings for the latter two studies would seem to suggest a symbol hierarchy for persons with cognitive impairments: color photographs, black-and-white photographs, and finally line drawings. This hierarchy should be viewed with caution, however, because of the paucity of research in this area.

Simple Line Drawings. Simple line drawings include any easily produced symbols or schematic representations of concepts. Although some of the commercial symbol sets mentioned above could fall into this definition (e.g., PCS, PIC), they will not be discussed here. One example of simple line drawings is **basic (simple) rebus**. The word *rebus* derives from a Latin word meaning "thing"

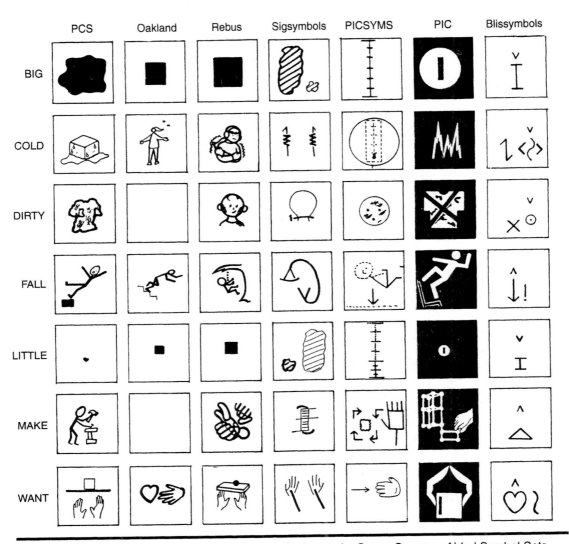

FIGURE 6.2 Representations of Selected Abstract Referents by Seven Common Aided Symbol Sets and Systems
From Vanderheiden, G. C., & Lloyd, L. L., 1986. Reprinted by permission.

(Woodcock, 1968), and there is a wide variety of rebuses in existence (Clark & Woodcock, 1976). One may remember the old television game show *Concentration*. The puzzles that made up the basis for that show were based on the rebus principle. The most common source of rebuses used in the United States today come from the Peabody Rebus Reading Program, a system that was originally developed to teach reading to young children without impairments. This reading program was

developed by Woodcock and his colleagues (Clark, Davies, & Woodcock, 1974; Clark & Woodcock, 1976; Woodcock, 1965, 1968; Woodcock, Clark, & Davies, 1968) and was originally distributed by American Guidance Service (AGS). There are actually two types of rebus symbols used with AAC systems today—basic (simple) rebus and expanded (complex) rebus. The only difference between the two is that the latter uses a semiphonic approach by combining alphabet letters, consonant clusters, syllables, and affixes to simple symbols to produce words (e.g., a picture of a baseball bat with the letters *tle* following it is an expanded rebus symbol for "battle") and therefore has more expansion capability. The same basic black-and-white symbols are used in both basic and expanded rebus. Expanded rebus will be discussed in more detail in a later section.

Basic rebus involves the use of the finite set of approximately 800 predominantly *pictographic* symbols from the Peabody Rebus Reading Program. In the formative years of AAC when few aided symbols were available, some clinicians/educators simply borrowed the rebus symbols from the reading program for use on communication boards (Vanderheiden & Lloyd, 1986). There are three types of basic rebus symbols: (1) iconic symbols, which depict objects and actions; (2) relational symbols, which typically depict locations or directions; and (3) opaque symbols, which are somewhat *ideographic* or *arbitrary* (examples of these symbols can be found in the third column of Figures 6.1 and 6.2). To avoid some of the more arbitrary and expanded rebuses and to make them more appropriate for persons with severe impairments, educators in the United Kingdom have developed other pictographic sets of rebus symbols (e.g., Chapman, 1982; Devereux & van Oosterom, 1984; J. Jones, 1979; K. Jones, 1972, 1976; van Oosterom & Devereux, 1982, 1985; Walker, Parsons, Cousins, Henderson, & Carpenter, 1985). Clark, Davies, and Woodcock (1974) have made similar revisions in the United States. Rebus symbols have been used successfully with persons having hearing impairments (Clark, Moores, & Woodcock, 1975), mental retardation, including Down syndrome (Apffel, Kelleher, Lilly, & Richardson, 1975; Pecyna, 1988), and autism (Reichle & Brown, 1986).

Most research involving rebus symbols has focused on comparative iconicity and short-term acquisition. Musselwhite and Ruscello (1984) found the transparency of rebus symbols to be equal to PICSYMS and better than Blissymbols for typically developing children and young adults. Bloomberg, Karlan, and Lloyd (1990) determined that rebus and PCS were more translucent than PICSYMS, PIC symbols, and Blissymbols for

adults without disabilities. Goossens' (1983/1984) compared the transparency of a small number of verb referents depicted by rebus symbols and Blissymbols for persons with moderate cognitive impairments. Verbs depicted by rebus symbols were significantly more transparent than verbs depicted by Blissymbols. The initial acquisition of rebus symbols and Blissymbols by preschool children without disabilities was studied by Clark (1977, 1981, 1984) and Ecklund and Reichle (1987). In both studies, the children acquired significantly more rebus symbols than Blissymbols. Similarly, Burroughs, Albritton, Eaton, and Montague (1990) found the short-term recall of rebus symbols to be superior to Blissymbols by preschoolers with language delays. Finally, Woodcock (1968) and Clark, Davies, and Woodcock (1974) reported that rebus symbols were consistently easier to learn than TO. Cumulatively, these data support the idea that rebus symbols are highly iconic and relatively easy to learn.

Core Picture Vocabulary. The Core Picture Vocabulary comprises a relatively small (approximately 160) commercially available set of symbols (black-and-white line drawings) depicting mostly concrete referents, including basic nouns, verbs, and adjectives. The symbols appear on cards, either single-sided for communication boards or double-sided for transparent displays such as eye transfer (ETRAN) displays made of plexiglass, or rotary scanning devices. Because of their limited vocabulary, they are typically not used exclusively but rather are used to augment symbols from other aided sets/systems. Don Johnston Incorporated recently made available the Core Picture Vocabulary Gallery, an icon gallery of about 300 color symbols for use with Ke:nx® on the Macintosh.

Picture Communication Symbols (PCS). Examples of **PCS** can be found in the first column of Figures 6.1 and 6.2. PCS is possibly the largest of all aided symbol sets. Designed by Roxanna Johnson (1981, 1985, 1992), PCS consists of more than 3,000 symbols grouped in three 3-ring binders. The first book contains approximately 700 symbols depicting basic vocabulary items in several categories:

people, food, clothing, grooming, animals, school, kitchen, health, time concepts, colors, body parts, vehicles, verbs, descriptive vocabulary, social, and miscellaneous. Book II expands on the vocabulary of the first book by adding over 1,000 new symbols representing topics such as religion, sexuality, computers, holidays, school, gardening, cleaning, and leisure. Generic face and head symbols can be customized to the user (e.g., the face symbol can be embellished with a mustache and eyeglasses to represent a specific person). Phrases used in typical conversation (e.g., "excuse me," "please repeat") are also included. Book III includes an additional 1,400 symbols depicting fast-food restaurant logos and food items, brand-name soft drinks, nursery rhymes and songs, story characters, and themes such as card playing, shopping, and watching television. In addition to the books, symbols can also be obtained in a wordless form (the symbols typically appear with their glosses), as adhesive stamps, and in Macintosh computer software (e.g., Boardmaker™, Speaking Dynamically™, and Communication Board-Builder 3.0) or IBM computer software (e.g., Windows Boardmaker™). Other teaching aids, including instructional books and materials, games, and symbol displays, can also be obtained from the Mayer-Johnson Company.

PCS were developed during Johnson's work with teenagers with mental retardation (Johnson, 1985). The primary objectives of the set were that they should (1) be easily learnable, (2) be appropriate for all age levels, (3) consist of simple, clear drawings for visual clarity, (4) be relatively inexpensive and readily reproducible on copying machines, (5) be easily separated into categories of symbols so that potential users need only use the appropriate symbols, and (6) be available in standardized sizes for easy placement in standardized grids. Many of the symbols are quite complex in their appearance, so hand drawing may not be an option (Musselwhite & St. Louis, 1988). Symbols are mostly pictographic, having a smaller proportion of ideographic symbols. For some concepts that are too abstract to depict by pictographs or ideographs, the English word is simply used instead of a symbol. The alphabet letters and numerals are also provided for individuals who are able

to spell out words that are not on their communication boards or devices. Although TO is used in these ways, there are no rules for the formation of new symbols, making PCS nongenerative (Whitley, 1985). As such, PCS are classified as an aided set. PCS have been used effectively with individuals exhibiting mental retardation (Mirenda & Santogrossi, 1985), cerebral palsy (Goossens', 1989), and autism (Rotholz, Berkowitz, & Burberry, 1989). Musselwhite and St. Louis (1988) suggest that PCS are also appropriate for use with persons having aphasia, apraxia, and postoperative conditions, although no known research has been conducted with these populations.

Research has not overlooked PCS. In a study involving cognitively average 3-year-olds, Mizuko (1987) found that symbols from PCS were more transparent than PICSYMS and Blissymbols. Mirenda and Locke (1989) determined that PCS were more transparent than Blissymbols for persons with cognitive impairments. Adults with cognitive impairments found PCS and PICSYMS equally transparent and easy to recall (Mizuko & Reichle, 1989). Finally, Bloomberg et al. (1990) compared translucency across five aided symbol sets and systems including PCS. They learned that undergraduate college students found PCS and rebus symbols to be the most translucent symbols, followed by PIC symbols, PICSYMS, and Blissymbols. PCS are, therefore, among the most highly iconic aided symbols.

Oakland Picture Dictionary.   Nearly 600 clear, realistic line drawings make up the Oakland Picture Dictionary (see the second column in Figures 6.1 and 6.2). The symbols are black and white and according to the author (Kirstein, 1981) are appropriate for all ages. A 3-ring binder houses the symbols, with alphabetical and categorical indexes provided for quick reference. Sample communication board layouts and grids are included to assist the clinician/educator in designing communication boards. Only one empirical investigation has included Oakland Picture Dictionary symbols. Francis, Nail, and Lloyd (1990) studied the transparency and translucency of Oakland, PCS, and rebus symbols depicting emotions for adults of average intelligence as well as adults with cognitive impairments. Results indicated that for this small set of referents, Oakland symbols are similar to PCS and rebus symbols in their iconic value.

Brady-Dobson Alternative Communication (B-DAC).   B-DAC symbols consist of black-and-white line drawings (Brady-Dobson, 1982). Approximately 1,250 symbols are arranged in 10 categories. Word glosses appear with their corresponding symbols but are upside down to the user (rightside up for the communication partner). A manual accompanies the symbols. The author has claimed that these symbols have been used successfully with individuals exhibiting aphasia, cerebral palsy, cognitive impairments, and other developmental disabilities. However, no research is cited to support this claim.

Pictogram Ideogram Communication (PIC).   PIC symbols were originally designed for persons with cognitive and/or physical impairments and include approximately 400 pictographic and ideographic symbols. PIC symbols are different than most aided symbols in that they utilize a white figure on a black background, which is opposite to most other symbols (see the sixth column in Figures 6.1 and 6.2). The designer (Maharaj, 1980) of this set used the white-on-black arrangement in an attempt to make the symbols more visually salient. However, several studies have indicated that a white-on-black background is not necessarily more visually salient than a black-on-white background (Bloomberg, 1984; Blyden, 1989; Campbell & Lloyd, 1986; Cooper & Fuller, 1994; Meador, Rumbaugh, Tribble, & Thompson, 1984). Nonetheless, PIC symbols have been used successfully with persons having severe/profound impairments (Leonhart & Maharaj, 1979; Reichle & Yoder, 1985) and autism (Reichle & Brown, 1986). Swedish and Portuguese editions of PIC symbols also exist (Beukelman & Mirenda, 1992). Other studies have been conducted using PIC symbols. Bloomberg et al. (1990), in a study of adults with average cognitive and physical abilities, found that PIC symbols were more translucent than Blissymbols although less translucent than rebus symbols and PCS. Leonhart and Maharaj (1979) determined that with no prior training,

short-term acquisition was quicker for PIC symbols than Blissymbols for adults with severe and profound cognitive impairments. These data indicate that PIC symbols are relatively iconic and easy to learn.

Mosman Sounds and Symbols.   The Mosman Sounds and Symbols set utilizes pictographic and ideographic symbols for organizing and retrieving vocabulary items from notebooks and other print media (Brereton, 1978a, 1978b; Brereton, Burnett, & Ivimey, 1979a, 1979b, 1979c). They are somewhat analogous to index tabs; in this case, they are used to separate categories of vocabulary (e.g., one symbol is used as the category organizer for foods, another for clothing). These symbols are not used widely in the United States, as they were developed in New South Wales, Australia. They are somewhat similar to subsequently developed **Minspeak**™ icons, where pictographs and ideographs are used as a mnemonic device for the storage and later retrieval of words, phrases, and sentences for speech output on an electronic communication device. Mosman Sounds and Symbols can be used as they were originally intended, or the pictographs or ideographs can be borrowed and used in conjunction with other aided symbols.

Other Commercially Available Symbols.   A number of commercial pictographic symbol sets is available. A sample of these is described below. (1) *COMPICS* (developed by COMPIC Development Association, Inc.) includes 1500 color-coded line drawings and is available in Ke:nx version for Macintosh (distributed by Don Johnston Incorporated). (2) *Kids in Action*™ (distributed by Don Johnston Incorporated) includes 400 color pictographs made for Ke:nx for Macintosh. (3) *Pick 'n Stick®* (developed by Cindy Drolet, C. Gilles-Brown, & Kelly Hume) includes 960 color-coded stickers in three packs including one fast-food pack. (4) *Picture Cue Dictionary* (distributed by Attainment Company) includes 350 color symbols for Macintosh and is TouchWindow™ compatible. (5) *Picture Prompt Cards* (distributed by Attainment Company) includes 576 color picture cards available as part of a picture prompt system. (6) *Self Talk* (developed by

Janice Johnson) includes 441 color and black-and-white stickers. (7) *Talking Pictures* (distributed by Crestwood Company) includes over 1,200 black-and-white cards in seven kits. (8) *Touch 'n Talk* (distributed by Imaginart Communication Company) includes 660 black-and-white stickers. Information about the developers, manufacturers, and vendors is provided in Appendix B-1.

Partially Picture-Based Symbols with Linguistic Characteristics

Table 6.1 shows that this category consists of PICSYMS, **Blissymbolics**, CyberGlyphs, and **Sigsymbols**. These symbols are taxonomically classified as aided-static-iconic systems. All four have a logic base for creating symbols beyond the original set. Practically any thought can be expressed using these symbols because of their excellent **expansion capability** and **representational range**. Therefore, these systems tend to correspond to the language of the community quite well. The symbols in these systems can also be technically referred to as pictures, but they are seldom referred to as such.

PICSYMS.   PICSYMS, a catenation of PICture SYMbolS, was created by Faith Carlson (1985) as a means of communication for young children who could not use speech to express their daily needs. She designed PICSYMS because she felt that most AAC symbol sets and systems lacked representations of concepts her students needed. Further, Carlson felt that as a whole, AAC symbols were too abstract for the level of cognitive sophistication her children exhibited. She thought that an effective way to provide an AAC system for an individual was to create symbols on the spot as her need arose. As such, she set out to design a system in which the symbols were relatively easy to produce by hand (even for the artistically challenged), highly recognizable, and open ended. The symbols were intended for use on communication boards (Carlson, 1981, 1985; Carlson & James, 1980; Carlson & Kovarik, 1985; Mizuko, 1987). Initial vocabulary was determined through her own clinical experience with young children with little or no functional speech, consultation with parents of her children, and inventory of several children's dictionaries. The result of her work is an alphabetically arranged dictionary of over 1,800 symbols (see the fifth column in Figures 6.1 and 6.2). In addition to the starter set of symbols, Carlson (1985) has delineated several principles to govern the system:

1. **Aesthetic appeal.** The symbols should be as attractive and appealing to the user and the general public as possible to promote their use.
2. **Developmental progression.** Carlson (1985) took into consideration the language abilities of her students in designing the system. Additionally, most PICSYMS appear in two forms—an immature and a mature form—for use depending on the individual's developmental level. The immature forms are more realistic in appearance, and the mature forms are more schematic.
3. **Level of abstraction.** More realistic symbols are created for concrete concepts such as objects. For more abstract concepts, less realism is used. For example, personal feelings and internal states are represented by a generic smiley face with facial expression changed according to the feeling. In addition, the forehead may be used as a billboard for symbolizing a concept (e.g., a bandaid is placed on the forehead to indicate "hurt"), or the face may be otherwise embellished to indicate a concept (see the PICSYM for "dirty" in Figure 6.2 in which the face is smudged).
4. **Semantic groupings.** PICSYMS is a semantically based system. In several instances, a generic figure is used to represent a class of objects. To illustrate, a rectangle with two doors in the lower left-hand corner is used to represent different types of buildings. The generic symbol is then customized by placing something in the building that is associated with it. For a bank (which conjures up various images to different people), a schematic dollar bill is placed in the generic building. For a school, a teacher and several students appear in the generic building. Buildings with features that are relatively well-recognized to the general population have their own distinct shape and form (e.g., "church" has its own form because most people recognize churches as large buildings with steeples). Generic people are symbolized by variations of stick figures, whereas specific people (e.g., characters and occupations) are more realistic.
5. **Customization of symbols.** PICSYMS depicting objects and people can be customized to fit the

user's experiential background. For example, if the user has an occupational therapist named Sue who wears a medic alert bracelet, a bracelet can be drawn on the generic woman stick figure's arm to create a customized symbol for "Sue."

6. **Creation of new symbols.** Carlson (1985) lists 28 rules that govern the creation of new symbols beyond the set of original vocabulary. These rules include the use of line contrasts such as solid and broken lines to differentiate **figure** from **ground**, a generic object indicator (a swatch of fabric to indicate a nonspecific thing), and function word indicators (e.g., a bag with a drawstring is used to indicate conjunctions such as "and," "but," and "or"), among others. The result is a system that has an excellent expansion capability and wide representational range.

Most PICSYMS can be drawn freehand, but tracing with the help of grids (which are provided in the dictionary) can also be effective for producing the symbols. Photocopying has somewhat disappointing results (Musselwhite & St. Louis, 1988). Word glosses typically appear with the symbols. A songbook (Musselwhite, 1985), materials for the teaching and use of PICSYMS, cardstock, and a computer software program (*Magic Symbols*, by Schneier Communication Unit) are available in addition to the original dictionary (Carlson, 1985). Although PICSYMS were developed for use with young children with little or no functional speech, Carlson has suggested that PICSYMS may have clinical value for children with language or learning disabilities, as well as for individuals with aphasia, apraxia, dysarthria, and cognitive impairments. However, she cautioned that until a broader base of research is accomplished, the true usefulness of PICSYMS with these populations is not known.

Most research using PICSYMS to date has focused on the comparative iconicity of PICSYMS to other aided symbols. Mizuko (1987) compared the transparency of PICSYMS, PCS, and Blissymbols for 3-year-old children of average intelligence. PICSYMS were not as transparent as PCS, but were more transparent than Blissymbols. Musselwhite and Ruscello (1984) investigated the transparency of PICSYMS, rebus symbols, and Blissymbols for persons of average cognitive abilities across a wide age range. Both PICSYMS and

rebus symbols were more transparent than Blissymbols; there was no statistically significant difference between PICSYMS and rebus symbols. Bloomberg et al. (1990) studied the translucency of PICSYMS, Blissymbols, PCS, PIC symbols, and rebus symbols using young adults without impairments. PICSYMS were less translucent than PCS and rebus symbols, but were comparable to PIC symbols and Blissymbols. Mirenda and Locke (1989) found both PICSYMS and PCS to be more transparent than Blissymbols for preschool children of average intellect and for school-aged and adult individuals with cognitive impairments. Finally, Morris (1986) compared the transparency of PICSYMS and PCS for 24 preschool children and found no statistically significant difference between the two. These data indicate that PICSYMS is a highly intelligible system.

Blissymbolics.   The history of Blissymbolics is interesting. Charles Bliss was born in Austria near the Russian border. He recognized early the misunderstandings that could result when people did not share the same language. His father was an optician and electrician, and Bliss himself became a chemical engineer. Through his own and his father's work, he was exposed to the logic and symbols these fields used. As a result of World War II, Bliss left Europe and resided in China, where he was intrigued by the ideographic system of Chinese writing. During the 1930s, the political climate in Europe had reinforced in Bliss the idea that all the strife in the world was due to the lack of a common language. He began to formulate a graphic system of communication that would transcend spoken languages. The influence of his father's and his own profession, as well as the logic of the Chinese system of writing, was clearly evident in the international communication system he called "Semantography" (which in Greek means a meaningful writing). His system was not widely accepted by the scientific community, so he published his own work in the book *Semantography* (Bliss, 1949, 1965). He continued perfecting his communication system despite little support from the scientific or political communities. At some point after the war, Bliss immigrated to Australia where he continued his work over two decades, hoping for the day it would be accepted as an international communication system. In 1971, Shirley McNaughton, an educator working at the Ontario Crippled Children's Centre in Toronto, discovered his system while working with an interdisciplinary team that was mandated to assist students with severe physical impairments to communicate. The team began teaching Blissymbols to children aged 4 to 6 years and immediately recognized the potential the symbols possessed as a communication system for persons with disabilities (Kates & McNaughton, 1975). The team members contacted Bliss and told him of the success of his system with the children in Canada. Although he had always envisioned his system as an international means of communication, he came to realize that Blissymbolics could make an important contribution to the lives of individuals with speech impairments. The Blissymbolics Communication Institute (BCI, now known as Blissymbolics Communication International) was established in Toronto in 1975. Bliss gave this organization a perpetual, nearly worldwide (except Australia) exclusive license to his copyright for supporting the use of the system by persons with communication, language, and learning difficulties. Use of Blissymbolics has expanded from Canada to 33 countries around the globe, including Brazil (Gill, 1985), France (Toulotte, Baudel-Cantgrit, & Trehou, 1990), Hungary (Collier, 1991), Iceland (Magnússon, 1990), India (Swartz, 1984), Israel (Seligman-Wine, 1988), Italy (Tronconi, 1990), South Africa (Shalit & Boonzaier, 1990), and Zimbabwe (Hussey, 1991). Examples of Blissymbols can be seen in the last column of Figures 6.1 and 6.2.

Blissymbolics is a semantically based, predominantly nonalphabetic symbol system in which the majority of the symbols are generated from 120 **key symbols** (Wood, Storr, & Reich, 1992), which are combined in various ways to produce a practically infinite number of composite symbols representing any concept imaginable. Figure 6.3 illustrates a small number of key sym-

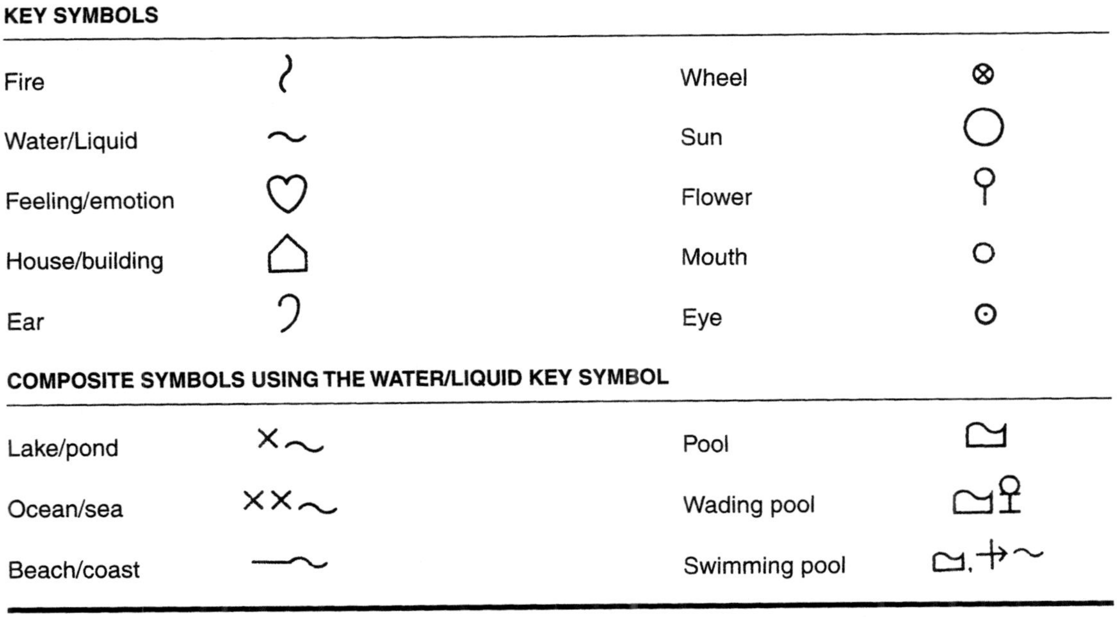

KEY SYMBOLS

Fire	⟨	Wheel	⊗
Water/Liquid	~	Sun	○
Feeling/emotion	♡	Flower	♀
House/building	⌂	Mouth	○
Ear	⟩	Eye	⊙

COMPOSITE SYMBOLS USING THE WATER/LIQUID KEY SYMBOL

Lake/pond	✕~	Pool	⌒
Ocean/sea	✕✕~	Wading pool	⌒♀
Beach/coast	—~	Swimming pool	⌒,+~

FIGURE 6.3   An Illustration of Key Symbols in Blissymbolics with Examples of Composite Symbols Using the Water/Liquid Key Symbol

Blissymbolics used herein with the approval of Blissymbolics Communication International (BCI). The symbols are described in the work *Semantography*, original copyright C. K. Bliss, 1949. BCI is the exclusive licensee, 1982.

bols with examples of how the key symbol for water/liquid is used to create composite symbols. The original vocabulary set published by BCI contained approximately 1,400 symbols with their word glosses (Hehner, 1980), but several updates have occurred over the years; the current standard vocabulary contains approximately 2,400 symbols (Wood et al., 1992). New symbols are evaluated by an advisory body, known as the International Blissymbol Panel, composed of more than 60 volunteers. Those symbols deemed acceptable are then submitted to an independent three-member Symbol Committee, which must approve each new symbol by majority vote (Wood et al., 1992). A provision is made whereby symbols needed for personal communication can be created by users through use of the combine strategy. These combined symbols can be submitted to BCI for review

by the International Blissymbol Panel and eventually the Symbol Committee.

As Figure 6.4 illustrates, there are four classes of Blissymbols: (1) **pictographs**, in which symbols resemble their referents, (2) **ideographs**, in which symbols are used to represent more abstract concepts, (3) **arbitrary**, in which symbols bear very little relationship to their referents, and (4) **international**, in which symbols have virtually universal meaning (some are borrowed from various disciplines such as mathematics). There can be simple and compound configurations of Blissymbols. A simple configuration involves a key symbol appearing alone to represent a concept. For compound configurations, key symbols can either be superimposed on one another, or arranged sequentially. The meaning of the elements is determined by several variables:

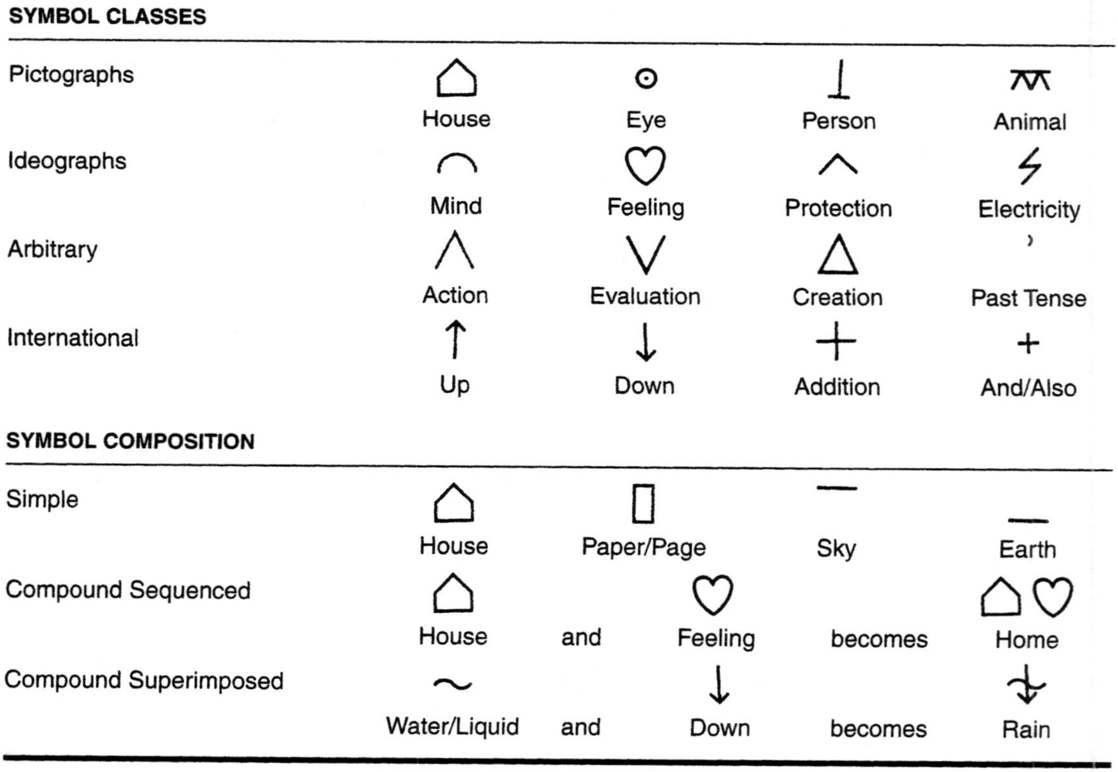

SYMBOL CLASSES

Pictographs	House	Eye	Person	Animal
Ideographs	Mind	Feeling	Protection	Electricity
Arbitrary	Action	Evaluation	Creation	Past Tense
International	Up	Down	Addition	And/Also

SYMBOL COMPOSITION

Simple	House	Paper/Page	Sky	Earth
Compound Sequenced	House and	Feeling becomes		Home
Compound Superimposed	Water/Liquid and	Down becomes		Rain

FIGURE 6.4 Classes and Composition of Blissymbols

Blissymbolics used herein with the approval of Blissymbolics Communication International (BCI). The symbols are described in the work *Semantography*, original copyright C. K. Bliss, 1949. BCI is the exclusive licensee, 1982.

1. **Changes in shape.** For example, a cross hatch (similar to the one used in a game of tic-tac-toe) can mean either "cloth" (if it is standing upright) or "number" (if it is slanted toward the right).
2. **Changes in size.** For example, a large circle can mean "sun" but a small circle can mean "mouth."
3. **Location.** A horizontal line at the top of the symbol space means "sky" but the same line at the bottom of the symbol space means "earth."
4. **Indicators.** Indicators are used to differentiate noun forms from verb (or action) and adjective (or descriptive) forms. There are indicators for verb tense and plurality as well.
5. **Orientation or direction.** To illustrate, the Blissymbols for both "happy" and "sad" are composed of heart elements, evaluation indicators, and arrows. The only difference is the orientation of the arrow (up for "happy" and down for "sad").
6. **Distance.** For example, both "near" and "far" consist of two parallel vertical lines with the evaluation indicator above. The difference in the two is the distance between the two vertical lines (they are farther apart for "far").
7. **Pointers.** These are used to indicate a specific part of a whole. For example, the meaning of "socks" is partially derived from a schematic stick figure of legs and feet with pointers at the front of the leg and foot to indicate where the socks are worn.

In addition to these (and other) variables, there are several strategies for changing the meanings of symbols. To illustrate, the "opposite-of" symbol can be used as follows: if an individual has the symbol for "hot" on a communication board, but no symbol for "cold," the concept of being cold can be communicated by pointing first to the "opposite-of" symbol and then to the symbol for "hot." This strategy saves space on the communication board by not displaying all opposite pairs. Blissymbolics has its own syntactic system, but the system can be adapted to the syntax of the greater community language as well as used telegraphically (Musselwhite & St. Louis, 1988). On initial observation, Blissymbols may seem a bit intimidating. However, once an individual understands the logic base, it becomes quite apparent that Blissymbolics is a very powerful aided symbol system.

Successful use of Blissymbols has been reported with persons having physical impairments (Kates & McNaughton, 1975), developmental delays (Harris-Vanderheiden, 1976; Song, 1979), aphasia (Saya, 1979), profound hearing impairments (Goddard, 1977), and multiple impairments (Elder & Bergman, 1978). McNaughton (1985) and Silverman, McNaughton, and Kates (1978) described three instructional models for the teaching of Blissymbols. These models are dependent on the language abilities and individual needs of the potential AAC system user and are not considered to be the only models for intervention. They include using Blissymbolics as (1) an expressive language to augment the individual's receptive native language, for symbol users who have reduced language experience rather than impaired language capability; (2) an expressive language concurrent with the development of receptive language; and (3) a medium providing communication at the surface level within a highly structured program that applies imitation and reinforcement techniques (Silverman et al., 1978).

The comparative research with Blissymbolics in regard to iconicity has been rather negative. Mirenda and Locke (1989) and Mizuko (1987) found Blissymbols to be less transparent than PCS and PICSYMS. Musselwhite and Ruscello (1984) determined that rebus symbols and PICSYMS were more transparent than Blissymbols. Bloomberg et al. (1990) compared the translucency of Blissymbols to PCS, PIC symbols, PICSYMS, and rebus symbols. Blissymbols were the least translucent of all. According to Mizuko (1987), PCS and PICSYMS are easier to learn than Blissymbols. Briggs (1983) found that PIC symbols were easier to acquire than either Blissymbols or TO. Rebus symbols appear to be easier than Blissymbols to acquire and retain (Burroughs et al., 1990; Ecklund & Reichle, 1987). Of all the studies known, only Hughes (1979) had a finding favorable to Blissymbols. In that case, they were found to be easier to learn than TO.

With the preponderance of data indicating that Blissymbols are less iconic than other AAC graphic representational sets/systems, the success of Blissymbol users must be explained by other factors. The original team that developed Blissymbolics for persons with communication disabilities emphasized the importance of an appropriate instructional approach and careful assessment to ensure that the learner was developmentally ready for symbols constructed of meaning-referenced components. Foremost among the many tips for teaching the symbols discussed in the *Handbook of Blissymbolics* (Silverman et al., 1978) are (1) explaining the symbol components and indicators in a manner appropriate to the learner; (2) relating to the families of symbols as illustrated in the *Blissymbol Reference Guide*, Section II, Finding Symbols by Meaning (Wood et al., 1992) and *Blissymbols for Use*, Finding Meaning Section (Hehner, 1980); and (3) introducing symbol strategies such as "opposite meaning," "combine," and "sounds like." All of these recommendations relate to the language, structure, and scaffolding that Blissymbolics provides. Vanderheiden and Lloyd (1986) have enumerated several strengths for this system: (1) the manner in which Blissymbolics was created is consistent with the processes necessary for reading and writing; (2) in the initial stages of training, the symbols can be introduced in a more simplistic form and then expanded at a later date; (3) because of its logic base, Blissymbolics has an excellent expansion capability and wide representational range; (4) the use of

principles and strategies allows users to communicate more than what is displayed on their communication boards or aids; and (5) BCI, the central resource service for Blissymbolics, offers extensive training and support materials. For example, there are dictionaries, an Independent Study Guide, videotapes, and other support media. Figure 6.5 illustrates a way of introducing Blissymbols to serve as a bridge from using pictures to beginning to use the language capabilities of Blissymbolics. Blissymbols have been embellished or enhanced to resemble their referents. The materials for this approach, *Picture Your Blissymbols* (McNaughton & Warrick, 1984), are available from BCI. Finally, in describing many Blissymbols as having a Type Two structure in which the component parts are sequenced and relate to each other semantically, McNaughton (1993) considers Blissymbolics as supportive to literacy learning through providing experience in "detecting graphic structural and lexical ambiguities, segmenting graphically represented symbols into smaller representational units, separating graphic symbols from their referents and making judge-

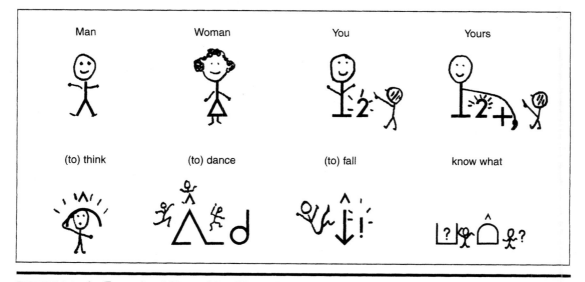

FIGURE 6.5   An Example of *Picture Your Blissymbols*

From McNaughton & Warrick, 1984; used by permission. Blissymbolics used herein with the approval of Blissymbolics Communication International (BCI). The symbols are described in the work *Semantography*, original copyright C. K. Bliss, 1949. BCI is the exclusive licensee, 1982.

ments about semantic and syntactic appropriateness by means of graphic markers" (McNaughton, 1993, p. 69).

As a final word, Blissymbols are available as an option on many commercially produced augmentative communication devices (BCI Catalog, 1995) and can be used for computer-mediated communication through software such as BlissNet (McNamara et al., 1994). The system, originally conceived as an international language in the 1940s and first applied to persons with communication disabilities in the 1970s, is having Bliss's dream realized in the 1990s through communication between AAC users and their partners from different language backgrounds around the world.

CyberGlyphs.   CyberGlyphs (formerly Jet Era Glyphs) were conceived in the early 1960s (Zavalani, 1991) for a similar purpose to that of Blissymbolics, that is, as a means of communication between people who do not share a common language. More recently, these symbols have been used by persons with severe communication disabilities.

The symbols are semantically based in much the same way as Blissymbols, but unlike Blissymbols, CyberGlyphs are intended to be hand drawn. The system is composed predominately of pictographs with a smaller proportion of ideographs and arbitrary symbols. Five basic rules govern the production and use of CyberGlyphs, making the system logical and expandable. Abstract thought in addition to concrete ideas can be represented by the symbols. Syntactic structure for CyberGlyphs has been adapted from the syntactic structure of English.

Sigsymbols.   Sigsymbols were designed by Ailsa Cregan (1982), an educator in Great Britain, as an alternative to the other primarily pictographic sets (e.g., PCS, PIC, rebus) in which some concepts or referents were too abstract to depict adequately. The name of the system is derived from the catenation of SIGns and SYMBOLS. It was created in a classroom setting for use with young persons with cognitive impairments, and has an initial lexicon of 390 symbols representing 352 different concepts (some concepts have more than one sym-

bol to represent them), housed within a 3-ring binder (samples appear in the fourth column of Figures 6.1 and 6.2). About half of the symbols are classified as pictographs and ideographs. A unique feature of this system, however, is the inclusion of 190 (184 different concepts) **sign-linked symbols**. Cregan realized that not all concepts could be adequately depicted using pictographs and ideographs. For these difficult concepts, symbols were linked to manual signs (i.e., unaided symbols). Basically, only the most salient characteristics of manual signs were depicted schematically in the sign-linked symbols. As an illustration, the Sigsymbol for "cold" appears in Figure 6.2. It depicts the sides of an individual's torso with jagged markings just below each armpit. The manual sign (from Signed English, an American pedagogical system based on American Sign Language [ASL]) for COLD is produced by making two *S* handshapes (i.e., fists), drawing the arms in close to the torso, and then shaking the hands vigorously as if shivering. In this case, the Sigsymbol is showing the action of the hands along the sides of the body.

Because Cregan was an educator in Great Britain, the sign-linked symbols were all originally based on manual signs from British Sign Language (BSL). Because sign languages are different from one another as spoken languages, the sign-linked symbols based on BSL were not applicable to Americans (or any other nationality) wanting to use the system. Lyle Lloyd met Cregan in the mid-1980s and was intrigued by the system. With her cooperation, he revised the sign-linked symbols to correspond to manual signs primarily from Signed English. There are now two editions of Sigsymbols—a British Edition (Cregan, 1982) and an American Edition (Cregan & Lloyd, 1990). Although some symbols in the two editions are similar (e.g., "afraid"), most of them are quite different (e.g., "Sunday") reflecting the differences in the manual signs used in the two countries (see Figure 6.6).

The discussion here focuses on the American Edition of Sigsymbols. The original lexicon of symbols for this edition was chosen according to the language of the school environment and the activities that take place there on a daily basis. Additionally, consideration was given to the earliest

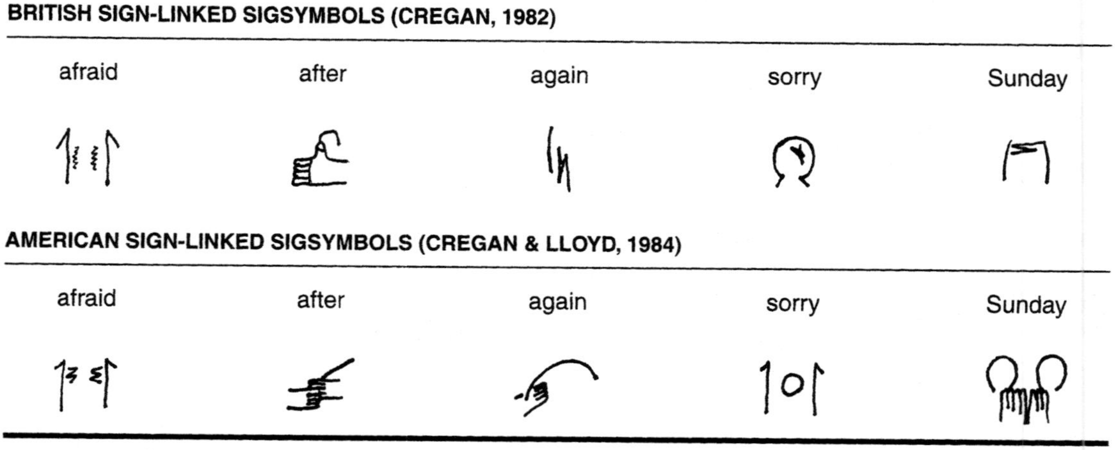

BRITISH SIGN-LINKED SIGSYMBOLS (CREGAN, 1982)

afraid	after	again	sorry	Sunday

AMERICAN SIGN-LINKED SIGSYMBOLS (CREGAN & LLOYD, 1984)

afraid	after	again	sorry	Sunday

FIGURE 6.6 Sample Comparison of British and American Sign-Linked Sigsymbols
From Cregan, 1982; Cregan & Lloyd, 1984. Reprinted by permission.

communication needs of individuals using manual signs (Fristoe & Lloyd, 1980). For the creation of Sigsymbols beyond the initial lexicon, Cregan and Lloyd (1990) list six criteria. These include

1. **Decodability.** Symbols should be as simple and as directly meaningful as possible to allow for maximum concentration of production. Composite symbols (such as those composing Blissymbols, TO, and other aided symbol systems) should be avoided.
2. **Avoidance of the abstract.** Symbols should relate to what is concrete within the user's experience. Concepts that cannot be depicted by pictographs or ideographs should be related to the user's concrete motor experience through the use of sign-linked symbols.
3. **Clarity.** Symbols should be as distinct from one another in size, position, and orientation as possible. Sigsymbols depicting opposite concepts should have a point of reference provided.
4. **Logicality/deducibility.** Rules should govern the design of Sigsymbols to assist in conceptual development. Logical design rules provide for the decoding of most ideographic Sigsymbols and the translating of sign-linked symbols into signs.
5. **Relevant available vocabulary.** Users should have access to a range of relevant vocabulary. The system should be easily expanded if needed.
6. **Reproducibility.** Symbols should be as simple to draw as possible with minimal reliance on artistic skill. There should be no need for any special equipment to produce them.

In addition to these design criteria, Cregan and Lloyd (1990) discuss 11 rules for creating new Sigsymbols. Rule 1 governs the entire symbol-creating process: "Distinctiveness of symbols, so they are clearly distinguishable one from another, is higher priority than absolute consistency" (Cregan & Lloyd, 1990). The other 10 rules are more specific to the addition of new symbols. For example, rules exist for the creation of pictographs, unspecified objects, pronouns, and personal Sigsymbols (e.g., a symbol to indicate the user or someone dear to the user). Other rules govern the depiction of numerals and the use of arrows. Rule 10 lists nine specific purposes for the use of red thick lines. Finally, Rule 11 delineates seven principles for creating sign-linked symbols.

Sigsymbols are similar to PICSYMS in the way the important information (i.e., the figure) is differentiated from the ground. PICSYMS uses solid and broken lines to differentiate figure from ground, while the Sigsymbol system uses thick red lines for the important information and thin black lines for the contextual information. The red and black lines can be produced on the spot in the classroom or clinical environment by using a thick red marker and a thin black marker. The thickness of lines is important; should the symbols be copied, the figure/ground differential will revert from red-versus-black to thick-versus-thin. In this manner, the critical relationship between figure and ground is not lost.

The logic base of Sigsymbols with its rules for the creation of new symbols makes it an open-ended system with an excellent expansion capability and wide representational range. To date, no known empirical research concerning characteristics of the symbols (either intrasystem or intersystem) has been published. There has been only one known published case study concerning the efficacy of using Sigsymbols with specific populations (Cregan, 1993). This case study with an adolescent male exhibiting severe mental retardation found Sigsymbols to be possibly facilitative in the development of spoken word combinations when used as part of a **multimodal approach** with manual sign production. Because Sigsymbols transcends the aided and unaided symbol domains, they are excellent possibilities for use in a multimodal approach in which the user may receive simultaneous training in graphic symbols and manual signs. This distinctive characteristic of Sigsymbols allows the system to be dually classified. Not only is it a partially picture-based system with linguistic characteristics, but the sign-linked symbols can also be considered aided representations of manual signs and gestures.

Primarily Picture-Based Symbols of Dedicated VOCAs

In recent years, symbols have been designed specifically for accessing vocabulary of VOCAs. To access vocabulary, many earlier devices relied on symbols external to the software controlling the vocabulary. In the earliest models, any type of symbol (e.g., basic rebus symbols, Blissymbols, PCS) could serve that purpose. With further advances in technology, however, new symbol sets/systems have been developed. Several VOCAs have been designed so that vocabulary could be accessed using **dynamic displays**. In contrast to earlier symbols, symbols on dynamic displays are an integral part of the vocabulary software. This section provides a brief discussion of two examples, DynaSyms and Lingraphica® Concept-Images (Figure 6.7). Although they have the representational function of other symbols, they do not appear in Tables 3.2 and 5.1 because they are not used independent of their respective devices, DynaVox® and Lingraphica. Minspeak icons (see Figure 6.7), an integral part of the Minspeak system of vocabulary/message storage and retrieval, are also discussed below.

SYMBOLS/ICONS		EXAMPLES		
DynaSyms				
Lingraphica concept-images				
Minispeak icons				

FIGURE 6.7   Illustrations of a Representative Sample of Primarily Picture-Based Symbols/Icons Dedicated to Use with Voice Output Communication Aids (VOCAs)

DynaSyms. **DynaSyms** were designed by Carlson (personal communication, 1995) as an extension of PICSYMS. There are approximately 1,700 symbols, which can be organized into several categories such as actions, amounts, attributes and feelings, buildings, categories (e.g., foods, clothes), objects, places/events, pronouns, questions, relationships, size, social, and time. Several symbols (predominantly verbs) are dynamic; their meanings are derived from movement within the symbol.

DynaSyms are used as an integral component of the DynaVox line of VOCAs by Sentient Systems Technology, Inc. The DynaVox communication aid utilizes a dynamic display to access vocabulary. The symbols can also be obtained as cut-and-paste sheets and stickers for use with low-technology aids such as communication boards. DynaSyms appear in color as part of the DynaVox dynamic display, but are available either in color or black-and-white in their graphic versions. A Ke:nx version for Macintosh is available through Don Johnston Incorporated.

Lingraphica Concept-Images. The vocabulary access system for the Lingraphica communication aid, designed by the Tolfa Corporation (Steele, personal communication), contains approximately 2,100 concept-images or icons. The icons were developed between 1984 and 1990 as part of the computerized visual input communication (C-VIC) system, an intervention program for persons with aphasia. Research and development was conducted by a host of professionals including specialists in neurology, speech-language pathology, linguistics, psychology, and computer science, at the Palo Alto VA Medical Center. Each icon can be assigned up to nine different concept assignments (e.g., sofa, couch, loveseat), which allows the symbols to be personalized to the individual user. Approximately 15% of the symbols are dynamic; these include mostly verbs and prepositions.

The Lingraphica prothesis uses Macintosh-based hardware, and vocabulary is accessed through dynamic displays. The entire system uses spoken and printed words, icons, and text processing. The U.S. Food and Drug Administration regulates it as a medical device, which means that it can only be dispensed by physician prescription.

Minspeak Icons. **Minspeak** icons, also known as Minsymbols, are an integral part of a vocabulary access system known as Minspeak (Baker, 1982), which is an acronym for Minimum Effort Speech. This system is used to access vocabulary stored in Prentke Romich Company products, such as the Touch Talker™, LightTalker™, DeltaTalker™, and Liberator™. In its most basic sense, Minspeak could be thought of as a mnemonic strategy to assist the VOCA user in remembering where vocabulary is stored. For example, Minspeak icons can be used to store and retrieve the message "What time are we going to eat?" The icons "question mark" and "apple" can be used to create that message. Then, all the user has to do is select the "question mark" and "apple" icons in the proper order to retrieve the message. As such, the user only needs to make two activations to retrieve a 7-word message. The icons are embued with color and are designed to be ambiguous so that different meanings can be derived by different people. When encoding messages, the icons should be used in reference to what meaning they hold for the VOCA *user*. A very small number (approximately 100) is used to access a very large vocabulary. Minspeak icons have not been listed in Tables 3.2, 5.1, and 6.1 because they were designed for stored message retrieval within the context of specific dedicated high-technology devices. Minspeak was the first semantic/conceptual encoding approach developed for AAC and is discussed further in Chapter 8 and is illustrated in Figure 8.7.

Aided Representations of Manual Signs and Gestures

As the category title implies, aided representations of manual signs and gestures are simply aided systems of communication that depict manual sign and/or gesture production. That is, the symbols are representations of how manual signs or gestures are produced. According to Table 6.1, this category includes Sigsymbols (i.e., the sign-linked symbols), pictures or illustrations of manual signs and gestures, Worldsign, Makaton symbols, HANDS, Sign Writing, and synthetic or animated manual signs and gestures. These symbols can be used in a multimodal approach in which graphic symbol and manual sign or gesture training occur simultaneously. They are typically used with selection-based communication systems for persons who are unable to produce manual signs or gestures directly (Vanderheiden & Lloyd, 1986). Symbols representing manual signs and gestures can take one of two forms—noncomputerized and computerized. Any of the symbols discussed below, however, can be easily computerized by scanning them into an appropriate software package. A major advantage of using aided representations of manual signs and gestures (whether noncomputerized or computerized) is similar to having TO as an analog of spoken communication; that is, the aided representations allow for **display permanence** (Vanderheiden & Lloyd, 1986).

Sigsymbols. Sigsymbols as a system is classified as partially picture-based with linguistic characteristics. The sign-linked symbols, however, can be further classified as aided representations of manual signs. This system was described thoroughly in an earlier section and will not be discussed further here.

Pictures or Illustrations of Manual Signs and Gestures.

Pictures or illustrations of manual signs and gestures are taken from various sign dictionaries and manuals. There are many books on the market, making an exhaustive list virtually impossible. However, some examples of these are illustrations from *User Manual: Hands On* (Watts & Llewellyn-Jones, 1984b), a sign dictionary based on BSL; *Music in Motion* (Wojcio, Gustason, & Zawolkow, 1983), based on signs from Signing Exact English (SEE-II; Gustason, Pfetzing, & Zawolkow, 1980), a pedagogical sign system based on ASL; and *Basic Preschool Signed English Dictionary* (Bornstein, Kannapell, Saulnier, Hamilton, & Roy, 1973) and *The Signed English Dictionary for Preschool and Elementary Levels* (Bornstein, Hamilton, Saulnier, & Roy, 1975), both based on Signed English, another pedagogical sign system based on ASL. Illustrations from various books can be used as graphic representations of manual signs during sign training. By definition, pictures of signs are taxonomically classified as aided-static-iconic sets. They are sets

in that they are limited to the number of concepts that are illustrated in any given sign dictionary or manual. Generally speaking, graphic representations or illustrations of manual signs may not be quite as iconic as most picture-based graphic symbols, but because they are graphic representations of manual signs, which have considerable iconicity, they are more iconic than the alphabet-based, phonemic-based, and arbitrary logographic aided symbols.

Worldsign. Developed by David Orcutt (1984, 1985, 1987), Worldsign includes gesture-linked symbols, pictographs, and ideographs in addition to sign-linked symbols. Orcutt described Worldsign as a multisensory communication system taking signed, written, and symbol animation forms. The symbols represent parts of whole concepts that are created to evoke that concept in the user's mind (Warrick, 1984). The original purpose of Worldsign was similar to that of Blissymbolics—that is, to serve as a communication link for persons who do not share a common spoken language.

The signing form of Worldsign is composed of about 700 basic manual signs, which can be combined to produce thousands of compounds. The signs are reported to be highly iconic, easy to produce, and conducive to graphic illustration and distinctive animation (Musselwhite & St. Louis, 1988). Signs were borrowed from ASL, Gestuno, North American Indian Sign, common gestures, and other sources. The written form includes the graphic symbols, which correspond to the manual signs. These symbols are pictographic and kinegraphic, where some aspect of how the sign is produced is illustrated. The graphic symbols corresponding to compound signs can be arranged in a sequential or superimposed (referred to as whole-writes) fashion. A variety of grammatical features is available with the symbols. Finally, the symbol animation form is similar to the written form with the exception of distinctive animation, or what Orcutt refers to as the symbol's kinetic signature. Animated forms can vary in time, space, and intensity depending on the context, and lend themselves well to multimedia production. The symbols can be animated though live stage performances, motion pictures, videotapes, and computer display. Although the animated symbols can be computerized, Worldsign as a whole is predominantly noncomputerized. Worldsign is illustrated in Figure 6.8.

Because the original purpose of Worldsign was as a means of communication for persons who do not share a common language, it is not an AAC set or system in the technical sense. This discussion has been provided here as a reference for clinicians/educators who may wish to consider its use for persons with severe communication disorders. The crossover between the aided and unaided domains makes Worldsign a possibility for individuals interested in a multimodal approach to communication training and use. The symbol forms of Worldsign (i.e., the graphic representations, not the sign forms) are classified as an aided-static-iconic set.

Makaton Symbols. The Makaton Vocabulary is a nine-stage educational program developed in Great Britain for teaching language and communication (Grove & Walker, 1990). As such, it is not an AAC system. When the vocabulary was

originally developed in the late 1970s, BSL signs were borrowed for the approximately 350 concepts. These signs were then taught in stages along with speech using a key word signing approach. Nearly a decade later, graphic symbols were designed to accompany the manual signs (Figure 6.9). Manual signs from SEE-II (Gustason et al., 1980) have been used in conjunction with the Makaton Vocabulary in the United States. Walker (1987) suggests that the Makaton training program can be used successfully with persons having cognitive impairments, autism, specific language disorders, multiple sensory impairments, and acquired neurological conditions.

The graphic symbols that correspond to the manual signs used in Makaton, referred to as Makaton symbols (Grove & Walker, 1990; Walker et al., 1985), fall into one of six categories: (1) pictorial (i.e., pictographic symbols), (2) relational (e.g., prepositions), (3) sign linked (showing some aspect of the manual sign), (4) abstract, (5) pos-

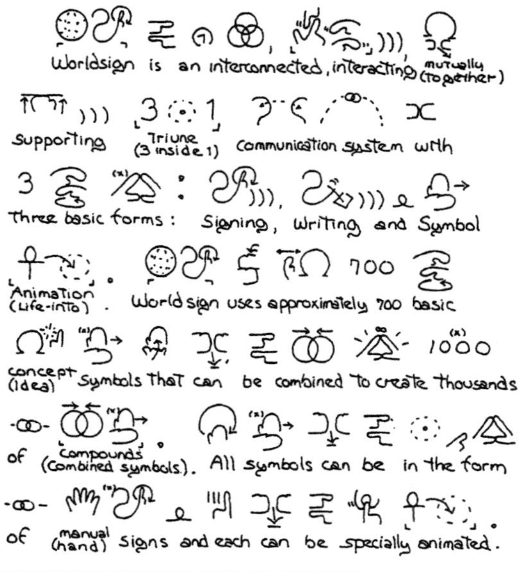

FIGURE 6.8 An Example of Worldsign

From Orcutt, D. (1985). Worldsign update. *Communicating Together, 3*(4), 24–25; used by permission.

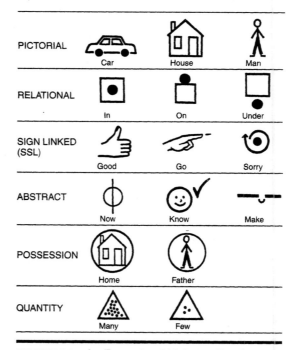

FIGURE 6.9 An Example of Makaton Symbols

From Grove, N., & Walker, M. (1990). Reprinted by permission.

session, and (6) quantity. A relatively small number of Makaton symbols are sign linked; the sign-linked symbols that do exist are based on BSL signs. For American use, these symbols may need to be replaced or adapted to ASL or signs from any of the American pedagogical sign systems. Makaton symbols can be used alone, with other aided symbols, or as part of the Makaton teaching program. The graphic symbols alone are taxonomically classified as an aided-static-iconic set.

HANDS. HANDS, a computerized system, is based on BSL (Llewellyn-Jones, 1983, 1984; Watts & Llewellyn-Jones, 1984a, 1984b) and is illustrated in Figure 6.10. This computer program allows the user three options for presenting sign-linked symbols with and without printed word glosses. As illustrated in Figure 6.10, for Option 1 the signs are arranged in the same order as they would be produced in BSL and appear without word glosses. Option 2 is identical to the first option except word glosses appear with the signs.

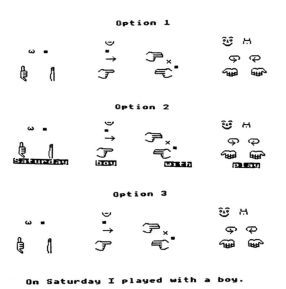

FIGURE 6.10 An Example of HANDS Based on Manual Signs from British Sign Language (BSL) Adapted from Watts, M., & Llewellyn-Jones, M. (1984b). *User manual: Hands on.* Nottingham, England: Signit Project, Arnold Derrymount School, p. 14; used by permission.

Finally, Option 3 provides a transliteration of the sign sequence; that is, a complete sentence interprets the message.

Sign Writing. Sign Writing is based on ASL (Sutton, 1981). It consists of computer-generated representations of manual signs illustrating locations, handshapes, and movements in a schematic form. Elements (i.e., locations and movements) are displayed sequentially. The composite representations are then separated from each other by vertical lines, with thick vertical lines delineating the beginnings and ends of sentences. Word glosses appear above the composite symbols, which are displayed in English syntactical word order.

Synthetic or Animated Manual Signs and Gestures. With computer technology becoming more sophisticated each day, synthetic or animated manual signs and gestures can now be produced by robotic hands, or hands on a computer monitor. These computer-controlled or computer-generated symbols have the same strengths and limitations as natural gestures and manual signs except that the user loses independence (Vanderheiden & Lloyd, 1986). This area is still largely in the developmental stage; at present synthetic or animated manual signs and gestures may be too expensive to be effective in an AAC system. Because the animation programs have not developed to the point that the handshapes, movements, etc., can generate manual signs or gestures, these symbols would be taxonomically classified as aided-dynamic-iconic sets. When any manual sign or gesture can be generated, they will be reclassified as systems.

Alphabet-Based Symbols

Although many alphabet systems exist worldwide, discussion in this text is limited to the TO of English and the modified orthographies based on English. From a technical standpoint, alphabet systems could be thought of as a form of augmentative communication; that is, they augment the spoken language of a community by providing a permanent record that can be referred to at a later date. Alphabet-based systems mimic the spoken language of the community, so they are open ended and extremely powerful in expansion capability. These systems include TO, modified orthography, Braille, Morse code, and aided representations of the manual alphabet (also referred to as fingerspelling). With the exception of modified orthography, these systems tend to be opaque. For example, the letters *d*, *o*, and *g*, when combined sequentially, produce the word *dog*, which in turn is used to represent the house pet that barks. However, *dog* does not look in any way, shape, or form like that animal, hence TO is opaque. The other orthography-based symbols (e.g., Braille, Morse code, and fingerspelling) are also opaque. The exception is modified orthography, which was originally designed to make TO more iconic. As such, TO, Braille, Morse code, and aided representations of the manual alphabet are taxonomically classified as aided-static-opaque systems. Modified orthography is classified as an aided-static-iconic system.

Traditional Orthography (TO).   English TO is based on the Roman alphabet of 26 letters. TO primarily serves as an augmentation to spoken language for persons without disabilities. In AAC systems, TO can be used in a variety of ways. For example, each of the 26 individual letters can be placed on a communication board or other display or device so that the user can spell out words using the letters. (This may be the only AAC system for some people, whereas for most others it may be only part of a system that includes others symbols.) In addition to the 26 individual letters, common cluster sequences (e.g., -*ly*, *th*, *ph*, *ck*) can be displayed to speed up the rate of communication (e.g., see the WRITE approach by Goodenough-Trepagnier, Tarry, & Prather, 1982). Either alone or in combination with letters and letter sequences, words and phrases can be displayed to improve the rate of communication even more (Beukelman, Yorkston, & Dowden, 1985). TO is typically used with other aided symbols as well. For example, word glosses usually appear with other graphic symbols (e.g., Blissymbols, PCS, PICSYMS, Sigsymbols) when they are displayed on a communication board or aid. TO is also an integral part of expanded (complex) rebus, as will be dis-

cussed in a later section. Finally, the individual letters of the alphabet may appear either alone (e.g., the Canon Communicator) or in conjunction with other graphic symbols (e.g., Minspeak icons on a Liberator) on electronic communication devices. When the alphabet is used as part or all of a communication system, the letters may appear in the QWERTY arrangement (especially for electronic devices), but the letters may also be arranged alphabetically from A to Z, or in the order of the most commonly used to the least commonly used letters (any player of the game show *Wheel of Fortune* is familiar with this strategy). For some individuals, a display of all 26 alphabet letters may be used to spell out entire words, whereas for those with dysarthria or apraxia, the letters may be used to assist the individual in gaining better intelligibility of speech. In this case, individuals typically point to the letter that corresponds to the first letter of each word they are speaking (Beukelman & Yorkston, 1977).

Not surprisingly, research involving the learnability of TO has been unfavorable. In comparison with other graphic symbol sets/systems (e.g., Blissymbols, Yerkish lexigrams, PCS, PIC symbols, PICSYMS, Premack symbols, and rebus symbols), TO has been consistently found to be the least iconic and most difficult to acquire over a short term (Briggs, 1983; Clark, 1977, 1981; Clark, Davies, & Woodcock, 1974; Kuntz, 1974/1975; Mirenda & Locke, 1989; Romski et al., 1985; Woodcock, 1968). To use TO to its best advantage, the user must know how to spell and read. In addition, there is not a one-to-one correspondence between letters of the alphabet and the sounds that are made by those letters. For example, two letters are sometimes required to represent a single sound (e.g., *ph* sounds like *f*). Conversely, a few single letters take on more than one sound (e.g., *c* can sound like either *k* or *s* depending on the context). This lack of a one-to-one relationship between letter and sound may create problems for some individuals when learning to read. The lack of iconicity only exacerbates the problem. Because of these problems, modified orthography and phonemic- or phonic-based systems may be an alternative to TO.

Modified Orthography.   **Modified orthography** systems were developed out of the problems experienced in trying to decipher the TO system. Modified orthography involves accentuation, elaboration, embellishment, or enhancement, of TO. Basically, the letters in words, or whole words, are modified to make them more visually salient or representative of their referents. There are several examples of modified orthography (e.g., Blischak & McDaniel, 1995; Devereux & van Oosterom, 1984; Fuchs & Fuchs, 1984; Hoogeveen, Smeets, & Lancioni, 1989; Jeffree, 1981; Marko, 1967; Tabe & Jackson, 1989; Wendon, 1979). Bannatyne (1968) described an approach in which such strategies as color coding of vowel phonemes is used to accentuate words. The *Diacritical Marking System* (Fry, 1964) and *Symbol Accentuation* (Miller, 1967, 1968; Miller & Miller, 1968, 1971) programs use accentuation or embellishments of words to make them more visually resemble the referents the words depict; for example, the word *cold* may be embellished by having icicles dangle off the letters. Modified orthography is similar to other embellished symbols (e.g., *Picture Your Bliss*, Figure 6.5). Once the learner understands the word with embellishments, the embellishments can be faded until only the word remains.

Braille.   The Braille system is actually one step removed from TO in that a series of raised dots are used to represent letters, which in turn are combined to form words to represent referents in the language. Invented by Louis Braille in 1824, the system is not an AAC system per se; it allows persons with visual or dual sensory impairments (DSI) to "read" English by feeling the encoded letters. Braille characters consist of six-dot matrices of two columns and three rows. For example, the letter *A* consists of only the dot in row 1, column 1 being raised. The letter *Z* is represented by raised dots in row 1, column 1; row 2, column 2; and row 3, columns 1 and 2. Other variations make up the other alphabet letters, parts of words, or in some cases whole words (e.g., *for* and *please*). There are three grades of Braille. Grade 1 contains no contractions, so that all words must be spelled out. Grade 2 uses some contractions, which speeds up

the rate of reading. Grade 3 is essentially a shorthand form. Of the three, Grade 2 is used most commonly in the United States (Beukelman & Mirenda, 1992). Braille has other applications besides as a means of reading English. It can be used as a music code, a Nemeth code (for using scientific notation in mathematics), and a computer code (Beukelman & Mirenda, 1992). Microcomputer-based devices exist that can automatically translate fully spelled-out text into Braille and that can translate Braille into regular text using TO (Vanderheiden & Lloyd, 1986). Since the Americans with Disabilities Act (ADA), Braille is seen now by the general community with greater regularity (e.g., in elevators, on candy and soda machines).

Morse Code.   International Morse code is also based on TO and is one step removed from it. In this case, a series of dots (called "dits") and dashes (called "dahs") are used to represent the alphabet letters, numerals, punctuation, and transmission signals (e.g., "error," "wait," "end"). The reader may remember being exposed to Morse code or even recall the familiar "••• --- •••" for SOS. When used with a Morse code emulator (such as WSKE (Words+ Software Keyboard Emulator) that provides full access to standard computer software, the dits and dahs can be signified by either the activation of two different switches, or by different periods of delay in the activation of a single switch. Clearly, Morse code is not used as an AAC system in and of itself, but rather is used with electronic devices that have Morse code input capability. As such, Morse code is an aided system. See Figure 8.9 for the use of Morse code in chart-based and display-based encoding. Morse code can also be used in unaided communication, as discussed in Chapter 7. Figure 7.8 provides the code.

Aided Representations of Fingerspelling.   As with aided representations of manual signs and gestures, the aided representation of **fingerspelling** allows for display permanence of the individual finger configurations. Because aided representations of fingerspelling are simply an analog of unaided fingerspelling, the symbols can be combined in a virtually unlimited number of ways to express any thought. Therefore, aided representations of fingerspelling have an excellent expansion capability and a wide representational range. Printed fingerspelling cards and other print media are quite common and can be easily obtained. Of course, to use a printed fingerspelling chart effectively, the sender must know how to spell and the receiver must know how to read. Animated fingerspelling (whether by computer, electronic glove, or robotic hand) is also an aided representation of fingerspelling. Because animated fingerspelling is better developed than synthetic or animated manual signs and gestures (i.e., all fingerspelling characters can be generated to produce any word), it is classified as an aided-static-opaque system.

Phonemic- or Phonic-Based Symbols

Rather than serve as an analog to TO, phonemic- or phonic-based symbols are direct analogs to the *acoustic signal of speech*. That is, the symbols of these systems are related to some extent to the sound of spoken language. Recall that a major shortcoming of TO is that there is not a one-to-one relationship between letter and sound. Phonemic- or phonic-based symbols serve to map onto the sound system, thereby improving the relationship between symbol and sound. As referenced in Table 6.1, examples of phonemic- or phonic-based symbols are expanded (complex) rebus, Visual Phonics, phonetic alphabets, and NU-VUE-CUE. These symbols are taxonomically categorized as aided-static-opaque systems.

Expanded (Complex) Rebus.   An earlier section of this chapter provided a thorough discussion of rebus symbols (Clark et al., 1974; Clark & Woodcock, 1976; Woodcock, 1965, 1968; Woodcock et al., 1968). Expanded rebus uses the pictographs from basic rebus (e.g., the pictograph for "tree" is used to represent a tree), but also uses a combine strategy and TO to produce more complex symbols with names that resemble the intended words or syllables in *sound*. For example, a grouping of logs and sticks is used to depict not only the noun *wood* but also the verb *would*. Because these two

words sound the same, the same symbol is used for both. Similarly, pictographs from the basic rebus set can be combined with each other, or with letters of the alphabet, to produce words. To illustrate, a combination of the pictographs for *table* and *spoon* becomes *tablespoon*. The basic rebus ideograph for the preposition *in* (a box with a big dot in it) becomes *pinch* when the letter *p* is placed to the left and the letters *ch* are placed to the right of the symbol. Likewise, replacing the letter *p* with the letters *f*, and *l*, will result in symbols for *finch* and *lynch*, respectively. Letters can be added to pictures to make different grammatical forms. For example, *s* can be added to the symbol for *run* to make *runs* and *ing* can be added to the symbol for *catch* to make *catching*. These aspects are illustrated in Figure 6.11. The symbols, then, are based on the sounds of the words and not on concepts. The addition of TO makes expanded rebus a system in which virtually any thought can be expressed.

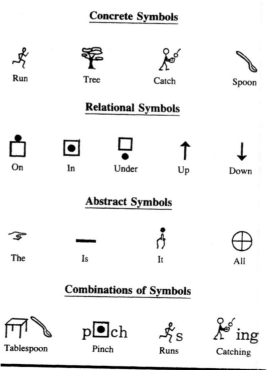

Concrete Symbols

Run   Tree   Catch   Spoon

Relational Symbols

On   In   Under   Up   Down

Abstract Symbols

The   Is   It   All

Combinations of Symbols

Tablespoon   Pinch   Runs   Catching

FIGURE 6.11   Examples of Expanded (Complex) Rebus

From Clark & Woodcock, 1976.

The original expanded rebus was used as a system for teaching children without disabilities to read. The learner would start the program by learning the pictographs, then the pictographs would be combined with each other and with TO to produce the expanded rebuses. Because expanded rebus relies on the sounds of words and not on words per se, the potential user must have adequate sound-blending skills to use the system effectively. The expansion of rebus using letters and rhyming is "limited to the level of language and cognitive development of the user" (Vanderheiden & Lloyd, 1986, p. 107).

Visual Phonics.   Visual Phonics transcends the aided and unaided symbol domains and therefore is multimodal. Created by a woman who had three children with profound hearing impairments (International Communication Learning Institute, 1986), Visual Phonics consists of 45 hand movements that look and feel like speech sounds. This part of the system is unaided. The aided portion consists of graphic symbols that resemble the hand in action along with pictures that are related to the hand movements. Visual Phonics has been used successfully with a wide variety of populations, including preschool and elementary-aged children without disabilities (as instruction for reading) as well as individuals with autism, Down syndrome and other cognitive impairments, physical impairments, hearing impairments, learning disabilities, and articulation disorders caused by cerebrovascular accident (Amend, 1987; International Communication Learning Institute, 1986).

Phonetic Alphabets.   Current and former students of speech-language pathology may recall learning phonetic transcription using the International Phonetic Alphabet (IPA). Because of the lack of a one-to-one relationship between letter and sound in TO, the IPA and other phonetic alphabets such as Fonetic English Alphabet, Goldman-Lynch Sounds and Symbols, Initial Teaching Alphabet (ITA), Ten-Vowel Alphabet, and UNIFON™ were created to provide systematic and unambiguous spellings of English words (Downing, 1963, 1970; Downing & Jones, 1966; Goldman & Lynch, 1971; Malone, 1962; Mathews, 1966; Rohner, 1966). For

example, in IPA the Greek symbol theta (θ) is used to represent the "voiceless th-" sound (as in "<u>th</u>imble," "too<u>th</u>brush," and "brea<u>th</u>"). Likewise, the symbol *k* is used to denote the sound in "Ira<u>q</u>," "<u>c</u>at," "blo<u>ck</u>," or "<u>k</u>iss," regardless of the letter or letters used as an analog to that sound. This allows each *sound* in the English language to be represented by a single symbol. In addition to the IPA, one of the best-known phonetic alphabets is the ITA (see Figure 6.12).

To enhance the rate of message transmission, letters can be chunked together into the most commonly occurring sound blends (e.g., chunking the *k* and *r* together into *kr* to represent the sound blend as found in "<u>cr</u>ispy" or "<u>Chr</u>istmas"). Goodenough-Trepagnier and Prather (1981) describe such a method (known as SPEEC), which is similar to WRITE, the chunking of letters in TO (a French form of chunking phonetic characters is

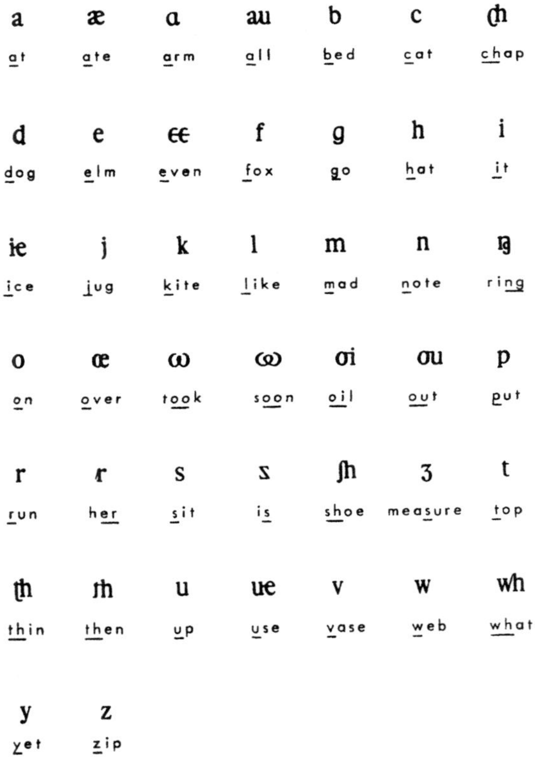

a	æ	ɑ	au	b	c	ch
<u>a</u>t	<u>a</u>te	<u>a</u>rm	<u>a</u>ll	<u>b</u>ed	<u>c</u>at	<u>ch</u>ap
d	e	ee	f	g	h	i
<u>d</u>og	<u>e</u>lm	<u>e</u>ven	<u>f</u>ox	<u>g</u>o	<u>h</u>at	<u>i</u>t
ie	j	k	l	m	n	ŋ
<u>i</u>ce	<u>j</u>ug	<u>k</u>ite	<u>l</u>ike	<u>m</u>ad	<u>n</u>ote	ri<u>ng</u>
o	œ	ω	ωω	oi	ou	p
<u>o</u>n	<u>o</u>ver	t<u>oo</u>k	s<u>oo</u>n	<u>oi</u>l	<u>ou</u>t	<u>p</u>ut
r	ɾ	s	ʃ	ʃh	ʒ	t
<u>r</u>un	he<u>r</u>	<u>s</u>it	i<u>s</u>	<u>sh</u>oe	mea<u>s</u>ure	<u>t</u>op
th	th	u	ue	v	w	wh
<u>th</u>in	<u>th</u>en	<u>u</u>p	<u>u</u>se	<u>v</u>ase	<u>w</u>eb	<u>wh</u>at
y	z					
<u>y</u>et	<u>z</u>ip					

FIGURE 6.12   The Initial Teaching Alphabet (ITA) From Clark & Woodcock (1976).

called Par lé si la b). Persons who may use phonetic alphabets exclusively or as part of a communication system must have internalized a good phonetic record of the sounds of the language. In most cases, the phonetic alphabet is used as a means of input for an electronic communication aid with speech output. In this case, the number of potential communication partners may be practically unlimited. However, if the individual uses a phonetic alphabet as *the* means of output, the size of the potential audience may be reduced.

NU-VUE-CUE.   Clark (1980, 1984) designed NU-VUE-CUE as a means of converting the phonetic sounds of English into an aided system. This can be accomplished by converting the locations and handshapes of Cued Speech (an unaided system; see Chapter 7) into graphic symbols, by placing phonetic characters on a chart in a color-coded order, or by using any of Clark's other strategies such as Nu-Script, Cue-Script, and Cal-i-Cue. Symbols can be displayed on an ETRAN, on the user's desk or laptray, or if the user and communication partners are well skilled, without an aided display in space. The user does not have to know how to spell to use NU-VUE-CUE, but must be able to sound out words phonetically. The user and all potential communication partners must understand the system to be able to use it effectively.

An illustration of the ETRAN display is provided in Figure 6.13. Consonant sounds are repre-

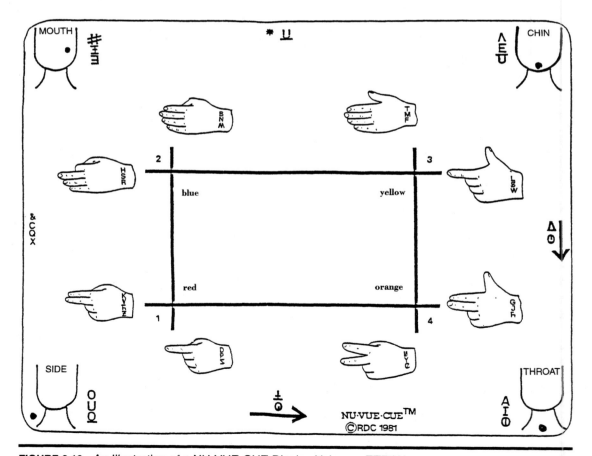

FIGURE 6.13   An Illustration of a NU-VUE-CUE Display Using an ETRAN
Original drawing by R. D. Clark, Inc. Used by permission.

sented by eight handshapes (each handshape could signal as many as four different consonants) located around the rectangular hole. The vowels and diphthongs (also appearing in groups) are placed along the outer edge. Color coding may also be used to indicate mouth configurations (e.g., bilabials, labiodental sounds) to assist in providing further cues. Support materials such as manuals, charts, sticker books, videotapes, and computer programs are available.

This system may be useful for an individual who uses phonetics instead of TO, but who has such severe physical impairments that eye gaze may be the only option for symbol access. Clark has reported that NU-VUE-CUE has been used successfully as a tool for developing reading skills through a heuristic approach. NU-VUE-CUE may offer affordability and portability for individuals with severe physical impairments who wish to communicate but do not have access to other, more expensive or nonportable symbol systems and/or devices.

Arbitrary Logographs and Shapes

Arbitrary logographs and shapes were originally born out of language research with nonhuman primates. The symbols from these sets were intentionally made as arbitrary as possible to circumvent criticisms that had been made against earlier research that used manual signs with chimpanzees (Gardner & Gardner, 1969). Critics argued that because many of the manual signs visually represented their referents (i.e., were iconic), the chimpanzees were not truly learning language but were simply influenced by the iconicity of the symbols. Later research with aided symbols addressed this criticism by arbitrarily assigning meaning to various graphic symbols and shapes. The two most commonly recognized arbitrary logographic symbol sets are Yerkish lexigrams and Premack symbols. These two sets are taxonomically classified as aided-static-opaque sets.

Yerkish Lexigrams.   Lexigrams were developed by Ernst von Glaserfeld (1977) as part of the Language Analog Project at the Yerkes Regional Primate Center in Atlanta, Georgia. The symbols

were designed as a part of research into the ability of nonhuman primates to acquire and use abstract language. The symbols and the language system used were termed *Yerkish*. The first subject was a chimpanzee named Lana (an acronym of the project name), and hence the symbols are sometimes referred to as Lana lexigrams. The symbols were eventually modified somewhat in subsequent research with individuals having severe to profound cognitive impairments.

Lexigrams are created from a set of nine basic elements that are used either singly or in superimposed combinations of two, three, or four to produce a vocabulary of 255 symbols. These nine elements and examples of composite symbols are illustrated in Figure 6.14. The basic elements were selected because they were easily distinguishable from one another individually and when superimposed. Typically, a single word (or in a few instances, a short phrase) is assigned to a single lexigram. Lexigrams have been used successfully with individuals with cognitive impairments (Adamson, Romski, Deffebach, & Sevcik, 1992; Brady & Saunders, 1991; Parkel, White, & Warner, 1977; Romski, 1989; Romski & Sevcik, 1989; Romski, Sevcik, & Joyner, 1984; Romski, Sevcik, & Pate, 1988; Romski et al., 1985; Romski, Sevcik, Robinson, & Bakeman, 1994; Romski, Sevcik, & Rumbaugh, 1985; Romski, White, Millen, & Rumbaugh, 1984; Sevcik & Romski, 1984). Facilitating Augmentative Communication Through Technology (Project FACTT), a program that uses lexigrams in conjunction with VOCAs, has also been successful with children having moderate and severe impairments (Romski & Sevcik, 1988b, 1992, 1993b). Because the assignment of meaning for lexigrams is arbitrary, the symbols and their referents need to be learned. This may limit the number of potential communication partners for the user. Therefore, the use of lexigrams as a symbol set by itself may be limited. Greater strength may be in its use as an input mechanism for VOCAs (Beukelman & Mirenda, 1992).

Premack Symbols.   David Premack (1971a, 1971b; Premack & Premack, 1974) invented Premack symbols to determine whether chimpanzees could learn language. The symbols con-

LEXIGRAM ELEMENTS

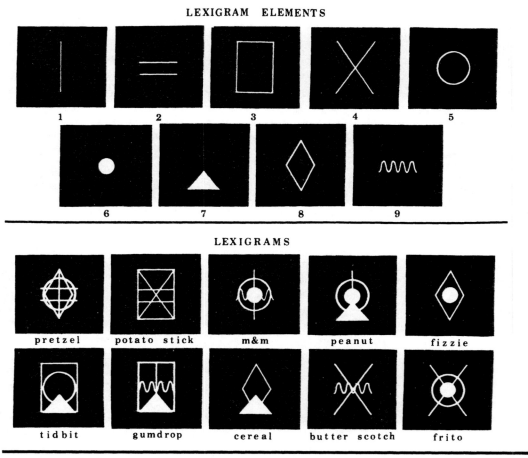

LEXIGRAMS

FIGURE 6.14 An Illustration of the Nine Basic Yerkish Lexigram Elements and Examples of Composite Symbols

From Romski, M. A., Sevcik, R. A., & Pate, J., 1988. Establishment of symbolic communication in persons with severe retardation. *Journal of Speech and Hearing Disorders, 53,* 94–107; used by permission.

sisted of various plastic shapes in different colors and sizes. The meaning of the shapes was arbitrarily assigned to circumvent the criticisms mentioned previously. Later, the shapes were used as part of the Non-Speech Language Initiation Program (Non-SLIP) (Carrier, 1976; Carrier & Peak, 1975) to teach young children language skills such as correct syntactic order (i.e., noun-verb-object). They were not used for communication as other AAC symbol sets typically are. Deich and Hodges (1977), however, made the arbitrary symbols more adaptable for use in communication by reshaping the symbols to be more representative of their referents (e.g., the symbol for "horse" was shaped like a horse). Premack symbols are now made of almost any durable material such as plexiglass, masonite, and wood. The Non-SLIP program has been used successfully with children exhibiting autism (McLean & McLean, 1974; Premack & Premack, 1974) and severe cognitive impairments (Hodges & Schwethelm, 1984; Premack & Premack, 1974), as well as with adults with global aphasia (Glass, Gazzaniga, & Premack, 1973).

Electronically Produced Vibratory/Acoustic Symbols

Electronically produced vibratory/acoustic symbols utilize either vibrotactile or acoustic output, or both. The systems in this category are the most sophisticated of all aided symbols because of their expansion capability and representational range. However, they are also the most arbitrary. This category includes vibrotactile codes, electronic-cued speech, and electronically produced speech, which are all taxonomically categorized as aided-dynamic-opaque systems.

Vibrotactile Codes.   Vibrotactile codes allow reception of speech by persons with profound hearing impairments. A number of electronic vibrotactile hearing aids have been developed and researched over the past few decades (Sanders, 1976), but to date these aids have demonstrated only limited success. In most cases, vibrotactile codes are used to transmit messages via another code such as Morse code. Vibrotactile, acoustic, or light output may also be used in attention-getting devices (e.g., to alert an individual with a profound hearing impairment that someone is at the door).

Electronic-Cued Speech.   Also being developed is a microprocessor-controlled device that will automatically analyze the speech of persons talking to a person with profound hearing impairment and then provide speech cues by way of special optics on the person's eyeglasses. The visual cues may be flashing light patterns that appear to float in space to either side of the mouth of the person to whom one is "listening." In this manner, electronic-cued speech would assist the individual in lipreading. Such technology already exists in aeronautics and in the design of some luxury automobiles.

Electronically Produced Speech.   Because natural speech is the standard by which all other symbols are compared, one may conclude (perhaps erroneously) that electronically produced speech would be just as powerful as natural speech. Although electronically produced speech has developed very well over the past decade or so, it still has problems. For example, although the highest quality electronically produced speech sounds fairly natural, it still does not have the ability to mimic the intonation or suprasegmentals of natural speech. Electronically produced speech can be digitized or synthesized, or can have qualities of both. The most natural-sounding electronically produced output is digitized or a combination of digitized and synthesized. These types of speech output are discussed in more detail in Chapter 10.

With aided symbol sets and systems discussed, the focus turns to symbols themselves. The clinician/educator should have knowledge of symbol characteristics so that symbols that maximize potential for acquisition and long-term memory can be selected and used during the intervention process.

AIDED SYMBOL CHARACTERISTICS

Several characteristics of both aided and unaided symbols have been identified by clinicians, educators, and researchers over the past several years. A discussion of the characteristics of unaided symbols will be discussed in the following chapter. This section is concerned with the characteristics of aided symbols identified as **iconicity, complexity, perceptual distinctness, size, level of abstraction, degree of ambiguity**, and number of messages that an individual can encode. Of these, iconicity has received the greatest amount of empirical attention.

Iconicity, also discussed briefly in Chapter 13, refers to the degree to which a symbol visually represents its referent or some aspect of its referent (Lloyd & Fuller, 1990). As an example, most people observing the various symbols for "bed" in Figure 6.1 would no doubt agree that they all look somewhat like a bed. Perhaps the Blissymbol looks least like a bed, and therefore it would not be considered as iconic as the other symbols. Those symbols that actually look like their referents, or at least depict some aspect of the referent that is recognizable, are easier to learn than symbols that have little or no resemblance to their referents. This has been referred to as the iconicity hypothesis (Fristoe & Lloyd, 1979a). For aided symbols, empirical research has supported the iconicity hypothesis overwhelmingly (Clark, 1984; Fuller, 1987/1988; Goossens', 1983/1984; Hern, Lammers, & Fuller, 1994; Luftig & Bersani, 1985; Mizuko, 1987; Nail-Chiwetalu, 1991/1992; Yovetich & Paivio, 1980).

Complexity is a second characteristic of aided symbols. Luftig and Bersani (1985) and Fuller and Lloyd (1987) have made attempts to operationally define complexity for Blissymbolics. Unfortunately, no data concerning the complexity of other aided symbols exist. Luftig and Bersani (1985) defined complexity according to the number of semantic elements (i.e., key symbols) that comprise Blissymbols (remember that Blissymbolics is composed of about 120 basic semantic elements or key symbols that can be combined to form composite symbols). They hypothesized that complexity increases as the number of semantic elements increases. Fuller and Lloyd (1987) defined complexity as the number of strokes required to produce a Blissymbol. Although they could have chosen semantic elements for a definition of complexity, they chose number of strokes because not all graphic symbols are composed of semantic elements in the same way as Blissymbols, making complexity research difficult to replicate. More graphic symbols can be analyzed using number of strokes. Silverman's (1995) definition of complexity, involving the relationship of figure information to the background of a symbol, is another possibility. According to his definition, the greater the separation of figure and ground, the lower the degree of complexity. For example, a symbol depicting a person reading a book against a white background has a lower degree of complexity than a symbol depicting the same activity against a background of shelves of books. Additional research is needed to further define complexity and its influence on symbol learning. Until complexity is better understood, clinicians/educators will have to rely on their own intuition and professional judgment.

Lloyd and Karlan (1983, 1984), Lloyd and Kiernan (1984), and Silverman (1995) identified other characteristics of aided symbols, including perceptual distinctness, which refers to the degree to which several symbols in a group seem obviously different or distinct from one another. As mentioned in the previous section, many aided symbol sets and systems have a proportion of minimal pairs, especially for concepts depicting polar opposites (e.g., hot/cold, clean/dirty, up/down). For some individuals, having symbols as visually distinctive as possible within the same group may be more conducive to the learning process.

Size can be an important characteristic to consider. The size of symbols should be just large enough for the user and communication partners to see, but small enough so that as many symbols as possible can be placed on a display (Silverman, 1995). An inverse relationship exists between symbol size and number of symbols displayed. The larger the symbol size, obviously, the fewer the number of symbols that can be displayed. However, the symbols must be large enough for all parties to see.

The amount of detail that is provided in the object or event being depicted in the symbol determines the level of abstraction (the figure as opposed to the ground; Silverman, 1995). Generally speaking, the less detail presented, the greater the level of abstraction, and vice versa. This may be an important variable to consider for individuals with cognitive impairments. Initial symbols may need to be as specific as possible, with much detail being given to the figure.

The degree of ambiguity describes the number of concepts a single symbol can represent (Silverman, 1995). The more meanings there are for a single symbol, the greater its ambiguity. For some individuals, this may be desirable. For most AAC users, however, symbols typically represent one word or concept.

The number of messages that an individual can encode is relevant to a group of aided symbols rather than a single symbol. Some sets of symbols allow an individual to encode more messages than others. Variables that influence the number of messages that can be created include the number of pictures in the set, the capability (or lack thereof) of **agglutination** (forming new concepts with the symbols in the set), and the capability of combining symbols meaningfully to create phrases and sentences.

SUMMARY

This chapter has thoroughly discussed aided AAC symbols by classifying and describing individual sets and systems. Additionally, various characteristics of aided symbols have been enumerated and elaborated on. Information about developers/vendors of symbol sets/systems can be found in Appendix B-1. The following chapter will discuss unaided symbols and their characteristics. Discussion regarding symbol selection can be found in Chapter 13. Brief discussions of symbols can also be found in Chapters 18 and 19, which deal with intervention strategies.

CHAPTER 7

UNAIDED AAC SYMBOLS

FILIP LONCKE AND HELEEN BOS

As stated in Chapter 3, **unaided communication** requires nothing more than the communicator's body as a whole or as parts that can be used as articulators. The vocal tract, the mouth, the tongue, and the lips are crucial for production of natural speech and vocalization. Hands, arms, facial expression, and body posture and movement are important for **manual signs** and **gestures**. The term *gesture* is used here and elsewhere in this text as nonlinguistic communicative behavior through body movement; facial expression; hand, limb, or eye movement; and pantomime. The term *manual sign* refers to the elements of either naturally developed sign languages or devised sign systems; that is, *manual sign* is the visual-gestural equivalent of *word* in spoken and written language. There are many other types of unaided communication (e.g., head shakes, pointing). Unaided communication is frequently combined with aided communication. For example, a voice output communication aid (VOCA) user (see Chapter 10) may combine electronic speech production with eye gaze, gestures, pointing, and vocalization. The following sections of this chapter (1) give the historical and theoretical background of sign languages and other unaided systems, (2) discuss the basic characteristics of unaided communication, and (3) classify and describe unaided communication symbols.

HISTORICAL AND THEORETICAL BACKGROUND OF SIGN LANGUAGES AND OTHER UNAIDED SYSTEMS

The use of unaided communication is not a recent phenomenon. Even before fingerspelling was introduced by Juan Pablo Bonet in the seventeenth century for use in the instruction of deaf children,

the **manual alphabet** (hand alphabet) was reportedly already in use (Savage, Evans, & Savage, 1981). In the second half of the eighteenth century, manual signing was considered to be the key to educating deaf children in France, and it spread over several countries of Europe and into North America in subsequent decades. Already the discovery of signing as a powerful tool to convey information had led to dramatic change in the way deaf individuals were perceived by the educational and academic community. Before, deafness had been equated with impossibility of education and inaccessibility to human language and culture (Lane, 1984). Interestingly, the use of manual signs for improving communication in hearing individuals with cognitive impairment was introduced as early as 1847 (Bonvillian & Miller, 1995).

However, in the second half of the nineteenth century, signing was largely abandoned throughout Europe and in many United States schools for deaf children. Signing had become generally assumed to be linguistically inferior to spoken language and believed to interfere with speech acquisition. At the Congress of Milan in 1880, educators of the deaf proclaimed that the so-called oral method was the only viable way of educating deaf children. Sign language was considered to be harmful to the objectives of spoken language acquisition and social integration in the world of hearing and speaking people.

Rediscovery of Sign Language

Negative assumptions about signing were discarded only during the last four decades, partially through major changes in the theoretical perspectives on language structure, language acquisition, and communication development. One important change was the recognition that language competence is different from language performance (Chomsky, 1965; Pinker, 1994), which fostered the idea that the connection between internal language capacity and salient language behavior might allow for variation. Hence, contrary to former beliefs, researchers began to ask whether the primary expressive modality of a language could be other than spoken. If this were true, sign communication within Deaf communities could be real languages. The first generation of sign language research showed that this was indeed the case. In their publication *The Signs of Language* (1979), Klima and Bellugi depicted **American Sign Language (ASL)** as a visual communication system with its own phonological and morphosyntactical rules. Today the full linguistic nature of the sign languages of Deaf communities in different areas over the world is no longer a matter of debate (e.g., Ahlgren, Bergman, & Brennan, 1994).

Reintroducing Sign as a Pedagogical Tool Through Simultaneous Communication

Although records indicate that small Deaf communities existed before the second half of the eighteenth century, the establishment of schools for deaf children at the end of that century was a catalyst in the development of communities of deaf people. Regardless of the educational policy, many deaf individuals continued to use signing as their vernacular language. Also, despite its negative image among educators, some schools and educational specialists kept using some form of signing as pedagogical tools. In the United States, a special situation has existed due to Gallaudet College (now Gallaudet University) in Washington, D.C., a liberal arts college founded in 1864 to provide higher education for students with hearing impairments. The policy of this university has always supported sign use and has been a training basis for deaf intellectuals throughout the United States.

Even in the typical orally oriented countries and areas, however, some educators proposed and experimented with the pedagogical use of signs.

These **artificial sign systems**, also called **pedagogical sign systems**, are designed for educational purposes and meant to be a gestural equivalent of spoken language. In most cases, each word is represented by a manual sign (often pulled out of a natural sign language). One of the earliest pedagogical sign systems was the British "A Systematic Sign Language," developed by Roger Paget in 1951 (Paget, 1951), which later became known in the United Kingdom as the Paget Gorman Sign System (PGSS) (Crystal & Craig, 1978; Paget & Gorman, 1968). PGSS is an entirely artificial sign system designed to represent the English language. It was used in several schools for deaf children as a visualization technique for English structures through the 1960s and 1970s (Kyle & Woll, 1985). Signing was also accepted as the most viable tool of communication for instruction of deaf children with additional cognitive impairments or other complicating factors (Moores, 1978).

Thus, although signing never completely disappeared from the education of deaf children, it was the discovery of the full linguistic nature of signs and sign languages that brought a new breakthrough (Stokoe, 1960). Gradually, educators in programs for students with hearing impairments felt pressure to reconsider the basic premises on which curricula and teaching methods were built, leading to the reintroduction of signing in schools and educational programs. Rejecting signs as being nonlinguistic turned out to be based on a myth.

During the late 1960s and the early 1970s, the use of simultaneous signing and speech in the education of deaf children became widespread in the United States and later in several European countries. **Simultaneous communication** aimed at facilitating the transfer of information in education as well as facilitating the acquisition of the structures of spoken language. The simultaneous presentation of sign and speech was intended to make spoken language structures more visually transparent and hence easier for deaf children to understand and acquire. The natural sign languages of Deaf communities were not used for this purpose, because the incongruency between the structures of sign language and spoken language makes simultaneous use of both impossible. For example, in general, the word order in a spoken language sentence is totally different from the sign order of its translation in a sign language sentence. Therefore, systems to allow better parallel production and processing of sign and speech were necessary. From the late 1960s on, several of these systems were developed to serve educational goals.

Bilingual Education for Deaf Children

The simultaneous use of sign and speech has been used in many settings and has conveyed messages in a fairly intelligible and consistent way if the message receiver was sufficiently acquainted with this form of message transmission. Fischer, Metz, Brown, and Caccamise (1991) found that students were able to process bimodal sign and speech information in learning situations, thus improving communication in educational situations. However, many of the basic assumptions about the effects of simultaneous communication have been challenged. First, the very possibility of parallel processing of sign and speech has been a matter of debate. Baker (1978) and Marmor and Petitto (1979) analyzed transcribed samples of bimodal use of sign and speech and found systematic deletions in the sign channel. Signing and speaking at the same time apparently leads to synchronization problems. Because the sign mode gives only a partial representation of the spoken channel in simultaneous communications, it does not seem to be reliable for accessing the structure of the spoken language. The debate about the very feasibility of simultaneously encoding spoken sentences into sign is still going on (Fischer et al., 1991; Mallery-Ruganis & Fischer, 1991).

Second, analyses of the signing behavior of young deaf children exposed to simultaneous communication showed the use of syntactical structures different from those of spoken language. Typical structures such as the use of spatial relations similar to those of sign language syntax (Engberg-Pedersen, 1993) appear in the signing of deaf children exposed to simultaneous communication (Livingston, 1983; Loncke, 1990; Mounty, 1986). This has lead to a growing movement to build the education of deaf children on a bilingual

basis and implies seeking direct access to a sign language to allow maximal development of linguistic skills and linguistic awareness. The spoken language is represented in speech, sign, and writing. Writing is acquired and learned in a more direct way (Ahlgren & Hyltenstam, 1994; Johnson, Liddell, & Erting, 1989).

Discovery of the Power of Modalities Other than Speech

The competence-performance distinction also led to the hypothesis that all language users have an underlying linguistic generative power that is shaped by environmental elements during language acquisition. Crucial elements are (1) the language the child is exposed to by individuals who serve as language models, and (2) the accessibility of the language model.

Within this framework, the essence of the developmental problem of deaf children is the discrepancy between access to the spoken language of the environment and the assumed linguistic potential. There is no reason to assume that deaf children are born with inferior basic language skills. Although access to the spoken language model has severe restrictions, deaf children often turn out to invest their linguistic potentials into visual communication. When a native sign language is accessible to the deaf child, it is acquired in a perfectly natural way. This is often the situation of deaf children of deaf parents. In these instances, the stages of acquisition mirror entirely the stages and the strategies of a hearing child acquiring a spoken language (Petitto, 1983). However, merely 5 to 10% of the population of deaf children have deaf parents. A much larger group does not have access to native sign language models. A number of studies has shown that deaf children in this larger non-native group can develop sign language skills if sufficient time is spent for peer group interaction and contacts with deaf adults during kindergarten and school years. Although the sign communication of non-native sign users may not have all the characteristics of a native sign language, it nevertheless shares many of its linguistic features, such as the typical sign language order and the use of sign inflections

(Gee & Mounty, 1991; Loncke, 1990; Maeder, 1994; Mounty, 1986; Nelson, Loncke, & Camarata, 1993; Quertinmont & Loncke, 1989). Research with deaf children without access to any signing model shows that even in their case an **idiosyncratic** gestural system with linguistic characteristics can emerge (Goldin-Meadow & Morford, 1985; Mylander & Goldin-Meadow, 1991).

More specifically in relation to **augmentative and alternative communication (AAC),** scholars have increasingly found that, when speech communication is not readily accessible, other modalities can assume many of the linguistic functions that speech has in typically developing or functioning individuals. For example, some hearing children with autistic characteristics may be better at processing linguistic and nonlinguistic symbols if they are presented visually. Therefore, a person may have trouble understanding and producing speech but nevertheless be able to acquire language if presented in a visual way (manual signs, traditional orthography [TO], or other graphic symbols).

Role of Gesture in Early Development

Before the onset of linguistic development, young children use gestures in symbol formation when they communicate and interact with their environment. Delayed gestural development can sometimes indicate delayed language development (Thal & Tobias, 1992). In many ways, gestural communication is one of the earliest spontaneously developing unaided communication forms. Because of its crucial role in development, the use of gesture has very strong potential for use as unaided communication either within gestural symbol sets or as a point of departure for developing linguistic communication through manual sign, graphic symbols, and/or speech.

Multimodal Nature of Communication

Even after linguistic development has matured into a good command of signed or spoken language use, gestures remain important in communication. Kimura (1990) has proposed a model that assumes gesture and speech production have a common underlying neuromotor basis. McNeill (1985, 1993) stresses that gesturing and speech function in a complementary and redundant way. The production of typical gestures appears to be triggered by the content of the message in the speech planning. Speakers who seek to emphasize a point, generally use much more pronounced gesturing. Also, when speakers struggle with a message, gesturing will generally increase. In other words, using gestures tends to enhance when speech requires support for message expression. This mutual support of gesture and speech illustrates well the multimodal nature of communication.

Multimodal communication is more the rule than the exception. Especially when the situation makes both visual and auditory reception possible, as in most face-to-face communication, communication partners tend to combine speech, gestures, pointing, and TO constantly. This multimodal functioning is highly natural. Generally communication partners are sensitive in selecting appropriate modes of communication to ensure maximal information reception (Lloyd & Kangas, 1994).

BASIC CHARACTERISTICS OF UNAIDED SYMBOL COMMUNICATION

Some fundamental characteristics of **unaided symbols** are partly related to the properties of human language discussed in Chapter 5; others are only relevant within an AAC context. The type and importance of various characteristics varies considerably both between and within symbol sets and systems. For example, a characteristic such as physical complexity varies from one unaided symbol set/system to another.

Naturalness

Many symbols develop in a totally natural way, as part of the human inclination toward communication. Complex symbol systems such as spoken or sign languages have never been designed in an artificial way. Natural languages strongly indicate that humans have an enormous capacity for developing communication symbol sets and systems.

The capacity of managing sets of symbols is mostly reflected by the enormity of the lexical content of the average natural language user. It has been estimated that a person can handle an internal lexicon of 50,000 elements. In addition, people can use the generative power of combination rules at different levels, to produce derived and inflected words, compound words, phrases, sentences, and discourse in a highly creative way.

Symbols and symbol sets can also be contrived, mostly as an explicit convention between two or more people, but also as an artificial design. For example, PGSS consists of made-up manual signs, whereas many other sign systems borrow most of the signs from naturally developed sign languages. Similarly, gestures can be chosen from culturally developed sets, or they can be made up and selected by one or more designers.

Conventionality

Because of the arbitrary nature of words, in principle any form can convey any meaning. However, to be able to communicate with each other, communication partners must use the same form to refer to the same concept. If not, communication will fail. All relationships between form and meaning of words rest on tacit conventions between the users of the same language. This also holds true for iconic signs. For example, whereas the sign CAT in ASL is a representation of the cat's whiskers, it could just as well have been another visual feature picked for iconic representation, such as the form of a cat's tail or its manner of walking. However, in ASL, the sign referring to its whiskers has become conventionalized. A comparison between sign languages also illustrates that symbols can be both iconic and conventional. For example, in ASL, the sign PIG is made with the downturned prone hand placed under the chin, illustrating the snout digging into the trough. In Belgian Sign Language (BeSL) PIG is made with the top of the extended index finger touching the side of the neck. This illustrates the typical way of stabbing a pig when it is slaughtered. Both signs are iconic but different because they have pulled the form of the sign from another image.

Physical Features

Certain unaided communication symbols have been introduced in clinical and educational settings and individualized education programs (IEPs), because of the physical ease of acquisition and production. Within unaided communication a whole variance in required motor control exists. When introduction of unaided symbols is considered, an improvement in motor performance is often one of the main facilitating communication factors. This issue has been analyzed in several studies, especially for manual signs. These parameters have been suggested to play a potential role in the relative physical ease of performance of signs:

1. **Touch vs. nontouch.** Several studies have shown that signs and gestures in which one hand comes in contact with the body or with the signer's other hand are more easily acquired. Probably these symbols allow the person a higher tactical and kinesthetical control while the symbol is produced (Doherty, 1985; Kohl, 1981; Lloyd & Doherty, 1983).
2. **Symmetrical vs. asymmetrical. Symmetrical** signs and gestures are those in which both hands perform the same pattern of movement. The movement of one hand can be the mirror image of the other or both hands can alternate the same pattern. Symmetrical signs are generally easier to learn and to perform than asymmetrical signs. The obvious explanation is that the symmetrical signs require a lower level of neuromotor organization: symmetrical signing allows the same neuromotor command to be spread over the two sides of the body, whereas **asymmetrical** signing requires activation of one movement for one hand and arm while inhibiting this movement pattern on the other side (Kohl, 1981).
3. **One-handed vs. two-handed.** In general, one- or two-handedness of a sign or gesture in itself is not a direct parameter of motor difficulty (Doherty, 1985; Lloyd & Doherty, 1983). Dennis, Reichle, Williams, and Vogelsberg (1982) suggest that the important factors are laterality (unilaterality/ bilaterality) combined with whether the midline of the body or face is crossed. For example, two-handed symmetrical signs can be easier to perform than one-handed signs that cross the body midline.
4. **Complexity of handshape and/or movement.** The configuration of the hand performing a sign or gesture is probably the most analyzed parameter (Boyes-Braem, 1982). Some handshapes are easier

to perform than others. Six basic handshapes have been distinguished; they are the ones that young children learn first in a natural way: the flat hand (or B-hand), the O-hand, the fist hand (or A-hand), the index hand, the C-hand, and the spread-hand (or 5-hand). Studies of sign perception under visual noise show that sign observers tend to reduce perception of the signal to one of these basic forms (Klima & Bellugi, 1979). Preference for signs and gestures with these basic handshapes are recommended in the selection or adaptation of signs and gestures for individuals with impaired motor and/or cognitive processing capacities. The more complex the movement pattern is, the more difficult it is to learn.

5. **Maximum topographical dissimilarity.** To be able to distinguish between symbols, they need to be sufficiently different from each other. The more features that are shared by symbols, the harder they can be to discriminate. Studies of naturally occurring errors in signing ("slips of the hands") (Klima & Bellugi, 1979) showed that users of manual sign communication sometimes confuse signs that are minimally different. So-called **minimal pairs** of symbols have all but one of the critical features in common. In Figures 7.1 and 7.2, two examples of minimal pairs from Sign Language of the Netherlands (SLN) are presented. In Figure 7.1, the two signs differ only in handshape. Figure 7.2 illustrates two signs that are identical except for orientation of the hand. Given that many AAC users have difficulties in visual processing and discrimination, minimal pairs in general should be avoided for early instructional activities.

6. **Visible vs. invisible.** A person who uses signs and gestures can visually monitor the hands and arms moving. Visual feedback can be an advantage for many users. While this is the case for signs and gestures, speech provides virtually no visual feedback to the speaker.

7. **One movement vs. two or more movements.** Unaided symbol production can vary in the degree of complexity that is required. Speech is considered a high-speed articulation process that is based on finely coordinated motor patterns (Levelt, 1993). On the other hand, many gestures require more peripheral movements. The less complicated these movements are, the more likely a person with limited neuromotor or psychomotor discriminatory capabilities will be able to learn them. For example, pointing is a fairly straightforward movement that does not require much coordination.

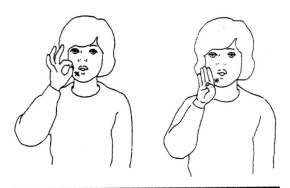

FIGURE 7.1 Two Signs from the Sign Language of the Netherlands (SLN), which Differ Only in Handshape. (Left) LIVE (SOMEWHERE) (RESIDE); (right) (VACATION).
From Schermer et al., 1991. Reprinted with permission.

Cognitive Difficulty: Degree of Iconicity or Arbitrariness

To understand a perceived symbol and to produce it in a meaningful situation, a person must be able to process it. The user must make a link between a form and its meaning. In general, spoken and written language can only be understood if the perceived symbol is interpreted by intervening linguistic processes. In general, through a phonologic or orthographic filter, the user looks for patterns that help to recognize the word. Psycholinguistic research suggests that language users have an internal mental lexicon that is readily ac-

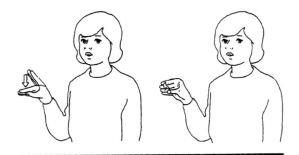

FIGURE 7.2 Two Signs from the Sign Language of the Netherlands (SLN), which Differ Only in Orientation of the Hand. (Left) DO; (right) TOGETHER WITH.
From Schermer et al., 1991. Reprinted with permission.

cessed when words are recognized or produced. Deaf users of a sign language process in similar ways when they sign (Klima & Bellugi, 1979). Understanding and producing language is an analytical, abstract process. Without this linguistic capacity, a person would be unable to develop and use fluently a lexicon containing 50,000 words.

Unlike spoken language words, several other unaided symbols can be processed through other less cognitively demanding ways. For example, many manual signs are considered to have a certain degree of meaning guessability due to some physical resemblance with the referent or an aspect of the referent. The manual sign HOUSE in BeSL is performed with two flat hands that roughly depict the shape of a roof and two walls underneath (Figure 7.3). The sign is made similarly in ASL. The only difference is the orientation of the hands. In ASL, the fingertips touch to suggest a roof.

Deaf and hearing users of sign languages largely ignore the visual relationship between a symbol and its referent while processing. They prefer a linguistic strategy, which implies that the manual sign recognition is based on analyzing the abstract configuration of the location, the movement, and other significant parameters. The reason is obviously that linguistic processing allows for a more direct and faster lexical decision and probably for a larger lexicon. However, several studies have shown that manual signs and other unaided symbols can be processed through association or visual recognition or an iconic strategy. Unaided symbols can vary in the degree that they allow access to meaning based on physical form recognition and thus are classed as either iconic or opaque. Symbols can be more or less iconic, depending on the ease with which new learners recognize aspects of the meaning of the symbol. One distinction in iconic signs is between transparent and translucent symbols. Transparency implies a direct recognition by most users who were not familiar with the symbol and can be defined operationally as "guessability." However, there are only a small number of transparent signs. Translucent symbols are those in which the learner can recognize the physical relationship between the form of the symbol and the referent when the referent is known. This relationship helps for later recognition and production.

Iconicity has been a central issue in the literature about manual signs and other aided and unaided symbols (Brown, 1977; Doherty, 1985; Fristoe & Lloyd, 1979b; Lloyd & Fuller, 1990; Luftig & Lloyd, 1981; Morrissey, 1986). Although iconicity is a generic term to cover a whole range of phenomena as well as certain processes of the user, there is strong evidence that iconic features increase the accessibility of the symbol by learners who have reached a minimal mental representational level.

Concreteness or Abstractness of Concepts Depicted

Although iconicity generally increases access to the meaning of the symbol through a perceivable relationship between aspects of the symbol and its referent, the referent might differ in the degree of concreteness. The designers of most initial symbol

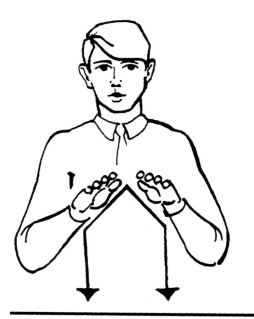

FIGURE 7.3 The Sign HOUSE in Belgian Sign Language (BeSL)
From Fevlado, 1983. Reprinted with permission.

lexicons carefully select symbols that refer to concrete and highly relevant elements in the daily lives of individuals with cognitive impairments. Contrary to former beliefs, abstract concepts can be conveyed just as well through symbols that do not require speech.

Grammar

Languages can be described as having a lexicon and a set of combination rules at different levels. The phonological level allows sounds to be put together into meaningful combinations such as syllables or words. The morphological and syntactical levels consist of rules to string these elements into phrases and sentences. Within the AAC literature, a similar but more general distinction applying to more than human languages has been proposed (see Chapter 4). A **grammar** provides a series of patterns that helps to produce combinations of language units. Grammars help the language user make decisions in the selection of symbols and in the order in which to combine them. Grammars are crucial in the production (speaking, signing, writing, pointing) of language as well as in its reception (understanding).

The use of symbol systems is not always generated by a grammar. For example, simply pointing toward elements in the immediate environment is usually not based on an underlying grammar. A number of symbol systems can be used within the grammar of the spoken language. For example, manual sign can be used to represent the structure of the spoken language (see section on manually coded languages). In such cases, the symbol system borrows the grammatical structure of the spoken language. However, the symbol system can also have its own grammar, as in natural sign languages.

Approximation to the Community Language and Communication

One important consideration in selecting symbols is how well they correspond to the **community language** and communication systems. Here, different elements are involved. One element is the approximation of the system structure. This is the degree to which the rules used to combine the symbols are the same as the syntactical rules of the community language. For example, manually coded languages have basically the same structure, whereas sign languages have a dramatically different structure from the languages of the hearing community.

Approximation to the community language and communication can also be seen from the standpoint of guessability and intelligibility of the symbols. This is a matter of accessibility to the meaning of the symbols by a nonuser. For example, some gesture sets may be easily understandable because they are part of the gestures generally used and understood within a culture. On the other hand, the meanings of most manual signs have low guessability for nonsigners.

In addition, approximation to the community language can be judged by the degree to which the symbols lend themselves to being simultaneously produced and processed with spoken language. For example, manual sign is often used simultaneously with spoken language. By producing both at the same time, the manual symbols are related systematically with the words of the (spoken) community language.

UNAIDED AAC SYMBOL CLASSIFICATIONS AND DESCRIPTIONS

A classification that points to crucial features of the different sets/systems of unaided communication can help indicate how the sets/systems can be introduced and used. The differences can help clinicians/educators make decisions about which sets/systems or what combination of them will be useful for a client.

One classification has been presented in Table 5.1 of this text. This classification is an attempt to order the symbol sets and systems from simple to more complex. An elaborated and slightly modified version of the unaided symbol sets and systems is presented in Table 7.1. A major distinction is made between nonlinguistic and linguistic symbol sets and systems. All the symbol sets/systems within each category share important features, but

TABLE 7.1   Classification of Unaided Symbols

CATEGORY	TYPE	EXAMPLES
NONLINGUISTIC		
Acoustic Symbols	Vocalization	
	Vocal message codes	
Visual Symbols	Common gestures	Pointing
		Yes/no headshakes
		Other common gestures
	Gesture sets	Amer-Ind
		Generally understood gestures
	Idiosyncratic gestures	
	Mime	
	Eye-blink codes	
LINGUISTIC		
Acoustic symbols	Natural speech	Spoken English
Visual Symbols	Natural sign languages	American Sign Language (ASL)
		British Sign Language (BSL)
		Sign Language of the Netherlands (SLN)
	Artificial sign sets/systems	Gestuno
	Manually coded languages	Signed English
		Signing Exact English (SEE-II)
	Key word signing	Makaton
	Alphabet-based symbols	Fingerspelling
		Morse code via eye-blink, gestural, and vocal transmission
	Phonemic- or phonic-based symbols (hand-cued systems)	Cued Speech
		Alphabet de Kinemes Assistes (AKA)
		Danish Mouth-Hand System
		Borel-Maisonny
Tactile Symbols	Alphabet-based symbols	Lorm Manual Alphabet
		Tactile Morse code
	Vibrotactile phonemic- or phonic-based symbols	Tadoma

may differ significantly in complexity and required cognitive processing load. For a number of set and system types, examples are given for illustration. These should not be interpreted as the most used or the most valuable.

Acoustic Symbols without Linguistic Characteristics

Vocalization.   Caregivers react and try to understand the vocalizations of babies, which are often part of the baby's general reaction to a state of well-being or frustration. These different states are reflected in different patterns of vocalizing. In many ways, vocalizing is a basis for more refined and distinctive communicative behavior, including speech. Through vocalizing and the caregiver's reaction to it, the baby will start to understand the essence of dyads in communication. Attending to spontaneous vocalizations, combined with aided or other unaided symbols, is a valuable part of intervention.

Vocal Message Codes.   Individuals with a communication disability may have little or no functional speech but nevertheless may be able to produce simple vocalized utterances. These may be limited to a few vocalization patterns that are familiar to and understandable by the larger public, such as the "uh-huh" for "yes" and "huh-uh" for "no." Obviously many more messages are possible, depending on the cognitive and discriminative strength of the user and the environment. A drawback of similar sets is the mainly idiosyncratic nature of these conventions, which most of the time cannot reach farther than the immediate environment of the user. Nevertheless, these sets can be highly useful for quick messages (Vanderheiden & Lloyd, 1986).

Visual Symbols without Linguistic Characteristics

Common Gestures.   As stated in Chapter 4, the term *gesture* broadly refers to nonlinguistic communication, including generalized body movement; facial expression; hand, limb, or eye movement; and pantomime. Gestures are largely used as nonverbal back channeling for spoken language. Although the use of gestures and their pragmatics differ from culture to culture, general patterns in each culture or group of cultures do make up a considerable arsenal of gestures that are commonly understood to bear a specific meaning.

Pointing is a specific gesture that occurs early in the development of children and is considered an essential part of early communicative development. Pointing can function as a fairly easily understandable symbol when the referent of the symbol is simply the object or the person being identified. However, pointing can also imply a more complex symbol-meaning relationship. For example, an individual might point to an empty chair to indicate the person who usually sits there. An even more complex use of pointing is in sign language, where it is used to mark a locus in the signing space. Pointing can thus be a manifestation of a straightforward symbol-referent relationship, but it can also be a part of a more complex system. In her study of sign language acquisition, Petitto (1983) found a dramatic difference between pointing in the early stages of development and pointing as part of the pronominal system of ASL. Contrary to what could be expected, the pronominal use of the signs YOU and ME was not fully mastered by deaf children acquiring sign language until the age of 3. Pointing is very powerful because it is both used separately and in combination with other aided and/or unaided symbols. It requires little motor abilities to produce, and it is generally easily understood.

Yes/no headshakes are widespread over and between different cultures, although variations in the way yes and no are actually marked do exist. They are generally easily understood and highly useful in AAC, mostly in combination with other aided and/or unaided symbols. If not combined with other symbols, the use of headshakes is rather limited. Their efficiency also highly depends on the questioning strategy by the communication partner. Because the up-and-down head movement is generally understood as *yes*, and the side-to-side movement as *no*, it is still a conventional gesture. In many cultures, (e.g., some parts of India), however, yes is a side-to-side head movement.

Other common gestures in different cultures include COME, DRINK, SLEEP, EAT, and GOOD-

BYE. The meanings of these gestures may be obvious for people living within a culture. A single gesture, however, can have totally different meanings in different cultures or regions (Morris, Collett, Marsh, & O'Shaughnessy, 1979). Nevertheless as these common gestures are generally easily understood within the same culture, their accessibility for persons with communication disabilities is often very good. They can be used as an initial phase or a partial component in the intervention plan to establish stronger communicative competence.

Gesture Sets.   **Amer-Ind** is a set of gestures based on those that the North American Indian tribes used for their intertribal communication. It is not regarded as a linguistic system but rather as a collection of signals or labels. The labeling expresses broader semantic fields than spoken words generally do. Amer-Ind has a limited lexicon of 250 signals, but the use of compound forms or **agglutinations** is recommended. For example, READ is actually a sequence of the gestures BOOK and LOOK (Tomkins, 1969).

Amer-Ind has been adapted for use with and by individuals with communication disabilities (Duncan & Silverman, 1977; Lloyd & Daniloff, 1983). Estimations of transparency vary from more than 80% (Skelly, 1979) to less than 50% (Doherty, Daniloff, & Lloyd, 1985), partially depending on the cognitive level of the learner. It is valuable for individuals with cognitive limitations for storing and processing a large vocabulary. An advantage of Amer-Ind is the low level of motor control that is required (Daniloff & Vergara, 1984).

Generally understood gestures is a set of gestures for use by and with persons with severe cognitive impairments (Hamre-Nietupski, Fullerton, Holz, Ryan-Flottum, Stoll, & Brown, 1977) . This set purposely has a limited number of gestures, and a high degree of intelligibility by the general public is assumed.

Idiosyncratic Gestures.   **Idiosyncratic gestures** are gestures that have been created by an individual or through the interaction between an individual and the environment. Gestures have a naturally augmentative and sometimes an alternative function in communication among persons without disabilities as well as persons with disabilities. McNeill (1985, 1993) describes the powerful role gestures have in structuring information. Although gestures are considered to be nonlinguistic, they can attain linguistic value through communication. The origin of several signs from sign language is nothing more than a gesture that has become conventionalized and has adopted the formal characteristics of manual signs. Mylander and Goldin-Meadow (1991) showed how idiosyncratic gestures tend to develop similar features as sign languages, including rules for sign formation, sign order, and sign combination. The use of idiosyncratic gestures can be a powerful help for an individual with communication disabilities. Gestures can be noted in a gesture dictionary, which can be a useful tool to record the expansion and evolution of an individual's use of gestures.

Mime.   **Mime** may be best described as a more elaborated form of gesturing. In general, mime includes the use of the whole body, whereas the principal articulators of gesturing are the hands, the arms, the shoulders, and the face. Although gesture use is typically discontinuous—each gesture is a unit in itself—mime is presented more as acting and has its strength in the continuous presentation of image-evoking movements and actions.

Mime can be helpful for individuals with specific impairments in language processing. For example, some people with aphasia are unable to understand or express spoken or written language (Poizner, Klima, & Bellugi, 1990). Nevertheless, they are sometimes able to communicate through mimed sequences. Mime can also be used as an initial technique before moving toward the use of gestures, signs, or other aided/unaided communication symbols (Silverman, 1995).

Eye-Blink Codes.   **Eye-blink codes** can be used for communication. Individuals learn to use eye blinking to convey a limited number of messages. By successively blinking a specific number of times or in a particular sequence, the user conveys a specific message, such as a need to go to the bathroom or a request for water (Adams, 1966).

Acoustic Symbols with Linguistic Characteristics

Natural Speech.   Natural speech is obviously the most common form of unaided communication. Individuals without disabilities are equipped with an amazingly sophisticated anatomical and physiological system that allows for quick productive and receptive processing of speech (Levelt, 1994). For many individuals with communication disabilities, processing of natural speech remains important either alone or when combined with one or more other symbol sets/systems.

The use of speech allows for variation that can affect dramatically its accessibility by individuals with communication problems. Rate adjustment, selective intonation patterns, careful selection of words, and syntactical structures can highly enhance the transparency of speech. In part, the adjustment of speech toward less proficient language users has been described as a natural phenomenon. Within speech and language therapy as well as in daily communication, the purposive monitoring of these variables is meant to improve significantly the access and learnability of speech and spoken language (Nelson, 1989).

Visual Symbols with Linguistic Characteristics

Natural Sign Languages.   Contrary to common assumptions, the sign languages deaf people use in their communities have not been designed in an artificial way, but are the result of a natural linguistic creation process. Because deaf individuals have a perfectly normal language capacity but a limited access to the spoken language of the community, they tend to invest their language with visual symbol formation. Because of its directness, signing is the most natural and obvious choice for linguistic development for deaf people. If other people with the same linguistic orientation are part of the environment, a sign language can emerge throughout daily conversation. Reportedly, sign languages started to develop when schools for deaf children were established, not so much because the education itself fostered sign language development, but because schools for deaf children met a crucial criterion for language to emerge: a community to use the language in social interactions.

A widespread misconception about deaf communication through sign is that one universal sign language exists. This is not so. Different countries use different sign languages, such as American Sign Language (ASL), British Sign Language (BSL), Danish Sign Language (DSL), Sign Language of the Netherlands (SLN), Taiwanese Sign Language (TSL), and Nicaraguan Sign Language (LNS). Sign languages differ from each other simply because they have developed in distinct Deaf communities, just as spoken languages have developed in distinct hearing communities. However, some similarities between sign languages from different countries do exist, which are the result of several factors. First, some sign languages are historically related. This has been largely documented for French Sign Language (FSL) and ASL. When the first school for deaf children was founded in 1812 in Connecticut, Laurent Clerc, a former student and teacher at the first European deaf school in Paris played a major role in its organization and curriculum development. The French manual signs, imported by Clerc, influenced the development of the emerging sign language communities in the first deaf schools in the United States.

Second, some correspondence may exist between sign languages at the lexical level as a result of iconicity; that is, different sign languages may have selected the same visual characteristic of the intended referent as the metaphoric base for the sign. Iconicity does not result in identical signs across sign languages, however. Sign languages may differ in the specific visual feature that is selected as the iconic base for the sign. For example, the sign CAT may depict either the cat's whiskers or the form of its tail, resulting in two iconic but different signs. Even when different sign languages have selected the same visual feature of a referent, the form of the resulting signs still may not be exactly the same (there might, for example, be differences in handshape and/or movement).

Finally and more generally, cross-linguistic similarities between sign languages may be the result of modality, the channel through which a language is perceived and produced. Spoken languages are perceived auditorily and produced orally; sign languages are perceived visually and (largely) produced manually. The structure of spoken and signed languages, at least to some extent, may be influenced by characteristics of auditory versus visual information processing and oral versus manual language production.

However, despite the analogies that may exist in the structure of distinct sign languages, they are largely unintelligible to each other. Users of different sign languages cannot communicate in sign language about topics that go beyond everyday life matters. Moreover, even when everyday matters are concerned, signers from different countries communicating with each other will not use their respective sign languages as such, but instead resort to other means of communication, such as mime.

The latter observation leads to yet another prevailing misconception that should be discarded. Many people think that there is a close connection between a sign language and mime, or even that these two are the same thing. This is quite clearly not true. A sign language is unintelligible for anybody who does not know it, which would not be the case if sign languages were a sort of mime.

The last myth about sign languages to be discussed here—one that probably is related to the misconception that signing is a kind of mime—is the belief of many people that signing is restricted to concrete concepts. This is also not true. In any sign language, signs exist for such abstract concepts as confidence, deceit, economy, and organization. Deaf people can have in-depth discussions about feelings or politics, or present a scientific lecture in sign language.

In the structure of sign languages, two main levels can be distinguished: (1) the internal structure of signs, and (2) the way signs combine into sign sentences.

The Internal Structure of Signs. Stokoe (1960) was the first linguist to point out that signs, just like words, are not unanalyzable wholes but instead are built up of smaller segments or building blocks that function in many ways similar to phonemes of

spoken languages. Stokoe distinguished these three basic types of building blocks, which in present sign language phonology are commonly termed the *parameters* of signs: location, movement, and handshape. Other linguists have expanded this description (Wilbur, 1979, 1987) and have added other parameters to make the description more accurate.

Location, or place of articulation, is the place at or near the signer's body where the sign is produced, for example, at the forehead, on the right cheek, at the left shoulder, or close in front of the signer's torso. All "citation forms" of signs are produced in the so-called signing space (i.e., in the area in front of the signer's upper body). A citation form of a sign is the way it is produced when someone is asked "what is the sign for . . . ?" In most sign dictionaries, signs are described in the citation form.

Movement refers to the pattern the hands describe in the space during execution of the sign, for example, a straight movement away from the signer's body, a circular movement with either one hand or both, and in the latter case either a simultaneous or alternating movement.

The **handshape** with which the sign is produced is the third parameter, for example, a flat hand with the fingers spread, a closed hand with only the index finger extended, or a closed fist. Figure 7.4 shows the handshapes that have been identified for ASL. Handshapes are traditionally named after the form of the manual alphabet that comes closest in resemblance (see Figure 7.7 for the American manual alphabet).

Orientation is the direction the palms and fingers are facing, for example, to the front, to the left, or upward. Orientation is sometimes considered to be a minor parameter of manual sign because it gives additional information about another parameter (handshape).

Nonmanual components are essential components of signs that are not expressed by features of the hands or arms. A substantial number of signs use certain facial expressions and/or some movement of the lips and/or the cheeks. European sign languages quite often have a mouth pattern produced simultaneously with the sign, corresponding with (part of) a word of the spoken lan-

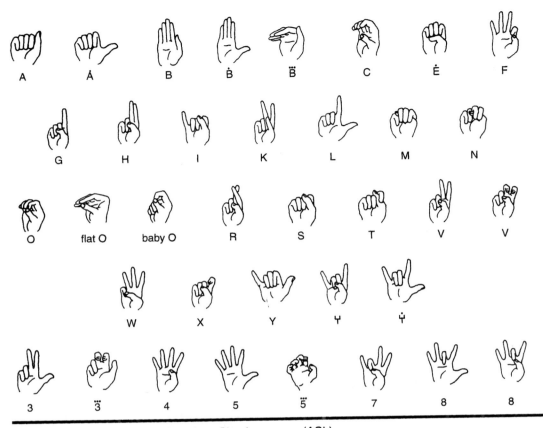

FIGURE 7.4   Handshapes in American Sign Language (ASL)
From Wilbur, 1979.

guage. For example, Schermer (1990) describes the sign MOOI (*beautiful* in SLN) as it is made with the mouth patterned to produce *m*.

Stokoe demonstrated that there are rules for the way these building blocks may be combined into signs; not all combinations are allowed. After Stokoe's pioneering research, other linguists have followed, at first mainly in the United States (e.g., Baker & Cokely, 1980; Fischer & Siple, 1990; Klima & Bellugi, 1979; Liddell, 1980; Lucas, 1990; Siple, 1978; Wilbur, 1979, 1987). Since the late 1970s, however, sign language research has also started in European and other countries (e.g., Ahlgren & Bergman, 1980; Ahlgren, Bergman, & Brennan, 1994; Kyle & Woll, 1985; Loncke, Boyes-Braem, & Lebrun, 1984; Prillwitz & Vollhaber, 1990; Tervoort, 1986). This research has not only elaborated on Stokoe's research on the

phonological system of ASL, but also extended to other areas of linguistic description, such as the way signs combine into sentences.

The Structure of Sign Sentences.   Within the context of this chapter it is not possible to discuss the characteristics of sign language sentences exhaustively. Therefore only some basic characteristics will be discussed, focusing on those aspects of sentence structure that might be especially relevant for the use of signs within AAC.

In all sign languages, the use of the space in front of the signer's body plays an important role in pronominal reference and verb agreement. The space in front of the signer's body is usually referred to as the syntactic signing space, and the grammatical usage of it is referred to as spatial grammar (Engberg-Pedersen, 1993; Padden, 1988).

Pronominal reference is realized by pointing to intended referents. These pointing signs are referred to as INDEXes. Reference to first person singular consists of an INDEX directed at the signer's own body and that of second person singular of an INDEX toward the location where the addressee is situated. Reference to third person singular referents is somewhat less straightforward, at least where nonpresent referents are concerned. Reference to third person singular referents who are present consists of pointing at their actual locations; for nonpresent referents, the signer often sets up a location in the signing space, which is called **localization**. The most common way to localize nonpresent referents is to produce the lexical sign for the intended referent (for example, a proper name sign such as PETER, or nominal signs such as MAN, GIRL, DOG, CAR), and to subsequently use an INDEX directed at some point in the signing space. At that moment an association has been established between the referent and its location in the signing space. This can be any location, as long as it does not coincide with the location of the signer or that of the addressee(s). When the signer and one addressee are directly opposite of each other, the signer will usually localize third-person referents who are not present at the left or right. The localization of nominals and their referents in the signing space is in many instances arbitrary, that is, it bears no relation to the real-world locations of referents in the situation referred to by the signer.

Having established an association between some point in the signing space and a referent, the signer can subsequently use this location for anaphoric (repeated) reference, without necessarily repeating the lexical sign for that referent. That means that the signer will use an INDEX directed at the location associated with the referent, much like the signer uses an INDEX directed at first and second person singular referents.

The locations of present and nonpresent referents play a role not only in pronominal reference, but also in the process of verb agreement. In all the sign languages so far studied, with respect to agreement, two classes of verbs exist (Bos, 1990; Engberg-Pedersen, 1986; Fischer & Gough, 1978; Friedman, 1975; Johnston, 1991; Padden, 1988;

Pizzuto, 1986): (1) verbs that can be modulated to agree with their subject and/or (indirect) object (agreement verbs), and (2) verbs that cannot be inflected for agreement (plain or nonagreement verbs). These will not be discussed here.

The function of verb agreement in sign language, just like in spoken languages, is to express the grammatical relations of who does what to whom. Verb agreement in sign languages takes the form of modulation of the citation form of verbs (Bos, 1993; Fischer & Gough, 1978; Padden, 1988). These modulations affect some of the building blocks of signs and are produced with respect to the locations of the signer, the addressee(s), and the nonpresent localized referents. In one group of verbs, the direction of the movement is altered for agreement. An example from BeSL is the sign SEND. In the citation form of SEND, the sign moves away from the body. When the sign SEND is made from the addressee to the signer, the meaning is "you send to me"; when the sign is made from the location of a localized referent to the addressee, the meaning is "he/she sends to you" (Figure 7.5). In another group of verbs, along with a change in the direction of movement, the orientation of the hand is altered (either of the palm or of the fingers), as, for example, in the ASL verb TEASE. In the citation form, the orientation of the palm is away from the signer. When the signer wants to express "he/she teases me," not only the direction of the movement but also the orientation of the hand is reversed: the back of the hand is oriented toward the localized third person referent, and the palm of the hand faces the signer.

Nonmanual Markers of Sentence Types: Affirmatives, Negations, and Questions. In sign languages, sentence types such as affirmatives, negations, and questions are marked by a fixed facial expression and/or a position or movement of the head. For example, Coerts (1992) demonstrated that in SLN, question-word questions (e.g., "how is . . . ?") are nonmanually marked by eyebrows down, chin up (see Figure 7.6). Raised eyebrows and head forward mark yes/no questions. Affirmatives and negations are marked by a nodding and a negative headshake, respectively. These nonmanual markings are produced simulta-

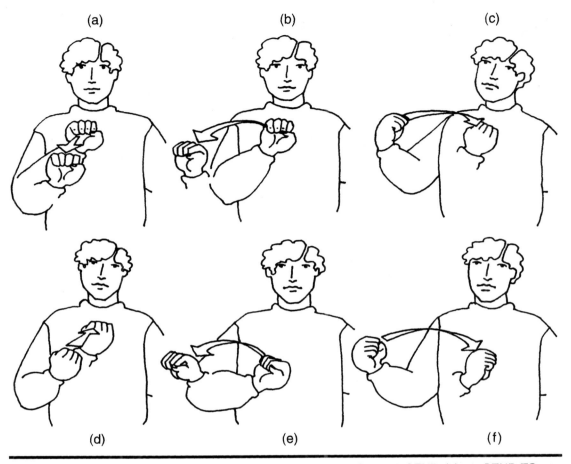

(a) (b) (c)

(d) (e) (f)

FIGURE 7.5 Agreement Forms of the Belgian Sign Language (BeSL) Verb SEND. (a) me-SEND-TO-you, (b) me-SEND-TO-him/her, (c) s/he-SEND-TO-me, (d) you-SEND-TO-me, (e) you-SEND-TO-him/her, (f) s/he-SEND-TO-you.

neously with the signs and are extended during the part of the utterance that is being affirmed, negated, or questioned. These nonmanual markings of sentence types are obligatory; without them, a sentence becomes ungrammatical or is not understood as a negation or a question. The use of lexical signs that may also mark these sentence types, such as negative signs in negations (NO, NOT), are optional. That is, one can have a negation without a negation sign but not without a no headshake. In example 1, there is a headshake and a negative sign. In example 2, however, there is only the headshake, and yet the sentence is grammatical and clearly denotes negation. The hori-

zontal lines above the glosses indicate the length of the nonmanual markings.

(1)
```
 _____ neg |
```
MY SISTER NOT ANGRY

"My sister is not angry."

(2)
```
 _____ neg |
```
PETER MARY ALSO LONG-TIME SEE

"Peter hasn't seen Mary for a long time either."

(These two examples are taken from SLN and represented in English glosses.)

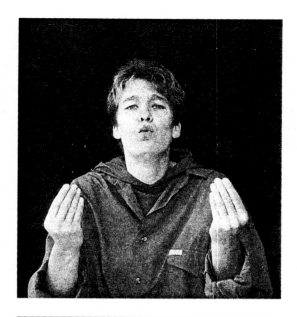

FIGURE 7.6 The Nonmanual Marking of Question-Word Questions in Sign Language of the Netherlands

From Coerts, 1992. Reprinted with permission.

Relevance of Sign Language Structure for Use within AAC. What is the relevance of sign language structure for the use of manual signs within AAC? First, professionals engaged in the use of manual sign in the AAC field must realize what sign language is in order to correctly appraise the nature of signing within AAC. They should be aware that within AAC, the use of signs is not synonymous with the use of sign language. Within AAC, the level of proficiency seldom will become so high that one is really justified to speak of the use of sign language. The signing ability of AAC users often does not go beyond the production of single sign utterances or very simple sign combinations, which implies that a sign lexicon, a set of signs, is used, but not sign language grammar. The same reasons that prevent many AAC users from acquiring adequate spoken language (for example, cognitive, linguistic, or motor abilities) may also hinder the acquisition of sign language, because sign language, just like spoken language, is complex and full-fledged.

Another reason signing within AAC is not the same as sign language is that signs are often combined into sentences according to the grammar of spoken language, not according to the grammatical rules of sign language. However, some aspects of sign language structure discussed earlier are relevant for the use of manual signs within AAC. This is quite clearly true for the internal structure of signs. Professionals should realize that signs are not unanalyzable wholes but instead are built up from smaller segments. When learning and producing signs, one should be aware of the building blocks needed to correctly produce signs. That is not to say that AAC users with motor problems should not use signs if they are unable to correctly produce them without adaptations. However, to be able to make these adaptations appropriately, one must know the internal structure of signs and the way the building blocks may and may not be combined. One should also be aware that when one changes one of the building blocks of a sign because of an imprecise execution, the result might be a nonexisting sign or another sign with another meaning.

Some aspects of sign language sentence structure that were discussed are also relevant for the use of signs within AAC. Fischer (1994) has argued convincingly that some linguistic aspects of sign languages in fact originate from certain characteristics of human communication in general. This holds quite clearly for the nonmanual markings of sentence types. Hearing people sometimes shake their heads or have an interrogative expression when negating or questioning something. The same line of reasoning also holds true for the use of space, the use of INDEXes, verb agreement, and role taking in sign languages. These and other aspects are to a greater or lesser extent also used by the overall human population. The important difference is that hearing people do not use these elements in a systematic way. That is, in the overall population, these characteristics are not part of the linguistic system; instead, they are extralinguistic behaviors. In sign language, however, these aspects of human communication have become systematic behaviors with a fixed linguistic function. As these sign language characteristics may in fact originate from human communicative behavior in general, it is only natural and logical to exploit them in signing with and by AAC users, thereby enlarging the naturalness and transparency of the communication.

Learning to use these sign language aspects is not easy. In many (especially Western) countries, however, one can enroll in sign language courses, usually given by teachers who are native signers. This helps professionals become more fluent, natural signers and allows them to learn those aspects of sign language structure that enlarge the expressive power of a restricted sign vocabulary and the quality of sign communication.

Artificial Sign Sets or Systems.   Only in the last few decades has the use of real sign languages for deaf children been considered part of a bilingual approach to education. For a long time clinicians and educators preferred the use of artificial sign sets/systems. These sets/systems are still the main option for hearing individuals with a communication disability for whom the use of manual communication is considered beneficial. The reasons vary: the lexicon of a sign set/system can be built up gradually and can be kept smaller or made larger depending on the needs and progress of the person; the vocabulary can be selected to allow maximal physical or conceptual accessibility; and signs can be used simultaneously with speech.

Gestuno (Rubino, Hayhurst, Guejlman, Madison, & Plum, 1975) is a set of signs that resulted from an attempt to facilitate communication among users of different sign languages. It was presented as an International Sign Language and was designed by a commission of the World Federation of the Deaf (WFD). The lexicon is mainly a selection of signs from ASL, BSL, and a number of other European sign languages. Reportedly the set has never found general acceptance among national and international Deaf communities for a number of reasons. First, Gestuno was mainly conceived in a time when little was known about sign language grammar and syntax. Therefore, Gestuno gives the false impression that a sign language mainly consists of a sign lexicon without many explicit grammatical (morphosyntactical) combination rules. Second, Gestuno overlooks the

phenomenon that language users prefer learning a second natural language to learning an artificial one. This has been observed for artificial spoken and written languages such as Esperanto (Tervoort, 1984), and it seems to be equally true for sign users.

Manually Coded Languages and Sign Systems. A basic characteristic of **manually coded languages** or sign systems is their reference to a spoken language. The systems usually use the lexicon of the sign language of the national Deaf community, without adopting the syntactical rules, because the signs are used to parallel spoken language grammar. Often, sign systems are elaborated by adding morpheme-referring signs, such as those corresponding to -s or -ing word endings. The most widely known English-referring systems are PGSS; Seeing Essential English, or SEE-I or SEE-1 (Anthony, 1966, 1971, 1974); Linguistics of Visual English, or LOVE, LoVE, or LVE (Wampler, 1971); Signing Exact English, or SEE-II or SEE-2 (Gustason, Pfetzing, & Zawolkow, 1980); Manual English (Washington State School for the Deaf, 1972); and Signed English (Bornstein, 1973, 1974; Bornstein & Saulnier, 1984).

The use of manually coded forms for grammatical morphemes of the spoken language makes the linguistic information conveyed by sign more complete. Although such a comprehensive use of manually coding spoken language may have the advantage of giving a more complete visual picture of elements of the spoken language and their order, it nevertheless has important drawbacks, too. The main problem is that because executing a manual sign takes about twice as much time as the spoken articulation of a word, combined use of speech and sign is bound to lead to synchronization problems for the signer/speaker. The addition of signs to represent morphemes makes the bimodal expression through sign and speech even more difficult. Studies show that signers/speakers can differ considerably in the way they succeed in simultaneously signing and speaking the same content in both modalities (Baker, 1978; Fischer, Metz, Brown, & Caccamise, 1991; Marmor & Petitto, 1979; Maxwell, Bernstein, & Mear, 1991; Wodlinger-Cohen,

1991). Also, some evidence shows that individuals who are exposed to these models mentally modify the structures they perceive into visual structures that more resemble those of real sign languages (Supalla, 1991).

Key Word Signing.   Instead of coding all lexical and most morphemic elements of the spoken message, manual coding may also be restricted to the most relevant content words in a sentence. This practice is known as **key word signing** and has been recommended for use with hearing individuals with little or no functional speech. Some systems that allow manually coded spoken languages have been purposely designed for key word signing. The rationale is that individuals who need a sign modality to supplement the spoken message will find it helpful if the flow of auditorily received information is broken down while some key elements are represented visually. One instructional approach based on this principle is Makaton (Grove & Walker, 1990), which uses only a core manual vocabulary of about 350 signs that the authors consider to be concepts. That is, the signs are much more than a translation of English words. They can often cover a much broader semantic field than the words do. For example, the manual sign HOUSE can be used for such words as house, villa, home, or apartment. A reduced lexicon might better meet the needs for structuring information by persons with cognitive impairments. Therefore, using a reduced Makaton lexicon may be more effective than using a greater number of different manual signs for English words that belong to the same semantic grouping.

Key word signing falls at the flexible end of the continuum of coding of the elements of the spoken message. Apart from the advantages of using a restricted vocabulary for processing by individuals with cognitive impairments, key word signing might favor the understanding and production of the message in other ways, such as the change of speaking rate when sign and speech are produced simultaneously. Windsor and Fristoe (1991) analyzed acoustic measures and listener judgments of key word signing utterances compared with spo-

ken-only utterances. They found that key word signing indeed forces a person to slow down the speech rate and changes the suprasegmental pattern; there were longer and more predictable pauses during speech.

Most forms of manually coded languages tend to be used in direct face-to-face communication through simultaneous or bimodal sign and speech communication. The strength of this practice may be that it allows a direct on-line combination of two semantically related linguistic symbols (manual sign and speech) resulting in a bimodal stimulus presentation. Apart from the combination of manual sign and speech, signs can also be combined with other symbols such as TO or other graphic symbols. To date, the Sigsymbol system (Cregan, 1982; Cregan & Lloyd, 1990; see also Chapter 6) has the advantage of providing the user with the means to intensify multimodal symbol formation in different environments. It offers the possibility of linking signs and words with graphic representations.

Alphabet-Based Symbols.   **Fingerspelling** goes back to ancient cross-cultural communication techniques (Savage, Evans, & Savage, 1981). It was used in attempts to educate deaf children individually in the seventeenth century and became more widely used in the nineteenth century, especially after Westervelt (Scouten, 1984) started to use it in a systematic way for language exposure and language teaching for deaf children in the Rochester School for the Deaf. This use of fingerspelling became known as the Rochester method. In the 1980s, fingerspelling was also promoted for deaf children who were thought to have specific problems in decoding lipreading. For them, fingerspelling was promoted as a useful tool that would allow them to better visually analyze sublexical units of the message (Van Uden, 1983).

Apart from this specific use in educational programs, fingerspelled words are often intermingled as loan elements in sign language communication, although in some sign languages more than in others. When a particular fingerspelled word is often used as a loan sign, it can become a sign

(Battison, 1978). For example, this is the case for ASL signs such as OK and NO.

Several manual alphabets are in use. Most of them differ among each other only minimally in a few handshapes. For example, the *t* in the American Manual Alphabet is a closed fist with the thumb between the index and the middle finger (Figure 7.7). Presumably because this hand configuration was considered to be obscene, it has been banned from most European manual alphabets. Instead of using a closed fist for the *t*, the middle finger, the ring finger, and the pinkie finger are extended. Although the American and several of the European manual alphabets (e.g., the Swedish Manual Alphabet) are one-handed, the British, Australian, and some others are two-handed (see Figure 7.7).

Morse code only uses two basic elements, the dot and the dash (Figure 7.8). This simplicity on the surface of the system is possible because of the underlying conventional combination rules (combinations of dots and dashes stand for a letter) and the underlying use of orthographic rules. For individuals with good cognitive and orthographic abilities, Morse code can easily be used as an unaided symbol system. The dots and dashes can be signaled by eye blinking, in a gestural way, or vocally, depending on the abilities of the user. Eye-blink Morse code can be done by contrasting short and long eye blinks (duration of eye closure). Gestural Morse code may imply either the production of a single gesture in two durations or the production of two different gestures. Similarly, vocal Morse code uses two different vocalization types (e.g., aaah and iiih) or two different vocalization durations.

One of the considerations in applying this system concerns the relatively high cognitive and orthographic-analytical abilities it requires, not only from the user but also from the communication partners.

Phonemic- or Phonic-Based Symbols (Hand-Cued Systems). **Hand-cued systems** have been designed primarily to improve and to complement the incomplete information obtained from seeing the speaker's articulation in order to make speechreading (lipreading) more reliable. For example, even experienced speechreaders cannot distinguish between voiced and unvoiced /d/ and /t/, or /b/ and /p/. The principle of hand cueing is to simply supplement this kind of invisible but crucial phonological information to clarify the spoken message.

Cued Speech is a system that was developed by Cornett (1967) and is actually used worldwide in different teaching programs for children with hearing impairments. Figure 7.9 gives an overview of the English version of Cued Speech. It can be used solely or in combination with other symbol systems. Périer (1987) suggests that a balanced combination of Cued Speech and a manually coded language (such as Signed French, le francais signé) offers excellent opportunities to expose the deaf child to visual information both on the phonological as well as on the syntactical level of the spoken language.

Research by Alegria, Leybaert, Charlier, and Hage (1992) shows that the frequent use of phoneme-based cueing can help the development of an internalized understanding of the phonological system. Contrary to the usual observations, they found that deaf children who have been regularly exposed to Cued Speech rated better in a series of phonological tests and performed better at reading tasks. This observation is congruent with other proposals to use hand-cued or other manual systems for establishing a better internalized relationship between graphemes and phonemes for beginning readers or for individuals with reading disabilities.

Alphabet de Kinemes Assistes (AKA) or Assisted Kineme Alphabet is a hand-cued system designed by Wouts (1987). The hand cues of the system are shown in Figure 7.10. As other cued systems, it facilitates speechreading but aims at strengthening the internalized visual-motor loop between phoneme perception in speechreading and phoneme articulation in speech. It partially goes back to the motor theory of speech production, which states that phoneme recognition is a result of speech production patterns. The cues are miniaturizations of the movement patterns used in

British Manual Alphabet

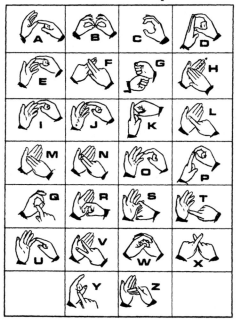

Swedish Manual Alphabet

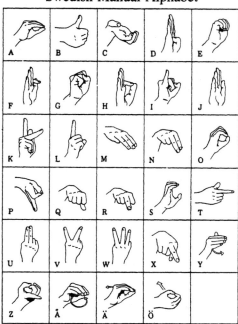

American Manual Alphabet

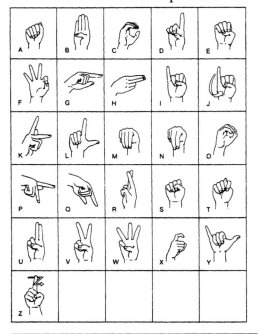

Lorm Manual Alphabet

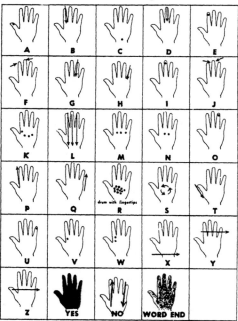

FIGURE 7.7 One- and Two-Handed Manual Alphabets
From Vanderheiden and Lloyd, 1986.

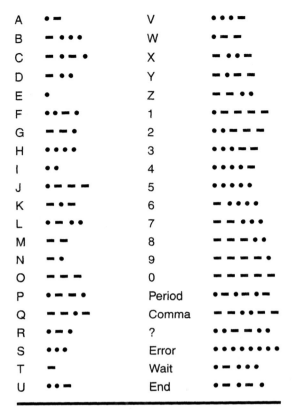

A	• ▬	V	• • • ▬
B	▬ • • •	W	• ▬ ▬
C	▬ • ▬ •	X	▬ • • ▬
D	▬ • •	Y	▬ • ▬ ▬
E	•	Z	▬ ▬ • •
F	• • ▬ •	1	• ▬ ▬ ▬ ▬
G	▬ ▬ •	2	• • ▬ ▬ ▬
H	• • • •	3	• • • ▬ ▬
I	• •	4	• • • • ▬
J	• ▬ ▬ ▬	5	• • • • •
K	▬ • ▬	6	▬ • • • •
L	• ▬ • •	7	▬ ▬ • • •
M	▬ ▬	8	▬ ▬ ▬ • •
N	▬ •	9	▬ ▬ ▬ ▬ •
O	▬ ▬ ▬	0	▬ ▬ ▬ ▬ ▬
P	• ▬ ▬ •	Period	• ▬ • ▬ • ▬
Q	▬ ▬ • ▬	Comma	▬ ▬ • • ▬ ▬
R	• ▬ •	?	• • ▬ ▬ • •
S	• • •	Error	• • • • • • • •
T	▬	Wait	• ▬ • • •
U	• • ▬	End	• ▬ • ▬ •

FIGURE 7.8 International Morse Code

the verbotonal speech training method for deaf children. Loncke, Feron, and Quertinmont (1992) found a significant increase in articulation intelligibility when deaf children used AKA.

The **Danish Mouth-Hand System** (Forchhammer, 1903; Holm, 1972) cues only consonants, because they are considered to be essential for disambiguation.

The **Borel-Maisonny** hand-cued system was developed in France (Borel-Maisonny, 1960) to be used in teaching grapheme-phoneme correspondence, especially for children who are suspected to have dyslectic problems or other learning disabilities. One of the symbols of the system is shown in Figure 7.11. Learning to read is supposed to be supported by the introduction of a gestural-motor component that has some physical resemblance with the form of the written letter or that refers to

features of articulation. The Borel-Maisonny system is largely used in Belgium and France.

Tactile Symbols

Vibrotactile methods are based on the observation that part of spoken information can be experienced through vibration recognition and through tactile exploration and observation of the speaker. Vibrotactile information for speech and auditory training goes back to old traditions in the rehabilitation and education of children with severe hearing impairments (Itard, 1801). It has been used most extensively in programs for individuals with dual sensory impairments (DSI).

Alphabet-Based Symbols.   Throughout the world, a number of manual alphabets have been used with blind persons holding their hand around the hand of the person producing the manual alphabet. This is the method that was used by the famous Helen Keller who was both deaf and blind. Some blind individuals have also had people trace the alphabet letters in their hands. Some specialized alphabets, such as the Lorm Manual Alphabet, involves a coding of the alphabet through a variety of repeated touches and movements on the fingers and hand (see Figure 7.7).

Tactile Morse code is another way of coding the alphabet (along with numbers and punctuation). Morse code has been mentioned several times with regard to both aided and unaided symbols. It is a relatively efficient coding of the letters of the alphabet in that the more frequently used letters require the fewest number of dots or dashes. Tactile Morse code uses long and short contacts.

Vibrotactile Phonemic- or Phonic-Based Symbols. The **Tadoma method** (Alcorn, 1932; Norton et al., 1977) is the best-known vibrotactile technique. The user places a thumb on the speaker's mouth to perceive the movements of the lips and to feel the air flow from the mouth. The other fingers are spread over the speaker's jaw and throat to feel simultaneously the vibrations and the movements in these speech articulators.

CUED SPEECH
English

CHART I
Cues for Vowel Sounds

	Side		Throat		Chin		Mouth	
open	ah	(father)	a	(that)	aw	(dog)	ee	(see)
	o	(got)						
flattened-relaxed	u	(but)	i	(is)	e	(get)	ur	(her)
rounded	oe	(home)	oo	(book)	ue	(blue)		

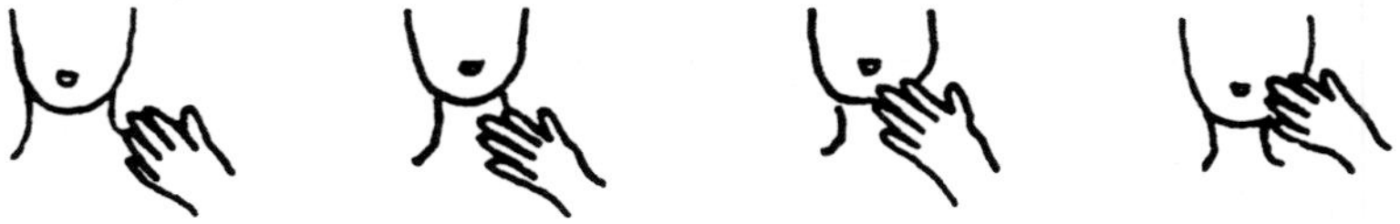

CHART II
Dipthongs

ie (my)   ou (cow)   ae (pay)   oi (boy)

CHART III
Cues for Consonant Sounds

t	h	d	ng	l	k	b	g
m	s	p	y	sh	v	n	j
f	r	zh	ch	w	tH	wh	th
					z		

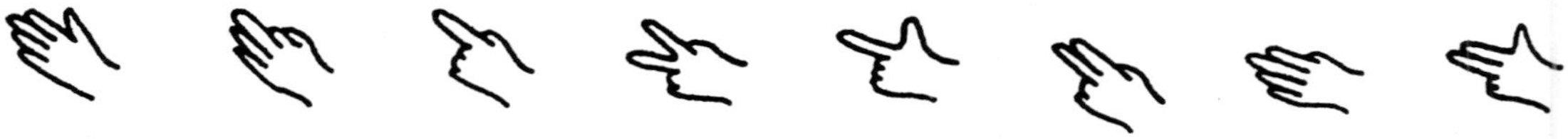

FIGURE 7.9 Cued Speech System
From Henegar and Cornett, 1971. *Cued Speech: Handbook for Parents*, pp. 154–155. Reprinted with permission.

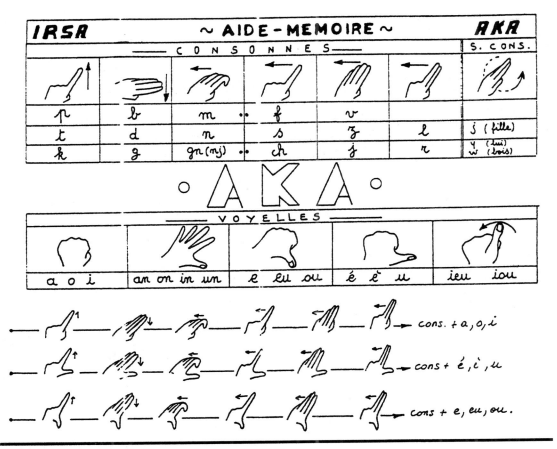

FIGURE 7.10 Alphabet de Kinemes Assistes (AKA) System
From Périer, 1987. Reprinted with permission.

OTHER CLASSIFICATIONS

Unaided communication symbol systems can be classified in different ways. One interesting way of classification is based on the levels of representation of the spoken language to which the system refers. For example, Morse code refers to the graphemic level. To be able to decipher and understand Morse code, a person must know the orthographic rules of the language. The cues of Cued Speech provide information at the phonological level, whereas the elements of most sign systems are on the lexical level. Some sign systems have manual codings of the morphological level as well, such as SEE-II, which has distinctive signs for prefixes and suffixes. Table 7.2 il-

lustrates how unaided systems operate at different levels.

Table 7.2 also explains how unaided systems differ in what they expect the user to do and the processing required for understanding and producing messages. For example, a person who mainly relies on Cued Speech for language reception receives phonological information that is complementary to information from speechreading. The cognitive effort to process this information starts from the phonological level and therefore implies mainly a bottom-up strategy. This means that the person proceeds by identifying the basic elements needed to form structures at a higher level (words, phrases), which again have to be identified (lexical access) to find a

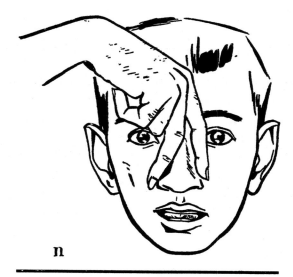

n

FIGURE 7.11 A Manual-Gestural Symbol from the Borel-Maisonny System

From Borel-Maisonny, 1960. Reprinted with permission.

higher meaning that covers wholes (words, phrases, sentences, contexts). If the sentence "I will arrive tomorrow" is presented to the listener in Cued Speech, both the unaided symbols (the cues) and the speech have no direct relationship with the meaning. The information from the cues can only be helpful if the receiver combines it with the significant articulation movements and positions of the mouth of the speaker. These movements and positions (articulemes) have a relationship with the phonological units (the phonemes) that are significant for word and sentence recognition. To make the synthesis of the phonemes into a form, a sufficient short-term memory is required. Presenting Cued Speech requires a cognitive effort from the receiver in terms of (1) a fair ability to combine the visual cues with the visual articulemes and identify them as representatives of phonemes, (2) an ability to synthesize these basic low-level elements into higher level meaningful units, and (3) an effective visual short-term memory. All the alphabet-based and phonemic-based symbol sets appeal to a strong

analytic-synthetic ability along with sufficient short-term memory.

On the other hand, a person who is mostly exposed to a manually coded spoken language will predominantly base language understanding on unanalyzed lexical wholes without much support in breaking up the elements into parts (i.e., phonemes). Individuals mainly exposed to key word signing need a top-down strategy, because the AAC system here provides content information in the sequential order of the main sentence constituents.

Clearly then, the symbols and symbol systems to which a person will be exposed have important implications for the processes that are likely to develop. For some individuals with AAC needs, using manual signs often allows for the development of a more extended internal lexicon. This often has opened tremendous new opportunities for people to learn to communicate in a linguistic way and to develop language skills. However, one disadvantage of manual signs is that they generally contain no information of the sublexical structure of the words. Insight in and access to this more basic language level is extremely important for developing literacy skills (see Chapter 23). This example also illustrates the importance of an advising team considering a strategic combined use of more than one aided and/or unaided communication symbol set or system (for a case example, see Blischak & Lloyd, 1996).

Still other classifications can be made. Von Tetzchner et al. (1996) suggest that it may be useful to know whether a code is nonlinguistic or linguistic and whether the language is primary or derived. Primary languages are those that developed in a natural way in a specific mode. For example, all spoken languages originated in speaking communities long before written forms were proposed. Written language is a typical example of a derived form. Morse code is a derived code to a second degree, because it is a recoding of orthography which is, in itself, a derivation of spoken language. Manually coded language is a derived form of spoken language, while natural sign languages are primary languages. These categories may help in

TABLE 7.2 Linguistic Levels of Language-Based Unaided Symbols

UNAIDED SYSTEM	COGNITIVE EFFORT FOR RECEIVER	LINGUISTIC LEVEL OF ACCESS TO LANGUAGE MODEL	COGNITIVE EFFORT FOR SENDER
Key Word Signing	Top-down strategy Context sensitivity	Syntactical	The sender must be able to identify the words in the sentence that carry most information.
Signed English	Top-down strategy Sufficient short-term memory	Lexical	The sender must be able to access and activate (speak and sign) words and manual signs simultaneously.
SEE-II	Strategy that requires the combination of low-level elements (morphemes) with lexical units (words) Sufficient short-term memory	Morphological	The sender must know and be able to identify and sign the morphemic elements (i.e., morphological mastery); must be able to access and activate (speak and sign) words and manual signs simultaneously.
Fingerspelling	Bottom-up strategy Mental storage of words as written entities Sufficient short-term memory	Orthographical	The sender must know the orthographic rules and be able to recode spoken language into orthography.
Cued Speech	Bottom-up strategy (analytic-synthetic skills) Sufficient short-term memory Phonological skills	Phonological	The sender must know and be able to identify and sign the phonological elements (i.e., phonological mastery).

understanding the cognitive and linguistic processes that are involved in the use of languages and symbol systems (see also Table 7.2).

SUMMARY

Unaided communication can be a powerful help for individuals with communication disabilities. Since the late 1960s, growing attention has been given to communication other than speech and writing. The discovery that modalities other than speech and TO could also contain linguistic meaning has been a breakthrough in exploring the possibilities of unaided modalities for individuals with communication disabilities. Probably the most dramatic development has been the study and recognition of sign language for use in Deaf communities throughout the world. The applications of this discovery have altered considerably the opportunities that are given to deaf persons as well as the way deaf people are perceived by the larger community.

The use of unaided symbols by and with hearing individuals with communication disabilities is also a substantial move toward activating otherwise untapped potential. Unaided systems exploit the natural tendency of humans (1) to invest communication in more than one modality (multimodality), and (2) to exploit other modalities more if one modality is less accessible.

A crucial aspect in developing unaided communication is the appearance of natural gesture in early development and how it may function partially as a substrate for language acquisition. In typically developing individuals, gestural communication remains important and keeps its communicative potential after language acquisition has reached an adult stage. AAC as a method seeks to activate this potential of so-called nonverbal communication in a systematic way.

A main distinction between types of unaided communication symbols is the dichotomy nonlinguistic/linguistic. This allows a further classification in visual symbols with linguistic characteristics (e.g., natural sign languages, manual sign systems), alphabet-based symbols (e.g., fingerspelling), and phonemic- or phonic-based symbols.

Other classifications can be used together with the one presented here. For example, unaided linguistic systems can be classified according to the linguistic level represented. Still another classification is based on whether access to information is visual or auditory, whether the system is nonlinguistic or linguistic, and whether the modality used is a primary or a derived code of the system. Because different classification systems are based on different perspectives and aspects of symbols and symbol use, the use of different classification systems can allow teams to make decisions about which symbol systems have the highest potential to serve an individual's needs.

CHAPTER 8

PRINCIPLES AND USES
OF TECHNOLOGY

RAYMOND W. QUIST AND LYLE L. LLOYD

The dictionary defines **technology** as "the science or practice of industrial arts" (*Webster's*, 1984). Other definitions refer to technology as an applied science. Traditionally, technology has referred to the use of machines or devices for specific purposes. For this text, however, the discussion considers the use of all materials (e.g., paper, board displays), mechanical devices (e.g., switch-operated toys, electric-operated scan devices), and computerized devices (e.g., computers, communication devices).

The application of technology to the general field of disabilities is referred to as **assistive technology (AT)**. The Technology-Related Assistance for Individuals with Disabilities Act (also known as the Tech Act, PL 100-407, 1988) defines an **assistive technology device** as "any item, piece of equipment, or product system, whether acquired commercially off the shelf, modified, or customized, that is used to increase, maintain, or improve functional capabilities of individuals with disabilities" (sec. 3.1). Technology (e.g., computer-driven artificial limbs, cochlear implants, Braille, image magnifiers, powered wheelchairs, or robotic assistance for feeding) has played an increasing role in enabling individuals with disabilities to participate in daily activities. The many cases demonstrating dramatic improvements in the lives of individuals using technology have led some people to conclude that technology will enable all individuals with disabilities to function as persons without disabilities. However, for the individual who has communication disabilities, technology is not a single solution to the problem; rather, the combined use of aided (mechanical, electronic, and computer*) and unaided approaches to facilitate communication and social participation provides the greatest opportunity.

In **augmentative and alternative communication (AAC)**, technology has taken on a major role in enabling individuals with little or no functional speech to communicate. In this chapter, discussion is focused on applying technology, characteristics, and feature matching as fundamental for the application of technology, descriptions of technology for individuals with communication disabilities, selection and transmission, laws for applying technology, and principles for using technology to provide a basis for further discussions on low technology (Chapter 9) and high technology (Chapter 10).

APPLYING TECHNOLOGY

In order to appreciate the role of technology, it is worthwhile to consider the range of technological applications (low to high), how technology connects the AAC user with the environment (interfaces), and some common myths that people have associated with technology.

Low and High Technology

Frequently, technology is discussed in terms of **low technology** and **high technology** (Church & Glennan, 1992; Cook & Hussey, 1995). Cook and Hussey, for example, refer to low technology as "inexpensive, simple to make, and easy to obtain"

---

*In this chapter, *electronic* refers to all devices that typically use transistors to control electron flow and *computer* refers to devices that operate on binary logic and use integrated circuitry.

(p. 577). Examples of low technology are head-pointers, communication boards, switch-operated toys, tape loops, and inexpensive tape recorders. Church and Glennen make a different distinction between low and high technology. For Church and Glennen, "low technology communication aids are simple devices that do not have printed or speech output" and ". . . have no vocabulary storage or programming capabilities" (p. 94). They define high technology devices as "computerized systems that are operated through special software" (p. 94). In general, this is a reasonable dichotomy, but there is room for confusion. The phrase *no vocabulary storage* is ambiguous. Church and Glennen intended it to mean no *computerized* vocabulary storage. Having words (or other graphics) on a communication board or in a communication book is a form of vocabulary storage but such boards/books are low technology.

These differences in definitions highlight the fact that most definitions are limited, potentially confusing, and open to debate. However, technology constantly changes and represents a *continuum* from low to high technology. The definitions in this text are similar to those of Church and Glennen in regarding high technology as being synonymous with computerized devices. However, rather than qualifying the definition in terms of software operation, high technology will be defined in terms of whether the device uses an **integrated circuit (IC)**. In this view, high technology is represented by any device that operates with an IC, but may not need additional software. This definition would include relatively inexpensive devices such as the MemoMate™ (a digital recorder that stores brief messages) as high technology. Although such inexpensive digital recording devices may resemble tape loops and may thus appear to be simple technology, their integrated circuitry is much more sophisticated and allows high sampling rates (11,000–22,000 samples per second) which assure high quality speech.

Technology as a Communication Interface

Interface refers to a surface that forms a common boundary between two parts of matter or space (*Webster's*, 1984). When a communication aid is attached to a computer or an electric appliance, an interface (e.g., a cable) is being used. In augmentative and alternative communication (AAC), the term *interface* also refers to the connection between the user and technology (e.g., a switch or an alternative keyboard that allows for the operation of a communication aid). An interface allows individuals with disabilities to transmit messages to a listener and control the environment (e.g., turn on a television set). AAC technology can be viewed as an interface because it allows a user to connect with the environment. Technological solutions include *both* communication and environmental control. The concept of an interface is useful in understanding the nature of communication in individuals with little or no functional speech. For a more thorough understanding of the role of the interface in communication, see the discussion on the AAC model in Chapter 3.

Technology Panacea Myths

Although high technology computer applications provide powerful communication prostheses, there is much more to meeting the communication needs of individuals with little or no speech. Individuals with disabilities desire to function in the same way as individuals without disabilities. For this reason, they often have high, even unrealistic, expectations whenever new technology becomes available. This ideal is reflected in the name of an organization, Closing the Gap (see Appendix B), which is dedicated to providing education and awareness of technological applications to all individuals with disabilities. Equalization through the use of computer technology may be a myth, however, because individuals without disabilities will also reap major benefits of savings in time and physical demand. The giant strides made by individuals without disabilities may further distance them from individuals with disabilities.

Because AAC service providers want what is best for AAC users, they often encourage selection of what appears to be the most powerful technology to meet the individual's needs. These desires may lead to the selection of technological applications that may be unnecessary, inappropriate, or too expensive. For example, AAC users may be able to point to a name on a communication board faster than they can type it out on a keyboard or even on one or two coded keys while waiting for the speech output. A laminated communication board can be easily used at the beach, whereas a computer is subject to damage from sand and water. As service providers consider applying high technology to meet the communication needs of AAC users, they must realize that it may play a major role, a small role, or no role. With further advances, it may become an increasingly important part of an individual's AAC system. However, low technology will always remain a part of the total communication spectrum.

CHARACTERISTICS AND FEATURE MATCHING

AAC service providers who have major decision-making responsibilities must have knowledge of the characteristics or features of a wide variety of devices. They also must understand the process of **feature matching** in which AAC devices are selected based on a match between individual strengths and needs and device features. Unfortunately, some professionals have considerable skill in operating specific devices (e.g., DeltaTalker™, DynaVox™, Wolf™), but know little about the underlying principles and features of the technology. Specific devices have changed during the past decade, with some no longer available and new models appearing, but the underlying principles have changed little. Some device features have improved (e.g., greater storage/memory, lighter weight, smaller size, easier programming), but they have not changed categorically. The AAC service provider must understand the features of the devices under consideration.

For almost three decades AAC researchers and clinicians/educators have delineated various features of symbols in an attempt to provide general guidelines for designing AAC systems. For example, Vanderheiden and Harris-Vanderheiden (1976) proposed six symbol selection considerations, noting that symbols should be: (1) compatible with the aid or technique, (2) nonrestrictive, (3) appropriate to the individuals' receptive and expressive abilities, (4) developmental and flexible,

(5) adaptable to clinical/educational approaches, and (6) acceptable to the user and others. Lloyd and Karlan (1983) reviewed the early work in this area prior to proposing these symbol selection considerations, and Lloyd and his colleagues have continued to develop them (see Chapter 13 for a further discussion of symbol selection). Many of these selection considerations are also applicable for technology (e.g., acceptability, initial cost, maintenance cost, and training). Subsequently, Vanderheiden and Lloyd (1986) presented a number of requirements for an overall multicomponent system (see Appendix A). Although these requirements apply to a total communication system, they apply equally to the selection and application of AAC technology. Quist and Blischak (1992) discussed many of these requirements as well as the features specified by Kraat and Sitver-Kogut (1991) and Galyas (1987). Galyas listed the following requirements for an ideal **voice output communication aid (VOCA)**:

1. Unlimited vocabulary
2. High-quality speech, including intelligibility and naturalness
3. Choice of voices (e.g., age and gender)
4. Choice of dialects and pronunciation
5. Appropriate rates for normal interaction
6. Flexibility (e.g., change of conversation)
7. True text-to-speech capabilities
8. Emotional expression (prosody)
9. Portability
10. Cosmetic appeal
11. Ease of physical access
12. Durability and ease of maintenance
13. Aesthetic appeal
14. Low mental and linguistic demands
15. Printed output and visual display
16. Access to computer/interfacing
17. Alternative inputs
18. Low cost

These characteristics or features should be considered when selecting a communication device. Although Galyas outlined these features with a VOCA in mind, with minor modifications these features are appropriate considerations for all technology devices. Successful use of communication devices depends on the extent to which such device characteristics or features match the strengths and needs of the AAC user. Chapter 14 discusses feature matching in more detail and includes a list of more than two dozen basic features considered by the Purdue-GLASS (Greater Lafayette Area Special Services) AAC Assessment Team during the feature matching process. To assist AAC service providers in systematically considering switch and communication device features, guides are provided in Appendix A.

TECHNOLOGY FOR INDIVIDUALS WITH COMMUNICATION DISABILITIES

Over the past 50 years, professionals working with individuals with disabilities have developed ways to facilitate communication through communication boards, amplification systems, artificial larynges, mechanical symbol selectors, modified typewriters, and computerized communication systems. The following sections briefly discuss these low and high technology developments.

Communication Boards and Materials

Historically, individuals with little or no functional speech have relied on gestures or pointing to objects and pictures. Typically, letters, words, pictures, or other graphic symbols have been arranged on paper, posterboard, oilcloth, an apron, or some other material according to predetermined categories or topics. Such arrangements are called communication boards. Communication boards are usually located so that the communication partner can easily see where the user is pointing. In many cases the picture or symbol has the printed word near it so that the communication partner can readily interpret the intended message. Although communication boards were used somewhat sparingly throughout the 1960s because of bias for spoken communication, they are used more frequently today as AAC service providers recognize the importance of using many communication modes to enhance the user's language development and inclusion in society.

When the AAC user is unable to point to a symbol, a variety of approaches can be used to facilitate communication. The communication partner, for example, can point to objects or symbols on a communication board and ask the user to indicate when the desired symbol is indicated (a form of scanning). For individuals with severe motor disabilities or with motor control limited to eye gaze, symbols can also be arranged on a clear piece of plexiglass that typically has a hole in the middle (e.g., ETRAN). The symbols can be arranged so that when the communication partner holds the ETRAN up and looks through the plexiglass, the symbols are facing the user. Because the symbols are placed in different quadrants of the ETRAN by category and word type (they also may be color coded), the communication partner can guess the intended word by judging the focal point of the AAC user's eyes.

Communication boards and ETRANs are examples of low technology AAC devices. They are typically inexpensive and often homemade. These materials or devices are easily modifiable, flexible, highly portable, durable, and readily available for instant communication. Often these advantages make them a highly preferred option for individuals with little or no functional speech. Chapter 9 provides a more extensive discussion of low technology.

Mechanical Communication Devices

Early technology consisted of using mechanical devices to assist individuals with little or no functional speech to communicate. For individuals who had lost use of their vocal folds or had them surgically removed (i.e., laryngectomized) but had intact articulators and motor control, a number of mechanical devices were available as alternatives or supplements for esophageal speech (i.e., speech involving the use of expelled air from the esophagus). Several of these devices are still in common use today. With a pneumatic device (e.g., Tokyo Reed artificial larynx, Figure 8.1a), a speaker generates speech by expelling air from the lungs via the tracheostoma through a trumpetlike mouthpiece. A plastic tube connected to the mouthpiece is inserted into the oral cavity. Once the sound is within the oral cavity, it becomes speech by movement of the articulators. An electrolarynx (Figure 8.1b) operates on the same principle. The sound source, however, is from electrical vibration rather than pulmonary air.

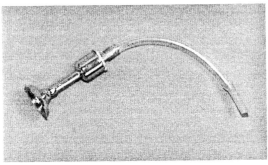

(a)

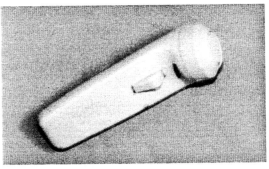

(b)

FIGURE 8.1 Mechanical Communication Devices. (a) Tokyo Reed Artificial Larynx, a pneumatic device that uses airflow from the lungs through a stoma to create a sound source for speech. (b) Western Electric Electrolarynx, a battery-operated artificial larynx that uses electrical vibrations as a sound source for speech.

Many professionals resisted the use of these devices throughout the 1950s and 1960s because the individual's own speech (i.e., esophageal speech) was considered most natural.

Because approximately two-thirds of the individuals who had laryngectomies did not learn to use effective esophageal speech, many of them benefited from the use of alternative methods (Salmon & Goldstein, 1989; Snidecor, 1962). For these reasons, mechanical devices became more acceptable and are frequently used today. Currently, the individual who has had a laryngectomy has many choices due to improved surgical techniques and prosthetic designs (e.g., the Blom-Singer Prosthesis). This shift in attitude allowed individuals to use alternatives to speech and also influenced many speech-language pathologists.

Many individuals unable to speak for a variety reasons (e.g., neurologically damaged vocal folds and/or articulators) used alternative communication modes, such as writing, printing, and typing. Some individuals (e.g., persons with cerebral palsy) lacked sufficient motor control to speak, write, or print, but they could strike the keys of a typewriter with a single finger, a headpointer, or mouthstick. In some cases, a keyguard was necessary to guide the finger or stick movement and prevent accidental activation of neighboring keys. For individuals with more severe motor impairments, however, more extensive modifications were necessary. For individuals with severe motor impairments who could not direct select, mechanical scanning devices were developed. Some of these scanning devices were homemade, and others were manufactured (e.g., Dial Scan™, Versa-Scan™). Pictures or words on these devices could be arranged so that the user could make selections by starting and stopping an electrically controlled rotating clock hand with a switch. Until the development of desktop and laptop computers, these devices were the state-of-the-art in AAC. Many are still used today and remain practical, low technology solutions for individuals with little or no functional speech.

Computerized Communication Devices

Over the years, computers have become less expensive, more portable, and more versatile. The Apple® computer, for example, was built with extra slots for inserting circuit boards, allowing expansion of power and function. This development facilitated the adaptation of computers for individuals with disabilities. Rehabilitation engineers quickly saw the potential and developed hardware and software for use with the Apple computer. The **Adaptive Firmware Card** (Schweijda & Vanderheiden, 1982), for example, made it possible to use commercially available software with alternate input devices (e.g., switches and expanded keyboards) and selection techniques. Although IBM® had a commitment to making computers more accessible to individuals with disabilities, its major emphasis remained in the development of business applications. Apple remained the preferred computer for use in schools for many years as rehabilitation engineers and programmers developed hardware adaptations and software. Now, however, IBM and IBM-compatible computers are more widely used with individuals who have disabilities, and software programs are written to work both with IBM and IBM-compatible machines (e.g., Dell, Epson, Gateway, Hewlett-Packard, IBM 486 series, NEC, Tandy, Zenith) and with Apple Macintosh® (e.g., Centris, Classic, Performa, Powerbook, PowerMac, Quadra).

SELECTION AND TRANSMISSION

Selection involves the retrieval of symbols (Fuller, Lloyd, & Schlosser, 1992; Lloyd, Quist, & Windsor, 1990). For most individuals, words are selected and retrieved mentally from a stored vocabulary in the brain (unaided). For individuals using AAC devices (aided), an additional physical step (e.g., pressing the symbol on a computer/communication device keyboard or pressing a switch until the appropriate symbol appears on the display) is required to select and send messages. Selection may be either direct (e.g., touching or eye gazing) or indirect (e.g., scanning).

Direct Selection

Generally, four types of **direct selection** are recognized: (1) pointing without physical contact (e.g., eye gaze, light pointers, head-controlled mouse); (2) physical pressure; (3) physical contact/proximity; and (4) voice/speech recognition. In the case of computers, most users press a key on the keyboard to select a given symbol (e.g., pressing *a* on the keyboard will place an *a* on the monitor). Other symbols (e.g., Blissymbols, pictures) can be placed on the keys so that pressing a symbol will result in its appearance on the screen. For individuals who have difficulty pressing or releasing keys in a timely manner, the computer can be programmed so that the keys and/or switches will be activated only when a predetermined amount of pressure is applied for a specified duration, known as **filtered/averaged activation**. Symbols can also be selected by touching them directly on a special touch screen (e.g., Powerpad) or on a touch screen that has been attached to a monitor. In this case no pressure is needed. Still further, symbols can be selected by interrupting a light beam (proximity). Finally, significant progress has been made in symbol selection and command issuance through the transmission of acoustic signals and speech (voice) recognition.

Scanning

Because direct selection is the most efficient and fastest form of input, it is preferred in cases in which an individual has reliable motor control. When a user has extensive loss of motor control, however, scanning selection techniques may be used. **Scanning** involves the movement of an indicator/highlighter (e.g., a person pointing, a cursor) across a display of symbols. When the indicator is positioned on the desired array, the user makes a selection. The speed and manner of control of highlighting choices can vary. Scanning may be done with a device by steps or automatically, or it may be partner assisted. **Step scanning** involves movement of the indicator each time the user activates a switch. Because movement is directly related to the depression or release of the switch, the user has direct control of the speed of selection. The high number of switch activations required to get to a target, however, can be fatiguing to the user. For this reason, **automatic scanning** is often used. In automatic scanning, one activation of the switch activates the highlighting of displays according to a preprogrammed rate and sequence. The user then only has to depress or in the case of **inverse scanning**, release the switch once at each stage (e.g., at the desired row and column for the desired symbol). This automation is much less fatiguing and allows the user to focus more completely on the selection task. The user must develop skill in anticipating when the indicator will reach the target so that the right amount of time can be allotted for switch activation.

In **partner-assisted scanning**, the AAC user watches as another person points to each choice of symbols (visual scanning) and then selects the desired symbol by signalling (e.g., nodding, eye blink). If the assistant speaks the choices, auditory scanning is being used. Most of the principles in the following discussion can be applied effectively to partner-assisted scanning as well as switch-operated scanning.

Scanning can be set up in many ways. The simplest ways are circular and linear, but they are the most time consuming. Multidimensional scanning approaches (e.g., group-item, row-column) are preferred when there is a large display (40–70 items) because individuals can access a target in a shorter period of time.

Circular Scanning. Devices for **circular scanning** (i.e., rotary scan) (Figure 8.2a) for an example) typically resemble clocks where a rotating hand points to a picture symbol or word as it moves either clockwise or counterclockwise around the circle. Circular scanning may also be accomplished using lights that go on as each choice is presented. The AAC user selects the symbol by pressing or releasing a switch to stop the hand or the light's movement. Circular scanning is a type of linear scanning (i.e., curvilinear).

Linear Scanning. **Linear scanning** involves highlighting one symbol at a time. The indicator typically moves left to right, one symbol at a time. In Figure 8.2(b) (partner-assisted scanning), an assistant points to each choice. In assisted scanning, the user indicates choice by vocalization, eye blink, or other gesture. In mechanical or electrical control of the scanning device, the user activates a switch when the desired symbol is highlighted. The direction of indicator movement (left-right, right-left, up-down, down-up) can be programmed according to user ability or preference. Linear scanning tends to be rather slow, however, as the user must move through each symbol in the designated sequence before choosing the desired symbol.

Group-Item Scanning. **Group-item scanning** is often called **block/group scanning** (Goossens' & Crain, 1992). Vanderheiden and Lloyd (1986) also refer to this as **multidimensional scanning**. Generally, this approach enables a user to reach a desired item faster by eliminating unwanted items from larger arrays. This also reduces the number of switch actions needed to select a desired symbol. One common approach to group-item scanning is to group items so the user is presented choices con-

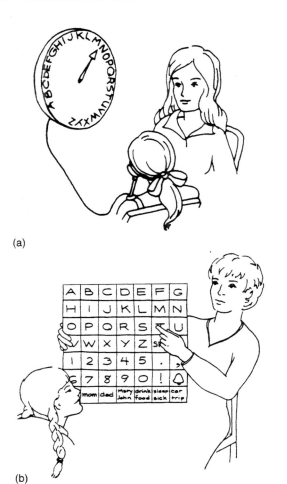

(a)

(b)

FIGURE 8.2 Scanning Approaches. (a) Circular (rotary) scanning with alphabet. (b) Linear scanning with alphabet. This illustration also shows partner-assisted scanning.
Copyright American Speech-Language-Hearing Association. Reprinted with permission.

taining a large number of items each time. Once the user selects the array with the desired item, items are presented in groups and/or individually until the final choice is made. This approach allows the user to reject large numbers of items first and then proceed to the desired item without wasting time proceeding through a number of unwanted items. In many cases the nature of an individual's disability dictates a minimal number of motor responses (e.g., unusually long response time). Figure 8.3 illustrates automatic group-item scanning, in which

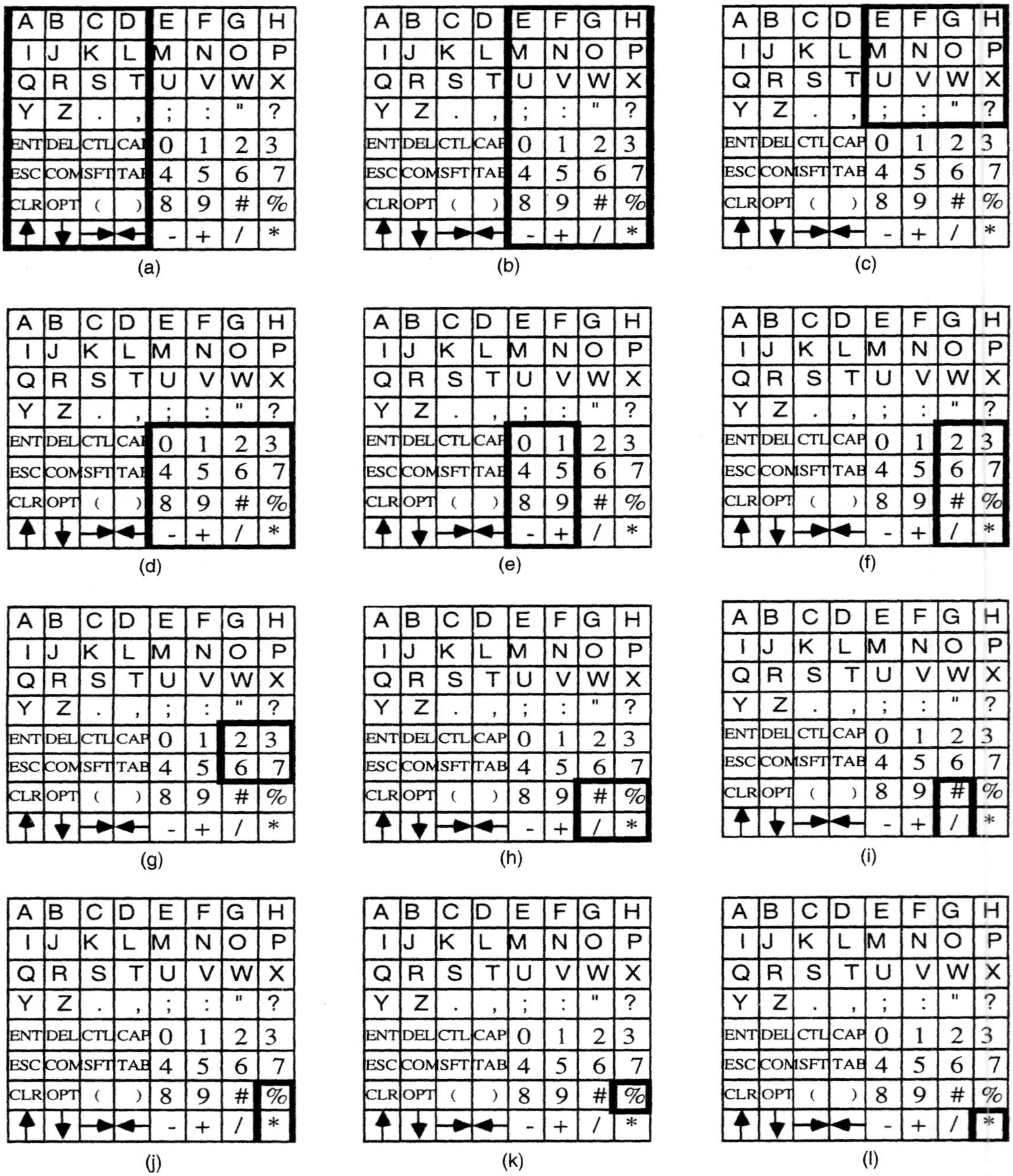

FIGURE 8.3 Group-Item Scanning. (a) First 4 × 8 array. (b) Second 4 × 8 array. (c) First 4 × 4 array. (d) Second 4 × 4 array. (e) First 2 × 4 array. (f) Second 2 × 4 array. (g) First 2 × 2 array. (h) Second 2 × 2 array. (i) First 1 × 2 array. (j) Second 1 × 2 array. (k) One-item display. (l) One target item.

the target item appears near the end of an 8 × 8 array. Initially, the first 4 × 8 array is highlighted (Figure 8.3a); if unselected by the user, the second 4 × 8 array is highlighted (Figure 8.3b). If the user selects this array, the top 4 × 4 array of 16 items is highlighted (Figure 8.3c) and then the bottom half (Figure 8.3d). If unselected, 2 × 4 arrays are displayed (Figures 8.3e–f), then 2 × 2 arrays (Figures 8.3g–h), then 1 × 2 arrays (Figure 8.3i–j), and finally single items (Figures 8.3k–l) until the target item is selected (Figure 8.3l).

The relative saving in time using automatic group-item scanning increases significantly when target items are near the end of the display and when the duration of the AAC user's response time is greater. For example, if the AAC user is given 2 seconds to respond to each presentation of the 64 items in Figure 8.3, by linear scanning (or item-by-item), it takes 128 seconds to reach the target item (asterisk). In row-column scanning, the time is reduced to 30 seconds. In group-item scanning, however, the time is reduced to 24 seconds. If the AAC user's response time requires displays lasting 8 seconds, the time required for reaching the target item is 512 seconds for linear scanning, 120 seconds for row-column scanning, and 96 seconds for group-item scanning. The savings are substantial with increases in the user's response time and the length of the array's display. There is a trade-off, however, in that the user must activate the switch 11 times in this illustration, as compared to once if the items were displayed one by one (i.e., linear scanning). This factor must be considered if the AAC user demonstrates significant muscle fatigue with more frequent responses. Group-item scanning can save even more time if the user misses a selection, inasmuch as less time is involved in waiting for the recycling of choices.

Row-Column Scanning.   **Row-column scanning** is a frequently used pattern in which an entire row is highlighted until the user selects the row in which the symbol appears. When the user selects the appropriate row, the highlighter then moves across columns one symbol at a time. The desired symbol is then selected by another activa-

	A	B	C	D	E	F	G
R	H	I	J	K	L	M	N
O	O	P	Q	R	S	T	U
W	V	W	X	Y	Z	SP	?
	1	2	3	4	5		
	6	7	8	9	0		
	+	-	=	x	-		

COLUMN

FIGURE 8.4   Row-Column Scanning

tion of a switch. Figure 8.4 illustrates the direction of the row and column movement in the process.

Directed Scanning.   **Directed scanning** involves the use of either a joystick or multiple switches, for which the user can control direction more precisely (up, down, left, right, diagonally) and can thus increase the rate of selection (Figure 8.5). Varying combinations of these different scanning

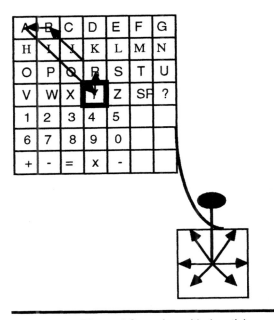

FIGURE 8.5   Directed Scanning with Joystick

techniques may be used to customize for the specific needs of the user.

Scanning Efficiency

Although scanning provides a method for a person with very limited motor ability to select symbols, in comparison with direct selection, it is very time consuming. Several strategies have been developed to decrease the time, thereby increasing scanning efficiency. One of these is group-item scanning previously discussed. Another strategy is to place the most frequently used symbols at the beginning of the scanning process. Decisions about frequency of use may be based either on actual observations of the symbols used by a given individual or on the frequency-of-occurrence data for letters/words (Beukleman & Yorkston, 1985; Pratt, 1939).

In text generation, the array may be arranged so that the most frequently occurring letters or letter combinations occur first. In circular or linear scanning, the most frequently used letters, E, T, A, O, N, I, S, H, R, would be the first nine letters. This scanning array would be much more efficient than using an alphabetical sequence as shown in Figure 8.2(a)–(b). In row-column scanning, the more frequently occurring letters would be clustered in the upper left-hand corner (see Figure 8.6).

If using symbols other than the alphabet, the same principles influencing strategic placement apply. If using words, the most frequently occurring words would occur early in the circular or linear scanning array, or in the upper-left hand corner of a row-column scanning array. Other types of fre-

quently used symbols (Blissymbols, pictographs, Sigsymbols) would be similarly arranged. Other display arrangements are discussed in Chapter 9.

In addition to selecting a pattern of scanning that is most efficient for the user, other variables can be arranged (e.g., setting different speeds or selection control techniques). A more in-depth discussion of switches is found in Goossens' and Crain (1992) and in Chapter 9. The activation of the switch itself may be through depression of the switch (down), release of the switch (up), or movement of a joystick (up, down, left, right, or diagonally). Although scanning can be programmed so that the highlighter (cursor or light) moves through the array of symbols more rapidly, thus reducing the time the user must wait between selections, motor and reaction times of the user must be considered carefully. Even individuals without disabilities find scanning to be a difficult task. With practice, however, users frequently develop considerable scanning skill.

Dynamic Displays

Computers, by their very nature, support the use of various types of **dynamic displays** (i.e., displays that change). In one type of dynamic display, part of the items for selection are displayed at a given movement, and then, with a further selection, additional items are displayed on the screen (e.g., Words+® and Talking Screen™). Dynamic displays enable the user considerable flexibility, as topics and specific items can be arranged so that the user can flip from page to page (levels). Another type of dynamic display actually involves the animation of a graphic symbol to represent action verbs (e.g., DynaVox™). A more in-depth discussion of dynamic displays can be found in Chapter 10.

Although scanning allows individuals with severe motor impairments to select and use symbols and thus participate in speech and writing activities, it requires considerable cognitive ability to attend to a variety of choices, plan selections, make decisions, and physically select in a timely manner. Because scanning involves the presentation and selection of choices at several levels, it can be a slow and tedious process, not only for the AAC user, but for the communication partner as well.

SP	T	N	R	F	B			
E	O	H	U	G	Q			
A	S	C	Y	J				
I	D	W	X					
L	P	K						
M	V							
Z								

FIGURE 8.6 Row-Column Scanning with Frequency of Occurrence Display

Encoding

In general, **encoding** is considered language formulation, the process by which a communicator formulates a linguistic message by retrieving selected symbols and symbol combinations from their areas of storage in the brain and arranging them in semantic categories and syntactical rule-governed order. The entire encoding process is usually completed instantaneously with little or no conscious thought about the complexities involved. For AAC users who communicate proficiently through manual sign (i.e., unaided AAC users), the encoding process of selecting and arranging is essentially the same as for individuals without disabilities who use natural speech. They retrieve selected symbols or symbol combinations, arrange them in logical order, and deliver them manually as a linguistic message. For AAC users who use assistive communication devices (i.e., aided AAC users), however, the encoding process takes on additional steps and involves additional elements (i.e., the aided symbols). In this case, symbols need to not only exist in the linguistic areas of the brain, but also in an external location (e.g., computer memory, on a communication board, on an ETRAN). For further clarification of the basic process of encoding and of the AAC processes and interface, see Chapter 3 and Figure 3.1.

In aided AAC, encoding includes the additional process by which messages are stored in association with a specific symbol or symbol sequence for later retrieval (Beukelman & Mirenda, 1992; Cook & Hussey, 1995; Musselwhite & St. Louis, 1988; Silverman, 1995; Vanderheiden & Lloyd, 1986). Encoding works in conjunction with either direct selection or scanning and serves to enhance the rate of communication (Vanderheiden & Lloyd, 1986). Encoding is a powerful secondary technique (Fishman, 1987) that allows an individual to code a smaller number of items to gain access to a more extensive vocabulary.

The following discussion describes several methods of encoding. **Memory-based encoding** involves memorization of codes. **Conceptual encoding** and **semantic encoding** involve the use of symbols that have a natural and/or taught association with their referents. **Visual-motor encoding** is a special case of conceptual and semantic encoding that uses visual representations that relate to motor components of manual signs or gestures that represent meaning (e.g., diagrams that illustrate hand movements). **Chart-based encoding** involves an organized chart or key for reference by the user during communication. **Display-based encoding** is similar to chart-based, except that the user responds to a display without any reference to a code. The best type of encoding for a particular individual depends on the size of the vocabulary and the cognitive ability of the user. Cook and Hussey (1995) discuss encoding under rate-enhancement techniques.

Memory-Based Encoding.   Memory-based encoding can be accomplished through color coding, combinations of letters or numbers, symbols (e.g., conceptual or semantic symbols), or Vois-Shapes™ (symbols associated with handshape, location, and movement, such as ASL signs).

Color coding is frequently used to facilitate organization and efficient retrieval of materials/information. Files may be tagged with blue markers to represent all items related to the budget and with yellow markers to indicate student files. In similar fashion, AAC users may organize the way in which messages are stored for use during conversation. Symbols displayed on blue, for example, may represent messages related to school, red area symbols may represent messages related to work, and yellow area symbols may represent messages related to recreational activities. Color coding is often used to categorize symbols on an eye-gaze board.

Alphabet encoding, sometimes referred to as **letter coding/encoding**, includes the use of traditional orthography (TO) or Morse code and occurs when one writes or sends a message. Alphabet encoding is discussed more thoroughly in Chapters 6 and 23. Decoding using TO occurs when one reads a message.

Abbreviation expansion uses typical or idiosyncratic abbreviations to code full words. Two approaches are truncation and contraction (R. W. Bailey, 1989). Truncation is an abbreviation approach in which a word is shortened (e.g., coop/cooperation). Contraction involves the omission of vowels (e.g., fr/for, vb/verb). Abbreviation strategies are often employed by individuals who use speed writing. Similarly, the AAC user can make effective use of such techniques to increase efficiency. For example, when the user inputs "conj," the output may be "conjunction." This elimination of seven keystrokes represents considerable savings in time, expended energy, and fatigue. If abbreviation is being used with word expansion techniques, the user often needs to instruct the communication device when the abbreviation is completely entered (i.e., a longer word is not intended). This may be done by inputting a special symbol when the abbreviation is completed (e.g., conj\). Some of the other encoding methods discussed in the following sections may also be considered abbreviation expansion techniques (Cook & Hussey, 1995).

Alphanumeric encoding uses both letters and numbers for retrieving messages. For example, H might be used to categorize humor, with numbers being used to categorize the jokes. The jokes could then be numbered so H1 is a knock-knock joke, H2 is a traveling salesman joke, and H3 is a shaggy dog story.

Numeric encoding, also known as **number encoding**, can be used alone, without letters. In these cases messages are numbered (e.g., 1 is a greeting, 2 is a joke, and 3 is a food item). Numbers can also be combined so that 1-2 is "hello," 1-3 is "what's up?," 2-1 is a knock-knock joke, 2-2 is a traveling salesman joke, 3-1 is "hamburger," and 3-2 is "pizza." This coding approach is useful when only a limited number of messages are needed. Because the associations between the numbers and messages are arbitrary, this approach can be taxing on the memory. For this reason, the messages are often displayed either on a computer menu or a chart.

Letter category encoding is used to develop categories of messages and then specific messages within the category (e.g., *D* for drinks, *E* for emotions or feeling, *F* for foods, *G* for greetings, *H* for humor). A second letter might be used for specific messages relating to the category. For example, one might use *H* (humor) + *K* to represent knock-knock jokes (i.e., *HK* would then represent a knock-knock joke for retrieval.) If one is a poor speller and has organized things phonetically, one

could use HN (nock-nock). Similarly, one might use *H* for humor + *T* for travel (i.e., *HT* would then mean traveling salesman joke). To retrieve a shaggy dog story, one might use *S* and *D* (i.e., *HS* or *HD*) to differentiate two different shaggy dog stories. If users organize their humor this way and have several jokes for each different type, they would need to use a third or even a fourth letter. Letters can also, of course, stand for sentences. The letters *D* for drinks and *C* for coffee could be used to retrieve the sentence, "How about a cup of coffee?"

Logical letter coding (LLC or LOLEC) uses letters of key words in a phrase to construct messages. For example, if the user wants a drink of water, the letters D and W might be used. If the user wants a drink of milk, the letters D and M might be used. A logical relationship exists between the letters used and the key words of the phrase or sentence. Beukelman & Mirenda (1992) use the term *salient letter coding* to refer to this approach.

Memory-based encoding strategies are useful in organizing symbols for easy storage and retrieval, and they capitalize on meaningful associations. A major disadvantage for some of them, however, is the limited number of possibilities before duplications in the code occur (e.g., because DW can mean either drink water or drink wine, two codes are needed). Another disadvantage is the need for the user to have an extraordinary memory to store and retrieve large numbers of messages. These limitations can be overcome in part with conceptual and/or semantic encoding (i.e., using icons that have natural and/or taught associations that can be used to reduce memory load).

Semantic and Conceptual Encoding. Minspeak™ (Baker, 1982) uses a semantic association approach. Semantic encoding involves associating multiple meanings with graphic symbols called icons. If the user associates specific symbols (icons) that are in some way related to the meaning of the message, recall may be easier. For example, in Figure 8.7, the icon in row 7, column G, on the Minspeak display can represent a lighting bolt or a ruffled french fry. The icon 6-C can rep-

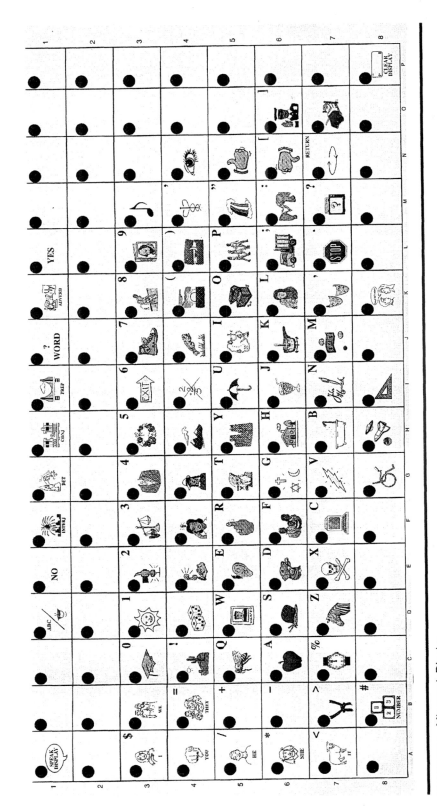

FIGURE 8.7 Minspeak Display
Courtesy of Prentke Romich Company.

resent apple, food, or the color red; the icon 5-I can represent umbrella or protection. This use of multiple meanings allows greater flexibility and expansion of programmed messages. For example, 7-G (lightning bolt) and 5-I (umbrella) can be programmed and used together to say "We are going to have a severe thunderstorm." When combining 7-G (french fry) with 6-C (food), one can program and retrieve the message "I want some french fries."

Minspeak was used on Prentke Romich communication devices such as the AlphaTalker™, DeltaTalker, and Liberator™ as well as on the IntroTalker™, LightTalker™, and TouchTalker™, which are no longer being manufactured. A variety of Minspeak Application Programs (MAPs) was developed for specific purposes and populations. Although still available, these MAPs, which were distinctly different in their icons and organization, have been replaced with the Unity approach designed to meet an AAC user's communication needs at varying stages of language development. Unity/AT and Unity/128 use the same icons at the same locations, thus providing for vocabulary growth without requiring the user to learn new associations. It also makes retrieval of messages more efficient by reinforcing motor patterns that lead to automaticity.

Subsequently others have developed conceptual association approaches. For example, the Words+ and Talking Screen allow the selection of symbols and the storing of language elements and commands that are associated with pictures and picture sequences rather than positions of symbols. A major advantage of this approach is that the AAC user can rearrange symbols without having to reprogram them (i.e., the language automatically goes with the symbol wherever it is placed).

Visual-Motor Encoding. Visual-motor encoding is a special case of memory-based encoding based on the major parameters of manual sign production (location, movement, handshape) rather than conceptual associations that have particular relevance in signing environments. An early computerized approach was HANDS, developed in the United Kingdom (Llewellyn-Jones, 1983, 1984;

Watts & Llewellyn-Jones, 1984a, 1984b). HANDS, based on British Sign Language, was developed using a general principles system for deaf, adolescent boys. More recently, VoisShapes™ (Shane & Wilbur, 1989) was developed using some of the general principles of American Sign Language (ASL). This system is based on visual representations that relate to the three major parameters of manual signs (or gestures) that represent meaning. The keyboard on VoisShapes (Figure 8.8) illustrates location, handshapes, and movement. A three-press sequence of these parameters retrieves prestored words corresponding to manual signs. HANDS and VoisShapes are examples of high technology visual-motor encoding. The use of sign-linked Sigsymbols is an example of low technology visual-motor encoding.

Chart-Based and Display-Based Encoding. Chart-based encoding, in which a chart remains visible throughout communication, is useful when the number of vocabulary items is particularly large, the codes are too complex or confusing, or the user has cognitive limitations. When such a chart is used, items are often arranged by category and/or color coded to make it easier and faster to locate items. Figure 8.9(a) illustrates the use of chart-based encoding. In this case, the user refers to the chart to send a message using Morse code. The code and meanings can be arranged to facilitate locating by the individual using the chart (e.g., the letter followed by the code).

Display-based encoding is identical to chart-based encoding except that the code is not apparent. In Figure 8.9(b), the user simply follows the line to select the appropriate letter through activation of a switch. Each switch activation needed to move the light to the designated letter will produce a dot or dash. The user does not need to know the code because by moving the light toward the target letters, the appropriate dots and dashes are selected.

Word Prediction

The AAC user can increase the efficiency of communication through a specialized technique called **word prediction**. Many software programs (e.g.,

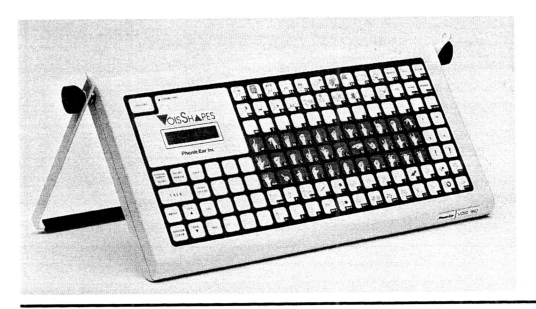

FIGURE 8.8   VoisShapes Keyboard Arrangements
Photo courtesy of Phonic Ear, Inc.

EZ Keys™ by Words+, and Predict-It™ by Don Johnston Incorporated) present menus of possible words each time the user types a letter. These lists are based on the rate or frequency with which the words are typically used by communicators and often are automatically adjusted by the software's program according to the individual's usage. For example, when the user types "lo," a menu of five numbered choices appears on the screen (e.g., look, loop, loose, lose, love). If the desired word appears, the user simply has to select the number of the choice. In this example, the user may save 1 or 2 keystrokes. Obviously, the savings in time and number of keystrokes is less for short words, but increases considerably with increased word length. One major advantage of word prediction techniques is that they do not require the user to remember codes.

LAWS FOR APPLYING TECHNOLOGY

Six general laws of assistive technology are applicable when considering technology use in AAC: (1) law of parsimony, (2) law of minimal learning, (3) law of minimal energy, (4) law of minimal interference, (5) law of best fit, and (6) law of practicality and use.

Law of Parsimony

The **law of parsimony** states that things should be as simple as possible. Because technological advances excite the imagination, one is tempted to consider elaborate systems for use with AAC users. The more elaborate the technology system employed, however, the more frequent and more serious drawbacks it may have, such as cost, excessive equipment to attach or transport, and potential for breakdown during use. AAC service providers should be stingy in selecting and applying technology, as long as the goals of communication can be met. For example, a great deal of communication can occur with gestures. Figure 8.10 illustrates an extreme violation of the law of parsimony.

Law of Minimal Learning

The **law of minimal learning** emphasizes that it is preferable to use an approach that does not need to be learned. Increased cognitive load (e.g., remem-

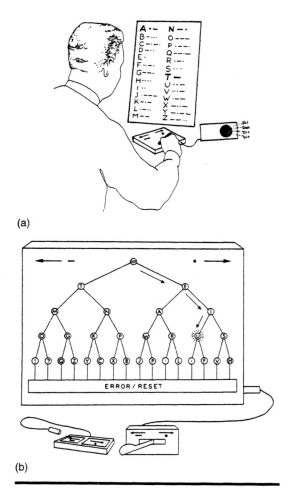

(a)

(b)

FIGURE 8.9 Different Types of Encoding. (a) Chart-based encoding. (b) Display-based encoding

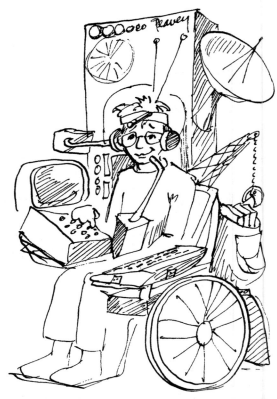

FIGURE 8.10 Law of Parsimony
Artwork by Gay Harris.

bering codes and key code sequences) may contribute to fatigue and interfere with the effectiveness of communication. An AAC device (e.g., picture communication board) that an AAC user can begin using without any training is ideal. When considerable training is needed, delays will occur in developing proficiency and reduce the likelihood of use of the device over time. This principle also applies to the general population. Many individuals are intimidated by technology. If they cannot immediately use technology, they tend to put it aside with good intentions to learn about

it later. All too often, good equipment for AAC users has ended up on shelves unused for months and even years. Device manuals must be clearly written, and workshops must be made readily available for individuals to obtain hands-on experience in using technology. The Assistive Technology Education Network (ATEN) of Florida and the Pennsylvania Assistive Technology Center (PATC) now known as Penn Tech are organizations that provide ongoing training for service providers and AAC users to facilitate the use of devices. The Tech Act (PL100-407, 1988) is intended to provide an extension of these types of services to all states. Many manufacturers and vendors provide training workshops for individuals who have purchased their devices and for their supporting personnel (e.g., speech-language pathologist or teacher, and family members). Most manufacturers also provide 24-hour hotlines to assist users, caregivers, and teaching staff in working through problems with operating the equipment. A need still exists, however, for service providers to be able to make immediate repairs and/or reprogram the device when needed. Otherwise, the user remains unable to communicate for a lengthy period of time. The user who is frequently unable to use the device is likely to feel increased frustration and reduced motivation. These problems argue for the need to have low technology backups available at all times.

Law of Minimal Energy

According to the **law of minimal energy**, an activity is preferred if it takes little effort and can be performed for long periods with minimal fatigue. Like most individuals, if AAC users have to expend too much energy to perform a specific act, they may tend to avoid the task altogether. A smile or movement of the eyes that requires minimal effort can be effective communication. If the switch prescribed for interfacing the AAC user with a device is either too hard to activate or results in frequent errors, the individual will likely use it on a very limited basis. AAC users who can speak but are highly dysarthric (virtually unintelligible) will often insist on using speech instead of their devices even when asked to repeat. AAC users may fall back on their devices to express their ideas, but often reluctantly, possibly because of the energy required to use them.

Law of Minimal Interference

The **law of minimal interference** emphasizes that whatever approach is to be used should not distract the user from an ongoing activity. If the AAC user has to think too much about how to use a device or how to retrieve vocabulary (cognitive load), there will be reduction in the efficiency in other tasks, such as work, school, and everyday communication (Lloyd & Belfiore, 1994). Any technology prescribed for an AAC user should fit into everyday functions as smoothly as possible. If using the device requires too much shift in the AAC user's thought processes or in physical movement, its effectiveness is reduced and it is not likely to be used. Related to this is the speed of the device. When too much time is required to type a message or to retrieve a prepared message, there is an artificial break in the flow of communication.

Law of Best Fit

Pursuant to the **law of best fit**, any technology prescribed for an AAC user should fit the personality and needs of the individual as much as possible. For example, for an adult female, a device that produces adult female voice output would be appropriate. Early speech synthesizers (e.g., Echo™ and Votrax™) used only male voices; consequently, females who used these synthesizers often experienced some difficulty in identifying with the output. However, newer, more sophisticated and costly speech synthesizers, such as DECtalk™, offer a variety of adult male and female, and child voice options.

For an individual with an ability to use a finger, a device with a keyboard may be a much better fit than one that requires a switch. Cosmetically, a device that looks like an attaché case when carried may be preferable to one with a more unusual design or one that is associated with disabilities. The law of best fit considers many factors, including communicative desire and interests of AAC users. It also considers the means to represent, the means to select, and the means to transmit.

Law of Practicality and Use

All of the above laws are meaningless, however, unless one considers how practical and available a device is. The **law of practicality and use** relates to all of the laws mentioned above and includes such considerations as the AAC user's environments, how the technology fits into these environments, and affordability in terms of purchase price, training, and maintenance. For example, for an individual who is highly destructive, use of a communication board that consists of symbols drawn on an oilcloth might be more practical and useful than an electronic communication device. Such a communication device can easily be taken into all environments, is inexpensive, and is relatively indestructible.

PRINCIPLES FOR USING TECHNOLOGY

The features for an ideal communication device that are applicable to AAC technology are incorporated into the following discussion of principles. References are made to the six laws on which they are based. All principles discussed consider the full range of options from low to high technology.

1. **Technology should contribute to the AAC user's full range of communication functions** (law of parsimony, law of minimal learning, and law of best fit). Although speech synthesis can be effective in summoning help from a distance, as well as facilitating the understanding of the message, many basic needs can be communicated through vocalizations, gestures, or a low technology communication board. A simple buzzer can be very effective for gaining attention. Visual displays and speech synthesis, on the other hand, do provide the user with more options for meaningful interactive communication. If the communication device interfaces with a computer, or the AAC user is using a computer, a host of electronic options is available (e.g., drawing, games, educational programming, information systems, and word processing). Whatever combination of approaches are selected, the user is encouraged to use all modes of communication to achieve the greatest flexibility in communication. A wheelchair-mounted table with communication symbols on it, for example, may be very functional in that it can be used as a communication board, food tray, and game board.

2. **Technology should be compatible with other aspects of the AAC user's life** (law of best fit). If the AAC user is mobile, the technological system should also be mobile. If the user is confined to specific positions, the communication system should be easily accessible to reduce fatigue. The system should be placed so as to encourage its use for communication and other functions, such as environmental control. Mounting a device on a wheelchair is a particularly demanding task because of the need to allow free access to a food tray and power controls, and to avoid too many controls (e.g., communication aid, environmental control, steering and speed of wheelchair). An overly outfitted wheelchair may resemble a mobile logistics command center! As impressive as such an arrangement might be, any communication technology should not interfere with other life functions. The more accessible the device and the more easily operated, the more the AAC user will be encouraged to integrate it into typical living patterns.

3. **Technology should consider the needs and communication patterns of the communication partner** (law of practicality and use, law of minimal interference, and law of best fit). The use of devices with speech synthesis, for example, allows the AAC user to communicate with individuals who are a distance away. It also allows the communication partner to be engaged in other tasks while still listening to the AAC user. Where earlier speech synthesizers were difficult to understand, current technology is quite good. There is much less guessing on the part of the communication partner. The improvement in understandability and in the ability to adjust the volume of the speech makes current high technology much more useful for interacting with strangers and speaking before groups of people. As useful as speech output is for communication, however, there is also a place for low technology options such as a communication board to convey more personal or confidential messages between the user and a partner. Having the visual backup also may be useful when the communication partner may have difficulty understanding speech.

4. **Technology should be usable in all environments and physical positions** (law of practicality and use, law of minimal interference, and law of best fit). More recent improvements in high technology communication devices have made them more portable (lighter, sleeker in design, easier to carry), more intelligible, and more easily adjusted in volume. Intelligibility and volume adjustment are critical if speech is to be understood in noisy environments, such as at the local mall or a basketball game. In addition, a communication device needs to be durable/rugged to withstand physical abuse, including exposure to sand (beach) and moisture (rain, snow, saliva). In these environments, unless a computerized communication device is constructed to be sandproof and waterproof, a low technology device such as a communication board may be a more effective option. Even though an AAC user may be able to operate a computerized communication system, eye gaze may be preferred at certain times (e.g., when fatigued or lying in bed). Multimodal communication should always be encouraged and usually will represent low technology, high technology, as well as unaided options.

5. **Technology should not restrict the topic or the scope of communication** (law of practicality and use, law of minimal learning, and law of minimal interference). Any individual with typical cognitive functioning is capable of constructing an infinite number of highly original and complex messages. Reducing available vocabulary to a set of pictures or prestored messages within a communication device or computer severely restricts the richness of communication. Ideally, a device allows the AAC user to determine the vocabulary for use and provides options so that the vocabulary can be expanded to express any idea needed in ongoing conversation. Blissymbols, TO, and text-to-speech synthesizers on communication devices, for example, allow for extensive vocabulary and generation of new ideas. However, this does not always imply the need for high technology. For example, the use of an alphabet card or board by an individual with severe dysarthria for the cueing of initial letters of words may assist a listener in understanding and help the user control the rate of interaction. A slower rate may also result in increased intelligibility.

6. **Technology should enhance the effectiveness of the AAC user's communication** (law of minimal interference, law of best fit, and law of parsimony). One advantage of the computer is its use to predict communication patterns and enhance rate. Because rate is always a major problem for AAC communication, any rate increase afforded by word prediction is helpful. Limitations still remain, however, because rate never approximates normal conversation. This is true both for the AAC user who is typing out messages and for the user who is activating a switch. Individuals using high technology devices often shift back and forth between prerecorded speech and typing out messages. The AAC user should be able to interrupt typing to ask or answer questions or make spontaneous observations. The capacity to express emotion in speech would also be desirable. All of this is desirable, of course, with minimal fatigue.

7. **Technology should allow and foster the AAC user's growth (e.g., skills in device usage and language)** (law of best fit, law of minimal interference, and law of parsimony). The device should fit the current skill levels of the AAC user so that it is rewarding to use, but it should also allow for the development of new skills (e.g., literacy) to enhance the effectiveness of communication. Inherent in the development of these skills is also the development of social, educational, and work skills to facilitate improvement in the overall quality of life.

8. **Technology should be acceptable and motivating for the user and significant others** (law of minimal interference). If the device is fun and effective in fostering communication, significant others (e.g., family, friends, co-workers) will be more likely to participate in communication and to actively encourage the use of the device. Factors such as the appearance of the device, ease of use and transport, and type and quality of output are important in the AAC user's (and family's) willingness to actively use the device in everyday living. Frequently AAC users prefer using their own speech, even if not intelligible. A combination of voice, speech, and gestures can enhance communication and increase motivation.

9. **Technology should be affordable** (law of parsimony, law of practicality and use). The cost of the device is an important variable in determining whether it will be made available to the AAC user. Although cost alone should not be the decisive factor in selecting a device, wise decisions consider a balance of cost and features in terms of an individual's needs. Although costs have come down considerably as computers and devices have been on the market, $1,500 to $7,000 still represents a great investment. Many families cannot afford such costly devices. Many insurers, schools, or other state agencies seriously question such a financial outlay due to budget constraints. The amounts cited represent the initial purchase; however, costs will also be incurred for training the AAC user to make effective use of the device and for maintenance costs, such as replacing the battery or electronic components throughout the life of the device. Finally, as the AAC user outgrows the device, or as new, more powerful devices come on the market, there will be additional costs for upgrading and/or replacement. The use of low technology that requires the ongoing use of an aide, however, can also represent considerable expense.

10. **Technology should be easily maintained and repaired** (law of practicality and use). Devices should be designed so that the user and caregivers can operate them and make simple repairs as needed. The availability of warranties is an important consideration in selecting a high technology device. Manufacturer's hotlines provide immediate access to information for solving problems in programming, simple maintenance, and repair. Often,

if repairs are needed, manufacturers will ship a loaner so that the user will have minimal downtime. Low technology devices are typically easily modified and easily replaced if necessary.

All of the above factors play a significant role in the selection and use of any communication technology. Technology is not to be applied with the expectation that it will be a miraculous solution. It is an important part of AAC and, when properly defined and integrated into the total plan for the AAC user, can increase the overall effectiveness of communication and improve quality of life.

SUMMARY

This chapter discussed the development of technology as it relates to AAC. Several factors must be considered when determining whether technological applications are appropriate for a given individual as part of the overall treatment for a communication problem. AAC may involve a combination of low technology (e.g., communication boards) and high technology (e.g., computer communication devices) approaches, selected for individual needs. A variety of scanning and encoding approaches have been discussed with a recognition of their roles both in low and high technology applications. A number of device features, 6 laws, and 10 general principles must be considered when selecting and using AAC technology. Generally, approaches that are simple, involve minimal interference with other cognitive and physical functions, and complement other aspects of the individuals' and caregivers' environments are the most appropriate. AAC systems should be motivating for the user to use, economical, and easy to learn, program, and use. In summary, the AAC system should be appropriate and meet the needs of the user.

CHAPTER 9

LOW TECHNOLOGY

CHARLOTTE A. WASSON, HELEN H. ARVIDSON, AND LYLE L. LLOYD

As noted in Chapter 3, **augmentative and alternative communication (AAC)** is frequently categorized as either aided or unaided. Unaided communication involves body movement and requires no equipment. Aided communication, on the other hand, uses some type of **assistive technology (AT)**. Although several taxonomies have been developed to distinguish between various types of assistive technologies (see Cook & Hussey, 1995), this text uses the **low technology/high technology** dichotomy discussed in Chapter 8 in which low technology and high technology communication devices are distinguished from one another due to the presence or absence of an integrated circuit (IC). Low technology communication devices are electronic or nonelectronic devices that lack an IC. The VersaScan™, a device containing a series of 16 lamps set up in circular fashion behind an overlay displaying symbols, is an electronic AAC device, but it is low technology because there is no IC. A picture or word-based communication book is an example of a nonelectronic, low technology device. Several examples of low technology AAC devices are illustrated in Figure 9.1.

Each low technology device has its own unique features. A communication necklace (Figure 9.1a), for example, promotes easy access and allows the hands to be free. Any of several types of symbols may be laminated and attached as individual entries. Similarly, a communication wallet (Figure 9.1b) can hold a variety of two-dimensional symbol options. Some AAC users who like a compact display may prefer a wallet because it can be put in a pocket instead of being worn in full view all the time. A communication board (Figure 9.1c) provides a display (e.g., letters, words, or numbers) that can be mounted on the wheelchair

tray for an individual who sits for long periods. Symbols can be displayed on a board in row-column or circular fashion that can be mounted for scanning. A communication wall chart (Figure 9.1d) allows several children in a classroom to make use of the same display. Wall charts can be put up in topic-specific areas (e.g., cooking, play, or snack). A calendar box (Figure 9.1e) displays whole or partial objects, miniature objects, or graphic symbols that represent activities scheduled across the day. Each portion of the calendar box typically represents one time segment. Upon completion of an activity, the symbol can be removed and placed in a "finished" area. A communication vest (Figure 9.1f) also allows for the display of a variety of symbol options. Vests that can be worn by both AAC users and communication partners (e.g., caregivers, paraprofessionals, or teachers) provide easy access to symbols for individuals who can direct select.

Although the demarcation between low and high technology AAC devices is distinct at the end points of the scale (e.g., a communication wallet is clearly a low technology AAC device, and a dedicated computer with high-quality speech output is clearly a high technology one), the boundaries become less discrete in the mid-range, and discerning what is high low-technology from that which is low high-technology is sometimes difficult. A tape player with a tape loop, for example, is considered low technology because the speech output is an analog recording that does not use integrated circuitry. The MemoMate™, however, is high technology because it uses a computer chip to make digital recordings. Although high technology can be a replacement for low technology (e.g., MemoMate can be used for the same purpose as a

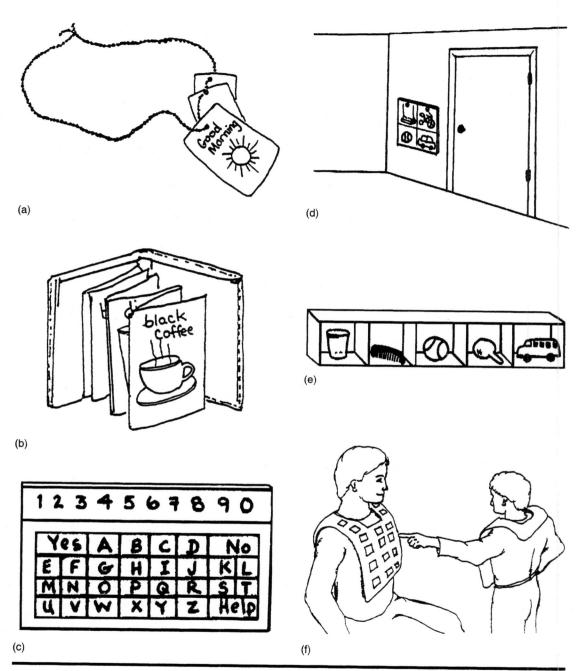

FIGURE 9.1   Low-Technology Communication Devices. (a) Communication necklace; (b) Communication wallet; (c) communication board; (d) communication wall chart; (e) calendar box; (f) communication vest.

tape loop), the advantages of low technology should not be underestimated.

Low technology applications in AAC support the development of communication systems that provide AAC users with opportunities for effective communication. Advantages and disadvantages of using low technology have been discussed by a number of authors (Blackstone 1993a, b, c; Mirenda & Mathy-Laikko, 1989; Parette, Hourcade, & VanBiervliet, 1993). These advantages and disadvantages should be considered within the larger realm of determining how a multicomponent communication system meets the functional communication needs of AAC users, because a single device will rarely, if ever, fit all needs.

One of the most obvious advantages of low technology is that it may facilitate early implementation of AAC services. Compared to high technology, start-up costs are often minimal. Once an individual's strengths and needs are known, the design and development of low technology may proceed efficiently. Low technology can be very portable, incorporating displays that can be easily customized, reorganized, and updated. Low technology devices can work well together. For example, an individual can easily use a combination of wallets, communication boards, and rotary scanning devices. Low technology can be useful to AAC users with a wide range of abilities in a wide variety of environments. It can help individuals with "gadget intolerance" make initial attempts at using AAC and lead to further development of a multimodal system.

Some of the disadvantages of low technology are that vocabulary storage may be limited and communicating abstract ideas beyond the here-and-now may be difficult. There may be heavy reliance on communication partners due to the lack of voice/print output, and AAC users may become passive communicators. The use of low technology sometimes leads communication partners to underestimate an AAC user's abilities.

COMPONENTS OF LOW TECHNOLOGY AAC DEVICES

Low technology devices have two physical components: **symbols** and **displays**. The combinations of symbols and display arrangements that are possible in low-technology AAC applications are almost endless. With innumerable possibilities, the decision-making process in selecting appropriate symbols and displays often presents serious challenges to AAC service delivery teams as do decisions regarding means of access and general strategies to facilitate maximal effectiveness and efficiency in communication.

Symbol Options

An important consideration in designing low-technology AAC is the selection of appropriate symbols. As discussed in Chapter 3, symbols may belong to a set or system. Sets include symbols, but have no specific rules for expanding the number of symbols beyond those in the original set. Systems, on the other hand, have rules and an internal logic that provide for the creation of new symbols that can be combined within a language structure. In Chapter 6, aided symbol sets and systems were classified according to physical similarity. Examples and descriptions were provided for symbols that were object-based, picture-based, representations of manual signs and gestures, alphabet-based, phonemic- or phonic-based, and arbitrary logographs and shapes. All of these types of symbols can be used with low-technology. Commercially available and custom-made low-technology symbol options are nearly limitless.

In addition to understanding how symbol sets and systems can be classified, however, clinicians/educators must have knowledge of symbol characteristics such as iconicity, complexity, perceptual distinctness, size, and degree of ambiguity so that symbols that best meet the needs of individual AAC users can be selected. Characteristics such as size and perceptual distinctness, for example, will be differentially important to individuals with and without visual impairments. Similarly, the importance of iconicity will vary depending upon an individual's ability to learn and use symbols that bear little resemblance to their referents. Appendix A-1 provides a symbol guide designed to be completed by clinicians/educators so that they can familiarize themselves with characteristics of various symbol options.

Symbol options in low-technology applications are many, but no given symbol set/system is likely to meet all the communication needs of an AAC user. Therefore, it can be advantageous to use symbols from more than one set/system (e.g., to mix photographs and Sigsymbols). Sometimes, however, no symbol will be a perfect representation of its referent and deciding to use one particular symbol over another will involve some compromise between what is wanted and what is available. Because the characteristics of symbols vary, a particular symbol or symbol type that offers one desired or necessary feature, such as high iconicity, may lack or rate poorly on another feature, such as degree of ambiguity. Decisions regarding symbol selection must be made with care and forethought. Chapter 13 discusses additional variables to be considered.

Display Options

Displays have been defined as objects onto which language is represented (Church & Glennen, 1992). Although the number and types of symbol choices for low-technology AAC applications are impressive, there are just as many options for displays. For example, low-technology displays may be large or small, portable or stationary, commercially purchased or custom made, or even electronic or nonelectronic. They may be similar in arrangement to other displays being used by the AAC user (e.g., a dedicated communication device), or unique.

Choosing how to display symbols is one more of the challenges of low-technology development. Display decisions must involve input from the AAC user and caregivers and be guided by issues of both effectiveness and efficiency (i.e., making the display work well for the AAC user with minimal time and energy expended). Several commonly used organizational strategies are discussed below. With few exceptions, most of them can be used when organizing displays such as those pictured in Figure 9.1.

Frequency of Use. When a display is organized according to frequency of use, the most frequently used symbols are placed in strategic positions,

which may be influenced by logic, visual/perceptual and motor needs, or both. When logic drives placement, symbols of high use are typically placed in the upper left corner of displays that are arranged in rows and columns to facilitate quicker access (e.g., communication boards). A left-right, top-bottom organizational system might then influence the placement of the remaining, less frequently used symbols (see Figure 8.6). Logical placement of high frequency symbols on a circular display would be where the scanning indicator begins scanning.

Displays that are organized by frequency of use in accordance to the visual-perceptual and motor needs of the AAC user will have symbols of high use placed in areas that can be most easily scanned visually and that require minimal energy to access (Koester & Levine, 1994). High use symbols are sometimes larger than other symbols on the display to facilitate access.

Taxonomic/Categoric. A frequently noted organizational system for low-technology displays, as well as for many high-technology displays, is that of taxonomy or category. In such an arrangement, symbols that have similar taxonomies or that belong to the same category (e.g., people, places, and actions) may be grouped in a similar area on the display. Such an arrangement may be effective whether few or multiple symbols are used. Many communication books and boards are arranged categorically, and the arrangement makes sense for many AAC users. It does not, however, facilitate expression of relational concepts or support syntactical development.

Syntactic. Communication displays that are organized syntactically often have a noun + verb + object organization. Such an arrangement (e.g., the Fitzgerald key) has been used to facilitate language development for individuals with hearing impairment and learning disorders for many years. When a syntactic arrangement is developed, symbols that are grouped according to their syntactic categories are often displayed on a background of the same color (e.g., nouns might be on red, verbs on green, and so forth). Syntactic arrangements (referred to as semantic-syntactic by

Blackstone) expose AAC users to the logic of generative language and afford communication partners rich modeling opportunities (Blackstone, 1993c).

Alphabetic/Numeric.   Frequently, when the letters of the alphabet are the selected symbols, arranging them in their *a* through *z* standard sequence is appropriate. Words may also be effectively arranged in alphabetical order. For some AAC users, however, a modification of the alphabet sequence facilitates effective and efficient use. These modifications might include grouping the vowels together, starting each line of a row with a vowel as illustrated here.

A B C D
E F G H
I J K L M N
O P Q R S T
U V W X Y Z

Placing the letters in the QWERTY arrangement as on a standard typewriter or computer keyboard is an option that has advantages for individuals with keyboarding experience.

If numbers are being used to code messages (e.g., "1-1" to convey "What did you say?" and "1-2" to represent "What time is it?"), the specific arrangement of the numbers on the display should be driven by the visual/perceptual, and motor skills of the user, as well as various other factors, for example, the presence of other symbols.

Schematic/Topic.   Sometimes arranging symbols in a schematic or topic manner is desirable. Such arrangements might, for example, display symbols for all items needed for a particular activity (e.g., snack time in a preschool classroom or packing for vacation) on one board. Such boards are often referred to as topic boards (Burkhart, 1993; Goossens', Crain, & Elder, 1992). Schematic displays may also show individuals participating in events (e.g., a fishing outing or graduation) or depict certain scenes (e.g., a living room or a baseball field). Although most schematic representations are not highly supportive of syntactical structures, they do offer representation, which may facilitate recall.

Partner Influence.   Blackstone (1993c) has noted that displays are sometimes organized to accommodate the needs of partners. In some instances, an upside-down or inside-out arrangement may be developed in the thought that the AAC user will quickly develop a sense of where symbols are, whereas the user's several partners may benefit from them being placed in a logical, easily viewed position. An example of such an arrangement is an ETRAN (i.e., eye transfer chart such as the one illustrated in Figure 9.2), which has the alphabet letters displayed in their correct orientation on the side facing the partner, and backward on the side facing the user. This arrangement, however, is appropriate only if the user is comfortable reading letters backwards. Another way that partners can influence displays is by their perception of most important and frequently used symbols. Additionally if a partner perceives that modeling the use of certain symbols is essential, then these symbol items may be strategically placed at the front or top of displays so the partner can access them quickly.

Personal Preference.   AAC users are as individual from each other as they are from others in society in general. When feasible, personal preferences for display arrangements should be adhered to, or at least meshed with other display choices. For example, when displays are schematically arranged and several displays are to be placed into a larger one (e.g., pages are put together in a com-

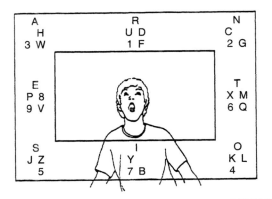

FIGURE 9.2   ETRAN Chart
From Vanderheiden and Lloyd, 1976.

munication book or folder), the AAC user should be given the choice of which pages should be at the front and which pages should be at the back.

Similarity to Other Displays.   An additional strategy for organizing a display is to replicate an arrangement that exists on a display being used in conjunction with the low technology. For example, if an individual is using a high-technology, dedicated communication device that has symbols displayed in a particular manner, a replication of that display may facilitate effective and efficient use of the low technology. A colored copy of an overlay can be made inexpensively at most copy centers. The identical size can be maintained, or the overlay can be enlarged or reduced as necessary. The low-technology display can serve as a back up for those times when the high-technology equipment might be malfunctioning, or it can serve as the display of choice when the speech and/or written output features of the dedicated device are not of benefit. Providing the AAC user with consistent displays diminishes the cognitive load required to effectively use multiple AAC systems that have varied arrangements (Goodenough-Trepagnier, 1994).

Access Options

Symbols on low-technology (and high-technology) AAC displays are selected, or *accessed*, by either **direct selection** or **scanning** (discussed in detail in Chapter 8).

Direct Selection.   If motor skills are adequate to support its use, direct selection is the preferred means of access with low-technology AAC devices because it places fewer cognitive-perceptual demands on the user than does scanning (Koester & Levine, 1994; Ratcliff, 1994). It is also faster and less ambiguous than scanning. The illustrations in Figure 9.1 are examples of low technology that can be accessed by direct selection. When direct selection is used, desired symbols are selected through a direct or assisted point, or touch. Various body parts (e.g., fingers and eyes as illustrated in Figures 9.1f and 9.2, respectively) or prosthetic devices (e.g., hand-held pointers or light beams)

can be used to accomplish these points or touches. Medical supply catalogs, as well as AAC-specific catalogs, provide an array of useful prostheses. Clear plastic, raised overlays that assist individuals in stopping directly on desired symbols may also be of benefit and may be used alone or in conjunction with prostheses.

Scanning.   When direct selection is not feasible, scanning can be used to select symbols from the low-technology communication display. Scanning is defined as "stepping through" (Church & Glennen, 1992) a set of symbols until the desired symbol is available and selected (refer back to Chapter 8 and Figures 8.2 to 8.6 for review). Low-technology, nonelectronic scanning can be accomplished via partner assistance. Here, an AAC partner highlights symbol choices in a logical and systematic manner until the AAC user produces some type of signaling response to indicate that the desired symbol (and message) has been reached. Piché and Reichle (1991) caution that care must be taken in selecting a teachable, salient, socially acceptable, and replicable signaling response.

Scanning can also be used as an access means with electronic, low technology devices. Figure 9.3 shows a rotary scanning device that turns on lights that are positioned near real objects. An in-

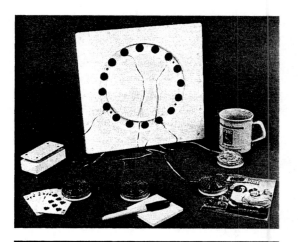

FIGURE 9.3   Rotary (Circular) Scanning Device with Rocker Switch and Remote Lights
Photo courtesy of Prentke Romich Company.

dividual makes a selection by pressing the switch when the light nearest the desired item comes on. Switches are typically used to make selections during scanning, and serve as highly effective interfaces between AAC users and their communication aids. Switches are used with both low and high technology. Because switches themselves do not have integrated circuitry, however, they are considered low technology.

Switches.

Switch Types. Numerous types of **switches** serve as interfaces between individuals and AT and/or AAC devices. A sample of commonly used switches appears in Figure 9.4. Switches can be classified in several ways. Switches that require some degree of force to be activated can be classified as pressure-sensitive switches. Specific examples include platform switches, membrane switches, leaf switches, treadle switches, cup switches, and grasp switches. Platform switches can be single or dual. The dual rocking lever (Figure 9.4a), for example, is a general-purpose dual switch. The mini rocking lever (Figure 9.4b) is also a dual switch, but smaller in size. The wobble switch (Figure 9.4c) is a single switch that can be activated by gross movements from any direction. The tongue switch (Figure 9.4d) is a dual switch that can be activated by minimal movement of the tongue, nose, chin, or finger. The joystick (Figure 9.4e) is a multiple switch that provides up, down, left, right, and diagonal control required for directed scanning. Pressure-sensitive switches vary in the amount of pressure required for activation, the amount of activation area available, and the time required to activate them.

Pneumatic switches are activated by air flow. Two examples of pneumatic switches common to AAC are sip-and-puff switches and pillow switches (Cook & Hussey, 1995). Sip-and-puff switches, which are held in the mouth during use, are controlled by the amount of air that is sucked in or puffed out (see Figure 9.4f). Sipping activates one switch, and puffing activates a second. Pillow switches are activated when air pressure is applied to the pillow or cushion housing the switch.

In addition to pressure-sensitive and pneumatic switches, several types of **piezoelectric crystal switches (P switches)**, which are activated by eye movements registered by the switches' electrodes, have been developed by various manufacturers for AAC. These can be used by individuals who lack the motor control necessary to use other types of switches.

Many individuals with multiple disabilities use switches not only to activate their AAC devices, but also to activate numerous assistive devices to gain control over their environments (Goossens' & Crain, 1992; Goossens', Crain, & Elder, 1992; Hanson & Hanline, 1985; MacNeela, 1987a, b; Schweigert & Rowland, 1992; York, Nietupski & Hamre-Nietupski, 1985).

Until recently, these individuals were frequently forced to use multiple controls (or switches) to operate their multiple pieces of assistive technology. Now, however, for many of these individuals, especially those using powered wheelchairs, integrated controls are effective. An integrated control is a single control system which allows management of several technologies. For example, by using a single sip-and-puff switch, an acquaintance of the lead author is able to operate her voice output communication aid (VOCA), wheelchair, lights, entertainment center, and computer.

Although it is certainly possible to construct switches (especially single switches), and the initial cost might be somewhat more economical than purchasing commercially available switches, many AAC professionals choose to purchase switches for the AAC users they serve. Commercially available switches tend to be more durable; better suited to an individual's cognitive, visual/perceptual, and/or motor needs; and more visually appealing. Repair and replacement costs which may be associated with homemade switches often result in them eventually being more expensive than vendor purchased switches. Commercially available switches are available from nearly every manufacturer of AAC devices, as well as from suppliers of durable medical equipment. They range in price from approximately $40 to $100. Because it is relatively simple to use various sized connectors to interface the switch with the tech-

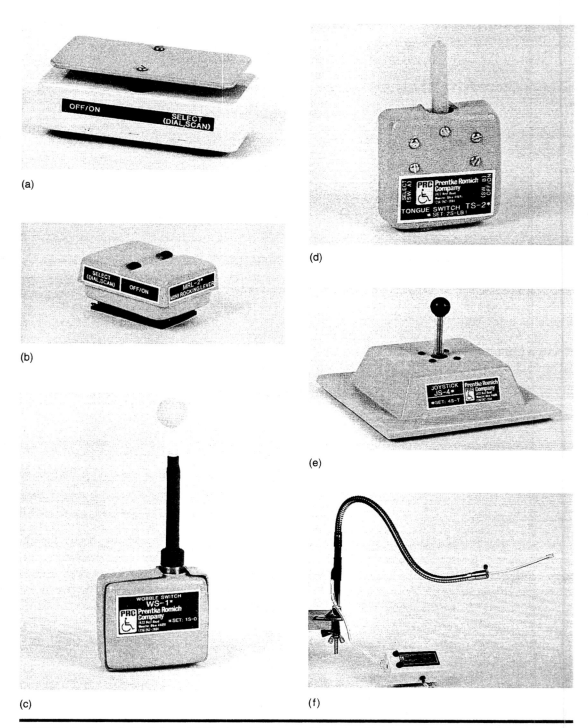

FIGURE 9.4   Sample Switches. (a) Dual rocking lever; (b) mini rocking lever; (c) wobble switch; (d) tongue switch; (e) joystick; (f) pneumatic sip-and-puff switch

Photos courtesy of Crestwood; Prentke Romich Company; and TASH, Inc.

nology it is to run, shifting from one manufacturer's switch to another's is not usually difficult.

Switch considerations. In choosing an appropriate switch several factors regarding the switch itself, as well as its intended user—usually an individual with severe motor impairment—must be simultaneously considered (Cook & Hussey, 1995; Goosens' & Crain, 1992). Of the factors associated with the switch, one of the most critical relates to its force, or the amount of energy which must be expended to bring it into action. A second factor relates to its size, in terms of two-dimensionality (length × width), and three-dimensionality (length × width × height), important considerations that relate to the motor impairments of the users. The switch's feedback (i.e., auditory, visual, tactile, kinesthetic, proprioceptive, and/or vibrotactile) requires careful consideration to promote accommodating the sensory needs of the AAC user (Goossens' & Crain, 1992). Also, the travel time, or the position the switch must move to before being activated, must be fitted to the individual user. Some of the newer pressure-sensitive switches have virtually no travel time because they require virtually no pressure, whereas some of the leaf switches have great travel time, but little activation force. A switch guide is provided in Appendix A-2.

Placement of the switch must be carefully selected. A number of control sites should be explored before determining the most advantageous one (Cook & Hussey, 1995; Goossens' & Crain, 1992). The switch should be placed to promote ease of access. The movement used to activate it should require minimal effort, be reproducible with each subsequent need, avoid promoting undesired muscle movements (e.g., asymmetrical tonic neck reflex or ATNR), and interfere minimally with ongoing activities (Goossens' & Crain, 1992; Silverman, 1995).

The Role of Play in Promoting Switch Use. Clinical judgment and emerging empirical data suggest that there is merit to providing intervention to individuals with severe, multiple disabilities that is focused on building communication within natural contexts; highlighting the physical, tactile, and affective relationships between individuals and their environments; teaching both horizontal and vertical cognitive skills within the context of naturally occurring routines; and alerting communication partners to be increasingly sensitive to often-subtle behaviors that carry communicative intent (Mirenda, Iacono, & Williams, 1990; Musselwhite & St. Louis, 1988; Siegel-Causey & Guess, 1989). For young AAC users, play may be the avenue of such intervention. Switches and switch-operated toys can facilitate such play.

Play is, after all, the business of childhood. It lays the groundwork for the emergence of more sophisticated skill development. Through play children can experience gross motor, fine motor, self-help, and social development. They can also learn important cognitive skills (e.g., object permanence and mean-ends relationships) that are closely associated with the development of language. Some children, especially those with severe, multiple disabilities, need assistance in learning to play. For many of these children, play can be taught effectively by providing switches to serve as interfaces between themselves and their toys (see Schweigert, 1989; Schweigert & Rowland, 1992).

Toys should be chosen according to their ability to fit a child's motor (whenever possible), sensory, developmental, chronological-age, and program needs. Commercially available toys may be adapted to meet all these criteria. Several adaptations that have been highlighted by Williams, Briggs, and Williams (1979) have applicability to toys. These include, for example, stabilizing the toy; enlarging or enhancing it or some of its most important features; or prosthesizing it (e.g., by adding handles to puzzle pieces, or even adding switches to run battery-operated toys). For toys to be effective tools of play, and for switches to be effective interfaces to promote play, they must be carefully selected and positioned. The switch and toy should be in close enough proximity to one another that the child realizes that activating the switch activates the toy. The play that is expected must often be demonstrated and elicited through coaxing and cueing. Once play routines have been established, a gradual shift in the play activity can lead to the addition of communication symbols.

SUMMARY

Low-technology AAC devices are those electronic and nonelectronic communication devices that do not have programmable vocabulary storage, programming capabilities, and speech and/or written output. They include devices such as communication books or boards, or simple rotary scanning devices that do not have an integrated circuit. Low technology is often introduced early to AAC users for a number of reasons. It can remain useful as a part of a multicomponent system, however, throughout the lifespan.

Because low-technology AAC devices, by their very nature, lend themselves to multiple symbol and display customization possibilities, symbol selection and organization often challenge service delivery teams. Sometimes AAC service providers choose symbols and arrange displays without AAC user involvement. Although such endeavors are probably initiated to conserve intervention time and accomplish a features-to-benefit match, this seemingly proactive stance may lead to unnecessary reactive revisions. To organize low technology effectively, service providers must study them from the viewpoint of the users, be flexible enough to periodically reorganize systems, and learn from each experience.

CHAPTER 10

HIGH TECHNOLOGY

RAYMOND W. QUIST AND LYLE L. LLOYD

In this chapter, high technology for **augmentative and alternative communication (AAC)** will be discussed in terms of (1) development of computers, (2) computer functions, (3) input devices and features, (4) output devices and features, (5) dedicated communication devices, (6) nondedicated communication devices, (7) software, (8) telecommunications, (9) environmental control, and (10) future applications. Understanding basic computer technology and operation is important for understanding high-technology applications for AAC. Today, because of the rapid integration of computers into daily living, any discussion of computers for individuals with disabilities is incomplete if it is limited to communication devices and adaptive hardware. Individuals with disabilities will increasingly be active users of computers in many aspects of their daily lives. Although many AAC devices are expensive, more economical options are now available. Reduced costs and an increase in the number of schools and third-party reimbursers paying for devices are making technology more available to individuals needing AAC.

In this chapter, some software programs and communication devices will be cited as examples, and selected software and devices will be described. However, because computer technology changes so rapidly it is a considerable task to keep current. Therefore, anyone concerned with technology for AAC users must make an effort not only to understand the terminology, features, and functions of technology, but even more importantly, understand the principles behind the use of technology. A commitment to ongoing research to expand the knowledge base regarding available technology is essential.

DEVELOPMENT OF COMPUTERS

Historically, a number of devices and events contributed to the development of today's computer, many of which are chronicled in *Understanding Computers: Computer Basics* (Time-Life, 1985), including the abacus, the Hollerith Tabulator, the Mark I, and the Electronic Numerical Integrator and Computer (ENIAC) which contained more than 17,000 vacuum tubes.

Although vacuum tubes enabled early computers to perform operations rapidly, the required number made computers extremely large and cumbersome. The heat generated within the vacuum tubes during operation frequently caused them to burn out. Because tube replacement was required often, there was considerable downtime. This problem reduced the reliability of function and increased the cost of operation.

Shockley's (1950) introduction of the first reliable juncture transistor in 1947 helped solve the problems related to vacuum tubes and led to the overall miniaturization of electronic devices needed for space exploration. This ultimately resulted in the development of the **integrated circuit (IC)** critical to the contemporary computer. One way of recognizing its significance to the development of computers is to compare the 30-ton ENIAC with the current 6.5-pound Macintosh Powerbook® (which has significantly more memory, speed, and computer power).

Although the initial development and use of computers was for military purposes (e.g., data collection and analysis, projectory tables), computers were valuable for a wide variety of operations. IBM® (International Business Machines

Corporation) became and remained a major developer and supplier of computer products for business and industry as the need for word processing and data collection, storage, retrieval, and analysis (spreadsheet, graphing, and database functions) has grown. Early use of computers, however, was limited to individuals who were highly trained in specialized business and engineering languages, such as COBOL and FORTRAN. The size and cost of the computers limited their use to businesses and organizations that could afford to buy or rent expensive equipment and pay the salaries of technicians to program and operate them.

During the mid-1970s, manufacturers began to develop computers that were smaller, less expensive, and more user friendly so that more people could use them in their everyday activities. Paul Allen and Bill Gates founded Microsoft® in 1975 and wrote a version of BASIC (Beginner's All-purpose Symbolic Instruction Code) for the Altair 8800 computer (Kinkoph, Fulton, & Oliver, 1994). Later, in contract with IBM, Allen and Gates developed MS-DOS® (Microsoft Disk Operating System), which became a standard of the industry and was the operating basis for a number of IBM-compatible computers (e.g., Epson®, Hewlett-Packard®, Radio Shack®, and Wang®) that emerged on the market. A variety of software for word processing, accounting (spreadsheet functions), and creating databases (information storage and retrieval) became readily available. Although software became more user friendly, users still needed to learn many coded commands.

In 1976, Steve Jobs and Steve Wozniak (Kinkoph et al., 1994) started a small company—Apple®—out of their garage with the idea of developing a computer that was more user friendly, less costly, and more portable. The result was the Apple computer, which was equipped with sound and color graphics. The simplicity of commands for operating Apple computers encouraged many individuals to begin using computers in their work and home activities. Whereas DOS commands required such configurations as *cd a:* (to change drives), Apple's commands relied on combining the Open Apple Key (command) with letters that stood for the functions, such as *C* for copy or *P* for print. Apple also was the first company to include

additional slots (buses) in their computer processing units to enable individuals to add more circuit boards (programmed functions).

Because buses allowed the easy connection of peripheral devices, many third-party developers were encouraged to develop adapters and add-on peripheral devices. Later, Apple developed the Macintosh®, a menu-driven computer that used a **graphic user interface (GUI)**. The user operated the computer by using a **mouse** to move a cursor to select graphic symbols representing commands, rather than typing a sequence of letters and symbols. These innovations made the Macintosh highly user friendly, and large numbers of individuals actually found the computer to be much easier to learn and fun to use. Many engineers, artists, and educators found the Macintosh to be highly compatible with their needs because the graphic interface lent itself to drawing or schematic functions. The emergence of Microsoft's Windows™ is an attempt to capitalize on the Macintosh GUI operating system's success and make computers more compatible in general.

Although IBM continued to focus primarily on business applications, Apple focused on encouraging the use of their computers in schools by offering many incentive programs. A wide variety of educational software was developed for use with the Apple computer. As a result, a large number of Apple computers are still used in educational environments today. Both IBM and Apple are to be commended for their concerted efforts to develop software and services for individuals with disabilities. IBM's Right to Read® (a software program to teach children to read) is widely regarded in educational circles. IBM and Apple have also developed information networks and resource directories for individuals with disabilities.

COMPUTER FUNCTIONS

Computers are simply devices that allow individuals to perform tasks in faster and more efficient ways. Speed and efficiency are relative dimensions clearly related to *how* an individual uses a computer. Computers do what people tell them to do and, therefore, need to be programmed in very specific ways to perform desired functions. If the information provided to the computer is insufficient or incorrect, the computer's output will be flawed. Although considerable strides are being made in artificial intelligence, where the computer "thinks" by forming associations among incoming data, individuals must always assume responsibility for what is input. Many current users are reaping minimal benefits from their computers simply because they are unaware of or too busy to learn their full capabilities.

Because computers can have enormous potential for empowering individuals with disabilities, professionals must have an understanding of their basic components and functions. Clinicians/educators have a major responsibility in assisting in the selection and programming of computer-based communication devices, and instructing in their effective use. Understanding memory, adaptive peripherals and connections, and software applications are important for effective evaluation and treatment in AAC.

The three major components of a computer are the **central processing unit (CPU)**, **input** (e.g., keyboard, mouse), and **output** (e.g., monitor, printer). These components and functions are generally discussed in this first section. Because input and output features all are significant to the operation of AAC communication devices, they are discussed in detail under separate headings.

The CPU is the "brain" of the computer that processes information. All computers have a basic circuitry made up of computer chips that provide its basic functions. These basic functions can be expanded by circuit boards (firmware) that can be inserted into slots to perform specific functions, such as providing sound output. Many, but not all, computers come with extra slots that allow expandability. IBM computers, for example, had these expansion slots housed within a closed unit, whereas the early Apple computers were designed with a cover that snapped off. It was this easy access to expansion slots that encouraged many rehabilitation professionals to design and use adaptive circuitry for individuals with disabilities.

This feature alone made Apple user friendly. As a consequence, in the early days a preponderance of adaptive firmware and **software** was designed for use with Apple computers.

Computer data are stored using **binary code**, which classifies all functions as either on (0) or off (1). The basic unit of **memory** for a computer is the **byte**, which is made up of 8 **bits** based on all possible combinations of 8 on-off switch positions. Currently, computer memory is measured in megabytes (MB) and gigabytes (GB). One MB is 1,048,576 bytes (approximately 8 million bits), the equivalent of 500 double-spaced pages of manuscript. One GB is 1,073,741,824 bytes (approximately 8 billion bits), the equivalent of 500,000 double-spaced pages of manuscript (Kinkoph et al., 1994). Memory is becoming more affordable. For example, the current cost for a 4GB internal hard drive is about $1,000.* These massive amounts of memory are becoming increasingly necessary as individuals use multimedia applications involving storage and manipulation of graphics and sound.

The internal memory of the CPU, which is programmed by the manufacturer and cannot be changed by the user, is called **read-only memory (ROM)**. There is a need, however, for a working memory within the computer that permits storage of data being used from a program and allows data to be added to it. This memory is called **random-access memory (RAM)**. Where in 1986 the IBM-compatible computers typically had 640K RAM, current computers typically have 16 MB to 32 MB RAM. The larger software programs now require RAMs of at least 32 MB, and users are being encouraged to increase their RAM. Upgrades now easily allow increases in RAM in excess of 500 MB to handle the huge memory requirements associated with multimedia programs.

Although the CPU processes information, it needs to get that information from somewhere (i.e., accept input) and, once having processed it, it needs to send it somewhere (either store it in temporary memory within the CPU or produce

---

*In the computer industry, however, the cost continues to drop as improvements occur, so it is quite possible that hard disk drives with even greater memory will be available at substantially less than $1,000 within the next few years.

output). Data (information) are kept on disks, which may be either hard disks (internal or external) or floppy disks. Floppy disks have changed dramatically over the past 10 years, both in size and type. They have changed in size from 10-inch to $3\frac{1}{2}$-inch—the standard size used in most computers today. Over the years the amount of data stored on these disks has changed from 256K (approximately 30 pages) to 1.4 MB (over 500 pages). Now, external disk drives with removable 100 MB cartridges are becoming available (e.g., Bernoulli™, Syquest™, Zip™). In addition, **compact disk read-only memory (CD-ROM)** has much greater storage capacity (typically about 600 MB) and increasingly is being used to store vast amounts of data, including graphics. For example, the entire Grollier's Encyclopedia is now available on one CD-ROM. Other CD-ROMs being marketed today include listings of over 91 million addresses and phone numbers for businesses and individuals within the United States. This technology promises to provide increased potential for the AAC user's access to and use of information, including extensive use of graphics. Recordable CD-ROM disks can now be obtained for about $20, and some recording CD-ROM drives are available for as little as $600. Because of the high memory demands of graphic information (e.g., pictures, movies), there has been a vast increase in favoring CD-ROM technology over floppy disks.

Information is transferred between the disk and the RAM of the computer via the disk drive. Disk drives may be installed as part of the CPU (hard disk) or may be external to the CPU and connected via cable. Information is stored on the disk in specific patterns (called tracks or sectors) and is retrieved by a magnetic or optical reading device, which then transmits the information to the RAM of the CPU. Because the disk is divided into well-defined sectors, the computer must be instructed in "addresses" so as to quickly locate and retrieve specific information. Computer users are increasingly storing information on the hard drive because of the convenience; however, because computer failures do occur, users are advised to back up their hard disk drive by storing on tape storage systems or external disks on a regular basis. Too many people have suffered serious data loss by failure to back up their hard drive frequently as they work. Also, because these addresses can become obscured, the hard drive should be periodically cleaned of data that can be stored on other disks or, preferably, on backup tape. Even the desktop (the display of files seen on the computer monitor) should be rebuilt every 30 days or so to ensure proper function in the organization and retrieval of data.

The speed of a computer is important, inasmuch as any time the user spends waiting is down time and can contribute to the user's frustration or loss of productivity. Anyone who has used the Apple+® or an earlier version of an IBM or IBM-compatible, such as the IBM 186™, can remember how slow these computers were (although they seemed pretty speedy at the time they were introduced). The speed in those machines has increased from 6 MHz up to 350 MHz on current computers with Pentium processors. These time differences are difficult to conceptualize, because they involve fractions of a second, but one way of appreciating them is to note that the early computers often placed messages on the screen during the processing time (e.g., "please wait, loading programs"). Today's higher speed computers literally perform the same function in a blink of an eye. As use moves toward interactive learning, speed becomes more important. Multimedia applications require rapid speeds for efficient, smooth operation because of the immense amounts of graphic and sound data being processed.

INPUT DEVICES AND FEATURES

The standard input device for all computers is the keyboard; however, other approaches include **optical input** and **speech recognition**.

Keyboards

Most personal and business computers use the capacitive (mechanical) keyboard. On these standard and extended keyboards (see Figure 10.1), a press of the key instantly completes a circuit with a soft clicking sound. Activation of these keys requires typical motor function from the computer user. A second type of keyboard, the hard contact or

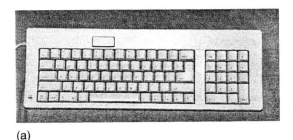

(a)

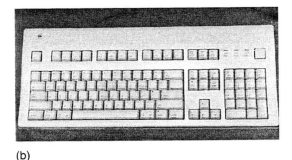

(b)

FIGURE 10.1 Types of Keyboards. (a) Standard keyboard. (b) Extended keyboard.

membrane board, is well-suited for use by individuals with disabilities who need adaptations to a standard keyboard such as modification of key size, pressure, or key activation time. Membrane keyboards protect the electronic circuitry from damage due to moisture. Because areas can be defined specifically on these keyboards, they are popular in restaurants, where the employee can bill the customer without knowing prices by pressing a key with a picture of a food item. These are frequently referred to as alternative keyboards. In a sense, they are electronic communication boards for individuals without disabilities.

Standard and Extended Keyboards. Standard and extended (sometimes referred to as enhanced) are two types of keyboards generally available for computers. The difference between the standard and extended keyboards is that the extended keyboard has additional function keys. These keyboards, patterned after the standard typewriter keyboard, are also called **QWERTY keyboards** because the letters QWERTY appear in the top left

row of keys. In 1932 the typewriter keyboard was rearranged by placing more frequently used letters in the home (middle) row of keys for the **Dvorak keyboard**. Although this keyboard is frequently used in Europe today, it never became widely used in the United States. It is available, however, for those who desire the increased efficiency afforded by this key arrangement (Kinkoph et al., 1994).

Because individuals with disabilities often cannot manipulate the keys on standard and extended keyboards, variations and adaptations have come on the market. For example, a person who has the use of only one hand can use a specially designed keyboard for single-hand use (e.g., the Bat Keyboard manufactured by Infogrip, Inc.) that has only seven keys that can input data through various combinations of keys, called chords. Keyboards are available for either right- or left-handed use. In other cases, users with motor problems may be unable to hit just one key at a time, either because of the size or proximity of the keys. A keyguard, which may be a plastic cover with holes, often is used to overcome these problems. The keyguard allows the user to use just the finger to press the key. The user cannot accidentally activate any keys by resting the hand on the guard or dragging fingers when making selections. Also, if the user has difficulty in pressing and releasing a key right away, it may repeat several times before the finger is removed. For this reason, time delays can be programmed for key action. If a user does not recognize or use letters, pictures may be appropriate. Although pictures can be pasted on top of the keys, they must be small and are thus difficult to see if the user has a visual impairment. For these individuals, a number of options other than a standard keyboard will provide access to a computer.

Keyboard Emulators. **Keyboard emulators** enable an individual to input into a computer directly without using a keyboard or altering standard application software. When keyboard emulators are used, the regular keyboard is said to be transparent because it behaves as if it does not exist. A commonly used keyboard emulator is the mouse, which enables a user to move a cursor across the monitor to selected points (e.g., words, icons) and make selections by clicking a button. The mouse was first designed in 1963 by Douglas Englebart at the Stanford Research Institute (Kinkoph et al., 1994). Later, it was used by scientists at the Palo Alto Research Center in the 1970s when they developed the GUI. During the early 1980s Microsoft added the mouse to its word processing program. Because MS-DOS was oriented toward text commands and the Macintosh was oriented toward graphics, the mouse became more closely associated with the Macintosh. Since the advent of Windows for IBM, however, the mouse has become standard fare.

The mouse plugs into an Apple Desktop Bus™ (ADB) port and provides input to the computer without interfering with keyboard functions. The user moves the cursor on the monitor's screen by moving the mouse across a plane surface. If adequate surface is not available, a trackball is useful. A **trackball** is like an upside down mouse—the user moves the ball within a stationary enclosure. Buttons on the mouse and the trackball enable the user to click on a choice once the cursor points to the desired word or icon. Trackballs have become popular with the new laptop computers because of their ease of use in a limited space. On the Macintosh Powerbook® and the Thinkpad®, the trackball is located in the lower center of the keyboard, whereas on the Gateway 2000®, it is located in a small slide-out drawer in front of the keyboard. The user who has motor problems may have difficulty accurately selecting keys on a keyboard. Also, over time the task may be fatiguing. For individuals with poor hand or finger control, trackballs may be preferable because the user can control movements with the whole hand or even part of the arm. Using a mouse or trackball to move a cursor on the monitor, however, requires good eye–hand coordination.

Many of the new personal computers (PCs) and Macintosh Powerbooks have replaced the trackball with a small sensitive square **trackpad** that can be activated by moving the finger across the surface. The touch-sensitive trackpad is also available as a plug-in accessory for both Macintosh and IBM-compatible computers. For some users, moving a finger, thumb, or knuckle across a sensitive pad may be easier than using either a mouse or a trackball.

The **joystick** is a special type of input device that is often used with fast-action computer games to control movement of an visual image, such as a car or plane, on the monitor. The joystick resembles the flight stick of an airplane. In scanning programs, it permits direct control (e.g., up, down, right, left, or diagonal). Often a pushbutton located on the side or top of the joystick allows the user to initiate the desired action. Some individuals with fine motor control difficulties may find the joystick easier to use; however, pushing the button while manipulating the joystick requires good thumb control.

One of the earliest keyboard emulators developed for individuals with disabilities was the **Adaptive Firmware Card (AFC)**, which was designed for the Apple IIe® and was marketed for Apple IIe and Apple IIGS® computers through Don Johnston Incorporated. The AFC computer card is inserted into a designated computer slot (usually #5) and attached by a cable to a small box that has two input jacks and a toggle switch. Clinicians/educators can program the AFC to adapt commands for selected software or to enable switch control for scanning and/or Morse code commands.

Ke:nx®, shown in Figure 10.2(a), is a keyboard emulator designed for the Macintosh. It is a multiple-access system that permits the user to operate standard software applications and to choose a number of different input methods, such as scanning, ASCII (American Standard Code Information Interchange), Morse code, and Access Window™ alternate keyboard and assisted keyboard. DADAEntry™ (Designing Aids for Disabled Adults) from TASH, Inc. is a keyboard emulator for IBM computers. **HeadMaster**™ (Figure 10.2b) is a keyboard (mouse) emulator that is available for Apple IIGS, Macintosh, or IBM-compatible computers. A cursor can be moved to a spot on the screen keyboard by an infrared beam controlled by head movement of the user and then activated by puffing, blowing, or sucking on a tube placed between the lips. Switch or hand activation is also possible. Madenta's Headmouse™, McIntyre's LipStick™, and Prentke Romich Company's (PRC's) JOUSE™ are other mouse emulators that provide alternate access for individuals with severe motor disabilities.

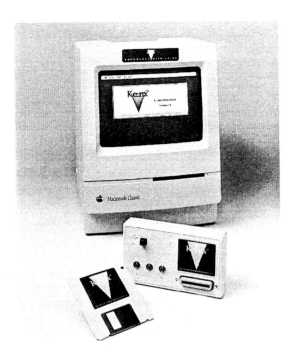

(a)

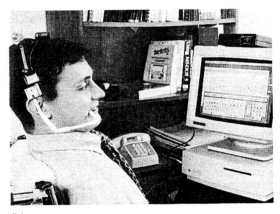

(b)

FIGURE 10.2 Keyboard Emulators. (a) Ke:nx keyboard emulator. Photo courtesy of Don Johnston, Incorporated. (b) Headmaster. Photo courtesy of Prentke Romich Company.

Expanded Keyboards. **Expanded keyboards** consist of 30 to 128 touch-sensitive membrane switches ($1'' \times 1''$) permitting reconfiguration of the keyboard so that keys can be grouped for a larger surface area. The **Unicorn Keyboard**™, one

example of an expanded keyboard, has several advantages: (1) the circuitry of the board is covered by the overlay and a sheet of clear plastic so that liquids (saliva, water) cannot damage it; (2) the board is larger than the computer keyboard, therefore accommodating the particular visual and motor needs of the AAC user; and (3) the board can be reconfigured so that pictures can be any size. If needed, the board can be configured to show only two pictures, or four pictures, and so on. The pressure and time needed to activate a square also can be programmed to the AAC user's needs. Particularly for younger children, who press the picture with the entire hand or continue to push on the symbol for several seconds, this configuration permits a functional use of the keyboard and eliminates accidental or unwanted responses. This type of keyboard is particularly useful for individuals who are unable to use a standard keyboard because of severe motor disabilities or limited cognitive functioning. Although the Unicorn Keyboard is no longer marketed by IntelliTools®, it has been described here because it is still used in many schools and clinics throughout the country.

Another alternative keyboard made by IntelliTools is the versatile IntelliKeys™ (Figure 10.3a), which connects with an Apple IIe (through the IntelliKeys IIe card), the Apple IIGS (directly through its keyboard port), the Macintosh, and the IBM computer. A major advantage of the IntelliKeys is that it can be run with any software that works with a standard keyboard and six accompanying preconfigured overlays. A setup overlay allows individual adjustment of many keyboard options, such as repeat rate and sensitivity. Software allows the user to create custom overlays. Some overlays are configured to work with MarbleSoft's Early Learning Series®. The availability of these preconfigured overlays makes this alternative keyboard very user friendly. TASH produces the Win King Keyboard™ (Figure 10.3b), an expanded keyboard that measures approximately $1' \times 2'$ and has large $1\frac{1}{4}''$ keys.

Mini Keyboards. Although expanded keyboards allow for a larger surface area, **mini keyboards** such as the Mac Mini Keyboard™ and the Win Mini Keyboard™ (Figure 10.3c) are much smaller

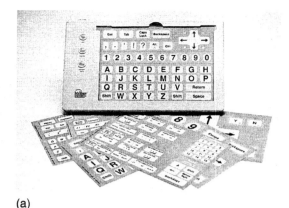

(a)

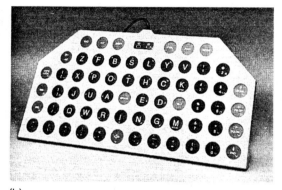

(b)

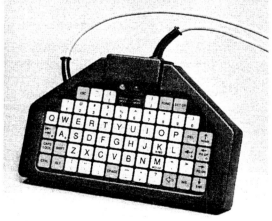

(c)

FIGURE 10.3 Alternative keyboards. (a) IntelliKeys. Photo courtesy of IntelliTools. (b) Win King Keyboard. Photo courtesy of TASH, Inc. (c) Win Mini Keyboard. Photo courtesy of TASH, Inc.

to accommodate individuals with limitations in range of motion. These keyboards may have 60 to 128 ($\frac{1}{2}'' \times \frac{1}{2}''$) membrane keys (switches) that can be reconfigured to specified surface areas. Individuals with limited range of motion in hand/arm or in head/neck movement (using a head/mouth stick) benefit from mini keyboards. TASH markets an IBM-compatible mini keyboard that measures about $4\frac{1}{2}'' \times 7\frac{1}{2}''$.

Keyboards also can be reconfigured to relocate keys to positions more appropriate to the needs of an individual with disabilities. Some individuals can use a standard keyboard if important functions are placed in a specific area they can easily access (e.g., the upper right quadrant of the keyboard). The AFC and Ke:nx, for example, are two of many keyboard emulators that allow designated keys to be programmed to perform specified command functions tailored to the capabilities of the user.

Touch Screens, Touch Pads, and Graphic Tablets.
The **touch screen** has been a popular input mode, particularly for use with children to encourage interaction with games and stories. For many young children, touching a screen is a more natural response than pressing specific keys. Children with finger dexterity problems may find pressing a spot on a screen with several fingers, a fist, or the palm of the hand much easier. The touch screen is actually comprised of three layers: a top mylar sheet with a transparent undercoating of metal, a second layer of a gel in which very tiny plastic balls are immersed, and a third layer of a glass with a metal coating on the surface. Under all three layers is a liquid crystal display (LCD) screen. As the finger or pen touches/moves across the surface of the top layer, the gel balls separate to allow the two metal coatings to touch, lowering electrical current. The computer notes the spot touched and turns on the corresponding **pixels** (dots) so that the user can see an image. Apple's Newton® represents an updated version of the touch screen/pad, which allows an individual to write or draw a schematic. These patterns are then read by the computer and transformed into digital data for computer filing. In many cases, these touch pads are also referred to as **graphic tablets**. Some resources for alternative keyboards are listed in Appendix C-1.

Optical Input

The two major approaches to optical input for operating computer devices are **optical character recognition (OCR)** devices (optical scanners) and light beam/light sensor devices. Optical scanners are used routinely with computers for digital picture reproduction. They are also routinely used with speech output for individuals with visual impairments. Another type of light scanner reads bar codes to input information into the computer (e.g., the bar code scanners typically used at the checkout counter in grocery and department stores). Light beams/light sensors provide an access means for individuals with disabilities to control their communication device and will be discussed in the section under communication devices.

Optical scanners are devices that permit pictures or text to be copied and stored digitally by a computer. Once converted into digital form, the data are generally displayed on the monitor so that the user can edit or print the image. Two types of scanners are generally used, a hand-held scanner and a flatbed scanner. Although the hand-held scanner is convenient and less costly, it often does not yield as clear an image due to surface movement irregularities during the scanning process. Material placed on a flatbed scanner, on the other hand, is fixed in position and can be uniformly scanned without irregularity; consequently, the image is much better. In either case, however, an art print program such as Adobe™ may be useful to touch up the image before filing or storing. Demasco, Mineo, Gray, and Bender (1994) have demonstrated the use of scanners for the computer customization of graphic symbols. An advantage is the capability of the computer to control variations in black and white or color in the representation of an object. Appendix C-1 lists a number of resources for OCR devices.

Speech Recognition

For some time people have considered the possibilities of controlling computers through the use of speech. This process is often referred to as either voice recognition or speech recognition. In this chapter, the term *speech recognition* will be used

because the computer is usually analyzing the speech spectrum in order to interpret the command.

The development and refinement of speech recognition techniques have moved individuals closer to operating computers with speech input rather than the more traditional inputs of the keyboard and mouse. Speech recognition involves the storage of speech data in digital form in the computer. When a speaker says a command (e.g., "open," "save"), the speech pattern is compared with the stored sample and, if they match, the computer initiates the command. Because no speaker repeats any word or command identically, the computer must first be trained by the speaker to recognize variations in the individual's speech patterns. The computer then learns to recognize and respond to an utterance despite slight differences. Such significant strides have been made in speech recognition software that it is now possible to obtain word processing software that can be operated by spoken commands. At one time such software was limited to specific patterns of a single speaker who had trained the computer, but now new software is designed so that the computer can quickly learn the pattern of new speakers. DragonDictate® is an excellent example of a functional speech recognition system integrated with word processing. Although considerable progress has been made, a great deal of practical research still needs to be done. The day individuals can truly converse with computers, however, may not be too far away.

Speech recognition is most useful for individuals who can speak but have motor limitations that hinder their operation of the computer, and it is much faster than using scanning techniques. A limited number of studies have explored speech recognition applications with individuals who have dysarthria (e.g., Raghavendra et al., 1994). Because the computer is taught to recognize unique speech patterns, distinctive dysarthric speech patterns can be input and the computer can be trained to respond to them. Although speech recognition offers exciting possibilities for helping dysarthric speakers with accompanying severe motor disabilities use computers in everyday activities, inconsistency in production remains a problem.

Some speech recognition systems are included in Appendix C-1.

OUTPUT DEVICES AND FEATURES

Output devices are essential components for ongoing access to the information being processed by the computer in a form that the user can modify according to needs. Output can be in the form of visual (monitors, printouts), acoustic (voice or other sound effects), and tactile (vibration) output for individuals who are unable to process either auditory or visual information (e.g., individuals who are deaf-blind).

Monitors

A computer monitor, a **cathode-ray tube (CRT)**, is a video display device that permits the user to observe input on an ongoing basis. Early computer monitors were monochrome (black and white) or other color combinations (e.g., amber or green) and had very low **resolution**. Today, most computer monitors are color. The vast majority of laptop computers, however, allow for color screens to be changed to monochrome through the computer's control panel. An advantage of using the monochrome option is that there is less drain on the battery. Other types of monitors include **light-emitting diode (LED)** and **liquid crystal display (LCD)**, both of which are used in portable/notebook computers. Earlier portables used a supertwist screen, which was limited in the extent to which it could be adjusted under varying light conditions. Most portable/notebook computers today have LCD monitors with back lighting.

Color monitors dominate the market today and are available for anywhere from $300 to several thousand dollars. Cost is related to the resolution, the number of pixels that can be displayed on the screen. Early color monitors were RGB (red, green, blue). The three main color monitors in use today include the CGA (color graphics adapter), EGA (enhanced graphics adapter), and VGA (video graphics adapter). CGA, developed in the early 1980s, has a resolution of 320×200 dpi (dots per inch) and can represent four colors. A later version, EGA, was able to display 16 colors

with a resolution of 640×360 dpi. Today's standard for color monitors, however, is the VGA. Three VGA monitors are commonly available that have resolutions of 640×480 dpi and higher. Color is a matter of preference, but for professional quality productions, high resolution is essential.

Printers

Printers provide a permanent display of the AAC user's communication efforts and are particularly critical for meaningful participation in educational and work environments. Users have a choice among dot matrix, daisywheel, thermal, and strip printers. More recently, because laser and inkjet printers have become more economical, they are more commonly used by computer users. Generally, printers are considered either impact printers or nonimpact printers.

Impact printers actually involve contact of the printhead directly with the paper. Two types of impact printers are the **dot-matrix printer** and **daisywheel printer**, which are becoming obsolete but are still used in businesses and schools because they are relatively inexpensive.

Nonimpact printers involve no physical contact of the printhead with the paper. Types of nonimpact printers are thermal, inkjet, and laser. **Thermal printers**, which were commonly used before laser printers became widely available, involved heat-sensitive paper that accepted a liquid ink spray.

Laser technology, initially very expensive, has become much more affordable today. The **laser printer** uses a laser to transform an image onto a drum that has been electrically charged. As the drum turns, dried ink is rubbed off onto paper and then permanently affixed by heat. **Inkjet printers**, on the other hand, involve drawing characters by spraying ink through a fine nozzle. Another version of the inkjet printer is the **bubble-jet printer** for personal use, which is typically a small, portable unit marketed for use with notebook printers. The bubble-jet printer involves the formation of "bubbles" of ink that burst from nozzles to spray dots on paper. Because these dots are very close together, the images are clear, although generally not as distinct as those produced by laser printers. Because inkjet and bubble-jet printers are generally available for less than $300, they are inexpensive options for personal use, particularly when portability is needed. Many of the portable devices (e.g., the Canon® bubble-jet printer, Apple Stylewriter®) can operate on batteries. Their size, light weight, easy portability, economical cost, and print quality make them viable options for the mobile AAC user. Certainly the quality of print is much better and is preferred for those with visual problems. Because these printers run much more quietly than dot matrix printers, they are less distracting when used in the classroom.

Speech Output

Speech output can be recorded (analog, digital) or synthesized (text-to-speech, phonetic or diphonic).

Speech Recordings. **Analog** and **digital** are the two major types of speech and music recordings today. Many are familiar with analog recordings (standard tape recorders and cassette tapes), which involve the arrangement of electromagnetic particles on tape that represent the entire pattern of sound waves. Digital recordings, on the other hand, represent sampled segments of sound waves that have been stored in binary code in the computer. Figure 10.4 illustrates an analog wave and digital sampling. Because the computer is programmed with information on the relationships among wave features (e.g., wavelength, maximum displacement), it is able to take the limited, stored information and faithfully reconstruct the sound waves. The result is **digitized speech** which has a superior sound that is free from distortion. Another advantage of digital recording is that it requires much less storage space than an analog recording. For example, a sampling rate of 11,000 bits per second (bps) would result in an understandable but low-quality speech, whereas most people's ears can detect the dramatic improvement when the sampling rate is increased to 22,000 bps. The superiority of this type of recording has influenced the recording industry so that, today, compact discs are rapidly replacing traditional tape recordings. In the context of this text, analog

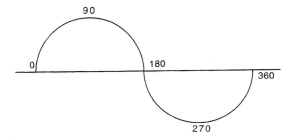

(a) Analog Wave

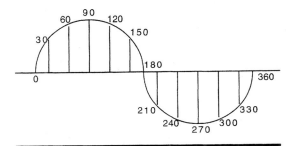

(b) Digital Sampling

FIGURE 10.4 Recording Samples. (a) Analog wave. (b) Digital sampling.

recordings are considered part of low technology and digital recordings are considered part of high technology. The use of the microchip in a number of devices such as the AlphaTalker™ (Figure 10.5a), MemoMate, and Parrot™ (Figure 10.6a) replaces tape loop technology. The integrated circuitry of the microchip provides higher memory capacity and allows the devices to be much smaller. Communication devices such as the AlphaTalker and Parrot have the added feature of miniature keyboard or switch access that allows selection of recorded messages. In the old tape loops, the listener had to listen to the entire loop in the recorded sequence. With the addition of devices that use CD-ROMS (such as the Pegasus™ [Figure 10.7a] and Pegasus Lite™), however, an almost unlimited number of auditory options has become available to AAC users.

The AlphaTalker (which replaces the IntroTalker™), Macaw™ (Figure 10.6b), and WalkerTalker™ (Figure 10.5b) are examples of low-cost

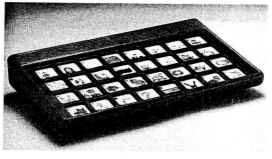

(a)

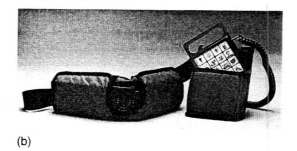

(b)

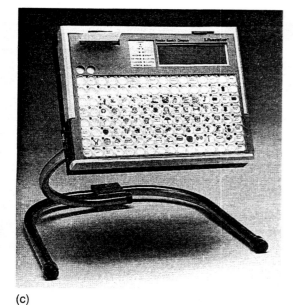

(c)

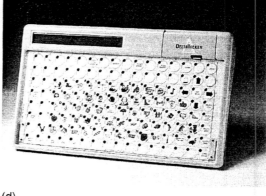

(d)

FIGURE 10.5 Prentke Romich Communication Devices. (a) AlphaTalker. (b) WalkerTalker. (c) Liberator. (d) DeltaTalker.

Photos courtesy of Prentke Romich Co.

voice output communication aids (VOCAs) that use digitized recorded speech. An advantage is the ease with which natural speech of familiar people can be recorded in designated areas on the VOCA and recalled by the AAC user. The devices allow recording at two different rates. The advantage of the slower rate is that more total speech can be stored so as to provide a more extensive, available vocabulary for the user. The downside of this, however, is that the available speech is of lesser quality and may at times be more difficult to understand.

Speech Synthesis. The Voder (Voice Operated Demonstrator), an early device that produced synthesized speech, was first demonstrated at the World's Fair in 1939 and 1940 (Borden & Harris, 1984). Colleagues at Bell Telephone Laboratories and Haskins Laboratory (Ralph Potter, Franklin Cooper, Alvin Liberman, and Pierre DeLattre) worked together to extend these principles to develop a speech perception and pattern playback system. Potter's sound spectrograph filtered and converted speech sounds into electrical energy that would, in turn, be represented by a visual display. These scientists reasoned that, if visual pictures of speech could be created, then tracings could be drawn and converted into electrical energy that could be transformed into speech. The direct, practical results of their success with these devices was the improvement of the telephone. The

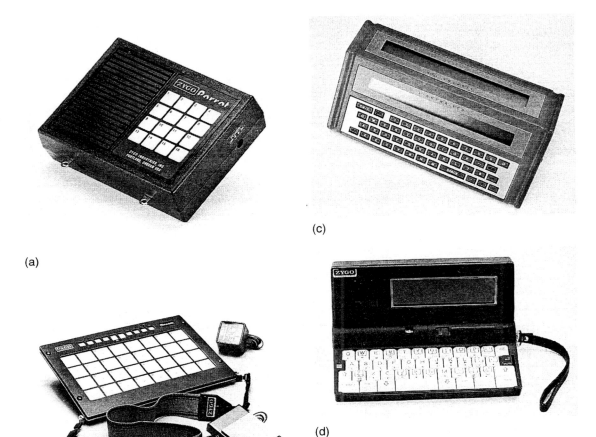

(a)

(b)

(c)

(d)

FIGURE 10.6   Zygo Communication Devices. (a) Parrot. (b) Macaw. (c) LightWRITER. (d) Polycom. Photos courtesy of Zygo Industries, Inc.

tremendous knowledge gained about the characteristics of sound and the increased understanding of the principles allowing the creation of speech through the design and application of electrical circuitry, however, clearly contributed to the development of today's speech output devices.

The quality and intelligibility of today's speech synthesizers is much improved over the primitive Voder. Improving speech synthesizers was a very expensive process; consequently, it was most available to the government and industry. However, during the early 1980s, Echo™ and Votrax™ were marketed for AAC users at a reasonable price ($100 to $500). Some of these devices were used first in talking toys, such as Texas Instru-

ments' Touch 'n Tell™. These speech synthesizers were very robotic due to limited inflection (pitch variation), somewhat choppy (due to lack of phoneme transition), and of generally poor intelligibility. But because of their low cost, these speech synthesizers were more accessible to most potential users and changed the lives of many individuals with disabilities.

Text-to-speech synthesis (Edwards, 1991) permits much greater flexibility in the use of a VOCA, because it allows the user to type words on a keyboard for conversion to speech. In text-to-speech synthesis, the computer program applies the rules for combining 44 phonemes to make intelligible speech. One of the problems, however, is

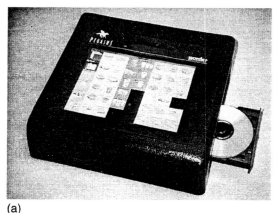

(a)

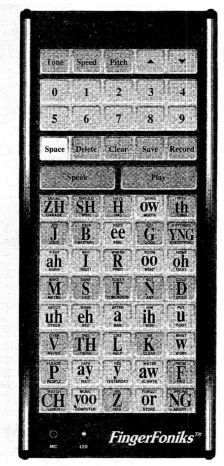

(b)

FIGURE 10.7 Words+ Communication Devices. (a) Pegasus. (b) FingerFoniks.

Photos courtesy of Words+, Inc.

that speech is an ongoing, continuous process in which phonemes are modified as they are combined. Early speech synthesizers did not consider, for example, the variations produced when phonemes combine in a process called coarticulation (e.g., when /p/ + /l/ combine, such as in the word *please*). The Echo did not handle these phoneme combinations; however, the clinician/educator could spell the word phonetically to accommodate the program's unique characteristics. Many of the newer VOCAs allow programmers to do this. Some include a procedure for storing the correct pronunciation of the word for correct auditory playback while retaining the correct spelling on the visual display. RealVoice™ includes storage and playback of diphones (phoneme pairs, blends) in accordance with phonological rules. The result is fairly natural, but somewhat choppy speech. Figure 10.8 shows the MultiVoice™ connected to a laptop computer. Features such as quality, rate, and pitch play a significant role in user/listener preference and can be significant factors in choosing a communication device. Another useful feature to consider is the extent to which a voice or speech pattern can be customized. Appendix C-2 lists resources for speech synthesizers.

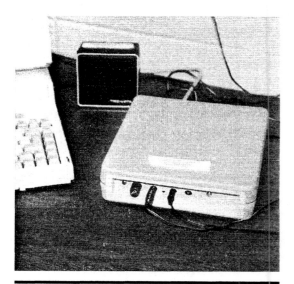

FIGURE 10.8 MultiVoice

Photo courtesy of Institute of Applied Technology, Boston Children's Hospital.

DEDICATED COMMUNICATION DEVICES

This section provides an overview of communication devices/programs specifically for use with individuals who have little or no functional speech. The fact that some devices/programs but not others are discussed should not be construed as selective endorsement. At the end of this chapter, some resource directories are mentioned to provide more complete information on device features, availability, and cost.

A communication device may consist of a computer operating with communication software or it may be a standalone device. In many cases, the keyboard of a communication device may interface with a computer keyboard (via a special cable or infrared or radio waves) to allow computer operation. A device made specifically for communication is called a **dedicated communication device**, because it is primarily limited to communication functions, although it may interface with a computer and perform limited environmental control functions. Computer communication systems are typically not dedicated devices, because communication is just one of many software functions that can be performed. In the past, the lack of portability of computers limited their use as communication devices, because they required users to remain in one place. Computers were fine in the workplace, but not very practical for everyday living situations. In the past, dedicated communication devices generally could be used only for communication and did not allow a user to perform other computer functions independently; consequently, they were more likely to be funded by third-party providers. As both traditionally dedicated devices and computers have evolved, the distinction between them is becoming blurred. Computers may become more readily funded in the future, however, for the following reasons: (1) technology laws are mandating their provision if needed for education or rehabilitation; (2) government-funded programs are placing an emphasis on making technology available for individuals with disabilities; and (3) providers are becoming more aware that a person with little or no functional speech has a need for an array of computer functions to have true access to education, employment, and recreational activities.

Prior to the availability of computers, mechanical or electronic scanning devices similar to the Dial Scan™, VersaScan™ (see Figure 9.3), and Zygo 16™ were workable and reliable for AAC users (see Chapter 9). These early low-technology scanning devices, however, were slow and limited the extent to which the AAC user could communicate (e.g., vocabulary, syntax, spontaneity). The increased availability of desktop and laptop computers provided a means for increasing the vocabulary available to AAC users, enabling them to access and/or create complex sentences for enhanced expression of ideas. In the early days, because computers were not portable and were difficult to mount with other equipment on an AAC user's wheelchair, they were used primarily in fixed workstations. This confined the AAC user to a given location. Workstations were functional for individuals who remained in a given position for long periods (e.g., lying in a hospital bed or working at a desk); but not for individuals who used wheelchairs or were independently mobile; therefore, the need for a truly portable communication device remained.

In solving the portability problem, developers designed devices that were similar to computers but were limited to specific tasks such as storage and retrieval of data (e.g., messages), word processing, speech output, and in some cases, printing. Because these devices were designed to perform highly specific functions (e.g., communication), they were said to be dedicated. Because they did not perform other functions associated with computers (e.g., word processing, database, spreadsheet), they could be made smaller and self-contained (i.e., not requiring disk drives and separate monitors). Improved technology also enabled these devices to run for considerable periods of time on relatively small and lightweight batteries.

Dedicated communication devices are like computers because they have integrated circuitry and installed software performs input, processing, storage, and output functions. They are unlike computers, however, because they are designed primarily for the function of communication. Specific communication software applications are installed in the device, and the user cannot insert program disks for other functions. In some cases, however, if a computer is configured so that its only function is communication (e.g., Lingraphica®), it becomes a dedicated communication device. Also, in some dedicated communication devices, the user can remove certain communication program chips and install others. Dedicated communication devices often are outfitted with computer-compatible keyboards, such as Prentke Romich's TouchTalker™, LightTalker™, Liberator™ (Figure 10.5c), DeltaTalker™ (Figure 10.5d), and Zygo's LightWRITER™ (Figure 10.6c), and can be used to operate computers through interfaces (cables) or infrared/radio frequencies.*

The AlphaTalker, introduced by Prentke Romich in 1993, represents an advanced design of the IntroTalker, a relatively inexpensive dedicated communication device that enjoyed considerable success from 1990 to 1993. The AlphaTalker is lightweight (under 3 pounds) and is capable of digitally recording up to 3 minutes of highly intelligible speech. The programmer can extend recorded speech to $5\frac{1}{4}$ minutes by pressing a button that results in a slower sampling rate and subsequent reduction in the quality of the speech. This time allows the storage and retrieval of between 100 and 200 words/phrases coded in Minspeak™. The keyboard of the AlphaTalker can be configured for 4, 8, or 32 locations. It can be accessed with optional devices such as optical headpointers and scanning switches. Like its much more expensive counterpart, the Liberator, the AlphaTalker uses **icon prediction**. Through a memory transfer interface (MTI), stored vocabulary can be transferred back and forth between the AlphaTalker and a computer. The AlphaTalker is also able to perform some computer functions (e.g., up to 32 commands can be sent to either an IBM or Macintosh).

The WalkerTalker is a highly portable communication device designed for use by ambulatory individuals with good motor control who either temporarily or permanently have little or no functional speech. It weighs 2 pounds and can be carried on a waist belt. The keyboard can be stored in a belt-held pouch, resembling a money pouch used by travelers. When needed, the keyboard (which has tiny keys) can be easily removed and used for generating digitized speech. The device permits storage and retrieval of 2 to 8 minutes of intelligible speech (approximately 60 to 400 words or phrases coded in Minspeak). The keyboard has a 16-location configuration. The WalkerTalker uses an MTI to allow computer storage of the programmed vocabulary.

The Lingraphica, earlier developed on a Macintosh portable computer, has been modified to work with the Macintosh Powerbook. Because the older Macintosh portable was unwieldy, this change represents a significant step toward making Lingraphica a viable communication option for the mobile user. This communication program is specifically designed for individuals with severe aphasia. The program makes use of icons arranged hierarchically to allow users to systematically search for and find words/phrases. For example, if a user wants to express a desire for an apple, the first selection might be from a group of icons representing objects, then foods, then fruits, and finally apple. Auditory feedback is provided, so each selection serves as a cue for the desired item.

Innocomp's Say-It-All™, shown in Figure 10.9(a), weighs $2\frac{1}{4}$ pounds and allows storage and retrieval of up to 846 user-definable phrases that can be combined with text-to-speech. A window permits a limited 2-line display of words for menu or speech choices. Its membrane keyboard consists of 58 squares that allow the use of up to 9 overlays. The Scan-It-All™ version (Figure 10.9b) has 96 1-inch squares with LED lights in all four corners to permit either direct selection or scanning. The squares can be reconfigured into larger squares. Phrases can be stored by scanning input, directly selecting input using the light pointer, attaching the included keyboard to a serial port of the Scan-It-All and typing the phrases, or using Voc-

---

*Although the TouchTalker and LightTalker are no longer sold—they have been replaced by the DeltaTalker—like several other communication devices, they are still described in this chapter because a number of them remain in active use. Clinicians/educators should be familiar with these devices.

Load software with an IBM or IBM-compatible computer. Say-It-Simply Plus™ (Figure 10.9c) is a touch pad that can be configured as one 12-inch × 12-inch active area, 4 squares, 9 squares, 16 squares, 36 squares, or 144 squares. It weighs $4\frac{1}{5}$ pounds and allows the programming of up to 762 user-definable phrases using 28 message levels. All three of these Innocomp devices can be used as transmitters for environmental control. All standard models use Clarity™ speech, which uses the Belgian Phillips Electronics PCF 8200 chip to produce either male or female voices in 10 different pitches. More recent Innocomp Gold models include DECtalk with the choice of child, adult male or female, and customized voices. Rate and volume of speech can be adjusted to the user's preference.

The VoiceMate4™, ScanMate4™, and ScanMate8™ (Figure 10.10) are small, lightweight devices that permit limited digital storage of phrases. The VoiceMate4 allows four phrases of up to 4 seconds each, and the ScanMate8 allows eight phrases of up to 4 seconds each. The SwitchMate4™ (not pictured) permits either direct selection or the use of one to four single switches.

Mardis Orac™ is a portable communication device (made in England) with a membrane board that can be configured in 2, 4, 8, 16, 32, 64, or 128 squares. It provides access through either direct selection or a scanning LED matrix for switch use. A variety of overlays can be used including letters, words, or other symbols. High-quality text-to-speech and digital speech (DECtalk™) is available in nine voices (four male, four female, and one child) in any dialect or language.

The BlissProcessor™ was developed cooperatively among the Blissymbols Communication Institute (BCI) in Canada, The Netherlands Bureau of the Handicapped, and the VOF Company and has received intensive field testing in institutions throughout Belgium and the Netherlands. Using a Bliss text program, a communication partner and user can select Blissymbols (or modify with a drawing program) to configure an electronic board that can be accessed either directly or through switches. Selections can be displayed on a computer screen, printed, or spoken (digitized or synthesized) in Dutch, English, German, or other selected languages.

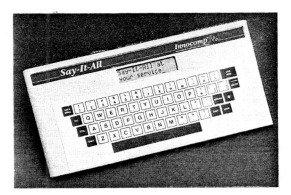

(a)

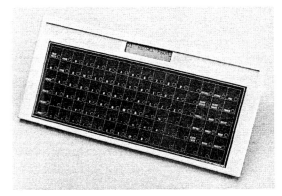

(b)

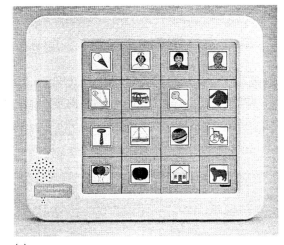

(c)

FIGURE 10.9 Innocomp Communication Devices. (a) Say-It-All. (b) Scan-It-All. (c) Say-It-Simply Plus. Photos courtesy of Innocomp.

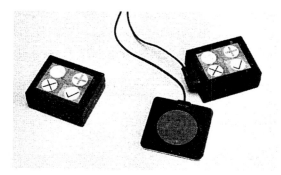

(a)

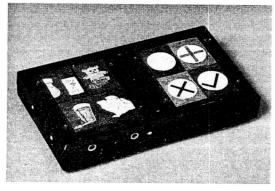

(b)

FIGURE 10.10 TASH Communication Devices.
(a) VoiceMate4 (left) and ScanMate4 (right).
(b) ScanMate8.
Photos courtesy of TASH, Inc.

Zygo has two models of the Macaw, which offer a range of functions from two enlarged keys to multilevel keys (up to eight levels) and key-linked messages. This design allows messages to be programmed according to eight categories (much like having access to eight communication boards). Messages recorded in different cells can be retrieved so they can be linked together in varying sequences. One model offers direct selection and the second offers both direct selection and scanning (including auditory scanning, manual linear step and directed scanning, automatic linear scanning, block-row-column scanning, row-column scanning, and multiswitch directed scanning). The standard membrane keyboard allows 32 active areas and can be modified for a variety

of configurations. Speech can be digitally recorded at two sampling rates (i.e., 16 Kbits and 32 Kbits), which allows 64 seconds of high-quality speech or 128 seconds of lower quality, but intelligible speech. The lightweight (2.7 pounds) and relatively small size ($8\frac{1}{2}'' \times 11''$) affords excellent portability.

Zygo's LightWRITERs SL 5 and 35 (see Figure 10.6c) are lightweight, flexible communication devices, both of which are unique in that they have two LCD displays, one facing the user and the other facing the communication partner. This arrangement facilitates the user's self-monitoring of the input. It also makes it easier for the communication partner to read the message while directly facing the user throughout the conversation. It can actually speed up communication because the partner can read the message as it is being typed and can frequently guess the message before completion. Either a rubber keyboard or a graphic (membrane) keyboard is available to fit the user's preference, and letters can be arranged in either a QWERTY or regular alphabetical order. The LightWRITER SL5 is a simple version allowing primarily visual display, whereas the LightWRITER SL35 provides options for text-to-speech synthesis, such as Articulate™, Eurotalk™, and DECtalk, which features choices from male and female adult voices, or a child's voice, as well as languages other than English. Other advantages of this device include 32K memory, text prompting, and its eight-function built-in calculator.

The Polycom™ (see Figure 10.6d) is another small communication device that has menu-driven programs containing 29 phrases that can be accessed with two keystrokes. It includes abbreviation expansion, text telephone for hearing impaired individuals, and a serial port for a printer. Synthesized speech is available in a variety of languages.

A much smaller, inexpensive, and functional communication device marketed by Zygo is the Parrot™ (see Figure 10.6a), which is a digital recorder-playback unit that allows storage and retrieval of up to 16 brief messages (32 seconds, 32KHz sampling rate). Its small size and weight ($5\frac{1}{4}'' \times 4'' \times 1\frac{1}{2}''$, 13 ounces) makes it highly portable and easy to use. Other small, functional

Zygo devices include the QED Scribe™ (a hand-held communication device with keys that can be activated with a finger or pointer, a 24-character visual display, and a memory of 26 messages) and the Secretary™ (which is similar to the QED Scribe, but with added features of 32 to 64 seconds of recorded speech and the capability of 52 memos of 256 characters each). Both devices also have a built-in printer that uses calculator-type paper. Words+ FingerFoniks™ (Figure 10.7b) uses both digitized and synthesized speech. Synthesized words and sentences can be produced by pressing keys representing phonemes.

DynaVox™, and DynaVox 2™ (Figure 10.11a), use a **dynamic display** that allows the user to change symbols (e.g., pictures, letters, words) whenever desired by touching the screen, thus eliminating the need for manually changing overlays. An added advantage is the capability to create and change both basic displays and subdisplays (that is, those displays that represent a subcategory of one of the symbols represented in the main display). DynaCards™, memory cartridges about the size of a credit card, insert directly into the device and can be customized to the specific needs of the user, eliminating the need to download from a computer. DynaCards include both symbol-based and alphabet dynamic display applications with abbreviation expansion, word prediction, and sentence templates, allowing progression from symbol-based communication to traditional orthography (TO). The basic system consists of 1,000 symbols (based on Faith Carlson's DynaSyms™) and can be expanded up to 1 million characters. The system is highly flexible for reconfiguring communication board arrangements and features high-quality voices by DECtalk. Another excellent feature of the DynaVox devices is the use of animation with graphic images to represent action or descriptive words. The DynaVox 2 is 4.5 pounds lighter than the original DynaVox and is thus more portable. The addition of color in DynaVox 2c adds both clarity and interest for the user. Sentient Systems Technology has recently come out with the DynaMyte™ that has all of the features of the earlier devices but at half the weight. It also makes the DigiVox™ (Figure 10.11b).

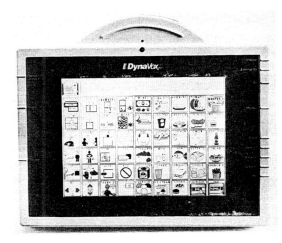

(a)

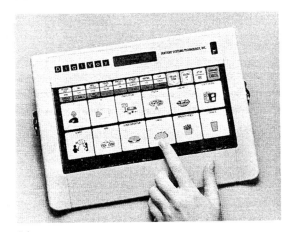

(b)

FIGURE 10.11 Sentient Systems Communication Devices. (a) DynaVox 2. (b) DigiVox.
Photos courtesy of Sentient Systems Technology.

The Pegasus™, by Words+ is a compact, self-contained communication device that includes a CD-ROM drive, built-in multivoice (DECtalk), and a built-in TouchWindow™. It contains Talking Screen™ for Windows, uses thousands of quality color symbols, and allows recording and playback of hours of sound. The Pegasus Lite™ is a smaller, lighter device that offers many of the basic features at substantially less cost.

DAC™ (Digital Augmentative Communicator) is a communication device that digitally records and plays back human speech, ranging from 2,000 to 8,000 words (18 to 72 minutes) and allows up to four levels of programming. Programming can be done with single pictures or picture sequences. An additional feature permits text-to-speech capabilities combined with the recorded human voice, spelling, or **abbreviation expansion**. A row of 16 function keys along the top enables the user to adjust volume and programming level. The remaining 128 keys can be reconfigured into a variety of key sizes and arrangements. The built-in 3½-inch disk drive provides a way to make quick copies of programs and transfer them from one DAC to another.

As these brief descriptions show, a high-technology communication device is essentially a communication board with the added capability of storing multiple messages for each symbol and outputting them in auditory and/or visual form. General principles for constructing low-technology communication boards apply equally to high-technology communication devices. Inexpensive communication devices operate much like a communication board and have the same limitations in vocabulary and flexibility when shifting topics. The advantage is the availability of voice output. Many of the more expensive communication devices, however, have increased flexibility because of the capability to store lengthy messages for retrieval at different levels and grouping words by category or theme. Because of these features, the AAC user has available a much more extensive vocabulary across communicative situations.

Input for Communication Devices

Keyboards. Communication aids have either standard keys or a membrane board with identified activation areas (squares or cells that may be modified in size according to the needs of the AAC user). One simple communication device is the Canon Communicator™, which has a keyboard consisting of letters, numbers, and arrow keys that allow users to edit messages and make mathematical calculations with printed output on a narrow strip of paper tape. Its light weight and small size make it a highly portable, convenient means of communication. A built-in guard over the keys

provides some support for individuals who may otherwise accidentally activate keys due to poor finger dexterity. For individuals with severe finger dexterity or visual impairments, however, the size of the keyboard may be problematic. The Canon Communicator comes in two models, one without speech and one that features recorded speech of up to 240 seconds. Currently, 26 keys allow the storage of up to 7,000 characters. The speech version allows both speech and printout on a narrow strip of tape, whereas the nonspeech version outputs only printed tape. Symbol overlays can be placed over the keys. Scanning is also possible with a single switch. Other small keyboards (under 6 inches) come with dedicated devices such as the Parrot (Figure 10.6a). The small size and light weight (under 1 pound) make such devices extremely portable. The Wolf™ (Figure 10.12) is another example of a lightweight, extremely portable communication device.

Some examples of medium-sized keyboards (8 to 14 inches wide) are found on LightWRITER SL-5, Macaw, Polycom, Say-It-All, VoisShapes™ (see Figure 8.8), VOIS 160™, and the Wolf. Large keyboards (over 14 inches and 10 pounds) come with such devices as Say-It-Simply Plus, and Steeper Communicator Teaching Aid™.

The Vocaid™ is a relatively inexpensive communication device that has a membrane board with a detachable plastic guard. It comes with

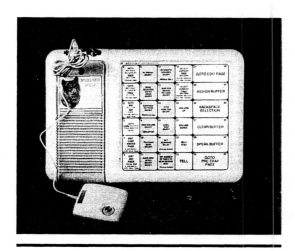

FIGURE 10.12 Wolf
Photo courtesy of ADAMLAB.

three overlays, each programmed for 16 words or short phrases that cannot be modified. The Vocaid uses an Echo speech synthesizer and is housed in the same casing as Mattel's Touch 'n Tell™. Some other relatively inexpensive but durable communication devices that use a membrane keyboard are the AlphaTalker and the Macaw. In each of these devices, the activation cells on the membrane board can be reconfigured to provide larger areas for picture display and to give the AAC user more surface area to touch (e.g., fist, palm of hand, or several fingers instead of just a finger).

ADAM LAB's Whisper Wolf™ and AIPS Wolf™ resemble the Vocaid (they are also housed in a Touch 'n Tell case), but they have more flexibility as communication devices. These devices come with a customized, preprogrammed vocabulary and have additional space available for user/teacher programming. Each of several overlays has 36 activation cells. The Whisper Wolf adds row-column and sequential scanning capability (single switch selection and auditory scanning that allows quiet playback of the selected message so the sender can hear it prior to playing for the receiver). The AIPS Wolf provides additional capability for scanning with up to nine switches. Each Wolf provides two options for synthesized speech. The Hawk™ is similar to the Wolf, but it is smaller (under 3 pounds and with only a 9-square touch panel). It records and plays back up to 5 seconds of speech for each activation area (a total of 45 seconds of speech and approximately 90 words).

ACS EvalPAC™, which is still in use in many places, includes a customized Epson HX-20™ laptop computer housed in a small, plastic attaché case and has a keyboard with 61 keys plus special menu keys that provide access to a number of functions (e.g., stored vocabulary, scanning). The flip-up portion of the case consists of rows of lights over which overlays can be placed. The AAC user can select symbols using a light pointer, either in direct or scanning mode. An attachable speech synthesizer (RealVoice™) adds speech capability to the device. Messages are stored using letter codes so they can be retrieved with a minimal number of keystrokes. The LightTalker and DeltaTalker are single units with membrane boards that have 128 1-inch squares with letters/symbols and light-emitting diodes that

can be activated by a light pointer. Other devices with membrane keyboards are Say-It-All Plus and Say-It-Simply Plus (Innocomp), VOIS 160 and VoisShapes (Phonic Ear), AlphaTalker and IntroTalker (Prentke Romich), and Macaw (Zygo). Standard keyboards are prone to the buildup of dust in recesses between the keys and have the potential for liquids to seep through and cause damage. With membrane boards, the circuitry is totally protected by the membrane; consequently, damage due to dust buildup and spilled liquids is minimal. Another major advantage of the membrane keyboard is the ease with which active areas can be reconfigured to the response capabilities of AAC users. Devices such as the TouchTalker typically allow 128 squares to be reconfigured into 2, 4, 8, 16, 32, and 64 active squares. This allows for the use of symbols of varying size to accommodate both the visual needs of the user and the motor needs as, for example, when the user needs to respond with the whole hand instead of a finger. Many of the keyboards for the devices listed may be accessed directly with a finger or headstick, LED sensor (LightTalker), or Lightpointer™ (LightTalker and EvalPAC). The AlphaTalker, Liberator, and DeltaTalker each makes use of icon prediction, a special technique that involves the emission of light beams only at the cells that are programmed. An advantage of this is that it cues the user to active cells holding the message and reduces the number of cells to consider in the recall of messages.

Many of the dedicated communication devices can be accessed through single or multiple switches adjustable for different types of activation. Switches for Special Friend™, for example, can be set for momentary switch action. The Zygo 100™ allows both momentary sustained switch and momentary step switch action. Combinations of all these switch actions are found in LightTalker, Macaw, and EvalPAC. The Scan Wolf™ uses only sequential scanning, whereas the LightTalker uses sequential group-item scanning. Directed, sequential, and group-item scanning are all available on the Macaw and RealVoice.

Scanning can be done in three modes—auditory, visual, and Morse code—all of which are available on the Whisper Wolf, DynaVox, and Talking Screen. Visual scanning is an available

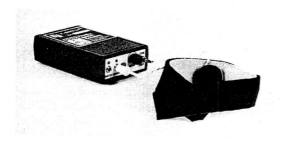

FIGURE 10.13   P Switch
Photo courtesy of Prentke Romich Co.

mode for the DeltaTalker, Macaw, LightWRITER, LightTalker, EvalPAC, and Scan Wolf. Morse code is used with RealVoice.

Scan Wolf, and Special Friend are accessible with one switch, whereas either single or multiple switches can be used with AIPS Wolf, LightTalker, Macaw SC, EvalPAC, Steeper Communicator Teaching Aid, and Zygo. Some specialized switches include the P switch (Figure 10.13) and Words+ IST™ (infrared, sound, and touch) switch. Programs working with switch configurations include Scanning WSKE II™, Say It™, and Screenkeys™. For more information on switches, see Chapter 9.

Optical Input.   A number of communication devices are operated through optical input, such as a light beam or infrared beam. The process is either a light-beam sensor for switch activation or optical scanning for OCR. Currently, most dedicated communication devices use switch activation (e.g., EvalPAC, LightTalker), but some use OCR (e.g., Tiger Communication's Magic Wand Keyboard™). A light pointer, which can be hand operated or fastened to the head, is typically used to activate a light sensor located on the input board (keyboard). The EvalPAC uses this approach. The procedure can also be reversed, having lights appear on the display area that can be sensed by a device worn by the user. The AlphaTalker, Delta-Talker, and LightTalker use this approach. In this case, the lights appear on the display (keyboard) one at a time in a sequence (e.g., left to right, top to bottom), and an individual light is made brighter (and the command activated) when the sensor is pointed at it. Because the sensor must be directed at the light on the display for a designated

period to activate it, there is less chance of unintentionally executing a command. Although users can see the light beam emitted with the light pointer, they cannot see any light beam with the head sensor; therefore, they must depend on the feedback provided by increased illumination of the selected light on the display. The Pegasus operates with a built-in ultrasonic head pointer.

Tiger Communication's Magic Wand contains pictures with bar codes that can be scanned to provide speech output with an Echo speech synthesizer. Picture storybooks also include bar codes, so the user can "read" stories using the scanning pen. Individual use can be cumbersome, however, and the pen must be moved across the bar code at a specified angle to be successful. This may be difficult for users who have problems with motor control.

VisionKey™ is a communication device that uses eye-tracking with a low-level illumination from an infrared LED reflected from the eye. This illumination is sensed by a photodetector. The 2-ounce eyepiece is mounted on a standard frame so that one eye sees a row-column keychart at what appears to be normal reading distance. The electronically determined focal point of the eye resembles a green flashlight. Because the chart has 49 keys, the user has access to a full-functioning keyboard. Selections are made through combinations of glances (quick looks) and gazes (over $\frac{1}{2}$ second). This system can be used with either a PC or Macintosh.

Output for Communication Devices

Visual Displays.   LEDs are used in a variety of communication devices. The LightTalker, Touch-Talker, DeltaTalker, and LightWRITER, have single-line displays. QED Scribe, EvalPAC, Say-It-All, Special Friend, and VOIS 160 have two- to nine-line displays. Most of these displays are visible only to the AAC user and may be difficult to read from other angles. The LightWRITER, however, uses two displays.

Speech Output.   Communication devices may use recorded analog, recorded digitized, or synthesized speech. Inexpensive devices using analog taped speech are adequate for immediate playback or playback of longer passages, but they do not have the efficient retrieval capabilities of other communication devices. Lower-priced devices, such as the AlphaTalker, Macaw, MessageMate™, and Parrot, use recorded digitized speech. Because digital recordings require considerable memory, these devices typically accommodate smaller vocabularies. Synthesized speech, on the other hand, requires significantly less memory and is included in such devices as DeltaTalker, LightTalker, LightWRITER, Polycom, RealVoice, Say-It-All Plus, Say-It-Simply Plus, Wolf, ScanWolf, Special Friend (D&S), Tiger Jr.™, and TouchTalker. VOIS 160 uses a speech synthesizer and allows programming of up to 14,000 words. SmoothTalker, a modestly priced speech synthesizer, is standard on such devices as the TouchTalker. For an additional cost, however, DECtalk can be installed to provide high-quality speech. The user can choose from a variety of different voices (e.g., child, adult male or female, and customized voices). Another high-quality speech synthesizer that uses DECtalk housed in an external device is the MultiVoice, which is marketed by Voice+. Speak It/Write™ also features a choice of a male, female, or child's voice.

Printers. Communication devices may have internal printers or they may be interfaced with computer printers. The Canon Communicator has a narrow strip of tape. Internal printers with calculator-sized paper are in such devices as the EvalPAC, LightWRITER, and the Liberator. Because the keyboards of the EvalPAC, TouchTalker, LightTalker, and the Liberator are full-function devices, the AAC user can access a computer through the serial port and use a number of word processing programs. Any type of computer printer can be used (e.g., dot matrix, daisywheel, thermal, inkjet, or laser).

Because dedicated communication devices are manufactured to be carried by the AAC user from one location to the other, they tend to be more rugged or durable than nondedicated devices based on computers. Typically dedicated devices are self-contained and housed within a rugged plastic casing to withstand bumping or dropping. Also, sealed cases and membrane boards protect the integrated circuitry within from fluids or debris (water, saliva, sand). For these reasons, dedicated communication devices are functional choices for young children and individuals who are active in a variety of environments. Appendix C-3 includes a listing of a number of assistive communication devices. Communication devices based on computers, on the other hand, may be more susceptible to damage or malfunction due to more sophisticated circuitry and less durable construction. Because of the greater memory and the capability of integrating communication functions with a wide variety of computer applications (e.g., word processing, database, graphics), computer-based systems are highly functional for older users who move from educational to work to recreational settings.

NONDEDICATED COMMUNICATION DEVICES

This section gives an overview of selected computer-based communication devices/systems currently on the market. Virtually all involve computer software programs that have been designed specifically for individuals with little or no functional speech. The major advantage is that the users have ongoing access to both communication and computer functions. Although these are software programs, because of their targeted purpose, they are discussed within the framework of communication devices. Later in this section a wide variety of software is discussed and some representative resources are provided for each category.

As indicated, a computer is not limited in functions. Communication is simply one of many jobs the computer performs for the user. The advantage for AAC users is the versatility; they are able to perform a number of work functions (database, spreadsheets, statistical calculations) and switch back and forth between these and communicating with peers. Early laptop computers, although they were lighter and more mobile than desktop computers, were neither lightweight nor small enough to provide true portability. They added convenience, however, in that they were small enough to fit with other mounted devices on a wheelchair. Individuals who had motor impairments found them too heavy to manage when they walked or tried to set them up (even with help from a caregiver) at a site (such as work or school). Earlier speech synthesizers and speaker systems often were attached to the computer through cables, which resulted in additional bulk and inconvenience. The advent of the notebook computer, because of its light weight (about 4 to 7 pounds) and smaller dimensions ($8\frac{1}{2}$ inches × 11 inches), has greatly expanded communication possibilities for AAC users. These computers have much greater memory, can handle speech synthesis, are easily carried, and require minimal effort to set up. An additional benefit is that most of these computers are more acceptable to AAC users because they appear "normal" (e.g., the notebook computer has come to be associated with status because busy executives often use them on airplanes to maximize productive use of time). Among popular notebook computers used today are the Macintosh Powerbook, IBM's Thinkpad, Gateway 2000, and Toshiba®.

A great deal of software has been developed for use with a computer to provide communication systems. As mentioned earlier, a major advantage of this approach is that, in addition to communication and environmental control, the user has available a full array of computer functions. Software updates also allow the user to take advantage of new developments.

Words+ is a major producer of computer software designed specifically for communication and adaptive computer access. A hallmark feature of its system is lifetime upgrades of software. Its comprehensive System 2000/Versa™ includes software combined with the NEC UltraLite Versa™ notebook computer with an option of a built-in touch screen. This device integrates all the noncomputer elements into a single unit that combines the advantages of a dedicated device with the power and versatility of the computer. The system comes with 4 MB RAM (expandable to 16 MB) and provides a choice of 120 or 250 MB internal hard disk drive. This system not only provides dynamic display of pictographic symbols (allowing user manipulation of the symbols and progression across categories and to subcategories), but also accommodates multimedia productions (sound and

video). A wide variety of input options (e.g., switch, joystick, mouse, touch screen) are possible. Words+ AAC software Equalizer™, EZ Keys™, Morse Code Equalizer™, Morse Code WSKE™, Scanning WSKE 11™, and Talking Screen can be used with any IBM-compatible computer.

Talking Screen is a pictographic, communication software program for Windows (IBM's graphic user interface). Because it is a dynamic graphic display system, the user can configure the display as desired (e.g., rearrange pictures, modify symbols, change background color, and create pages with single or multiple symbols). This software allows AAC users to import Picture Communication Symbols™ (PCS) and symbols from clip art and symbol collections. CD-ROM libraries also allow users to import photo-quality images and preprogram pages. Other features allow users to enlarge symbols and play video segments. Auditory scanning is also available, as well as magnified visual scanning. High-quality speech is available from text-to-speech synthesis (Vocalite™ and MultiVoice both include male, female, and child voices by DECtalk) and by digitally recording any speaker's voice.

Speaking Dynamically™ is a communication software program marketed by Mayer-Johnson for use with the Macintosh Powerbook. It is designed to work together with another software program, Boardmaker™, which enables the user to construct communication boards using vocabulary from the Mayer-Johnson library of PCS. The communication board can be constructed in a variety of configurations, and speech can be added for any symbol. In addition, the program comes with preconstructed communication boards with speech. The user, therefore, can copy any parts of an existing communication board (including speech) to a board that is being designed, thus saving the user considerable time. The dynamic display allows the user to move from page to page sequentially to facilitate natural conversation. The synthesized speech output of the Powerbook (MacinTalk™) is easily understood; however, the recording capabilities of the Powerbook also allows users to attach any voice to a symbol. Speaking Dynamically will also work with such speech synthesizers as Multitalk™ and Infovox™. A variety of access methods may be used to select the symbols. See Appendixes B-1 and B-2 for a sample listing of developers/distributors and software respectively. See Appendix C-3 for a list of representative assistive communication devices.

SOFTWARE

Although the software programs just discussed were developed specifically for individuals with little or no functional speech, adaptations for access, built-in speech synthesizers, and computer graphics make it possible for a great deal of the software available for the general public to be modified to accommodate the needs of individuals with disabilities. AAC users, for example, can make use of programs for word processing, databases, and spreadsheets used by the general public. This may afford greater employability. They can also use generally available software for educational purposes independently or in structured situations. Clinicians/educators use many of these programs to assist AAC users to develop specific skills in communication. Some clinicians/educators use programming software, for example, to develop interactive lessons.

Authoring/Multimedia

Currently, a number of authoring programs enable a person to create software packages (e.g., interactive training packages and animated stories). At one time, creating individual software was a formidable task because it required programming skills. HyperCard® is an economical, multipurpose authoring program that is essentially an electronic index card file. It is a particularly powerful and highly flexible program because it can be used in a wide variety of ways (e.g., database, flashcards, animated stories, multimedia presentations, and interactive learning programs). A person can create defined areas on each card that link one card to another, allowing the user to click the mouse when the cursor is on the defined area to move between cards. This method can be used for controlling external devices, such as slide projectors and VCRs. HyperTalk®, the programming language for HyperCard, is user friendly. Another program

similar to HyperCard that has extended capabilities and more vivid color is Supercard®. Both of these programs work with Macintosh.

Two relatively easy programs similar to HyperCard, but designed for the Apple IIGS, are HyperScreen 2.0® and HyperStudio®. Both of these software programs allow users to design self-booting and self-instructional lessons on the Apple IIGS and Macintosh. The programs include capability for sound, graphics, and video. As with HyperCard, the user can also control external devices such as VCRs. The great flexibility and relative ease of programming makes these programs highly useful clinical and educational tools. IBM Linkway Live™ and IBM Linkway V2.01™ are two similar multimedia authoring programs for IBM-compatible computers.

Programs incorporating graphics, sound (speech and music), and video require vast amounts of memory. For this reason, CD-ROM is essential if one is going to do a great deal of computer-based multimedia instruction. For sophisticated multimedia programs, authoring software such as Macromedia Director®, Authorware®, and the upper-end Linkway is suggested. These programs are more expensive, but they have extensive editing capabilities that yield highly professional results without the extremely high cost of movie studio productions. Representative authoring/multimedia programs are listed in Appendix C-4.

Word Prediction and Expanded Abbreviation

One of the major difficulties for AAC users is the slow rate of communication. A number of software programs have been developed to enhance rate through word prediction and abbreviation expansion. Word prediction is a technique for inputting words while minimizing the total number of keystrokes. Normally, the AAC user would have to hit nine keys to spell the word *important*. If, however, the user is presented a menu of five numbered, possible words on typing *imp* (e.g., *important, importance, imported, importing, imports*), the number of keystrokes can be reduced to a total of four when the user types the number of the desired word. Predictions can also be based on word sequences. For example, if the user types the phrase "I went to," the computer program might present a menu with the five choices *a, an, many, some, the*, which represent highly probable grammatic sequences. This can result in a significant savings in time over the course of typing a sentence. Obviously, a greater amount of time is saved when larger words are supplied (e.g., fewer keystrokes are needed). When small words are supplied, the user may do just as well typing the word especially if the user is a good speller and can type reasonably well. In addition to increasing the comfort of the listener who would generally spend less time waiting for the completion of the message, word prediction allows the user to expend less energy and experience less fatigue. When long-term or uninterrupted activity is demanded (e.g., on the job), these are important considerations. Word prediction techniques are valuable approaches not only for speeding up communication; they can help the user improve both spelling and writing skills as well (Newell et al., 1992).

Abbreviation expansion, which includes various encoding techniques, is discussed in Chapter 8. Many software programs allow users to create macros so that a single keystroke will initiate a series of commands or complete the spelling of entire words or phrases. Often these approaches are combined with word prediction techniques in the same software. Abbreviation expansion, unlike word prediction, requires memory skill on the part of the user. Some rate enhancement software programs are listed in Appendix C-5.

Braille and Text Enlargement

Braille and text enlargement are two means by which individuals with visual impairments are able to use computers. Although text enlargement is available simply by using larger monitors or by using enlargement devices that can be attached to the computer screen, the extent of such enlargement is fixed. Because visual acuity may vary at different times of the day and according to level of fatigue, programs that will provide more flexibility in degree of magnification are generally more desirable. The best degree of magnification is provided through a combination of hardware and software (e.g., using closed-circuit television in combination with soft-

ware). This combined approach is more expensive. Inexpensive options include software programs designed for managing image size.

At the simplest level, most general-purpose software for word processing, database, and spreadsheet use allows for adjustment of font size. Special software, however, is available that will allow considerable flexibility in adjusting image size and in moving the cursor around the screen. CloseView®, a software program for the Macintosh, allows both text and graphic enlargement. It also provides a means for the user to scroll around the screen. Another program that is compatible with the Macintosh is InLarge®. However, such increased enlargement may cause the user to lose orientation. Some other programs (e.g., Vista™) provide designated areas on the screen (windows) to help the user determine location. Many software programs that are designed for individuals with visual impairments include Braille output capabilities as well as text enlargement. Some of these total software programs are included in Appendix C-6.

Keyboard Emulation and Adapted Access

Earlier in this chapter, several keyboard emulator programs were discussed. A great deal of the software allows the user to adjust key functions (e.g., sequences, combinations) to accommodate specific needs. Because many functions require activating combinations of keys simultaneously (e.g., capital letters require the user to press and hold the shift key and then the letter key), individuals using a stick or single finger are restricted in their use of the keyboard. Software, such as Easy Access®, adapts key action so that the user can accomplish these sequences either by slowing down activation time so that keys can be hit separately, or by programming macros (one key is programmed so that it commands a specified sequence of key hits).

The mouse and trackball are convenient alternatives for many individuals whose motor difficulties preclude the use of a keyboard. Through an on-screen image of the keyboard and selection of commands and keys by a mouse-driven cursor, many individuals can operate a variety of standard software programs. These types of keyboard emulators are referred to as virtual keyboards by Cook and Hussey (1995). Some examples of adapted access and keyboard emulator programs are listed in Appendix C-7.

Scanning and Switch Use

In Chapter 8 as well as earlier in this chapter, different scanning approaches were discussed in relation to specific communication devices. Because the ability to scan requires good visual perception and tracking skills coupled with sufficient visual-motor coordination, a number of software programs are marketed to train these skills. Also, many arcade games can provide an enjoyable means for learning these important skills. Appendix C-7 lists several programs that provide access by switches or scanning and can be used to train scanning and switch use.

Cause and Effect

Cause and effect refers to an individual's ability to see a relationship between two events (e.g., pressing a switch causes an image to appear on a computer monitor). In AAC, a child must be able to see these relationships to develop the ability to use computers for language and communication. A number of software programs are designed to teach cause and effect. A Cause & Effect Public Domain Package (Technology for Language and Learning) consists of eight programs that can be used with the Apple IIe or IIGS and the AFC. Cause 'n Effect (MarbleSoft) involves four activities that the student can initiate, change, or stop by pressing a key. This program also is used with Apple IIe and IIGS and is compatible with Echo, Cricket™, Touch Window, IntelliKeys, and single switch input. Another DOS-based cause and effect program (Judy Lynn Software) is designed to produce either a sound or a graphic whenever the child presses a switch. Appendix C-7 includes a sample of some programs for training cause and effect.

Motor Training

Once an individual has learned the relationship between pressing a switch and an action on the computer (appearance of a sound or graphic), the individual must then learn switch control. A number of motor training games are available for this purpose. Don Johnston Incorporated markets a collection of 14 motor training games that use single switch input for developing skills that can be transferred to use Ke:nx or the AFC with single switch configurations. Computers to Help People also makes a 14-game motor training program to develop switch control skills. Both of these programs require an Apple IIe or Apple IIGS. A third motor training series (CLASS Adaptive Technologies) that also teaches single switch action requires HyperCard 2.0 for the Macintosh. AFC Setups for Sharon's Program trains the use of multiple switches. Another program containing 13 games is Early and Advanced Switch Games; it can be used with Macintosh and IBM-compatible computers. This program is available through shareware (software available without cost or for a minimal voluntary fee). Because shareware is frequently made available on bulletin boards of computer networks, it is often called public domain software. Appendix C-7 lists examples of programs for motor training.

Customizing Communication Boards/Overlays

Typically, clinicians/educators have constructed communication boards by selecting and using pictures from a dictionary of symbols, such as PCS, PICSYMS™, or from catalogs and magazines. Cutting, arranging, and pasting symbols on a communication board is time consuming. The development of software programs that can select, arrange, and print specified configurations has been a significant, practical advancement in AAC. IntelliTool's Unicorn Overlay Express™ (Apple IIe and IIGS), Mayer-Johnson's Boardmaker (Macintosh), and Ke:nx are all examples of programs that enable an individual to design and construct a custom overlay for a communication board. These programs allow the user to select the number and size of squares and to print in black and white or color. Boardmaker International™ (Macintosh or PC Windows) is a version of the Boardmaker that can use the same symbols with printed words in one's choice of 10 languages. Used in conjunction with the program Speaking Dynamically or Talking Screen, Boardmaker allows users to instantly create and redesign communication boards with auditory output. Several software programs have been developed, including AccessBliss™, a HyperCard stack that contains all the approved Blissymbols and is distributed by BCI. The user can select any Blissymbol and copy it to the clipboard for use in word processing or drawing programs. Prentke Romich's Therapy Material BUILLDer is a software program that allows users to make overlays, flashcards, and stickers with the Unity icons in several sizes. A number of programs for constructing communication boards/overlays are listed in Appendix C-8.

Literacy

There is a growing interest in approaches for developing literacy in individuals who have little or no functional speech. Although software has been developed to foster literacy skills in children with reading/language problems, a great deal of it is applicable for all children learning to read. Generally, literacy software can be categorized as story experience software, reading readiness software, vocabulary development software, and Cloze software. These categorizations are artificial, however, because many features may be found in each of them. For example, all four types of software really involve an overlap in components of emergent literacy and skill development. For a more in-depth discussion of literacy and principles of software use, see Chapter 23.

Story Experience Software. Story experience software allows nonreaders to interact with a computer while "reading" a story. Many of these stories are now on CD-ROM and have excellent graphics and voice output. They usually appeal to children who already have some interest in reading books, but are not yet independent. The Living Book Series™ (Brøderbund) are interactive stories on CD-ROM for either the Macintosh or IBM computers. Reading Magic Library™ (Tom Snyder Productions) is a problem-solving program that

encourages both child and parent to share stories on a computer highlighted with graphics. The series includes branching, which allows users to select story directions. This software is designed for either IBM or Macintosh and includes such stories as Peter Pan™ and Jack and the Beanstalk™. Follow the Reader™, a Disney product that is IBM-compatible, is a delightful talking reading sequel to Mickey's ABC™ in which children can create sentences and stories and have them read aloud or printed. The open-ended nature of these stories enables the child to choose where Mickey goes by selecting from options provided. The software, which requires Sound Blaster 16™, has excellent sound and speech.

Reading Readiness Software. Reading readiness software teaches specific skills needed for reading (e.g., matching pictures to words, identifying words that rhyme, knowing the alphabet, and differentiating uppercase and lowercase letters). The Reader Rabbit™ software programs (Learning Company) have been used for several years to develop and improve reading skills in children. Reader Rabbit II™ is an updated, extended version. Each of four games (e.g., crystal word mine, a vowel pond, a match patch, and a wacky barnyard dance) focuses on teaching specific language skills. Reader Rabbit Ready for Letters™ has exploratory activities to teach letter discrimination. Reader Rabbit's Interactive Journey™ also teaches basic letter-recognition skills through a variety of scenes and activities. There are over 100 skill-building activities. On CD-ROM, it contains 540 interactive electronic reading books and uses 3,000 lifelike speech and sound effects. The Muppet Word Book™ teaches letter discrimination, initial consonants, and word endings using large text and colorful graphics. It also contains a mini word processing program to allow children to practice spelling names. Bailey's Book House™ (Edmark) also helps develop reading skills by teaching letters, sounds, and basic vocabulary. In addition, this program allows children to compose their own stories and print both greeting cards and personalized storybooks. Both of these software programs can be used with either IBM or Macintosh.

Vocabulary Development Software. Vocabulary development software focuses primarily on teaching vocabulary. Laureate Learning Words and Concepts I, II, and III™ teach sets of 50 nouns in different ways (e.g., vocabulary, categorization, word identification by function, and word association). Word Attack 3™ (Davidson & Associates) includes four vocabulary-building activities for 675 words and has an editor to allow the user to add words. Word Attack 3 is available for Macintosh, IBM, and Atari™ computers. BlissLiteracy™ is, in essence, a vocabulary development program that teaches elements of Blissymbols and how they are combined to form new words.

Cloze Software. Cloze software is intended to increase children's awareness of the relationships of letters to words and words to sentences by presenting text with letters or words missing. M-ss-ng L-nks: Young People's Literature™ (Wings for Learning/Sunburst) is a good example of this software. Text is derived from young people's literature where letters and words have been purposely deleted. There are 500 different puzzles at nine different levels of difficulty. In the Apple version, the teacher can make up versions for practice. A/V Concepts makes two programs that use cloze techniques to teach reading comprehension skills: CLOZE Thinking™ and CLOZE Vocabulary and More™. Similar programs include Cloze-Plus™ and Clozemaster™. Cloze Clues™ and Clozemaster allow children and parents to share their stories on a computer with the use of graphics. Word (lexical) prediction programs are based upon this relationship of letters to words and provides a means to speed many word processing and communication programs. For example, the user can type the first letters of a word (such as *comp*) and the computer program automatically provides a choice of words that most likely represent the intended word (e.g., *complain, complete, computer*). This scheme is based on frequency of occurrence of the next letter or word according to usage in the prescribed context and saves keystrokes and time. The efficiency of this approach is even greater because many programs store the user's most frequently used words in a dictionary. Appendix C-9 includes a small sampling of the many programs available for the development of language and literacy skills.

Blissymbols. BlissProcessor and BlissLiteracy are two other useful programs. Bliss Literacy facilitates the learning of Blissymbols within the context of a story by teaching the logic of the system (i.e., elements and how they are combined to form various words). Appendix C-9 includes some resources for Blissymbol programs.

Cognitive Rehabilitation

Brain injury may result in a variety of conditions that have a profound influence on language and perceptual functioning. Aphasia (loss of ability to associate meanings with symbols), apraxia of speech (loss of voluntary motor control for speech), and **traumatic brain injury (TBI)** are among conditions resulting from brain injury. These conditions have increased significantly as a result of today's high number of accidents (e.g., cars, sports) and the improved medical techniques that are saving lives and keeping people alive longer. Difficulties in the use of language and speech are associated with aphasia. With TBI, people experience reduced organizational skills, poor short-term memory, short attention span, difficulties in problem solving, and problems related to visual skills, all of which affect an individual's ability to use **assistive technology (AT)**. A number of software programs are available for cognitive rehabilitation and are listed in Appendix C-9.

TELECOMMUNICATIONS

Interest in the information superhighway or phone network is growing rapidly. With the introduction of interactive televisions, cable television companies are competing with telephone companies to capture the communication market, inasmuch as telecommunications is seen as the next major development of the century. Although people have been able for many years to connect a computer to a modem to transmit and receive data, those people have been primarily a select number of computer-literate individuals. For many years, universities have allowed professors to connect with a mainframe on campus and, through the university telephone, connect with a computer on another campus anywhere in the world. Now the general public is being enticed into this communication world. Although access to computer and communication networks is important for all individuals, its impact on individuals with disabilities is likely to be substantial.

Traditional telephone access for an individual with disabilities is difficult. Dial and touch-tone buttons can be very difficult to manipulate. For individuals who have little or no functional speech, the use of a telephone is problematic because listeners often hang up thinking there is no one there, or that it is a prank call. Computers have helped in these cases by using a prerecorded message to alert the listener to the circumstances. With automation and the increasing number of businesses using recorded messages with instructions to press specific numbers for specific services, individuals with disabilities are being faced with increasingly frustrating circumstances. One challenge of the future is to design telephone equipment and tailor services to facilitate use by individuals with disabilities. Although many environmental control programs include automated dialing features, existing programs may have to be modified to accommodate the systems used by companies for processing their calls. The ability of an AAC user to respond within the prescribed timelines set by the company or agency called is critical. Designers of telephone systems and computer programs for companies/agencies will have to consider such variables as response time, memory span, order of presentation, ability to control sequence or repeats, and ease of escaping or quitting the program.

As communication networks are established, individuals will have increasing access to information of all kinds through a variety of services. A modem, a computerized device that transforms all data into ASCII form for transmission across telephone lines, is needed to gain access to these networks. Because ASCII is the universal computer language, individuals with different computers (e.g., Macintosh and IBM) can communicate with each other. Newer modems allow for a transmission speed of 28.8K to 33.6K bps. The advantage of higher bps rates is less on-line time to process messages.

A number of good communication software programs are currently available (e.g., Crosstalk™ for Macintosh and Windows, Geoport™ for Power Macintosh, AppleTalk® remote access, and Smartcom™, Comm Works™, and Wincomm Pro™ for Windows). Available for Macintosh also are Smartcom, Sitcom™, and White Knight™. A good communication package is included as part of Claris Works' integrated software package (available for both Macintosh and Windows). Additional programs that provide faxing capability are Delrina Fax™, Winfax™, and Fax Works™ for IBM-compatible computers and Delrina Fax Pro™ and Fax stf™ for Macintosh. Currently, a number of communication services are being marketed to enable an individual to communicate via modem with other computers (e.g., America Online®, CompuServe®, Genie®, Prodigy®). Through these services, an individual can obtain information on stocks, purchase airline tickets, exchange information on bulletin boards, read magazines or newspapers, obtain articles from libraries, and shop. People can even become acquainted with other individuals who have similar interests. An individual with a disability who has access to a computer can access the same wide array of services available to individuals without disabilities. Specialized services exist for individuals with interests in disabilities. In addition to the Trace Center (Madison, WI), which serves all states, each state has an assistive technology project through funding of the Tech Act. Appendix C-10 lists a sample of telecommunications software programs.

ENVIRONMENTAL CONTROL

Although communication is a significant need for many individuals with disabilities, it is only part of an overall issue of quality of life. Any person with limited mobility (e.g., confinement to a bed or wheelchair) may be restricted in access to the environment. The person may be unable to operate devices such as a remote control for a television set or a CD player, or to use a telephone. Technology now provides ways for these persons to access and enjoy their environment in the same way as their peers without disabilities. The use of technology for controlling devices in a person's environment is called environmental control.

Environmental control involves the use of **infrared rays (IRs)** or **radio frequencies (RF)** to operate an electrical device, such as a kitchen appliance, a VCR, or a television set. A transmitter sends signals (codes) to the device to activate it in specified ways. For RFs, information is transmitted within specific bandwidths (a range of frequencies). **Medium frequency (MF)** bandwidths are generally used for AM broadcasting, whereas **very high frequency (VHF)** bandwidths are generally used for FM broadcasting. VHF is now frequently used for mobile communications, such as car cellular phones. Because VHF bandwidth frequencies are now so heavily used, increasing the chance for interference, more mobile communication is beginning to rely on **ultra high frequency (UHF)** bandwidths.

A major advantage of RF systems is that the signals can travel freely throughout the environment without electrical wires. This allows the AAC user to control a variety of devices from a central location. The system's simple design allows for efficient control of devices in situations where individuals can move around. It is not without some limitations, however, in that devices must operate within a fairly small radius (50 to 200 feet) of the control unit. Also, signals can be picked up by other devices and result in turning other, unwanted electrical appliances on and off.

Environmental control units (ECUs) with infrared rays are frequently used to operate electrical devices. These rays are invisible outside the visible spectrum for human sight. A transmitter generates digital commands that are converted to infrared signals and sent to a receiver, which interprets the codes to activate the device. This highly flexible system provides the AAC user with many options to control electrical appliances in the environment. One problem with these systems is that there can be no obstruction between the transmitter and receiver. Consequently, the AAC user cannot control devices located in another room.

Ultrasound ECU systems use UHFs that are beyond the range of human hearing. Because these sound waves are nondirectional, they tend to bounce off the walls until detected by a receiver that then converts them into control commands that operate a device. Unlike IRs, ultrasound waves are not affected by obstructions between transmitter and receiver; consequently, the transmitter can be located anywhere without interference of signals. However, ultrasound waves do not pass through walls, so the ECU can only operate devices within the same room. This means that devices in other rooms cannot be accidentally activated. The small size of UHF transmitters, however, allows for portability.

Another type of ECU system relies on the AC wiring existing within a house. This can be a practical and relatively inexpensive way to provide for environmental control. A control center sends signals directly to a power line that can be interfaced with a computer. A second unit, the base receiver, is plugged into an electrical receptacle. The base receiver can be configured to receive either IR or RF signals. This allows an individual to operate devices inside and outside the house from a single control center and therefore avoids many of the limitations of using only IR or only RF signals.

As with all AAC systems, service providers must carefully analyze the potential user's needs as they relate to everyday living within the environment in order to devise a truly useful environmental control system. Providers need to know the person's movement patterns throughout the house to determine what devices are used, as well as how they are used. A careful analysis of the layout of rooms and receptacle locations is needed to determine placement of units. Also, service providers must consider the cognitive capacity of the potential user, as well as sensory limitations and mobility requirements. A person with severe cognitive limitations, for example, may be able to control single on/off switches; however, that person may experience considerable difficulty with more complex operations, such as controlling all the functions of a television set and VCR. AAC users with severe visual impairments may need voice output to accompany their switch selections. For an individual who has severe motor impairments, providers may need to analyze specifications for device input and match appropriate switches.

The consideration of environmental control along with AAC needs can contribute greatly to the overall quality of life for an individual. Both require careful consideration of the needs of the individual and other significant communication partners in everyday life patterns. Many systems are now available. Although some clinicians/educators may not have the technical knowledge to design a system, a knowledge of the options can at least make the potential user aware of what is available and how it can be obtained. A number of programs for environmental control are included in Appendix C-11.

FUTURE APPLICATIONS

Each day brings new technology that yesterday was either unimaginable or a part of science fiction. Each new item of technology reinforces recognition of what is possible. Innovations in computer technology not only offer the average individual exciting new forms of education and entertainment, but also suggest possibilities for enhancing the lives of individuals with disabilities. Virtual reality has already become the theme of many motion picture and television dramas. Although expensive, certain features are available in computer programs now. Three-dimensional imagery is available in a number of computer games, and some drawing programs, such as Vision 3D™ and Logomotion™. Virtus VR™ and Virtus Walk Thru™ are 3D interior design packages that provide a more realistic appearance of rooms or scenes (i.e., play directors can obtain an idea of what a scene might look like). As the realism of computer sound and images becomes more dramatic, virtual reality may provide individuals with disabilities a real opportunity to be immersed in the sensations of life experiences. Through the power of interactive programming in virtual reality, individuals with disabilities may be able to practice responses to real-life situations and gain enriched exposure to situations that foster good interactive communication skills.

Already, electrodes have been planted on the optic nerve to enable some individuals who are blind to sense changes in lights and shadows detected by their retina. Cochlear implants allow some individuals who are deaf to sense changes in the rhythmic patterns of speech. Some day in the not-too-distant future, perhaps electrode sensors

along the motor pathways will enable the activation of either the speech musculature or input mechanisms to a speech synthesizer so that typical rates of speech may be attained. This is truly an exciting era. As technology continues to advance, individuals with disabilities may discover newfound capabilities that change their lives.

TECHNOLOGY RESOURCES

During recent decades, a number of resources related to both technology and other aspects of AAC have been developed. Appendix B provides addresses and other relevant information about (1) manufacturers and vendors, (2) software, (3) organizations and resource centers, and (4) periodicals and newsletters. Two extremely valuable technology resource directories are as follows:

1. *Closing the Gap: Resource Directory*, published annually as the February/March issue, provides a comprehensive listing of communication disorders and special education hardware and software solutions.
2. *Hyper – ABLEDATA + DOS – ABLEDATA*, by the Trace Research & Development Center, is a directory of AAC products, available as an on-line bulletin board service, as well as on an IBM disk or CD-ROM database.

SUMMARY

Computers, peripheral and adaptive devices, dedicated and nondedicated communication devices, and AAC software are becoming increasingly important to AAC users. The AAC specialist should have a working knowledge of basic terminology, how computers function, how computers can be adapted for use by individuals with disabilities, and the features of dedicated and nondedicated communication devices. Rapid advances in today's technology guarantees that new devices are emerging on the market at an exponential rate. The resources listed at the end of this chapter and in Appendix C provide more complete information on devices and software. Practicing AAC specialists who use the technology should be consulted for their recommendations, as they have the opportunity to truly assess daily performance and durability.

CHAPTER 11

AAC ASSESSMENT PROCESS

CHARLOTTE A. WASSON, HELEN H. ARVIDSON, AND LYLE L. LLOYD

Augmentative and alternative communication (AAC) service delivery involves such a close relationship between **assessment** and **intervention** that at no particular point does one end and the other begin. Even when an assessment seems to have come to logical closure, assessment will most likely be renewed numerous times. The multiple communication needs of individuals with severe communication disabilities seldom go away, but they do change. Thus, AAC assessment needs to be ongoing. This chapter overviews the purposes, principles, and practices in this assessment process. Throughout the chapter, the term **AAC users** is used to refer to individuals who are the focus of AAC assessments, because it is assumed that individuals arrive at the assessment process already using some form of aided or unaided communication. See Lloyd and Blischak (1992) or Chapter 4 for further clarification of terminology.

AAC ASSESSMENT PROCESS AND PURPOSE

Assessment is a process during which information is gathered to make management decisions (D. B. Bailey, 1989; Tomblin, 1994; Yorkston & Karlan, 1986). It is an essential and fundamental activity of AAC service delivery. Although numerous authors have suggested varying purposes for AAC assessment (e.g., Beukelman & Mirenda, 1992; Blackstone, 1994; Silverman, 1995; von Tetzchner & Martinsen, 1992; Yorkston & Karlan, 1986), this assessment has four primary objectives: (1) to determine the functional communication needs of the individual with little or no functional speech and/or writing; (2) to increase or maintain the individual's opportunities for participation in communication interactions by meeting those communication needs—today, tomorrow, and in the

future; (3) to monitor change within the individual; and (4) to measure and evaluate the effects of intervention (Beukelman & Mirenda, 1992; Mirenda, Iacono, & Williams, 1990; Reichle, 1991). The assessment process involves gathering information related to four specific components of the Lloyd, Quist, and Windsor (1990) AAC communication model: (1) AAC user, (2) communication partners, (3) communication environments, and (4) AAC system (see Chapter 3).

The model in Figure 11.1 shows that assessment components are integrally related, with each holding the potential to exert influence and change on the others. Quite often, modification of any one component will necessitate at least some modification in some or all of the other three. Consider, for example, Ashley, a teenage AAC user who is in a shopping mall, interacting with a best friend—a typical and supportive communication partner—using a voice output communication aid (VOCA)—a typical and supportive communication tool. Although in a quieter and less congested environment, Ashley, her VOCA, and best friend might work together to produce positive communicative exchanges, in this scenario, the noise and confusion of the environment may diminish both the quality and quantity of Ashley's VOCA-based communication turns, and she may choose to use manual signs and gestures. The AAC service delivery team may assist Ashley in assessing which of multiple communication options best match the environments and partners encountered.

Also consider Andrew, an 8-year-old AAC user with moderate cognitive impairment, who has recently developed proficiency in using manual sign. He proudly and effectively uses sign in several environments where he encounters familiar communication partners but is devastated when

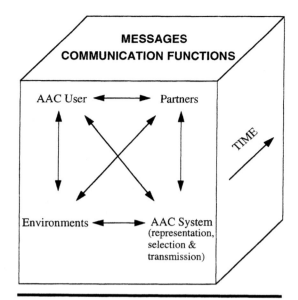

FIGURE 11.1 Components of an AAC Assessment

workers at a fast-food restaurant fail to respond to his signed order for a cheeseburger, french fries, and soft drink. Now, although the AAC user, communication mode, and environment may all appropriately support Andrew's typical communication, the inability of infrequent partners to understand manual sign necessitates assessment of other AAC modalities. Again, the assessment team may assist in evaluating which of several communication options will best support Andrew in multiple environments with multiple partners.

An important component in Figure 11.1 is the influence of the passage of time. Even when AAC users, their partners, their environments, and their systems remain relatively static, the passage of time may have an effect on any or all of the four components of the model. (This model is not meant to replace the AAC model developed by Lloyd, Quist, and Windsor (1990), but is intended to provide a diagrammatical representation of critical components of AAC assessment and intervention.) Adam, an AAC user with amyotrophic lateral sclerosis (ALS), provides an example of the effects of the passage of a short period of time. Early in the day, Adam directly selects graphic symbols on his VOCA using either index finger; by

day's end, however, he is too motorically fatigued to continue this method of direct selection. Thus, without an alternative access method (e.g., an optical pointer for direct selection or a switch for scanning), engaging in VOCA-based communicative exchanges late in the day, even in the familiar surrounding of his home with familiar partners, may be virtually impossible.

The effects of the passage of a long period of time often relate to AAC users' changing communicative needs due to modifications in social, educational, and vocational programs. For example, as Courtney, a young AAC user, approaches dating age, a chosen communication device and its vocabulary may not be as well-suited to her needs as when first developed. Effects related to the passage of a long period of time also emerge with changes in the pathophysiological conditions of the AAC user. Adam, the AAC user with ALS, for example, may eventually become unable to use touch at all as a means of accessing his communication device.

AAC ASSESSMENT PRINCIPLES

Growing out of and relating directly to the purposes of AAC assessment are a number of principles that reflect a current philosophy of service delivery (e.g., Beukelman & Mirenda, 1992; Blackstone, 1994; National Joint Committee for the Communicative Needs of Persons with Severe Disabilities, 1992; Silverman, 1995). Although several journal articles and book chapters have focused either directly or indirectly on these AAC assessment principles, much of what has emerged is built on clinical judgments that have been borrowed primarily from the more general area of speech-language pathology. The following principles are not yet well-grounded in AAC-specific theory (Jones, Jolleff, McConachie, & Wisbeach, 1990), because, as noted by Burkhart (1993), "the art and science of augmentative communication is still a developing field" (p. 22), and there is not yet a plethora of published studies of AAC assessment practices.

Still further, Records and Tomblin (1994) have suggested that even in speech-language pathology, "there is minimal empirical information available regarding how speech-language pathologists use information from several sources to arrive at a diagnostic decision" (p. 144), and that principles related to assessment decision making are based primarily on an implicit rule system that is passed from one professional generation to another. Records and Tomblin have called for empirical studies of diagnostic decision making in communication sciences and disorders to develop explicit assessment standards. AAC's future, similar to that of speech-language pathology, should include investigations of theoretically sound, explicit standards, along with refinement of implicit standards specific to AAC. In the interim, the following assessment principles to clinical decision making provide a foundation.

Principle 1. AAC assessment is based on the premise that everyone can and does communicate. All individuals display behaviors that carry communicative intent. Individuals with severe communication disabilities often possess some repertoire of both linguistic and nonlinguistic speech and gestures. Individuals, in general, communicate through a variety of modes. This is no less true for AAC users. Individuals with little linguistic competence, for example, may exhibit excessive or problem behaviors that carry communicative intent. Donnellan, Mirenda, Mesaros, and Fassbender (1984) have suggested that all excessive or problem behaviors that occur in the presence of others may be thought of as attempts at communication.

Principle 2. AAC assessment must be consumer responsive. Recently there has been an increased use of the term *consumers* when referring to individuals with disabilities (e.g., Franklin, 1993; Jinks & Sinteff, 1994). This has grown out of a recognition that individuals with disabilities (e.g., individuals with little or no functional speech) and their families should be the stakeholders of their own service deliveries —consumers of services provided by various members of their service delivery teams. This text generally uses the term *AAC user* instead of consumer to suggest that individuals with severe communication disabilities are using AAC. The important point is that responsiveness to the needs of AAC users/consumers and their families is a requisite for effective AAC assessment and total service delivery. Blackstone (1994) emphasized the importance of user/consumer

input when she suggested that AAC users should be trained and encouraged to lead their own service delivery teams.

Principle 3. AAC assessment must involve a team of individuals who have a shared agenda and common goals. Primary to success of AAC service delivery is team involvement in both assessment and intervention (Yorkston & Karlan, 1986). The communication and related service needs of AAC users can only be addressed when various professionals join with AAC users, their family members, and peers to design, implement, and evaluate comprehensive, coordinated service delivery that views communication as a basic human need and right (Mirenda et al., 1990), while addressing related services as well. Yet consensus within a team is often lacking. For example, in a severe disabilities survey study involving occupational therapists, parents, physical therapists, special education teachers, and speech-language pathologists, Giangreco (1990) discovered that team members often disagree on such critical issues as the roles of related service professionals, the criteria used for making related service decisions, and the authority for making decisions. In fact, separate disciplines were noted to sometimes make critical service delivery decisions even before informing family members and other professionals. Giangreco noted that balancing consumer empowerment and professional authority continues to challenge group decision making and quality service delivery, and that team conflicts result in "(a) gaps in service, (b) overlaps in service, (c) contradictory recommendations by persons from various disciplines, and (d) services that do not match student or family needs" (Giangreco, 1990, p. 29). AAC team members must avoid these serious dangers by working collaboratively throughout the assessment process. Using a transdisciplinary approach can minimize these dangers.

Principle 4. AAC assessment must include information about typical routines, collected in natural settings and multiple environments. Most individuals have rather typical lifestyles that change somewhat, but often not dramatically from day-to-day and week-to-week. Most individuals communicate with a core of close communication partners. The same is just as true, if not more so, for the majority of AAC users. With the aim of assessment being to identify communication needs and develop, enhance, and maintain participation opportunities, it is crucial to gather thorough information about typical routines. At least a portion of the AAC assessment should be carried out in familiar settings during activity routines that are naturalistically representative. A number of observational analyses can be used along with guided interviews to obtain realistic information regarding the typical communication needs of and opportunities for the AAC user. Activity routines occur in different environments. Information should be gathered from multiple environments, which can include home, school, work, and community.

Principle 5. AAC assessment must be comprehensive, focusing on the functional limitations and disabling influences of pathologies and impairments, not just on the pathologies and impairments themselves. Although it is important to understand the individual's pathology/impairment, understanding the functional aspects of the impairment relative to the specific individual is more important. In some cases, professional efforts have focused far too extensively on the pathologies and impairments that result in severe communication disabilities, while focusing far too little on the functional limitations and disabling influences of these pathologies. Assessment teams can guard against taking such a narrow view of disabling conditions by balancing their assessments across the components of the AAC user, partners, environments, and AAC system.

Principle 6. AAC assessment must focus on communication strengths as well as communication weaknesses. The participation model (Beukelman & Mirenda, 1992; Mirenda et al., 1990; Rosenberg & Beukelman, 1988) provides a framework that allows service providers to identify an AAC user's abilities and opportunities. At the same time, the model focuses service providers' attention on identifying and modifying barriers that may impede the development and maintenance of maximally effective communication interactions. The participation model recognizes that strengths and weaknesses are both intrinsic and extrinsic; that is, some strengths and weaknesses lie within AAC users whereas others are shaped by AAC partners, environments, and systems. All these strengths and weaknesses require scrutiny if

overall AAC service delivery is to be effective and efficient.

Principle 7. AAC assessment must involve feature matching. Because AAC assessment centers on meeting the communication needs of individuals with severe communication disabilities, the assessment process must involve finding the best AAC system available for each individual. To do this, assessment teams must match features of no technology, low-technology, and high-technology approaches to the current and future needs of AAC users. Typically, no one device has enough of the desirable or necessary features. Therefore, both aided and unaided modes, and both low and high technology must be melded together to create a comprehensive communication system that meets an AAC user's needs across partners and environments. Feature matching applies to multimodal communication and not just technology.

Principle 8. AAC assessment must adhere to the law of parsimony. Although AAC assessment is an extremely extensive process involving the AAC user, communication partners, environments, and a multimodal AAC system (with the various means to represent, select, and transmit), one must be guided by the law of parsimony. There is elegance in simplicity, or as Einstein said, "One must attempt to make all things as simple as possible, but no simpler." Because of the number and type of assessments that typically need to be made, it is important to simplify the process and minimize the amount of effort the AAC user must put forth without sacrificing quality. Additionally, it is important that clinicians/educators do not become involved with so many aspects of assessment that they have difficulty synthesizing information.

Principle 9. AAC assessment must be ongoing, often occurring in conjunction with intervention. As previously noted, the communication needs of AAC users typically do not go away, but they do change. As communication needs change, ongoing assessment is appropriate and essential. Predictable time lines change an individual's communication needs, so more assessment may be needed to minimize the impact of such changes. For example, as an AAC user moves from one educational level to another, changing communication needs should be anticipated and assessed. Ongoing assessments may also be necessitated by changes in the AAC user's pathophysiological condition (e.g., progression of a degenerative disease such as ALS or improved motor control in an individual recovering from a closed head injury). Still other assessment may be initiated because of advances in technology, changes in team members' knowledge of technologies or strategies, changes in the number and types of environments, or changes in the number and types of communication partners. In other words, to promote, maintain, and enhance functional communication, AAC assessment must examine the interrelationship among AAC users, partners, environments, and systems on an ongoing basis. Assessment may promote immediate and initial success by addressing the needs of today, while continued investigations of the needs of tomorrow are conducted (Beukelman & Mirenda, 1992).

Principle 10. AAC assessment should result in positive change. Accountable service delivery encompasses a balance between assessment and intervention that is so interwoven as to often seem inseparable. The service delivery plan should undergo constant scrutiny and, when new information is uncovered, logical modifications should be made. These modifications may involve, for example, adjusting the AAC user's seating and positioning, shaping the use of more effective communication strategies, or identifying and breaking down various policy or attitudinal barriers. Assessing the service delivery plan may also identify a need for new or modified low- and high-technology communication devices to allow best feature matching for the user. All four components in Figure 11.1 must be subjected to fine-tuning to meet the communication needs of the AAC user.

AAC ASSESSMENT PROCEDURES

AAC Assessment Team

As indicated, AAC assessments are team-based endeavors involving AAC users, their family members, friends, and peers, as well as representatives of various professional disciplines. AAC assessment teams can be found in local settings (e.g., schools or vocational service centers), in center-based settings (e.g., university or hospital clinics), or in specialized assessment centers. Increased awareness of and competencies in AAC service delivery, along with a shift toward functional on-site assessment and intervention, have resulted in a growing number of locally based teams.

The American Speech-Language-Hearing Association (ASHA) (1991) has determined that "the provision of augmentative and alternative communication services is within the scope of practice of speech-language pathologists and audiologists" (p. 8) and has charged speech-language pathologists to lead the planning and coordination efforts of AAC teams, as well as conduct direct speech-language assessments (ASHA, 1989). Speech-language pathologists must possess the skills and competencies of AAC service delivery that have been set forth by ASHA (1989). They must also have extensive knowledge about the AAC user and the user's educational and/or vocational program. In some cases, other professionals are more appropriately designated as the AAC assessment team leader. Locke and Mirenda (1992), for example, note that special educators are often called on to execute the administrative and case-management tasks of AAC team leadership. In other cases, social workers serve as team leaders.

Beyond discussing the duties of a leader, minimal guidelines exist for the involvement of other professional team members. Logically, team membership is determined by the unique needs of the individual being assessed, the availability and expertise of personnel, and a number of other logistic factors such as transportation and scheduling (Beukelman & Mirenda, 1992; Reichle, 1991). Typically, members who will most frequently and extensively be involved in AAC assessment, service delivery development, and implementation form a core team. The professional core members of the Purdue-GLASS (Greater Lafayette Area Special Services) AAC Assessment Team, for example, include (as a bare minimum) a speech-language pathologist, a special educator, and an occupational or physical therapist. Other professionals become core members as appropriate. For example, an AAC user with a visual impairment may need an orientation and mobility (O & M) specialist as a core team member. The ophthalmologist at a distant assessment center, on the other hand, might serve a less central role. Although results of ophthalmologic assessments are critical to the outcomes of overall service delivery, the ophthalmologist might be minimally, if at all, involved in the daily implementation of service delivery. On the Purdue-GLASS team, students involved in preservice professional training have less central roles. Appendix D provides a listing along with descriptive information related to responsibilities of potential team members.

Models of AAC Service Delivery

In some settings, AAC services (assessment and intervention) are provided by professionals from one discipline (e.g., speech-language pathology) within the context of a **unidisciplinary model**. Because AAC requires the expertise of several disciplines, however, models involving more than one discipline are preferred. Professional members of AAC assessment teams most often work together using one of three generally recognized service delivery team models: multidisciplinary, interdisciplinary, or transdisciplinary (McCormick, 1990a). Locke and Mirenda (1992) found these three models of service delivery to be comparably represented, at least in educational settings.

A chosen model is specifically influenced by the team's demographic characteristics, its administrative charges, and its professional training and preferences, as well as by the characteristics and needs of the individuals to be assessed. In the **multidisciplinary team model**, although guided by a team leader, each team member functions rather independently in assessment, decision making, and intervention. In the **interdisciplinary team model**, members, also governed by a team leader, often use information shared by other members to guide their decision making and intervention, even though they usually engage in independent assessments. In the **transdisciplinary team model**, the team forms a partnership under the guidance of the team leader to jointly share in information gathering, diagnostic decision making, and program development (Locke & Mirenda, 1992; Yorkston & Karlan, 1986). Transdisciplinary team members thus have mutual investment in the as-

sessment and intervention design (McCormick, 1990a). Team members participate in **role release** (Locke & Mirenda, 1992; McCormick, 1990a), giving up traditional territorial roles. Sometimes they take on some of the roles and responsibilities of other professionals or yield their own to team members who carry out the most significant proportions of the service delivery plan (e.g., the special educator or speech-language pathologist). The type and amount of role release is determined on a case-by-case basis to result in effective integration of assessment and intervention services. Teams participating in role release must adhere to any and all legal and ethical guidelines specific to their professional areas of training (ASHA, 1991; McCormick, 1990a).

As AAC service delivery becomes more responsive and individuals with disabilities are included increasingly in educational, vocational, recreational, and social settings, the transdisciplinary model should become the model of choice, because it is most adept at supporting collaboration, not fragmentation (McCormick, 1990a; Zangari, Lloyd, & Vicker, 1994). For many professionals, learning to work as part of a transdisciplinary service delivery team will entail the development of new attitudes, skills, and tools. For further information on these models and other aspects of service delivery, see Chapter 21.

Approaches to AAC Assessment

Because AAC assessments are tailored to individual AAC users, assessment teams must carefully select which multiple life and communication areas need investigation and to what extent. Although they may use a variety of procedures, the assessment team typically evaluates individuals' current capabilities using one of two basic assessment approaches: **comprehensive capability profiling** or **criteria-based profiling** (Beukelman & Mirenda, 1992; Lloyd & Kangas, 1994; Mirenda et al., 1990; Yorkston & Karlan, 1986). During comprehensive capability profiling, maximal information is gathered by pertinent team members in each of several chosen target areas. For example, a comprehensive physical examination of an AAC user with cerebral palsy might involve gathering information about the individual's range of motion, skeletal deformities, skeletal alignment, muscle tone, reflex patterns, postural control, and voluntary muscle movements (Cook & Hussey, 1995). Even though having such extensive information is often preferable, gathering maximal detail in so many areas may actually yield irrelevant information, tire the AAC user, and consume considerable time.

Criteria-based profiling involves judging the AAC user's abilities in certain critical target areas against a set of criteria considered essential for skill development in these areas. For example, assessing an AAC user's potential using manual sign might not be necessary if using a communication board is considered to be more appropriate than using manual sign. Although criteria-based profiling obviously saves assessment time, the team must clearly understand the standard against which the AAC user is being judged and must guard against overlooking critical areas of assessment. Due to time constraints and the team's mission to conduct functional assessments that quickly lead to positive outcomes, criteria-based profiling is often the assessment approach of choice. It is also chosen because it can help predict success with particular devices or strategies and assess changes over time. When used as a predictor, it may be termed *predictive profiling* (Beukelman & Mirenda, 1992; Lloyd & Kangas, 1994; Mirenda et al., 1990).

AAC ASSESSMENT COMPONENTS

AAC assessment and overall service delivery has changed rather dramatically over the past several years. As noted by Mirenda et al. (1990), the AAC field has witnessed "(a) a shift in assessment procedures from those designed to identify appropriate candidates for augmentative communication to those based on the inclusionary principle that improved communication is possible for *all* persons with severe intellectual disabilities (Kangas & Lloyd, 1988); (b) a shift in the goal of intervention from the development of specific, isolated speech and language skills to the development of integrated, functionally relevant communication abilities (Romski & Sevcik, 1988a); and (c) a shift toward an increased understanding of the multi-

modal nature of communication (Reichle & Karlan, 1985)" (p. 3).

Even with this needed and timely shift to more functional AAC assessment and service delivery, many areas of the traditional assessment process remain valid, because communication disabilities can only be truly assessed when considered within the framework of the individual's overall physical and psychological capabilities and disabilities (Bristow, 1993). Thus, potential target areas of AAC assessments remain as numerous or more numerous than they were during AAC's early years when traditional, clinic-based assessments prevailed. For now, although many of the traditional assessment areas continue to warrant investigation, assessment of the AAC user's strengths and needs against the backdrop of natural environments must surely be added. AAC assessment areas, therefore, include the AAC user, partners, environments, and AAC system (Arthur, 1989; Beukelman & Mirenda, 1992; Blackstone, 1994; Mirenda et al., 1990; National Joint Committee for the Communicative Needs of Persons with Severe Disabilities, 1992).

Assessment of AAC User

The following AAC user assessment areas may be considered during the assessment process:

- Etiology
- Cognition and psychological functioning
- Language comprehension and production
- Oromotor structure and functioning
- Motor functioning
- Sensory acuity and processing abilities
- Academic and literacy abilities
- Communicative desire
- Present communication abilities and needs
- Future communication needs

Etiology. The assessment team should gather information regarding the pathologies or disorders (impairments) contributing to the communication disabilities as well as any other impairments the AAC user may have (Silverman, 1995; Vanderheiden & Yoder, 1986). Such information, as part of either an initial or an ongoing assessment, may be obtained from medical members of the team, from the AAC user and family, or from record reviews, and should be intermittently reviewed for currency and accuracy. The condition(s) should be considered for degree of impairment as well as for time of onset and progression (e.g., congenital, acquired, progressive, or temporary) (Vanderheiden & Yoder, 1986), because such information may yield knowledge regarding the expected course and consequence of the condition (Blackstone, 1994). For example, an adult with ALS may be expected to progressively lose muscle function, whereas an individual with traumatic brain injury (TBI) may be expected to continue improving in several areas of overall functioning. In some cases, the neurologist on the assessment team may be called on to complete a cranial nerve examination (by testing the motor and sensory function of various body parts served by each cranial nerve) and/or a motor system examination (by inspection, palpation, and passive and active motion testing) to yield further detail for the pool of etiologic information.

Cognition and Psychological Functioning.   Although there has been a shift away from candidacy models that viewed certain sensorimotor and cognitive skills as necessary prerequisites for AAC services (Kangas & Lloyd, 1988; McCormick & Shane, 1990; Mirenda et al., 1990; Reichle & Karlan, 1985; Silverman, 1995), it is still valid to examine the AAC user's cognitive and psychological status, because such examinations establish a baseline of cognitive functioning for future comparisons (Sevcik, Romski, & Wilkinson, 1991). Cognitive assessments should not result in excluding individuals from AAC service delivery based on assumptions that they do not possess the skills necessary to benefit from intervention programs; rather, assessments should contribute to an understanding of individuals' abilities to apply certain mental processes to nonlinguistic and linguistic behaviors to accomplish effective communication (Reichle & Karlan, 1985; Silverman, 1995). According to ASHA (1988), "cognition and language are intrinsically and reciprocally related both in development and function" and "an impairment of language may disrupt one or more cognitive processes, and, similarly, an impairment of one or more cognitive processes may disrupt language" (p. 79).

Because AAC intervention is most productive for individuals who show evidence of means-ends relationships and causality (Jones et al., 1990; Reichle, 1991), these and other Piagetian sensorimotor skills are frequent areas of cognitive investigations during AAC assessments with individuals who function at early cognitive levels (Snyder-McLean, McLean, & Etter, 1988). Sensorimotor intelligence is defined as those complex mental behaviors related to responding and adapting to sensory information to accomplish problem solving (Bailey & Rouse, 1989; French, 1964; Langley, 1989; McCormick, 1990a; McCormick & Shane, 1990). Sensorimotor assessments consider the range and variety of the sensorimotor behaviors, as well as the general level of competence within each area. Thus, information regarding the horizontal competence within each level of development, as well as the vertical hierarchy of sensorimotor skill development, is significant and may be gathered by examining the individual's ability to apply six schemes to mental processes: (1) **object permanence**, (2) **means-ends relationships**, (3) **causality**, (4) **spatial relationships**, (5) **imitation**, and (6) **object concept** (Langley, 1989).

Object permanence relates to the ability to understand that an object exists even when it is not immediately perceptible. Assessment of object permanence usually entails presentation of varying search tasks to assess an individual's ability to attend to objects, to organize an efficient search for objects, and then to deduce appropriate responses (Langley, 1989). Means-ends relationships involve an understanding that the problem-solving process (i.e., the means) is distinct from the problem-solving goal (i.e., the ends). Development of means-ends skills has long been thought to be closely associated with the development of language (McCormick, 1990a). Assessment of this scheme often involves ascertaining an individual's success in using someone or something as a tool to acquire another (e.g., using a caregiver to reach a toy or using an AAC symbol to request an actual object). Development of causality reflects an individual's ability to search for the source behind a problem or realize that a relationship exists between a problem and its solution, and is also thought to be closely related to effective language use. Causality assessment typically involves examining an individual's ability to choose a correct solution to a problem from an array of potential choices. Existence of spatial relationships skills reflects an understanding of the three-dimentionality of objects and may be assessed by evaluating the ability to discriminate foreground from background and to make judgments regarding the spatial limits and relationships of objects. Imitation is reflected by an ability to copy vocal and/or gestural behaviors of people and events. This scheme is frequently assessed by examining social attention and interaction, and the application of these behaviors from situation to situation. Finally, object concept is reflected in an individual's ability to apply appropriate behaviors to objects according to their perceptual properties. Assessment of object concept may be accomplished through evaluation of the extent and range of object manipulation behaviors.

Assessing the degree and quality of any or all these sensorimotor skills may provide insight into an individual's current abilities to effectively use AAC strategies and techniques, because communication is a behavior that employs both the processes and products of certain mental behaviors (ASHA, 1988). Advocating assessment of sensorimotor functioning, however, should not imply that a causal relationship exists between certain sensorimotor skills and the ability to benefit from AAC intervention (McCormick & Shane, 1990; Reichle & Karlan, 1985; Silverman, 1995). In fact, to provide AAC services to *all* individuals who possess severe communication disorders is in keeping with contemporary philosophies of service delivery (Mirenda et al., 1990). However, this service delivery may include providing an appropriate AAC system to the AAC user and then teaching various sensorimotor schemes as initial intervention targets in a test-teach-test paradigm (McCormick & Shane, 1990; Paget, 1989; Reichle & Karlan, 1985).

For individuals functioning beyond the sensorimotor stages, numerous other areas of cognition, such as cognitive operations, principles, processes, and strategies warrant assessment (Haywood & Switzky, 1986; Paget, 1989). These cognitive functions pair with nonintellectual factors such as attitude, motivation, and habits to support the learning needs of an individual. Assessment of these intellectual and nonintellectual factors may, therefore, be appropriate targets of the AAC assessment and may provide invaluable assessment information. For instance, the team may be able to predict the AAC user's ability to (1) acquire, retain, and use various AAC symbols and devices; (2) apply problem-solving skills to select and use appropriate communication modes in particular environmental settings with particular communication partners; and (3) repeat successful communication exchanges and avoid unsuccessful ones (Gerber & Kraat, 1992; Iacono, 1992).

Cognitive functioning levels are difficult to ascertain, and some AAC users, regardless of intellectual potential, may display variability in their cognitive profiles because of experiential deficits. AAC users who have not had access to appropriate AAC systems and training, for example, may present with artificial cognitive deficits that will subside or disappear soon after appropriate AAC service delivery has begun. Ongoing assessment is a must.

In many cases, accurately profiling the AAC user's cognitive skills will also be challenging due to a lack of appropriate test instruments for use with individuals with severe communication disabilities. Conjoining standard and nonstandard testing, observational analyses, and interviews, however, can contribute to developing a general profile of cognitive skills. Several assessment tools, developmental scales, and checklists that may be considered by the AAC assessment team to inventory sensorimotor and cognitive skills are listed in Table 11.1. Some of these examine cognitive functions that are present and intact, whereas others identify functions that are weak, deficient, or absent. Using assessment instruments that cross both areas will produce a profile of the AAC user's cognitive strengths and weaknesses. If standard test instruments are employed, test adaptations will often be required. Such adaptations, and their cautious interpretation, are discussed later in this section.

In addition to cognitive factors, the AAC user's psychological status such as general mental health, disability adjustment, and overall interper-

TABLE 11.1   Sample of Sensorimotor and Cognitive Assessment Instruments

INSTRUMENT	CHRONOLOGICAL AGE	AREA ASSESSED
The Arthur Adaptation of the Leiter International Performance Scale (Arthur, 1952)	3 to 7 years	Cognitive structures. No verbal response is required.
Assessment in Infancy: Ordinal Scales of Psychological Development (Uzgiris & Hunt, 1975)	Infancy	Sensorimotor development in visual pursuit and object permanence, means-ends relationships, causality, gestural imitation, focal imitation, construction of objects in space, and object relations.
Bayley Scale of Infant Development (Bayley, 1969)	Birth to 30 months	Mental, psychomotor, and social domains; several items related to visual and auditory abilities (often cited as most frequently used scale of sensorimotor intelligence). Many items can be scored from observation.
Generic Skills Assessment Inventory (McLean, Snyder-McLean, Rowland, Jacobs & Stremel-Campbell, 1985)	2 weeks to 30 months	Object relationships, comprehension, imitation, expressive interaction. Many items can be scored from observation.
Kaufman Assessment Battery for Children (K-ABC) (Kaufman & Kaufman, 1983)	$2\frac{1}{2}$ to $12\frac{1}{2}$ years	Cognition; focuses on information-processing and problem-solving style.
McCarthy Scales of Children's Abilities (McCarthy, 1972)	$2\frac{1}{2}$ to $8\frac{1}{2}$ years	Intellectual level with specific testing in verbal, perceptual-performance, quantitative, memory, and motor skills.
Hiskey-Nebraska Test of Learning Aptitude (Hiskey, 1966)	3 to 16 years	Cognition can be administered via pantomime. No verbal response required. Normed on deaf children.
The Stanford-Binet Intelligence Scale (Terman & Merrill, 1973)	2 years to adult	Intellectual abilities in verbal reasoning, abstract/visual reasoning, quantitative reasoning, and short-term memory.
Wechsler Preschool and Primary Scale of Intelligence (WPPSI) (Wechsler, 1967)	4 to $6\frac{1}{2}$ years	Intellectual functioning in verbal and performance areas. Requires approximately 1.5 hours to administer, so fatigue is a concern.
Woodcock-Johnson Psychoeducational Battery (Woodcock & Johnson, 1977)	3 years to adult	Cognitive skills related to educational capabilities.

sonal skills should be considered (Bristow, 1993). Similar to cognitive status, psychological status may be determined by direct testing, observations, interviews, and record reviews. Information regarding the AAC user's psychological status should be periodically reassessed to ensure that it remains accurate.

Although some AAC users have rather static cognitive and psychological profiles across the life span (e.g., individuals with mental retardation), others may experience declines in cognitive and mental health status (e.g., individuals with cerebral arteriosclerosis, dementia). Because cognition and language are interrelated, still others may show significant positive cognitive and psychological changes as better AAC strategies and systems are provided. Information regarding the AAC user's cognitive and psychological status should, therefore, be updated at appropriate intervals. Additional information regarding cognitive and psychological issues relevant to AAC users with developmental disabilities and acquired disorders is provided in Chapters 18 and 19.

Language Comprehension and Production. The National Joint Committee for the Communicative Needs of Persons with Severe Disabilities (1992) has recognized that all individuals, including those with little or no functional speech and other severe disabilities, possess some level of communicative proficiency. The committee has advocated that individuals with severe disabilities be examined comprehensively for a full range of extant communicative abilities in receptive and expressive form, content, and use gathered through repeated measures. This part of an assessment should be guided by team members who are experts in the structures and functions of language with input from other team members who are familiar with the AAC user's functional communication uses and needs. As part of the assessment, the team must consider the mutual influences of psychosocial, motoric, and cognitive functioning on the individual's attempts and abilities to communicate.

Language has traditionally been thought of and assessed in terms of its reception (comprehension or understanding) and expression (production) and along its three primary components:

form, content, and use. **Language form** relates to the elements of language, including its sounds and sound systems (phonology), its units (morphology), and its structures (syntax). **Language content** (semantics) relates to the meaning or mental representations of language (semantic knowledge), as well as rules for linking meaning with language units (semantic relations). **Language use** (pragmatics) relates to the understanding of and ability to use the social exchange dimension of communication (e.g., knowing why, when, where, and with whom to use language) (McCormick & Schiefelbusch, 1990). Pragmatic aspects encompass (1) varying language use to accomplish different functions, (2) using contextual information to guide decisions about which functions to use to achieve intended goals, and (3) using social skills to initiate, maintain, and terminate interactions (Lahey, 1988). (See Bloom and Lahey [1978] and Lahey [1988] for a comprehensive review of language development and language disorders.)

Romski and Sevcik (1993a) have suggested that far too little attention has been directed at understanding the role of language comprehension in the total AAC service delivery process. Some aspects of the AAC user's language comprehension (receptive language) can often be examined using several tests or test portions. Table 11.2 overviews various standard receptive and expressive language assessment tools and also lists examples of AAC-specific instruments. These standard receptive tests should be supplemented with interviews and environmental assessments that have been conducted in settings where demands and opportunities for communication exist. When adapted administration of standard tests is not feasible, informal assessments and observational analyses may replace them (McCormick & Shane, 1990; Mirenda et al., 1990; National Joint Committee for the Communicative Needs of Persons with Severe Disabilities, 1992; Sternberg, Ehren, Lefferts, & Eloranta, 1988).

Although receptive language tests and test portions can provide information about the individual's understanding of speech and/or writing, such tests, when considered alone, will contribute little to investigating the AAC user's ability to understand forms of communication that are not spo-

TABLE 11.2   Sample of Receptive and Expressive Language Assessment Instruments

INSTRUMENT	CHRONOGLOCIAL AGE	AREA ASSESSED
Assessment of Children's Language Comprehension (Foster, Giddan, & Stark, 1973)	3 to 6 years, 11 months	Picture identification, object manipulation, parent report, best choice
Assessment of Phonological Processes—Revised (Hodson & Paden, 1991)	Any age, norms for 2 to 5 years, 11 months	Phonological skills by object naming
Birth to Three Developmental Scales (Bangs & Dodson, 1979)	0 to 3 years	Observation, direction following, verbal imitation, motor imitation, naming, parent report
Communicative Evaluation Chart (Anderson, Miles, & Matheny, 1963)	3 months to 5 years	Observation, direction following, verbal and motor production, drawing, question answering
Environmental Language Inventory (MacDonald, 1978)	1 year, 1 month to 4 years, 9 months	Expressive semantics and grammar forms and structure; evaluated through imitation and play
Expressive One-Word Picture Vocabulary Test (Gardner, 1979)	2 to 11 years, 11 months	Expressive vocabulary skills
Infant Scale of Communicative Intent (Sacks & Young, 1982)	Birth to 1½ years	Prelinguistic skills; assessed by checklist of observed behaviors
INteraction CHecklist for Augmentative Communication: INCH (Bolton & Dashiell, 1984)	Any age	Interactive behavior: initiation, facilitation, regulation, termination
Lifespace Access Profile (Williams, Stemach, Wolfe, & Stanger, 1993)	Any age	Physical resources, cognitive resources, emotional resources, technology support resources, environmental analysis
Preschool Language Scale—Revised (Zimmerman, Steiner, & Pond, 1979)	1 to 6 years, 7 months	Responses to pictures; object manipulation; picture identification; direction following
Receptive-Expressive Emergent Language Scale (Bzoch & League, 1970)	1 month to 3 years	Emerging receptive and expressive language skills; parent report

ken. This area can best be examined using informal procedures and even AAC symbols during environmentally based evaluations (Romski & Sevcik, 1993a). In many instances, exposing the AAC user to symbols is a prerequisite to using them to document receptive language skills.

Several areas of expressive language assessment are essential to profiling the AAC user's current level of language form, content, and use. Because many AAC users have some speaking abilities, an inventory of phonological and/or articulatory skills may be appropriate. Some speaking AAC users may further develop or recover use of natural speech; some may maintain speech at its current level; others will experience deteriorating speaking abilities. Bodine and Beukelman (1991) surveyed 17 AAC specialists and found that they used personal opinions or clinical intuitions to predict speech recovery or loss, because few empirical studies are available to guide accurate prognoses.

Although phonological assessments evaluate whole processes or sound patterns involved in speech sound production, articulatory inventories examine individual speech sounds as they occur in initial, medial, and final word positions across single word, phrase, and continuous speech production boundaries. Those phonological patterns noted to detract most significantly from the intelligibility of natural speech production include stopping sounds that should be continued and omitting syllables, final consonants, or parts of sound clusters. Similarly, although sound distortions and sound substitutions certainly impede intelligibility, sound omissions are noted to be the most deviant articulatory error (McReynolds, 1988). Several standard phonological and articulation tests that contain real or miniature items or large, colored, line drawings may be used with minimal adaptations to assess phoneme productions at word, phrase, and sentence levels, and a speech sample can be analyzed to assess sound productions as they occur in longer units. In addition to completing these standard articulation assessments, the intelligibility of articulation as judged by various familiar and unfamiliar partners will help determine the functionality of speech.

Because many AAC users have central and/or peripheral nervous system motor impairments (as influenced by injuries or diseases), and yet possess some degree of speech production, they must be evaluated for the presence and severity of **apraxia** and/or **dysarthria**. Apraxia refers to difficulty in executing volitional movements (Cumley & Jones, 1992; Hayden, 1994). Several types of apraxia exist, including buccofacial (or oral) apraxia, ideomotor (or limb) apraxia, and apraxia of speech. In apraxia of speech, sound breakdowns occur, affecting the intelligibility of speech production. These speech sound breakdowns usually consist of sound substitutions or omissions. Although the errors are noted to be inconsistent, they generally are more predominant on initial sounds in words, in clustered speech sounds, and in longer speech utterances. For a thorough review of the assessment of developmental apraxia, see Hodge (1994), Hodge and Hancock (1994), and Hayden (1994).

Dysarthria relates to muscle weakness, dyscoordination, or paralysis. Although there are commonly agreed upon types (related to site of involvement), dysarthric speech, in general, is often described as slow, labored, and imprecise. The speech-language pathologist on the AAC assessment team should rate the speech of the individuals with motor speech disorders in the areas of articulation, phonation, prosody, resonation, and respiration to determine which of these five subsystems are disturbed and to what degree (Dworkin, 1991). The work of Yorkston and colleagues (e.g., Yorkston, Beukelman, & Bell, 1988) is recommended as a reference to the assessment and management of dysarthria. Dworkin (1991) offers a comprehensive treatment guide to both apraxia and dysarthria.

Along with assessing the presence or absence of apraxia or dysarthria, it is a good idea to investigate the occurrences and purposes of extraneous vocalizations or sounds. Such vocalizations may be used to call attention or may carry other specific message intents (e.g., a vowel produced with rising intonation may consistently be used to request a positional change) (Bristow, 1993).

The AAC user's language form, content, and use must be examined beyond speech production (National Joint Committee for the Communicative Needs of Persons with Severe Disabilities, 1992). Expressive language assessment may make use of all or parts of standard tests or test adaptations, but is most validly conducted as part of repeated measures of communication in natural environments so that it becomes evident what forms and functions various symbolic and nonsymbolic behaviors serve. Such assessments should even include establishing the purpose of behaviors expressed in socially unacceptable ways (see Chapter 24; Baumgart, Johnson, & Helmstetter, 1990; Musselwhite & St. Louis, 1988; National Joint Committee for the Communicative Needs of Persons with Severe Disabilities, 1992; Silverman, 1995). AAC-specific instruments may be particularly useful in validly assessing the AAC user's various language strengths and weaknesses.

Oromotor Structure and Functioning.   Because the individual being assessed has a severe communication impairment, a comprehensive, thorough evaluation of the structure and function of the oromotor system is essential. Several areas of this assessment may contribute to the differential diagnosis of speech apraxia or dysarthria or of a swallowing/feeding disorder (i.e., dysphagia) and its severity.

Dysphagia may exist in the presence or the absence of speech impairment. Its assessment requires the skills of several professionals. Using appropriate instrumentation (e.g., videofluoroscopy or electromyography), speech-language pathologists and physicians assess the phase of swallowing that is affected, ascertain the degree of involvement, and determine appropriate dietary and compensatory training strategies. The occupational therapist may lead the assessment of the need for adaptive feeding equipment, the physical therapist may lead the assessment of the need for seating and positioning devices to promote safe feedings, and the dietitian may develop appropriate diets to accommodate the individual's special feeding and swallowing needs.

In addition to evaluating the structure and function of the oromotor system, AAC service providers should assess the various oral reflexes. Reflexes are automatic, stereotypic, involuntary responses to stimuli. Individuals with severe speech impairments related to neurological damage may display abnormal reflexes that negatively affect the production of functional speech. Some of these include jaw thrusting, tongue thrusting, and tonic biting (Alexander & Bigge, 1982). Evaluation of the type and extent of abnormal oral reflexes warrants careful attention because the persistence of abnormal reflexes provides essential prognostic information regarding the potential for development, recovery, and/or maintenance of functional natural speech (Bodine & Beukelman, 1991; Shane & Sauer, 1986; Silverman, 1995; Vanderheiden & Lloyd, 1986). Assessment of oral reflexes can be conducted within a framework of motor examinations in areas such as general muscle tone and movement and can be accomplished through informal measures of functional oral tasks (e.g., eating and speaking) or specialized tests, such as videofluoroscopy studies. Several detailed oral-peripheral examination protocols are available in speech-language pathology texts (see, e.g., Kent, 1994).

Motor Functioning.   Evaluation of both fine and gross motor functioning is a critical part of the AAC assessment process, aimed primarily at identifying an individual's positional and ambulation status as related to effectively using AAC devices, as well as assess status related to direct selection or scanning choices (Enstrom, 1992; Mirenda et al., 1990; Musselwhite & St. Louis, 1988; Ratcliff, 1994; Silverman, 1995; Yorkston & Karlan, 1986). Although many AAC users have motor impairments requiring positional adaptations to maximize communication and other life functions, few specific guidelines are offered to assist the team in motor evaluations (McEwen & Karlan, 1989; Mirenda et al., 1990). An indepth discussion of AAC and motor function is provided in Chapter 17.

Guided by the skills and knowledge of the occupational therapist, physical therapist, and/or rehabilitation specialist, the AAC team should conduct motor assessments to identify functional positions that will best support the use of AAC devices and overall attempts to communicate. For most individuals being assessed, appropriate seating positions must be sought prior to and throughout motor assessment to allow for proper trunk support and accurate evaluations of overall motor capabilities (Campbell, 1989; Rainforth & York, 1987; York & Weimann, 1991). The function of the head and neck should be assessed for range of motion, control, and endurance (Bristow, 1993; Lee & Thomas, 1990). Because most individuals will need several functional positions across a day's time, the effects of positional changes will frequently require evaluation. For individuals who are able to ambulate independently, maximal ways to transport devices should be sought, whereas consideration of seating, AAC device mounting, and mobility will be key aspects of the motor assessment for individuals who are unable to ambulate independently (York & Weimann, 1991). Fishman (1987) has suggested that both portability and mounting factors can be evaluated along parameters of accessibility, independence, and flexibility.

Until recently, the degree of motor impairment was thought to directly affect the ability to access communication devices (MacNeela, 1987a, b; York, Nietupski, & Hamre-Nietupski, 1985). Although individuals with less severe motor impairments were noted to have multiple access options and, thus increased expectations for their efficient use, individuals with severe and multiple motor impairments were thought to have diminished access to and use of options. Several recent works, however, have documented that individuals with severe and multiple disabilities are able to access microswitches and microtechnologies when appropriate supports are provided (see, for example, Goossens' & Crain, 1992; Goossens', Crain, & Elder, 1992; Hanson & Hanline, 1985; Schweigert & Rowland, 1992).

Typically, the muscles most desirable to augmentative communication access, aided communication systems, and certainly unaided communication systems are those of the upper extremities (Lee & Thomas, 1990; McEwen & Lloyd, 1990b). Assessment of arm placement; hand function; eye–hand coordination; upper extremity tone, strength, and endurance; and reflexes helps establish the functional capabilities of the upper extremities. Lower extremity muscles may also be used for direct selection and/or scanning and should thus be assessed for range of motion; coordination; tone, strength and endurance; and reflexes. Evaluation of pertinent muscle groups and the ability to function with accuracy, speed, and force (pressure) should be investigated, as should fatigue of motor functioning. If scanning and a switching mechanism (i.e., an alternative input device) are being considered, the type of switch and the anatomical switch site must be evaluated. Fatigue inventories with the switch may be completed to yield prognostic information.

Identifying the appropriate size, location, and mounting of the augmentative communication device and/or switching mechanism is an additional area of the motor control assessment. If the AAC user is to use direct selection, team members must evaluate the user's range of motion, marking optimal access areas on the display. If the user is being considered for a scanning system accessed via a switch, size and location of the device remain important considerations, because visual-motor coordination and head control will be involved. A recent investigation by Ratcliff (1994) identified several factors that should be considered along with motor functioning when scanning is being considered. These included memory and cognitive load and the visual and visual-perceptual load unique to this access mode.

Motor coordination and head control are of concern for individuals using eye gaze. The eye-gaze communication board should be positioned so that the user can gaze with maximal accuracy and minimal fatigue. A guide to other pertinent motor issues can be found in Chapter 17.

Sensory Acuity and Processing Abilities.   The ability to process incoming information may influence the ability to maximally benefit from certain AAC modes (Mirenda et al., 1990; Silverman, 1995). Therefore, AAC teams must assess vision, hearing, and tactile skills, especially because individuals with severe disabilities are three to four times more likely to experience sensory acuity and sensory processing disorders than individuals from the general population (Batshaw & Perret, 1992; Kinney, Ouellette, & Wolery, 1989). According to Sobsey and Wolf-Schein (1991), six factors affect this increased occurrence:

1. The same factors that cause other physiopathological conditions may also cause sensory impairments.

2. The same syndromes that cause other disabilities may have a high association with sensory impairments.

3. Attempts to treat one condition may actually result in the development or worsening of a sensory impairment.

4. Failure to recognize and appropriately manage early signs of an impairment may result in a more pronounced or different form of the impairment.

5. Appropriate management of a sensory impairment may be withheld, or at least offered less aggressively, for individuals with more severe and multiple disabilities.

6. Decreased expectations for performance may result in reduced sensory stimulation and an eventual overall worsening of a sensory impairment.

Early detection and management of both auditory and visual impairments are crucial because auditory and visual deprivation may result in functional or physiological atrophy of neural channels (Kinney et al., 1989). Some sensory acuity and processing assessment procedures may be carried out in their usual form to provide valid measures of assessing individuals with little or no functional speech. Other assessment procedures will require adaptation or modification.

In addition to completing assessments that are legally and validly within the domains of the core AAC assessment team, conducting indepth evaluations of hearing and vision may often require the assistance of specialists (e.g., audiologists or ophthalmologists). Because these specialists may have had minimal previous experience in working with individuals with severe communication disorders, members of the core AAC team may provide them with valuable insights into how they can prepare for the assessment.

Members of the team should watch for overt signs typically associated with hearing or vision impairments. For example, individuals with hearing impairments may give wrong or inconsistent responses to auditory stimuli, exhibit passive or aggressive behavior, tire easily, mouth breathe, turn toward a sound source, and/or watch a speaker's mouth intently (Alpiner & McCarthy, 1993; Kinney et al., 1989; McCormick, 1990a). Individuals with visual impairments may be unable to coordinate eye movements, may be able to turn toward a visual source but unable to track with the eyes only, squint, fail to reach directly for objects, or engage in eye-pressing behaviors. Physical symptoms suggestive of vision impairment typically include excessive eye tearing, rapid, involuntary eye movements, crusty or reddened eyelids, and absent or impaired response to light and sudden movement (Jan & Groenveld, 1993; Kinney et al., 1989; McCormick, 1990a). Because many of these auditory and visual characteristics are also typical of individuals with severe disabilities, differential diagnoses must be made. In addition, auditory and visual acuity and processing assessments must be repeated frequently throughout the life span because both senses demonstrate change over time. Chapter 16 provides detail regarding other hearing and vision assessment issues.

Assessing the AAC user's tactile perception is important, because impaired tactile perceptions may modify and distort cognitive mapping of the environment in general, and of components of the AAC system specifically (McCormick, 1990a; Mirenda et al., 1990). "Unfortunately, systematic procedures for assessing this modality are noticeably lacking in the literature" (Mirenda et al., 1990, p. 7). This area may benefit from application of the test-teach-test paradigm in which various tactual enhancements are offered and periodically assessed for their benefit. York, Nietupski, and Hamre-Nietupski (1985) have suggested evaluating and adapting AAC switches and devices for tactile and kinesthetic feedback, as well as for the more traditional auditory and/or visual feedback.

Although individuals who have auditory and visual impairments may be at greatest risk for tactile impairments because of sensory impairment concurrence, they can benefit significantly from tactual enhancements of components of AAC systems. Locke and Mirenda (1988), for example, reported the successful use of tactually enhanced computer keys by a young male with profound visual and cognitive impairment.

Academic and Literacy Abilities. If the AAC user is of school age or is nearing school age, the assessment team may choose to sample the academic skill areas of reading, mathematics, and written language through one of the multiple academic assessment tools available to most special educators. Several of these assessment tools may need to be adapted, but they can serve as a basis for sampling particular academic skills such as reading and spelling. An alternative to using standard instruments is to develop informal inventories that facilitate a response through an aided or unaided AAC mode, thus minimizing task frustration. Additionally, the use of questionnaires, interviews, observations, and error analyses may broaden the team's knowledge about the AAC user's current and projected academic abilities (McLoughlin & Lewis, 1986). During the assessment, the AAC team may discover that devices need to be created or modified to enhance the AAC user's opportunities to participate in academic endeavors.

Considerable attention has been focused recently on the emergent literacy skills of AAC users, and numerous assessment procedures are now being suggested and tested. Chapter 23 suggests some emergent literacy assessments for preschool to early elementary AAC users, as well as older elementary AAC users.

Communicative Desire.   Assessment of the AAC user's desire to communicate must be given tremendous weight in the total assessment process. Individual differences in intrinsic motivation are strongly associated with effective and efficient learning, and this intrinsic motivation is largely a learned disposition that is, at least in part, shaped by past experiences (Bailey & Wolery, 1989). Therefore, assessment of communicative desire must be considered within the framework of communicative demands and opportunities (related to partners and environments), because individuals who have something to say and have expectations for performance in place are more socially charged to communicate (National Joint Committee for the Communicative Needs of Persons with Severe Disabilities, 1992).

Individuals with little or no functional speech are often passive communicators with little history of communicative success (Reichle, 1991). Beyond lack of communicative demands and opportunities, a myriad of other factors may contribute to low communicative desire or learned helplessness behaviors (Guess, Benson, & Siegel-Causey, 1985; National Joint Committee for the

Communicative Needs of Persons with Severe Disabilities, 1992). Such factors include the type and extent of the impairment, the time of the condition's onset, the potential for speech recovery or development, the ability to be mobile in and across environments, the type and success of previous communicative attempts, and even the type and extent of previous communication intervention (ASHA, 1989; Calculator, 1988a; Musselwhite & St. Louis, 1988; Silverman, 1995). No standard test batteries will validly or completely assess communicative desire. This area is most accurately assessed through interviews and repeated observations conducted in environments natural to the AAC user (National Joint Committee for the Communicative Needs of Persons with Severe Disabilities 1992; Reichle, 1991).

Present Communicative Abilities and Needs. Due to their interrelatedness, the present communication abilities and needs of the AAC user may be jointly examined and may also be evaluated concurrently with AAC partners, environments, and devices, because these latter components influence the user's communication successes and establish what communication demands and opportunities exist (ASHA, 1989; Blackstone, 1994; Fishman, 1987; Kraat, 1986; McCormick & Shane, 1990; Reichle, 1991; Shane, 1986; Vanderheiden & Lloyd, 1986). Some insight into the AAC user's present aided and/or unaided communicative abilities can be gained by examining four competencies, which were first suggested by Light (1989): (1) **linguistic competence**, (2) **operational competence**, (3) **social competence**, and (4) **strategic competence**. Refer back to Chapter 1 for a summary of these competencies.

Future Communication Needs.   The ability of the AAC assessment team to assist the AAC user and partner in anticipating future communication needs is critical to positive outcomes. When a team has validly met current needs, transition to needs of the future should be relatively easy and feasible (Beukelman, Yorkston, & Dowden, 1985; Yorkston & Karlan, 1986). In many instances, the information gathered in the initial AAC assessment will enable the team to generate a list of valid future needs. At other times, however, such predictions may be virtually impossible. Even when valid prediction is feasible, the future communication needs certainly may change; change is, after all, a part of the life experience, and often a sign of progress. For example, as Beukelman and Mirenda (1992) noted, "once an AAC user has mastered a device or system for today, parallel training and practice can begin to prepare for one that is even more accurate, efficient and nonfatiguing for tomorrow. Once these new skills are acquired, today becomes yesterday, tomorrow becomes today, and planning can begin for a new 'tomorrow!' " (p. 156).

Tools and Procedures for AAC User Assessment.
Knowing how to assess is just as important as knowing what to assess. AAC assessment teams may use the assessment tools and general procedures described below to varying degrees. Team members with extensive AAC experience and acute observational and interview skills may, for example, use informal techniques as much as or more than standard assessment tools (Beukelman & Mirenda, 1992; Blackstone, 1994; Mirenda et al., 1990). Formal, standard instruments may, however, be used to provide essential baseline data or to provide the objective data necessary to justify AAC service delivery funding.

Standard and Nonstandard Tests. A number of standard and nonstandard test instruments have varying degrees of merit for assessing AAC user capabilities. A few norm-referenced tests can be administered to individuals with little or no functional speech according to their standardized procedures. Beukelman and Mirenda (1992) note that "there are certainly situations in which educational or similar agencies require standardized test administrations in order to verify client eligibility for services" (p. 122). Other tests, however, require adaptations. When deviation from the standardized administration of norm-referenced tests is permissible, they may be useful tools for gathering information, because they contain critical content. Mirenda et al. (1990) noted that "scores obtained under carefully modified conditions compare favorably with those obtained using standard test

protocols" (p. 6). Modifications that significantly deviate from procedures outlined in a test's manual should be reported and fully explained in written or spoken documentations of the test proceedings (Morse, 1987). See Morse (1987) for a review of barriers in using norm-referenced and criterion-referenced assessments with individuals with severe disabilities.

Lahey (1988) defined nonstandardized assessments (e.g., criterion-referenced assessments) as elicitations that sample "low-structured, or naturalistic, situations" to allow observation of spontaneous behaviors (p. 131). She notes that nonstandardized elicitations represent less observer-imposed structure than do standardized test administrations, yet more structural control than is present in naturalistic observations, because certain tasks and probes are intentionally introduced in an attempt to elicit particular responses. By their low-structured nature, several nonstandardized elicitation procedures are useful AAC assessment instruments. Team members choosing to employ nonstandardized assessments must possess a firm understanding of the criterion being imposed. See Tables 11.1 and 11.2 for several standardized and nonstandardized instruments that may be useful to the AAC assessment team.

Test Adaptations. Many standardized tests can be desirable assessment instruments, yet procedures of administration minimize their usefulness as AAC assessment tools. Assessment teams may frequently choose to modify or adapt recommended test procedures and use the tests for their content information (Allen & Collins, 1955). Modifications are often made to "ensure that information is more adequately received (e.g., namely, increasing visual and auditory attending, ensuring proper positioning, ensuring adequate lighting, eliminating glare, and minimizing extraneous sights and sounds)" (Morse, 1987, p. 120). Adaptations or modifications that deviate from the researcher's expected administration, however, must be fully reported to avoid misrepresentation of test results. Following are several suggested test modifications that may be used alone or in combination to obtain significant information. Because these deviate significantly from standard administrative procedures, however, their use precludes norm-referenced scoring.

1. **Alter test instructions and feedback.** Sometimes the instructions from the test manual need to be paraphrased using simpler, less complex directions and tasks to be performed need to be demonstrated. Having to halt the test during its initial tasks due to a lack of understanding would be unfortunate. Although most standardized tests permit only neutral feedback (e.g., "I like the way you're listening"), better performance may be obtained by offering task-specific feedback to confirm correct or incorrect performance. Along with this feedback, positive reinforcement may sustain performance.

2. **Allow an alternative response type.** Alterations in response types do not significantly change the outcomes of assessments (Mirenda et al., 1990; Morse, 1987). Wagner (1994), for example, administered the Peabody Picture Vocabulary Test-Revised (PPVT-R) (Dunn & Dunn, 1981) to individuals with severe communication and motor dysfunctions by permitting use of a binary yes/no response mode while scanning through the four choices. Although no modifications were made in the test stimuli or in the stimuli's visual presentation, test subjects were permitted to use any response mode (e.g., speech approximations or cessation of activity) to communicate yes and no, thus indicating which test plate was felt to contain the stimulus item. Results from the binary presentation and standard administration were highly correlated.

    Cauley, Golinkoff, Hirsh-Pasek, and Gordon (1989) adapted testing procedures to support use of materials that would elicit a forced-choice response from children with motor involvement. Other alternative selections might come from the use of eye gaze to replace a more usual finger point, the use of a number line to indicate test plate choices, or the use of a switch-driven rotary scan.

3. **Alter test stimuli.** Useful alterations of test materials include enlarging materials, enhancing materials (e.g., adding tactual features), or substituting one type of material for another (e.g., using miniature manipulative items instead of pictured items) (Morse, 1987).

4. **Alter the position of test stimuli.** Frequently, the AAC user may have visual acuity and/or processing deficits that result in preferred visual tracking patterns. If such patterns exist (e.g., a vertical scan over a horizontal scan, or a rotary scan over a horizontal scan), test stimuli can be positioned to ac-

commodate them (Morse, 1987). The position of test stimuli may also be altered to accommodate motor patterns.

5. **Adapt testing time.** Some individuals being evaluated for AAC needs will perseverate (i.e., repeat a previous answer or behavior). Others will require additional response time related to their motor and/or sensory processing impairments. Still others will simply fatigue during the assessment, especially if similar activities continue over several minutes. The AAC assessment team should watch for signs of perseveration and fatigue and adjust testing procedures appropriately. Such adjustments could include shifting from one activity to another and/or breaking the assessment into several segments.

Observation.   Observation can serve to corroborate information gleaned from reports and interviews (Wolery, 1989). Observations can also provide rich information not available through tests, because the interrelationships among AAC users, partners, environments, and systems can be examined concurrently. Periodic directed observations may, in fact, be of more assessment value than any test administration, because observation of how the AAC user performs in day-to-day environments is, after all, the real test of the functionality of communication (Blackstone, 1994).

Observation supplies specific information about the AAC user. For example, the AAC user's activity level, attention to task, perseverance, and need for reassurance can all be validly assessed through observation (Buzolich, King, & Baroody, 1991; Calculator & Bedrosian, 1988). Additionally, the critical area of pragmatics (i.e., the ability to use communication to serve various functions) is elucidated through observation. A guide to analyzing the presence and success of these communicative functions (for either symbolic and/or nonsymbolic behaviors) is provided in Table 11.3. These may be coded as present, absent, or emerging (if they can be elicited). Behaviors may also be coded as being successful. The success of a communicative attempt often lies in the ability of the communication partner to recognize the communicative attempt and act on it.

Additionally, information regarding the appropriateness of the AAC symbols, displays, ac-

TABLE 11.3 Observational Analysis Coding Sheet

COMMUNICATION FUNCTION	VOCAL, NATURAL SPEECH	AIDED	UNAIDED
Comment	P A E S	P A E S	P A E S
Direct attention	P A E S	P A E S	P A E S
Express feeling	P A E S	P A E S	P A E S
Greet	P A E S	P A E S	P A E S
Initiate turn	P A E S	P A E S	P A E S
Interject	P A E S	P A E S	P A E S
Label	P A E S	P A E S	P A E S
Question	P A E S	P A E S	P A E S
Refuse	P A E S	P A E S	P A E S
Request	P A E S	P A E S	P A E S
Request action	P A E S	P A E S	P A E S
Request clarification	P A E S	P A E S	P A E S
Request object	P A E S	P A E S	P A E S
Signal for attention	P A E S	P A E S	P A E S
Terminate turn	P A E S	P A E S	P A E S

Note: P = behavior present; A = behavior absent; E = behavior emerging (may be elicited); S = behavior successful

cess means, strategies, and output can be borne out in typical environmental observations. Still further, observation of partners interacting with the AAC user can provide information about the availability, clarity, and duration of communicative cues, and a survey of the environment can provide information about its ability to support meaningful interactions.

Data can be collected during environmental assessments in a number of ways (McLoughlin & Lewis, 1986; Wolery, 1989). Some of these include anecdotal records, running records, and permanent products. Although anecdotal records and running records are both comments on events being observed, running records are usually specific to a particular episode (e.g., ordering in a fast-food restaurant). Permanent products can be analyzed after an event has occurred (e.g., the printout of a computer-based AAC system used in a community outing). Other observations can be guided by checklists similar to guided interview forms (e.g., Calculator & Bedrosian, 1988; Schuler, Peck, Willard, & Theimer, 1989). Re-

gardless of what type of real-time procedures are chosen for analyzing an observation, the events should be audio and/or video recorded. Records and Tomblin (1994) lauded the use of well-controlled videotapes as a means of providing both process and product information during diagnostic investigations.

Two observation approaches that have recently been applied extensively to AAC assessment and intervention include (1) completion of ecological inventories and (2) assessment of opportunities for participation (i.e., the participation model). Both approaches are briefly described below.

Ecological Inventories. First proposed by Brown et al. (1979) as an environmental assessment especially well-suited to presenting a socially valid perspective on the communication needs and opportunities of adolescents and young adults with severe disabilities (Noonan & Siegel-Causey, 1990), an **ecological inventory** has since become a respected and broadly used informal tool for functional AAC assessment with a wide range of individuals with AAC needs. As noted by Sigafoos and York (1991), an environmental assessment is an informal survey that analyzes the domestic, recreational/leisure, educational/vocational, and community domains of the AAC user to identify (1) communication demands, (2) communication opportunities, (3) communicative intents to meet those demands and opportunities, (4) vocabulary needs, (5) communication mode needs, and (6) natural cues and consequences. Assessment of these six factors should subsequently lead to intervention plans that meet these needs, with the specific intervention being of a skills-cluster format rather than isolated skills instruction. An ecological inventory, by its very structure, assesses pertinent AAC user, partner, environmental, and system components.

Developing an assessment tool to use throughout an ecological inventory is a relatively easy yet time-consuming task; the inventory should be tailored to a specific AAC user. First, the team should identify meaningful natural environments and develop a list of competencies required for maximal participation in those environments. Within each large environment, there may be several subenvironments that require different competency sets. The list of competencies necessary for full participation in each environment and subenvironment should be broken into steps (task analysis). The AAC user can then be judged on ability to complete areas of each task independently or with varying degrees of assistance. Participation, then, would not be withheld until appropriate skills were mastered on each step within the task analysis. Instead, the AAC user would be permitted to complete the task as independently as possible, while being provided with necessary supports in areas where independence was not yet feasible.

Participation Model. Originally described by Rosenberg and Beukelman (1988), the **Participation Model** has been expanded by Beukelman and Mirenda (1988, 1992). The basic philosophy of the model is that AAC assessment and intervention must meet the needs of today, tomorrow, and the future, and AAC users should have opportunities to functionally participate on a level commensurate with chronological-aged peers. The Participation Model assessment is built around (1) assessing patterns of participation and communication need (similar to an essential phase of an ecological inventory), (2) assessing opportunity barriers, and (3) assessing access barriers.

To assess participation patterns and communication needs, the AAC team should complete activities inventories. These inventories, similar to daily schedules suggested by von Tetzchner and Martinsen (1992) and others, identify typical daily or weekly events of importance to the AAC user. Patterns of participation and needs for communication are further examined by comparing the participation patterns of peers in the environments with those of the AAC user. Judgments of the level of independence of participation are made along the following parameters: independent, independent with set-up, verbally assisted, physically assisted, and unable to participate.

Assessing opportunity barriers consists of identifying obstacles that prevent the AAC user from having full participation opportunities. Specific opportunity barriers are extrinsic and might, for example, include policy, practice, attitude, and skills (Beukelman & Mirenda, 1992). Access barriers, in contrast, are intrinsic, because they concern "capabilities, attitude, and resource limitations" of the AAC user (Beukelman & Mirenda, 1992, p.111). Specific barriers regarding the AAC user relate to current communication capabilities and limitations as well as to cognition, mobility, and sensory functioning. Once the three informational strands are gathered (i.e., participation patterns and communication needs, opportunity barriers, and access barriers) consensus among team members is needed to implement intervention strategies that maximize change in extrinsic and intrinsic factors that are inhibiting full participation of the AAC user. Because peers of the same chronological age are used as the standard of comparison, the participation model should serve teams well when fuller inclusion is implemented.

Interviews. Interviews are powerful assessment tools that can be used to corroborate information in case histories and reports, information gathered during formal and informal test administrations, or from observational analyses. According to Emerick (1969), an interview "is a purposeful exchange of meanings between two persons, a directed conversation that proceeds in an orderly fashion to obtain data, to convey certain information, and to provide release and support" (p. 3).

Ericksen (1979, as referenced in Larson & McKinley, 1987) has delineated six interactive dimensions associated with traditional diagnostic interviews: (1) people, (2) places, (3) purposes, (4) problems, (5) processes, and (6) products. An additional dimension that may be added is *time*. Because individuals from varying cultures may have distinct preferences regarding the specificity of several of these dimensions, a thorough understanding of the cultural implications of interviews must be sought. Several excellent resources on cultural diversity and service delivery are currently available and should help the AAC team conduct culturally valid interviews (see, for example, Battle, 1993, or Chapter 22).

The *people* involved in an AAC assessment interview will likely include one or more professional team members (i.e., the *interviewer*) along with the AAC user and/or one or more family members (i.e., the *interviewee*). The interviewer is responsible for setting the mood of the interview, demonstrating active listening and genuine positive regard, and also sharing control of the interview with the interviewee. Although many excellent interviews may be conducted between only two people because such intimacy often promotes comfort, in some instances the interviewee will feel more at ease when in the company of a larger number of individuals. Interviewees should be asked whom they would like in attendance. Some decisions regarding whom and how many people should be involved will also be guided by the intended outcome of the interview.

The *place* where an interview is conducted may significantly affect the outcome. Although the interview environment should be private and free of auditory and visual distracters (Flynn, 1978), some AAC users and family members may prefer their home settings. In these cases, the interviewer will have little control over the auditory and visual environments. The room arrangement should generally allow relatively close proxemics between

the interviewer and interviewee. Having a desk or large piece of furniture as a barrier between the interviewer and interviewee is not advisable. Places and proxemics should be adjusted to fit the cultural needs of the interviewee. When the interview is to be held outside the home, school, or work settings that are easily accessible to the interviewees, the AAC user and/or family members may need assistance in planning for the travel and travel expenses (Larson & McKinley, 1987).

The *purpose* of an interview, according to Emerick (1969), is to gather and give information. The specific purposes of interviewing as a part of AAC assessment do not differ from these general purposes, even though the type of information gathered and given is somewhat unique. During an initial AAC interview, the interviewer may be gathering information not available through other assessment modes or may be corroborating information already available. During interviews conducted as part of ongoing assessment, information sharing may be related to examining the functional outcomes of intervention programs that have been implemented.

The *problem* dealt with during the interview is the AAC user's severe communication disabilities and/or related disorders, and their impact on functional communication and life involvement. To ensure that interviewees develop trust and respect for the interviewer and thus share full and essential information related to the problem, the interviewer should present less personal questions first (e.g., "Could you tell me about a typical day at home?"), and hold questions related to attitude and feelings until later (Larson & McKinley, 1987).

The *process* of an AAC assessment interview should have a recognizable beginning, middle, and end (Ericksen, 1979). The beginning of the interview sets the tone of the discussion. If the interviewer senses mistrust during this initial phase, adjustments of verbal communication styles, body movements, and/or the physical arrangement and proxemics of the interview site are strongly suggested. The middle phase of the interview analyzes the severe communication disabilities. Use of open-ended questions and encouragement to thoroughly explore thoughts and feelings may assist the interviewee in sharing significant information.

Finally, the end of the interview summarizes the information that has been shared between the interviewer and interviewee and may often lead to discussion of necessary service delivery. Either a directive or nondirective approach can be used during the interview process.

The *product* or outcome of the interview should be meaningful information both gathered and given. Ericksen (1979) has urged that interviewers reflect on each interview at its conclusion to identify its strengths and weaknesses, thereby prompting the interviewer to further develop interview skills.

Another dimension of the interview, *time*, should accommodate the schedules (e.g., school or work) of interviewees as much as possible. If interviewees are dissatisfied about the time (or place) of an interview they may provide less information than if they were satisfied. Some flexibility within the general time frame of the interview's beginning is also recommended. In some cultures, for instance, arriving near the scheduled time is perceived as being on time (Sue, 1981). An additional issue is planning for the length of the interview. Many interviewees will prefer knowing ahead of time how long the interview is expected to last.

Yorkston and Karlan (1986) have proposed that an AAC interview can be used as a needs assessment serving four distinct functions: (1) generating and prioritizing a list of communication needs and then comparing that list to currently available AAC options (i.e., feature matching); (2) gathering information to develop specific intervention goals; (3) building consensus regarding the service delivery program; and (4) educating the AAC user and family members about appropriate AAC system components and services. To structure this phase of an AAC interview, Schuler et al. (1989) have developed a checklist questionnaire that allows interviewees to reflect on the communicative functions of various symbolic and nonsymbolic behaviors, for example, intents to seek attention, request action, protest, or comment.

Due to its unique characteristics as an informal means of information gathering, interviewing can be used on an ongoing basis during total AAC service delivery. To use interviews effectively, however, interviewers should avoid the following errors (Emerick, 1969; J. Taylor 1992): (1) talking too much; (2) asking questions that allow yes/no answers, as opposed to eliciting expanded information; (3) biasing answers by the wording of questions; (4) accepting superficial answers to in-depth questions; (5) responding negatively to information provided by the interviewee; (6) eliciting too much information in one interview; (7) providing specific service delivery information prematurely; and (8) failing to document the activities of the interview through note taking and/or audio or videorecording.

Assessment of Communication Partners

The National Joint Committee for the Communicative Needs of Persons with Severe Disabilities (1992) has noted the importance of identifying communication partners who are most critical to various communication environments. Typically, the AAC user will have closest affiliation with family, friends, and frequent caregivers. No AAC assessment is, therefore, complete unless it has viewed AAC users' partners as major components in the AAC assessment model.

Perhaps the most critical assessment issue regarding communication partners is to determine whether they contribute to the development and continuance of learned helplessness or to the development, recovery, or maintenance of functional communication (Beukelman & Mirenda, 1992; Blischak, 1995; Fishman, 1987; Reichle, 1991). The National Joint Committee for the Communicative Needs of Persons with Severe Disabilities (1992) identified several areas of functional environmental assessment, five of which relate specifically to individuals serving as partners. The committee charged assessment teams to (1) identify critical partners in each essential environment, (2) measure communication opportunities provided by those partners, (3) compare communication opportunities provided by partners from different environments, (4) determine the number of communication acts responded to appropriately and inappropriately, and (5) identify partners who might be most facilitating to the further establishment of communication demands and opportunities. The energies of these partners would be used extensively during early stages of intervention.

Several other partner parameters, however, also bear investigation. Intrinsic factors include cognitive and communicative abilities, along with sensory acuity and processing abilities. Extrinsic factors include partners' availability in terms of time and setting.

Because an intrinsic and reciprocal relationship exists between language and cognition (ASHA, 1989), AAC partners who have cognitive impairments may have limitations in language comprehension, and therefore limitations in their ability to support the communicative attempts of AAC users (Morse, 1987). Even though they may be AAC users themselves, unless they have familiarity with the AAC systems of individuals for whom they are serving as partners, the opportunity for communication breakdown certainly exists. In close association to these cognitive factors, individuals who have communication disabilities of their own have impoverished communication systems to offer to individuals for whom they are serving as partners (Fishman, 1987).

The sensory acuity and processing abilities of AAC partners also affect the success of communicative exchanges. For instance, older communication partners and communication partners with other impairments will frequently have auditory and/or visual impairments. Although sensory impairments may have a negative impact on interactions involving natural speech, the risk increases dramatically when AAC systems are used. In a recent study, for example, Wasson (1994b) found that older individuals both with and without hearing impairments achieved significantly lower listening scores on passages centering on everyday themes when they were presented with synthetic speech than when they were presented with natural speech. Even for individuals with normal hearing acuity, processing of the synthetic speech signal was impaired. Additionally, individuals from both groups were less confident in their abilities to listen to synthetic messages than were younger adults who performed the same listening tasks.

The "cautious factor" (i.e., the tendency to say "I don't know" rather than take the chance of guessing incorrectly) of older individuals has also been documented in listening research not involving synthetic speech (Cox, Alexander, & Rivera, 1991).

In regards to the extrinsic factor of time, use of most AAC is time intense! Some AAC partners have limited time to devote to communicative exchanges with AAC users, or have time availability that varies across the day. Take, for example, George, a schoolbus driver who is busily trying to board several children while Scott, who is using a VOCA, is trying to tell about an exciting event from the evening before, or consider Scott's mother who is trying to rush her four children off to school, just as Scott is attempting to ask permission to buy a present and attend a birthday party across town. Because of the slow nature of using a VOCA, neither partner is able to devote enough time to support Scott's communicative attempts. If Scott also has extensive or unusual needs from caregivers, yet another time factor comes into play. Under such circumstances, even when time may be available to Scott's mother, she may put minimal weight on communication needs, viewing needs such as feeding and toileting as higher priorities.

Partner settings also need investigation. A partner who is unable to make communication demands and provide communication opportunities in one setting may be quite able (and willing) to do so in others. For example, perhaps George, Scott's bus driver, lives in the same neighborhood. While in his "on duty" setting, he may rarely be able to be a supportive partner for Scott, but on a Saturday, when he sees Scott on the way to the store with his mother, he may willingly ask about the exciting events in Scott's life.

Assessment of partners' abilities to make communication demands and opportunities is complex, with multiple factors contributed by the AAC user, partners, environments, and AAC system. Assessment of partners can best be accomplished through interviews and observations. Repeated measures are suggested to further document validity.

Assessment of Environments

Interest in environmental AAC assessments has been spurred by the move toward functional service delivery to individuals. Search for a goodness of fit between AAC users and their environments requires assessment of (1) the cognitive, communicative, and social demands and opportunities provided in various environments, and (2) the physical demands and opportunities that exist (D. B. Bailey, 1989). Environmental assessments of both aspects may be accomplished through interviews, checklists, and observational analyses.

When assessing the many cognitive, communicative, and social dimensions of the AAC environment, the assessment team will find an ecological approach with situation specificity essential. This ecological approach calls for evaluation of AAC users in each significant environment that influences their cognitive, communicative, or social functioning. Environmental assessments, then, should be designed to measure "the degree to which different environments invite, accept, and respond to communicative acts" by individuals with severe communication impairments (National Joint Committee for the Communicative Needs of Persons with Severe Disabilities, 1992, p. 4).

An essential facet of this sociocommunicative assessment should be to determine the AAC user's typical schedule of events. Knowing a typical schedule will allow the AAC team to determine the ability of the AAC user and system to survive the communication demands and opportunities of the situations. Von Tetzchner and Martinsen (1992) have suggested developing a **day clock** to serve as a visual representation of a typical day's routines. This clock can be completed either by observation, interview, or record review. Determining what typical weekly events take place (e.g., eating out on Thursday and attending church on Sunday) is also essential.

The environmental assessment should focus on opportunities for participation and the communication needs of the AAC user in various environments. Beukelman and Mirenda (1992) developed a systematic method for identifying environmental barriers as part of the Participation Model discussed earlier. They used the Activity/Standards Inventory to determine levels of participation for both the AAC user and peers, discrepancies in participation, and opportunity and access barriers. Beukelman and Mirenda (1992) described five opportunity barriers imposed by society and the environment.

1. *Policy barriers* are the result of legislation, regulations, and administrative policies that limit the full participation of AAC users. School policies that segregate AAC users and/or limit the use of communication devices purchased with school funding to classroom use are policy barriers.

2. *Practice barriers* result from the precedents, procedures, and common practice within a school or other environments that are not actual policies or laws, but limit the full participation of AAC users. For example, a school may not have a written policy that prevents an AAC user from taking a school-purchased communication device home, but because no one else has taken devices home, the staff believes there is a policy and therefore decides not to allow the device to leave the classroom.

3. *Attitude barriers* result from individual opinions and beliefs that affect the AAC user's full participation. For example, if an individual feels that allowing an AAC user in a schoolroom or other group setting will have a negative impact on the other members of the group, an attitude barrier has been established. Another example is an individual's opinion that tests should never be adapted for AAC users (or for other individuals with disabilities).

4. *Knowledge barriers* result from the lack of knowledge about AAC intervention and use options. For example, the family, professionals, and/or administrators may not be aware of the wide variety of AAC strategies and the related assistive technology available to meet the needs of a given individual. There may also be misinformation about the difficulties of using some symbol systems and/or technology that would be appropriate for a given AAC user.

5. *Skill barriers* are related to the limits of the technical and communication knowledge and skill of those responsible for the AAC assessment and intervention plan. In other words, "skill barriers" refers to the skills of the individuals who assist AAC users.

In addition to these five barriers, opportunity can be limited by what might be referred to as *structural barriers* that include, for example, inappropriately designed workstations that do not accommodate a wheelchair into the seating arrangement of a group. Another example is an extremely noisy environment that prevents effective communication with VOCAs. By law, such barriers should not exist, but they do. Professionals must assess the environments of the AAC users to ensure that if any such barriers exist, they can be eliminated.

Physical environmental factors such as space, safety, temperature, lighting, and noise may affect AAC users and their communication attempts and successes. To assess some of these factors, the team may draw information from schematic diagrams of the environment's physical space, checklists that survey the presence or absence of essential physical features, or interviews conducted with individuals knowledgeable about the physical environments in question. The Home Observation and Measurement of the Environment Inventory (Caldwell & Bradley, 1972) is an example of a quantitative and qualitative assessment of a home's physical environment. Additionally, it surveys opportunities and demands associated with aspects of social, emotional, and cognitive well-being (Bailey, 1989).

Assessment of an AAC System

As noted previously, the individual with little or no functional speech will often have one or more aided or unaided means to communicate in place at the time of assessment. Before their initial assessment, these may be as simple as signals for attention or common gestures, or as sophisticated as communication books or boards developed by family members or service providers who initiated intervention. For individuals participating in ongoing AAC assessments or AAC assessment updates, any range and/or combination of aided and unaided AAC including low- or high-technology devices may require evaluation. In general, whether aided or unaided, commercially made or homemade, system components are evaluated to determine their ability to meet the multiple communication needs of the AAC user. Assessment of the functionality of an AAC system as a whole is accomplished by evaluating each of its major components, as well as how the components interrelate. Thus, systems should be evaluated in areas of their major components: symbols and displays, transmission techniques, strategies for effective and efficient use, and output (Beukelman & Mirenda, 1992; Vanderheiden & Lloyd, 1986). When a new or adapted AAC device is introduced into the system, a valid assessment can be made only after the AAC user has had time to practice using it.

Vanderheiden and Lloyd (1986) have developed two tables to determine the functionality of an AAC system's components and subcomponents (see Appendix A-4 and Appendix A-5). The first table (Appendix A-4) provides a checklist for determining the ability of an overall multicomponent system to meet the communication needs of individuals being assessed. The second table examines an individual AAC system along the broad dimensions and subdimensions of functionality, availability, and acceptability. Both tables can be used by the assessment team as a rating scale for judging the functional efficiency and effectiveness of single and multicomponent AAC systems currently being used by the AAC user (Silverman, 1995). These rating scales could use numbers, such as 1 for "low ability" and 5 for "maximal ability," or adjectives ranging from "highly ineffective" to "highly effective." The AAC assessment team might also use these tables to project how components might meet future communication needs by evaluating matching features. See Chapter 14 for a discussion of feature matching.

System functionality can also be judged by posing a series of assessment-based questions (see, for example, Reichle [1991]). Although some questions are specific to communication demands and opportunities, others relate directly to the ability of components to support these demands and opportunities. Inquiries regarding devices might, for example, question the type, size, and display of symbols; the vocabulary represented by symbols; and the selection technique associated with symbols (Hux, Rankin, Beukelman, & Hahn, 1993).

Although "virtually no research has been conducted about how different assessment tasks—receptive language labeling, visual matching, question and answer, and requesting—relate to various levels of symbol use" (Beukelman & Mirenda, 1992, p. 135), the assessment team must make choices of symbols and displays, access or transmission strategies and techniques, and output in an effort to design an AAC system to match individual needs. Locke and Mirenda (1992) have suggested that assessment of symbolic representation is closely related to assessment of an AAC user's cognition. Numerous other areas of assessment are likewise interconnected and should be considered within the context of feature matching.

The work of Beukelman and colleagues (e.g., Beukelman, McGinnis, & Morrow, 1991; Beukelman & Mirenda, 1992; Beukelman, Yorkston, Poblete, & Naranjo, 1984), in addition to Chapter 12, should assist the AAC team in making specific vocabulary suggestions during initial and ongoing AAC assessments. Church and Glennen's text (1992) is an excellent resource on both low- and high-technology devices and may be useful during assessment of AAC systems. Chapter 9 on low-technology devices, Chapter 10 on high-technology devices, and Chapter 14 on technology selection may also assist teams in assessing the functionality of current and future AAC systems.

FLOW OF AN AAC ASSESSMENT

To facilitate smooth progression throughout an AAC assessment (especially first-time assessments), a flowchart similar to that in Figure 11.2 may be useful. As can be noted, significant background information must be obtained prior to initiation of some forms of the assessment. Therefore, the AAC team generally sends a referral packet to the AAC user, family, or referring source prior to gathering other information (Enstrom, 1992). The referral packet might include, for example, a case history form to elicit past and current educational, vocational, medical, motor, sensory, communication, residential, recreational, and social information. The packet might also include consent forms to allow solicitation of reports from

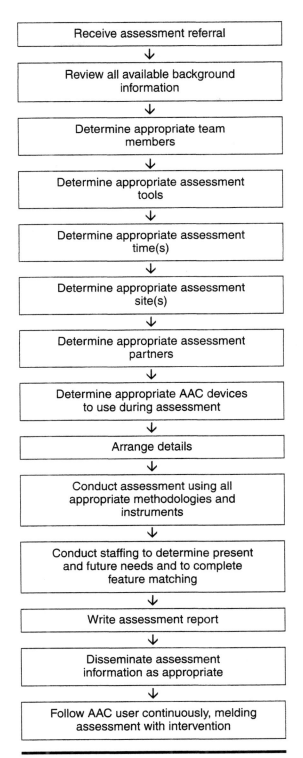

FIGURE 11.2 AAC Assessment Flowchart

other sources as well as permission to videotape assessment procedures. A call to the AAC user and family may facilitate making arrangements for conducting interviews and carrying out various portions of the assessment.

The assessment team may also use an assessment guide that identifies the multiple components or domains of the assessment process. Such a guide based on the items in Lifespace Access Profile: Assistive Technology Planning for Individuals with Severe or Multiple Disabilities (Williams, Stemach, Wolfe, & Stanger, 1993) and domains of assessment outlined by Costello and Shane (1994) is provided in Table 11.4.

TABLE 11.4   AAC Assessment Domains

Client-Centered

- Goals
- Priorities
- Expectations

Medical

- Etiology
- Current status
- Medications

Sensory

- Auditory
- Visual
- Tactile

Motor

- Seating and positioning
- Ambulatory status
- Muscle tone
- Coordination/control
- Fatigue
- Force
- Range of motion
- Resolution

Speech

- Intelligibility
- Consistency
- Endurance
- Voice

Language

- Comprehension
- Expression

Communication Modes

- Nonverbal behavior
- Natural speech
- Aided AAC
- Unaided AAC

Cognitive

- Attention
- Memory
- Problem solving
- Judgment
- Intelligence measures

Behavioral

- Communicative behaviors
- Medically related behaviors

Educational

- History
- Current status
- Learning style

Vocational

- History
- Current status

Family and/or Support

- Emotional
- Technical

Financial

- Personal resources
- Private funds
- Government programs

Staffing

A critical element of the assessment process is sharing information with other members of the team, including the AAC user, family members, caregivers, and perhaps close peers. A formal meeting will often be called. Participants will be affected by the type of team (i.e., multidisciplinary, interdisciplinary, or transdisciplinary) and by such factors as schedules and distance. For example, the team that has followed a multidisciplinary approach may submit written reports to the team leader, who may then sit down with the AAC user and family to share the written information from multiple disciplines. The interdisciplinary team may meet to engage in joint decision making, even if separate disciplines have conducted separate assessments. The transdisciplinary team, on the other hand, will nearly always meet because joint assessment and joint decision making are features of the approach.

Regardless of the team structure, the meeting should follow a structured format and time frame. The assessment team leader, who will often serve as chair or coordinator of the meeting, will work to maintain order. Relevant information shared by team members should be expressed with clarity and lead to the development of intervention plans that yield immediate and future results (McLoughlin & Lewis, 1986).

The physical environment of the meeting should provide comfort and promote eye contact. The AAC user, family members, caregivers, and peers who may be in attendance should not feel overwhelmed by the number of professionals on the team. Therefore, the team leader should avoid an arrangement where all professionals sit on one side of a table, with the AAC user, family members, caregivers, and peers on the opposite side. The meeting should be announced well in advance by written and spoken invitation. Arrangements for transportation may be necessary.

Assessment Report

The assessment team should always generate a written report to document the assessment activities and to set forth intervention goals (Wolery, 1989). Although writing assessment reports is a skill that often requires considerable work and practice, the assessment team must strive for a valid and meaningful report even in its first AAC assessment. Publication of a thorough, accurate, objective, and detailed report can spur team members into collaborative, functional service delivery. Even the chosen display of the assessment information can influence immediate and future service delivery. Recent work in the psychological sciences, for example, has documented that the form, organization, and sequence of information display can lead to changes in decision making (Kleinmuntz & Schkade, 1993).

A rather traditional form, organization, and sequence framework for report writing is suggested for assessments conducted with students with special needs (McLoughlin & Lewis, 1986; Shipley & McAfee, 1992). Key components of this framework include (1) identifying information, (2) reason for referral, (3) relevant background, (4) behavioral observations, (5) assessment results and discussion, (6) discussion and conclusions, (7) recommendations, and (8) appendices and data sheets. Within these standard areas, the team can report information gained through standard and/or informal assessments, interviews, and observational analyses.

ASSESSMENT ACROSS THE LIFE SPAN

Maximal AAC service delivery should be the mission of the AAC team. The team must, therefore, possess flexible styles of service delivery because the needs of AAC users will change across the life span. Although some AAC users may eventually discard their systems due to the development or return of functional natural speech, the majority of AAC users will need lifelong AAC.

Infants or toddlers considered for AAC assessments are likely to have conditions that put them at risk for developing natural speech. They will require extensive family involvement throughout assessment and intervention so that effective communication opportunities can be recognized, reinforced, and shaped toward developing more sophisticated communicative behaviors. The AAC team serving the multiple needs of school-aged children will need to frequently assess and update vocabulary to promote maximal inclusion in whatever educational setting is selected.

As children mature, AAC teams must monitor and assess changing communication needs and opportunities. Adolescence is widely recognized as a difficult developmental period for most youth. It may be particularly challenging for youth with little or no functional speech and other severe disabilities. Issues such as self-esteem, friendship, and dating may take precedence over vocabulary survival in academic subjects.

The young and middle adult years for AAC users should see them move into the mainstream of work and recreational opportunities. Many adult AAC users will marry and take on the roles and responsibilities of parenting. Changes in AAC systems will surely be in order.

Geriatric AAC users present unique challenges to the AAC assessment team, partly because they comprise a group about which little is known and partly because they have multiple service needs. As is well documented, the world's population is aging. By the year 2025, 20% of the U.S. population will be over 65 years of age. Between the years 2010 and 2030 the number of individuals over age 65 will increase by 73%, whereas the population under 65 will decrease by 3%. Many AAC users who were offered some of the earliest AAC services are joining this aging population. Many other individuals who manifest acquired or progressive disorders are becoming new AAC users. The occurrence of communication disorders is highest in older individuals (Hirdes, Ellis-Hale, & Hirdes, 1993). Still further, individuals with mental retardation and developmental disabilities demonstrate the effects of aging more quickly than individuals from the general population, so they may be considered to be elderly at a much younger chronological age (Carlsen, Galluzze, Forman, & Cavlieri, 1994; Solomon, 1988). Jacobson, Sutton, and Janicki (1985), for example, suggested that these individuals be considered elderly at the age of 55.

To assist aging AAC users in maintaining an optimal quality of life well into late adulthood, specialized AAC assessment procedures that are sensitive to their increased medical, social, and communication needs will be necessary. AAC teams must also recognize that sensory and cognitive capabilities show age-related decline and that depression is a common condition of late adulthood. Older AAC users who may already have experienced significant mobility limitations are likely to acquire more. Given factors such as restricted mobility, increased use of medication, fewer life choices, restricted or changing social roles, decreased sensory abilities, and declining overall health, aging adults who also experience severe communication disabilities may suffer great psychological distress. Far too little research has targeted the needs of aging AAC users, but much is certainly in order. The team that is sensitive to the challenges of older AAC users will ensure that assessment procedures identify their unique communication needs.

SUMMARY

Nothing to date has indicated that AAC assessments are, should be, or ever will be quick and easy. The AAC user's communicative behaviors are, like their overall behaviors, "relative, conditional, complex and dynamic. Accordingly, clinical assessment must be relative, contextual, process-oriented and dynamic" (Muma, 1978, p. 211).

AAC assessment focuses on an individual, not on isolated clusters of behaviors exhibited by that individual. The team that has exercised prudent judgment throughout the assessment process will have completed a balanced assessment resulting in a valid profile of the AAC user's strengths and weaknesses, as well as identification of the most facilitating multimodal AAC system that will meet the communication needs of the AAC user within the context of supporting environments and communication partners.

CHAPTER 12

VOCABULARY SELECTION

HELEN H. ARVIDSON AND LYLE L. LLOYD

Communication takes place when one individual, the sender, formulates an idea, encodes, and transmits it as a message to a second individual, the receiver, who transduces, decodes, and responds. This dynamic interaction, described in Chapter 3, involves the exchange of messages between partners through one or more modes of communication. Symbols (e.g., gestures, manual signs, photographs, line drawings, enhanced words, and speech) provide the means to represent. The modes (e.g., body movement, communication boards, and voice output communication devices) provide the means to transmit. Selecting vocabulary provides a link between the creation and conveyance of messages.

Vocabulary selection is frequently taken for granted by typically communicating individuals. Unless trying to communicate in an unfamiliar language, for example, individuals with no communication disabilities usually retrieve and produce words needed to create and convey messages with little or no effort. They typically have a store of words, phrases, and sentences that they can easily retrieve and produce. Individuals with severe communication disabilities, on the other hand, cannot create and convey messages as effortlessly, because words may be difficult to retrieve and/or produce. Their communication disabilities may be receptive and/or expressive, related to cognitive and/or physical factors. Knowing the factors involved and understanding how they influence an individual's ability to communicate are critical to providing appropriate **augmentative and alternative communication (AAC)**. Critical to the effective use of AAC is the selection of functional and motivational vocabulary.

Vocabulary selection is a team task requiring the sensitivity and skill of many individuals who take into consideration many characteristics and criteria. This chapter provides background information on typical early lexicons and linguistic changes across the life span. It then suggests characteristics to consider in the individualization of vocabulary and discusses different sources and methods used in vocabulary selection. The chapter concludes with a case example and questions to consider in evaluating the adequacy and appropriateness of selected vocabulary.

EARLY LEXICONS AND LINGUISTIC CHANGES

Infants

A number of papers relate to the development and composition of early **lexicons** in children (Benedict, 1979; Beukelman, Jones, & Rowan, 1989; Fried-Oken & More, 1992; Fristoe & Lloyd, 1980; Karlan & Lloyd, 1983; Lieven, Pine, & Barnes, 1992; Wilson, 1980) and to the vocabulary and linguistic changes that occur in conversational speech as individuals mature and age (Berger, 1967; Cannito, Hayashi, & Ulatowska, 1988; Emery, 1986; Hipskind & Nerbonne, 1970; Kynette & Kemper, 1986; Stuart, Vanderhoof, & Beukelman, 1993; Ulatowska, Hayashi, Cannito, & Fleming, 1986). Benedict (1979) looked at the receptive and expressive vocabularies of infants, studying the relationship between comprehension and production. She confirmed the findings of previous investigators who reported that comprehension of words outdistances production when infants are beginning to learn language. When she analyzed the grammatical categories that appear in an infant's first 50 words, however, she did not confirm previous findings. Previous investigators suggested that early vocabularies contained only one category of words, although they disagreed as to whether this one category was made up of ritualized game words, action words, or object words.

Benedict (1979) looked specifically at the first 50 words produced by eight firstborn children of white, middle-class, English-speaking families. She found that although a higher percentage of nominals (61%) existed in the earliest lexicons of typically developing infants, all major classes of words including action words (19%), modifiers (10%), and personal-social words (10%) were represented. These findings have significance for individuals responsible for selecting vocabulary for very young AAC users. If typically developing children use a variety of word classes when they begin to speak, then young AAC users should be provided with a similar selection. Vocabularies that contain only nouns or verbs, for example, may be too restrictive.

Children

Holland (1975) reported that early one-word utterances of typically developing children are predominately nouns or attributes of nouns. She pointed out, however, that these nouns are not just used as labels. Holland considered language to be more than labeling or matching pictures to words. She regarded language as an active, dynamic component of communication, and believed that the utterance of a single noun may have multiple meanings. "Cookie," for example, may not just mean "This is a cookie." The child may intend "Cookie" to mean "I want a cookie" or "I dropped my cookie." Holland suggested, however, that initial lexicons for use in language intervention with children should contain not only nouns, but rather a variety of parts of speech. Table 12.1 is an alphabetical list of 35 words or types of words that Holland suggested for a lexicon that could be used in language intervention for young children. These words allow a child to indicate greetings, specific individuals, selected playthings, ownership, location, affirmation, negation, emotions, likes, and dislikes.

Lahey and Bloom (1977) also suggested that an initial lexicon for use in language intervention should contain a variety of parts of speech. They suggested including substantive words (nouns) that refer to persons, places, and objects and relational words (adjectives, prepositions, and verbs) that refer to relationships among persons, places, and objects. Both types of words can be either general or specific to a child's environment. If the number of words in a lexicon must be limited, Lahey and Bloom recommended selecting general substantive and relational words that can be used in many situations. For example, *money* would be preferred to *quarter*, because money can be used in more contexts. Similarly *give* has more potential for use than *throw*.

Lahey and Bloom did not agree, however, with some of the words suggested by Holland (1975) for an initial lexicon. They recognized the value of including *no*, but questioned the value of including *yes*, because yes is often implied and does not need to be said. Lahey and Bloom also questioned the importance of including pronouns in an initial lexicon. They suggested waiting until a child has an average length of utterance of 2.0 morphemes. They also suggested waiting to teach a word that codes an internal state such as love until after teaching a more tangible word such as kiss that codes the manifestation of the state. Lahey and Bloom supported early teaching of a few general adjectives, but discouraged teaching polar opposites and colors. Note that they were actually planning initial lexicons for intervention with speaking children. Many of their ideas, however, are relevant to the selection of vocabulary for AAC users.

Fristoe and Lloyd (1980) considered the suggestions of Holland (1975) and Lahey and Bloom (1977) in planning an initial sign lexicon to aid in the communication of individuals with mental retardation and other individuals with little or no functional speech. They examined 20 sources of sign vocabularies, looking at the cognitive and functional aspects of vocabulary and the linguistic and physical aspects of sign production. They considered categorization, iconicity, whether signs were made with one or two hands, and whether the hands touched each other or the body. Fristoe and

TABLE 12.1   Core Lexicon for Language Intervention with Children

Allgone	Gimme (Wanna)	Names of significant others*
Ball†	Go	No
Beads†	Hate	Scared
Big†	Hi	That
Block†	Kiss	There
Car†	Least favorite food*	Up
Child's own name*	Little†	Very angry word*
Clinician's name*†	Loved activity*	Wash
Doll/stuffed cuddly toy*†	Me (I)	Yes
Down	More	You
Favorite food*	My (mine)	Your

*The specific words will vary from child to child.

†These words represent typical words used in therapy.

Adapted from Holland (1975).

Lloyd also considered how well the 50 or so signs that appeared most frequently in the 20 vocabulary sign lists met the criteria that Holland and Lahey and Bloom used to select vocabulary to teach children with delayed language. Fristoe and Lloyd suggested a number of vocabulary items to guide vocabulary selection for an initial sign lexicon. These words are not presented as the specific words to be included, but rather as exemplars. The basic list of suggested signs and recommended additions appears in Table 12.2. Signs that can be deleted appear in parentheses.

A number of investigators have studied the vocabulary words used by typically developing children. Marvin, Beukelman, and Bilyeu (1994) tape-recorded conversational samples of two groups of children at their preschools and at their homes to study vocabulary use patterns. Vocabulary analyses of the words used in both settings revealed that approximately four-fifths were content words and one-fifth were structure words. Content words included nouns, verbs, adjectives, and adverbs that provided specific information. Structure words included pronouns, auxiliary verbs, conjunctions, and prepositions that provided the grammatical construction of utterances. Of the

words used only at preschool or at home, approximately 98% were content words, illustrating the impact that environment can have on vocabulary.

Moe, Hopkins, and Rush (1982) studied the oral language of 329 first-grade children over a period of 7 years to determine vocabulary usage. They conducted individual, structured interviews in quiet surroundings familiar to the children. They asked the children to answer questions about favorite games, television shows, and exciting events. They also asked the children to tell a story. The children produced a total of 286,108 words, which included 6,412 different words. The most frequently occurring word, *and*, appeared 6.78% of the time. The vast majority of different words, however, appeared less than .01% of the time, illustrating that many words are used infrequently.

Adults

Berger (1967) provided information about the characteristics of conversation and composition of vocabularies of adults by collecting and analyzing a sample of 25,000 words taken from unguarded conversations of businesspeople, white-collar workers, and skilled laborers, which took place

TABLE 12.2 Basic Exemplars for an Expressive Sign Lexicon*

APPLE	DOG	ON
BABY	DOOR	OPEN
BAD	DRINK	PANTS
BALL	EAT/FOOD	PLAY
BATHROOM/TOILET/POTTY	FATHER/DADDY	(RED)
BED/SLEEP	GIRL	RUN
BIRD	GIVE	SCHOOL
(BLUE)	GO	SHIRT
BOOK	GOOD	SHOE(S)
BOY	(GREEN)	SOCK
CANDY	HAPPY	SPOON
CAR	HAT	STAND
CAT	HELP	STOP
CHAIR/SIT	HOT	TABLE
(CLEAN)	HOUSE	WALK
COAT	IN	WASH
(COLD)	LOOK/WATCH	WATER
COMB	MILK	(WHAT)
COME	(MONEY)	(WHO)
COOKIE	NAME SIGN (I, ME, YOU)	(WORK)
CRY	(NO)	(YELLOW)
CUP	NOW	YOU
DIRTY		

ADDITIONAL EXEMPLARS

AFRAID	GET	SAD
ALL-GONE/USED-UP/FINISHED	HAVE/POSSESS	T.V.
ANGRY/MAD	HEAVY	THIS/THAT/THOSE
BIG	KISS	THROW
BREAK/BROKEN	MAKE	UNDER
BRING	MAN	UP
DO	MORE	WOMAN
DOWN	NEGATIVE	
FALL	PUT	

*Signs that appear in parentheses can be deleted.

From Fristoe & Lloyd (1980). © American Speech-Language-Hearing Association. Reprinted by permission.

mostly in restaurants. Berger noticed a simplicity in the samples of adult conversational speech, both in syllable length and vocabulary usage. He discovered that 24 of the 25 most frequently occurring words were monosyllabic. In Berger's sample, 2,507 of the 25,000 words were different.

Hipskind and Nerbonne (1970) replicated Berger's investigation and obtained similar results. The words *I* and *you* were the most frequently used words in both studies. Additionally, the nine most frequently occurring words were the same in both studies. Nearly half of the most frequently occurring vocabulary words in the two adult studies were also the most frequently occurring words in the study of first graders (Moe et al., 1982). Table 12.3 lists the 25 most frequently occurring words in all three studies of conversational samples. None of these 25 words are nouns, which indicates a shift from the frequent use of nouns by typically developing infants to the less frequent use of nouns by children and adults. Studies of conversational samples of elderly individuals have revealed further reduction in the use of nouns and referencing (Cannito et al., 1988; Ulatowska et al., 1986).

Ulatowska et al. (1986) looked at impairment of referencing, the occurrence of fewer proper nouns, reduced variation of noun types, and an increase in frequency of pronouns to the point of ambiguity in the speech of elderly individuals (64 to 92 years). The impairment in referencing began to emerge in the discourse sample of individuals in the younger elderly group (64 to 76 years) and became more pronounced in individuals in the older elderly group (77 to 92 years), suggesting a lifespan continuum of referential decline. In addition, words of greater specificity were found less frequently than more general nouns and pronouns, especially in the conversation samples of the older elderly group.

Cognitive decline may be one reason for changes in syntax and semantics over the life span (Cannito et al., 1988). Other possible reasons for these changes include changes in the beliefs of individuals of different ages about the extent of shared knowledge between the speaker and the listener; differences in the purpose of discourse, which may have changed from information sharing to social closeness; and stylistic variations in

TABLE 12.3 Most Frequently Occurring Words in Conversational Samples (in decreasing order)

MOE, HOPKINS, AND RUSH (FIRST GRADERS)	BERGER (ADULTS)	HIPSKIND AND NERBONNE (ADULTS)
And	I	You
The	You	I
I	To	The
To	The	It
A	A	That(s) Thats
It	It	A
You	That(s) Thats	To
He	Is	Is
Then	And	And
They	What	Know
In	Have	Have
Was	Of	This
On	Do	Oh
My	We	What
That	Are	Yea
Got	This	No
We	In	In
Of	Don't	Here
One	On	Don't
She	Get(s)	One
Like	For	They
All	Was	On
Get	Going	Of
This	All	Are
There	Not	Do

discourse, which may be due to low-level auditory and visual sensory impairments.

Understanding typical vocabulary development and changes that occur across the life span is important, because the information can guide vocabulary selection. AAC service providers should recognize the difference between the vocabulary suggested for an initial lexicon for individuals with delayed language, which includes a majority of content words, and the vocabulary used most frequently by children and adults with typical language skills, which includes a majority of structure words. If AAC users were restricted to a vocabulary of 25 words, they might be able to communicate specific ideas with the words on the suggested initial lexicon, but they would not be able to communicate them grammatically. They would require more of the structure words used by typical communicators. Individual AAC users have different vocabulary needs from one another. If vocabulary is to meet the needs of individuals with different abilities, it must be individualized (Yorkston, Honsinger, Dowden, & Marriner, 1989). If AAC users do not have access to vocabularies that provide success and satisfaction in their communication with others, they may become discouraged and choose not to communicate with words at all. The following section discusses considerations for individualization of vocabulary, which in this chapter refers not only to words, but also to phrases, sentences and longer utterances.

INDIVIDUALIZATION

Developmental Aspects

Cognition. The level of cognition is a personal attribute that should be taken into consideration during vocabulary selection. Many individuals with little or no functional speech, for example, have typical cognitive abilities, even though they may not have been able to demonstrate them. Other individuals have developmental delays. Depending on the extent of delay, individuals with cognitive impairments may exhibit reductions in the number and types of words they are able to comprehend and express. They may be able to use concrete words such as *blanket* or *money* effectively, but be unable to use more abstract words such as *comfort* and *wealth*. Additionally, individuals with developmental delays may have difficulty sequencing words. They may be able to sequence two or three words such as "want kitty" or "I like toys," but not yet be ready to create longer utterances or sentences such as "I want to hold the kitty" or "I like to play with toys." An AAC user may, however, be able to use a longer utterance if it can be retrieved and produced by accessing one or two locations.

Musselwhite and St. Louis (1988) suggested that vocabulary selection is especially important for individuals who are not yet using a great variety or number of words. They outlined several criteria they considered important to vocabulary selection. Vocabulary words should (1) be of high interest to the individual, (2) cover a range of semantic notions or pragmatic functions, (3) reflect the "here and now," and (4) have the potential for frequent and multiword use. Additionally, they recommended considering ease of production and interpretation. Musselwhite and St. Louis suggested that consideration of these criteria could aid in generating an initial lexicon that is functional and motivational. They discouraged using communication boards for AAC users with cognitive impairments that include only words such as *eat, drink,* and *toilet,* because they may be neither functional nor motivational. When basic needs are taken care of whether individuals use these messages or not, the messages serve no real function and individuals may have little motivation to use them. If, on the other hand, individuals are given words for choosing different foods and drinks, the vocabulary would serve a function, and the individuals might be more motivated to communicate.

The criteria that Holland (1975) proposed for evaluating vocabulary to be used in teaching oral language to children with language delays can also be used to guide vocabulary selection for AAC users. According to Holland, vocabulary selected for children should come from the language of children (i.e., include words that are actually important to children). Holland also suggested that vocabulary should focus on objects that are present and events that are happening. Additionally, vocabulary should be selected with regard to the function that it can offer during actual communication exchanges and not for the opportunities that it might provide for the practice of language skills out of context (Yorkston & Karlan, 1986).

Lahey and Bloom (1977) also recognized the importance of these criteria, adding three additional criteria. Other factors they consider important when selecting vocabulary for instructing children with language delays include (1) the ease with which a concept can be demonstrated in context, (2) the potential usefulness of the vocabulary words to a child, and (3) the way in which these words can be organized according to the ideas that can be encoded.

AAC service providers should select vocabulary for individuals that is neither too difficult and demanding nor too simple and restrictive. Many individuals who use AAC, for example, have only physical disabilities. Their language may be delayed, not because of any cognitive impairment, but because they may not have had exposure to the same language stimulation that individuals without physical disabilities have had. They may be quite capable of learning expressive language skills if given the opportunity. Consider, for example, an adult with typical cognitive skills who is not communicating because of severe dysarthria secondary to cerebral palsy. Providing a limited vocabulary of just nouns and verbs would be inappropriate. This individual should be provided not only with content words, but also with structure words that provide for grammatical messages. Care must be taken to evaluate cognitive abilities so that appropriate vocabulary can be provided and communicative potential is not limited.

Age.   Age is another attribute to consider in vocabulary selection. Young children vary in their use of words, but differences become even more apparent by adolescence when latent differences in conceptual development emerge and the range and number of life experiences increase (Corson, 1989). Adolescents have quite different vocabulary needs than young children. In addition to needing vocabulary to create more complex constructions, adolescents may desire vocabulary to communicate popular expressions, which may be important in promoting self-esteem and acceptance by peers. Consideration of age can be just as important as consideration of cognition. If the cognitive abilities of two 15-year-old boys differ, for example, such that one has the cognitive abilities of a typical 5-year-old and the other of a typical 15-year-old, vocabularies should be selected not only with regard to cognition, but also with regard to age. The individual with cognitive impairment should not be restricted to vocabulary used by a typical 5-year-old,

but rather be given vocabulary more typically used by an adolescent. Adolescents who use AAC may be more likely to engage in communication exchanges with their peers if they can do so using the language of their peers.

Just as adolescents have different vocabulary needs than young children, middle-aged adults have different vocabulary needs than adolescents. Similarly, elderly adults have different vocabulary needs than middle-aged adults. Elderly adults, for example, have long and varied personal histories, which they may enjoy sharing through story telling. If they are telling about things from the past, they need vocabulary from the past (Stuart et al., 1993). They may need to include names of prominent persons and places from an earlier time. AAC users who have not been provided with historical vocabulary will be at a disadvantage.

Literacy Levels.   Level of literacy is yet another consideration in the selection of vocabulary for AAC users and is especially relevant when using traditional orthography (TO). An individual's literacy level may be related to cognitive status, but it may be quite independent. Beukelman and Mirenda (1992) describe individuals as being preliterate, nonliterate, or literate.

Preliterate individuals have not yet learned to read, write, and spell but appear to have the cognitive skills to do so if given the time and opportunity to learn. Preliterate individuals include young children who have not yet had the time to learn to read, write, and spell and also older individuals who have not yet had the opportunity. Preliterate individuals need two different types of vocabulary. The first type, **coverage vocabulary**, includes a limited number of recognizable messages that enable an individual to cover a wide range of topics. Coverage vocabulary becomes more specific when it is divided into topics and put on different pages of communication boards or different locations of electronic communication devices. AAC users may have an overlay containing coverage vocabulary useful in the grocery store that includes words and phrases such as "Meat" and "Please weigh these" and another overlay containing vocabulary for a game with friends that includes "You start," "Your turn," and "Checkmate."

The second type of vocabulary appropriate for preliterate individuals is **developmental vocabulary**. It includes vocabulary that individuals are learning, but are not yet able to recognize or read. Developmental vocabularies encourage communication skills by adding words such as adjectives and adverbs to modify nouns and verbs so that two or more words can be combined. Selecting and including *new* and *fast* to a vocabulary that already includes *car* and *goes* enables an AAC user to say "new car" and "goes fast," which can then be strung together to create "new car goes fast." Prepositions and conjunctions should be added to developmental vocabulary to encourage the expression of relationships and more complex utterances. Developmental vocabularies enrich communication. Adding such words as *collie* and *beagle*, for example, to a vocabulary that contains the word *dog* facilitates the richness of language and may even influence cognitive development.

Nonliterate individuals have had the time and opportunity to learn to read, write, and spell but have not succeeded. Nonliterate individuals may be able to recognize sight words that they have memorized, but they are not actually reading. The development of reading, writing, and spelling skills are typically not the main considerations in the selection of vocabulary for nonliterate individuals. Rather, vocabulary is selected more for its value in facilitating functional communication. Care should be taken, however, not to limit vocabulary. The possibility that reading, writing, and spelling skills may still develop should not be dismissed (see Chapter 23 for additional discussion).

Literate individuals can read, write, and spell, so considerations for vocabulary selection are often quite different than they are for preliterate and nonliterate AAC users. Literate AAC users have the advantage of being able to use letters to create novel messages. They are typically not restricted by vocabulary that has been selected for them. One might argue that the importance of vocabulary selection would be diminished, but this is not necessarily the case. Spelling out every word during a communicative exchange, for example, can be not only fatiguing for an individual with limited motor skills, but also time consuming (Beukelman, McGinnis, & Morrow, 1991). Even if

AAC users have the time and energy to spell out every word, not all listeners will take the time to receive messages that are delivered letter by letter. It is often advantageous to have whole words accessible. Literate AAC users can write their own words.

Sending messages word by word, however, may also be fatiguing and time consuming. Yorkston, Beukelman, Smith, and Tice (1990) studied communication samples from 10 AAC users to explore the benefits of selecting sequences of words for storage and retrieval in AAC devices. They found that sequences of three to five words occurred so infrequently that coding them to be retrieved with single or few keystrokes would do little to improve communication efficiency. Coding frequently occurring sequences such as "I have," "I was," and "to be," however, did suggest keystroke savings and accompanying communication efficiency. Yorkston et al. (1990) did not rule out the possible value of coding longer multiword utterances, however. When longer utterances are individualized for the unique needs of AAC users and retrieved in their entirety with a single keystroke, significant improvement in speed of output results. Retrieving and producing whole sentences is useful for messages meant to be delivered in a hurry. For example, the message "Yay, they won the game" is functional and effective if delivered at the appropriate moment. It has much less value when it comes 5 minutes after the game is over. AAC users often require messages that can be expressed quickly.

Interests.   Interest is a key factor to consider in the selection of vocabulary for children (Carlson, 1981; Fristoe & Lloyd, 1980; Holland, 1975; Lahey & Bloom, 1977) and adults (Stuart et al., 1993). If vocabulary does not provide for communication on topics of interest, AAC users may have little motivation to communicate. Interests may be related to cognition, age, literacy level, or all three. On the other hand, they may be related to none. Baseball, for example, may be a topic of interest for individuals of various cognitive abilities, ages, and literacy levels. A 5-year-old boy with typical cognitive abilities who is learning to read, for example, may be just as interested in baseball as a 40-

year-old man with cognitive impairment who has never learned to read. Care should be taken to determine just what topics are of interest to AAC users. Care should also be taken to consider what topics are of interest to communication partners. If partners are not interested in what the user is able to communicate, the user will again be at a disadvantage.

Social Aspects

Vocabulary should also be selected and individualized with sensitivity to social aspects such as culture, gender, and social status.

Culture. Culture should be taken into consideration in vocabulary selection, because AAC users may want to speak in a manner similar to individuals from the same cultural background. If vocabulary is selected by an individual from a cultural background different from that of the AAC user, the meanings of words and expressions may be confused, and communication will be less than effective. Words and expressions that have clear meanings in one culture may not in another (Wolfram, 1986). The role that cultural background plays in communication is discussed in Chapter 22.

Gender. Gender should also be considered when selecting vocabulary for AAC users. Manufacturers of some voice output communication aids (VOCAs) have taken gender into consideration by providing a choice between male and female voices. Individuals involved in vocabulary selection for AAC users should show similar sensitivity to gender differences. Speech and language related to gender has become a popular area of investigation that has provided considerable insight into the similarities and differences in vocabulary and word usage of male and female speakers (Wolfram, 1986).

Social Status. Social status is yet another aspect to consider when selecting vocabulary for AAC users. Vocabulary and expressions used by individuals of one educational and economic status may be quite different and even inappropriate for individuals of another. Vocabulary should not, however, be limited by sensitivity to social aspects. AAC users need vocabulary appropriate for use with a variety of communication partners across a variety of settings.

Communication Contexts

Partners. Wilson (1980) discussed the importance of vocabulary selection with regard to communication partners. In addition to having vocabulary for communicating about topics of interest with a variety of partners, AAC users should have vocabulary appropriate for interacting with communication partners at different levels of formality. Children, for example, typically communicate on a different level with other children than they do with adults, and adults typically communicate on a different level with other adults than they do with children. Similarly, adolescents are likely to speak differently with young children than they do with adults or with other adolescents. A phrase such as "No way" might be appropriate to use when communicating with a peer, but inappropriate when communicating with someone in authority. Similarly, phrases appropriate for communicating with familiar partners may be inappropriate for communicating with unfamiliar partners.

Settings. Although many vocabulary words are functional across settings, some words are specific to certain settings. Vocabulary selected for use by an AAC user at home, for example, might include vocabulary related to areas of the home, daily chores, and leisure activities. Vocabulary needs, however, may be quite different if the home is a private home, a group home, or an extended care facility. Vocabulary for use at school must be specific to the school and might appropriately include vocabulary words related to names, classrooms, and daily assignments. Similarly, vocabulary for use in the workplace must be specific to tasks in the work environment. An individual whose work is putting bows in bags will need the specific words *bows* and *bags* in additional to general phrases such as "I need more" and "I'm done." AAC users who go out in the community need vocabularies that allow them to communicate at a variety of locations (e.g., a grocery store or a bank) and at a variety of events (e.g., a concert or a ball game). AAC users also need vocabularies to communicate emergency situations and medical needs.

Purposes. Vocabulary should be selected according to the communication purposes of the AAC user. Light (1988) proposed that an individual communicates to (1) convey wants and needs, (2) establish social closeness, (3) express social etiquette, and (4) transfer information. AAC users need vocabulary for these purposes just as typical communicators do. The sentence "Please get my math book, so I can study for a test," conveys wants and needs and also transfers a certain amount of information about the academic life of the user. "Thanks for visiting with me" serves to establish social closeness and express social etiquette. Vocabulary can be selected that accomplishes these purposes in a certain way. For example, individuals may want to transfer information in such a way that it is not a passive response but rather an active warning or directive. For example, they may want to have the vocabulary to say "Look out" or "Be careful." AAC users may want to demonstrate a certain amount of power and control through communication. They may also want vocabulary that allows them to supervise or manage.

METHODS OF VOCABULARY SELECTION

Informants

Several methods have been proposed to aid in selecting vocabulary. One of the most basic involves simply asking **informants**. Knowledge of vocabulary that is important to AAC users can come from a variety of individuals (Beukelman et al., 1991). Peers, friends, family members, caregivers, professionals, and others who interact with AAC users can be invaluable in supplying words, phrases, sentences, and even longer utterances that are important to AAC users. These individuals may also provide ideas about topics and vocabulary to support conversation that they themselves find interesting so that they can engage in conversation about these topics with AAC users. Care must be taken, however, not to include vocabulary that partners feel are important at the expense of

what AAC users want. Every effort should be made to include AAC users in selecting their own vocabulary (Yorkston et al., 1989). AAC users can be presented with suggested vocabulary and then asked for a final decision as to whether individual words, phrases, or sentences should be included.

Vocabulary Lists

Vocabulary lists are well-recognized and frequently used sources from which to select vocabulary for AAC users. **Core vocabulary** lists include words with universal utility that occur with high frequency across individuals. They are typically small and include many commonly used structure words that form the framework or grammatical structure for the sentences used in conversations. They provide the stable words that change little from context to context (Yorkston, Dowden, Honsinger, Marriner, & Smith, 1988).

Fried-Oken and More (1992) compiled a single-word core vocabulary list designed to stimulate expressive language and communicative interaction for 3- to 6-year-old preliterate children with severe communication disabilities. Ninety word lists were generated from suggestions made by parents of speaking children and from language samples of speaking children to form a pool of words from which to select a core lexicon. The lists generated were quite diverse with no one word appearing on all 90 lists. The most frequently occurring word, *mom*, appeared on 85 lists. Only 46 words appeared on more than half of the lists. The core list that was compiled contained 211 words that appeared on 18 or more of the 90 lists. The 25 words that appeared on the most lists included a variety of parts of speech.

An investigation by Yorkston et al. (1988) compared and contrasted 11 standard vocabulary lists from a variety of sources including lists derived from natural speakers, teaching English as a second language, source vocabularies designed for use with individuals with disabilities, and AAC users. All of the lists contained relatively simple words, but again, considerable diversity existed among the words on each of the lists. The study concluded that although one vocabulary list may not be particularly appropriate for any one individual, composite lists can be useful, because they provide a larger number of diverse words from which to select.

A subsequent study investigated the advantages of using individualized lists compared with standard vocabulary lists for 10 linguistically intact AAC users (Yorkston, Smith, & Beukelman, 1990). Communication samples were collected from these individuals every day for two weeks in natural settings. The data suggested that relatively short lists of words could be derived for each individual that would meet urgent and personal/ social communication needs that are communicated frequently in many settings. The authors concluded that focusing on the environments, needs, and vocabulary use patterns of individual communicators afforded the selection of individualized vocabularies that were more efficient than vocabularies selected from standard vocabulary lists. They did not, however, recommend abandoning standard vocabulary lists. Rather, they suggested using them as a base from which to select the most appropriate vocabulary, eliminating the words that are unnecessary for individual AAC users.

Vocabulary words that provide for specific, individual communication needs have been referred to as **fringe vocabulary** (Beukelman & Mirenda, 1992). In contrast to core vocabulary, which contains a relatively stable number of words useful to a large number of individuals, fringe vocabulary contains user-specific words that allow AAC users to express themselves as unique individuals. Many words in a fringe vocabulary are not used frequently, but are highly desired for personal expression. Fringe vocabularies are most successfully developed from interviews and environmental and ecological inventories (Yorkston et al., 1988).

Environmental Inventory

Carlson (1981) developed a format for conducting an **environmental inventory** that identifies vocabulary to reflect the activities and interests of children in meaningful, observable contexts. Parents are asked to identify how their children spend their time, and the children are then observed in the identified settings. Parents observe how their children's lack of language affects their participation and note whether their children's activity was observatory or participatory. They then create categories of words that they believe would enable their children to participate more fully. Educators identify which words are at or below the children's developmental levels. These words and others that may be above children's developmental levels are selected for inclusion.

This environmental inventory method can be adapted for use with older individuals who have more fully developed language skills by using structured interviews instead of observations (Yorkston et al., 1989). Questions asked during interviews could include how much time an individual spends in a particular environment, the objects and people who are in the environment, and what usually happens there. An understanding of the communication environment allows team members working on vocabulary selection to generate lists of useful words. AAC users should be encouraged to verify or refute the appropriateness and desirability of the vocabulary that is generated.

Ecological Inventory

A similar method for determining vocabulary needs is the **ecological inventory** (e.g., Sigafoos & York, 1991). This method identifies current and future environments in which an individual with severe communication disabilities is expected to function. A task analysis is done in which activities are broken down into small steps. The steps are written on an assessment form, and an observer notes whether the steps were performed independently, with prompts, or not at all. A discrepancy analysis is done by comparing the participation of the individual being assessed with the participation of a peer.

An ecological inventory provides information on the communication demands in different environments and generates vocabulary that enables tasks to be completed. Inventories often reveal that tasks require a wide range of vocabulary and communication skills. Going to a movie, for example, may require that AAC users communicate to the ticket seller exactly which movie they want to see and how many tickets they want to purchase. If AAC users want to buy refreshments, they must be able to communicate at the concession stand. If the AAC user speaks first to ask for the tickets and refreshments, the messages are initiations. Therefore, AAC users must have the vocabulary to initiate. Too often, AAC users assume passive roles and simply respond to questions asked of them. AAC users, however, must also have the vocabulary to make spontaneous responses. Many times, initiations bring about responses from communication partners, but these responses are actually questions. For example, an AAC user may initiate a request for buttered popcorn, but instead of getting the buttered popcorn, the AAC user may be asked "What size?" The AAC user must then have the vocabulary to respond with the desired size before the communicative exchange can come to a natural close.

Daily Routine Diary

Glennen (1989) suggested keeping a **daily routine diary** to identify activities in which children participate. Parents and teachers fill out a form noting activities as they occur throughout the day. They are encouraged to be specific in their notations. For example, if a child watches a television program or plays a game, the recorder is encouraged to indicate which show or which game. The time spent engaged in these activities and an indication of the communication interaction that occurs is noted to facilitate prioritization for **scripting**. Scripting involves breaking the activity down into small steps and recording what words and expressions are needed. The script should include words from a variety of parts of speech and expressions that serve a variety of communication functions (Millikin, 1997). Children should be consulted as to specific vocabulary preferences. In this way, vocabulary that would be appropriate and desired can be determined.

Dialogue Method

Baker (1986) suggested using the **dialogue method**, which adapts techniques from second language acquisition, to create messages for inter-

action and dialogue. He outlined five considerations.

1. **Age and cognitive appropriateness.** A starting place in determining appropriateness of vocabulary for an AAC user is to think of what vocabulary and language is appropriate for an individual of a similar age who does not have disabilities. Although adjustments may need to be made for differences in cognition, care should be taken not to select a vocabulary at a level so low that it might deprive an individual of the opportunity to develop language skills.

2. **Colloquialism.** Vocabulary and messages provided for AAC users sometimes sound stilted and/or formal, perhaps because writing an utterance is often one of the steps in vocabulary selection. Baker suggested that changing a spoken message to a written one may prompt the writer to make it more formal or grammatical. Although "Will you please come with me" looks good on paper, the more colloquial expression, "Come on," may be just as understandable and even more acceptable for spoken communication.

3. **Vocabulary richness.** Baker recognized the value of standardized word lists as a guide for selecting vocabulary, but pointed out that AAC users need a wide variety of both common and uncommon words or a special vocabulary. Although space for vocabulary may be at a premium on communication boards and in some high-technology communication devices, the value and impact that special vocabulary may have for an AAC user or communication partner can be significant.

4. **Reusability.** Baker recognized the value of being economical with board space and electronic device memory. Although memory for storing vocabulary in high-technology devices is becoming more available and affordable, structuring phrases and sentences so that they are reusable with different communication partners across a variety of contexts can still be helpful. For example, an AAC user can effectively use the sentence, "What time should we go to the football game?" only in the context of finding out when to be ready to go to a football game. "What time should we go to the ball game?" would have applicability to more kinds of ball games. However, "What time should we go?" might be most economical, because it can be used on many more occasions.

5. **How utterances sound as synthesized speech.** Even with the high-quality voice output available on

many VOCAs today, unfamiliar listeners some-times experience difficulty understanding synthe-sized speech, especially utterances of single words and long sentences. Baker suggested creating a con-text by providing a cue to prepare the listener about what might be coming. "Remember what we talked about earlier today?", for example, serves to direct the listener to an earlier conversation, thereby re-ducing the chance for communication breakdowns.

Baker (1997) emphasizes the importance of using vocabulary selection methods designed to benefit not just a specific population, but a broad range of AAC users. He recommends providing a variety of words that can do more than just label (e.g., helping verbs, pivot words). He suggests that if vocabulary does not allow individuals to create and organize word combinations, it poses barriers to personal expression. Baker encourages the se-lection of vocabulary that promotes interaction, language learning (see Chapter 18), and literacy (see Chapter 23).

Vocabulary Selection Protocol

Many variations to the general approach of look-ing at environments, tasks, and routines to select vocabulary for AAC users have been used by prac-titioners. The Purdue University Technical Assis-tance Team developed an inventory protocol for use with schoolchildren. It outlines eight specific steps for selecting vocabulary for use in any one particular environment. These steps should be re-peated for each targeted environment.

1. Identify the environments in which an AAC user participates. A protocol that lists a variety of po-tential environments can be developed and used for many AAC users, or individual lists can be devel-oped for each individual user. General categories such as home, school, work, and community should be listed along with more specific environ-ments listed beneath. For example, *own home, par-ent's home*, and *friend's home* could be listed under the general heading of *home*. Various classrooms and more informal settings such as playground, cafeteria, and hallway could be listed under the general heading of *school*.

2. Note the amount of time spent in each environment per week. Although time spent in each environ-ment will vary from day to day, less than 2 hours,

2 to 10 hours, and more than 10 hours per week provide good general measures to indicate where the AAC user spends time.

3. Select the environment that is highest in priority using the information from the previous two steps. Ask for input from the AAC user and communica-tion partners when making the determination.

4. Record vocabulary required for a wide range of sit-uations and communication functions within the selected environments. Include, for example, vo-cabulary related to actions, objects, and people within emergency and social situations. Include vo-cabulary for such functions as complimenting, apol-ogizing, expressing appreciation, and exercising communication control that comes with the ability to initiate, maintain, and terminate conversations. As noted earlier, vocabulary refers not only to words, but also to phrases, sentences, and longer utterances.

5. Prioritize vocabulary by rating each entry from most important to least important using a scale from 1 to 4. Consider potential frequency of use and power (level of interest and motivation of the user).

6. Highlight the vocabulary items being selected ini-tially. Highlight additional items as they are incor-porated into intervention.

7. Select the most appropriate means of transmission for each vocabulary item. For example, vocabulary for "people" might be communicated through sign-ing or pointing to graphic symbols on a communi-cation board. Apologies might be communicated through voice or written output from an electronic communication device.

8. Make notes that will aid in vocabulary revisions. Vocabulary will need to be individualized and pos-sibly made more colloquial to meet the needs and accommodate the preferences of individual AAC users.

CASE EXAMPLE

Ethel is a 75-year-old female who resides in an ex-tended care facility 5 miles from her home. Nine months ago she had a stroke, which left her with very little functional speech. Ethel can recite sev-eral passages that she memorized years ago, but they are virtually unintelligible because of severe dysarthria. Ethel does not currently create novel, intelligible messages.

The AAC team charged with selecting vocab-ulary for Ethel's VOCA began by interviewing individuals close to her to gain information about topics of interest. Grandchildren, children, spouse, and friends related a variety of topics that they knew had been of interest to Ethel, ranging from handwork to family gatherings. These informants worked with members of the team to write down words, phrases, and sentences that would facilitate a dialogue about these topics. The team members wrote scripts that could be used in conversations between these individuals and Ethel. A sample script developed for an exchange between Ethel and her daughter appears below.

> **DAUGHTER:** Remember when you had the birthday party for the twins?
> **ETHEL:** No, which one?
> **DAUGHTER:** When Sam and Sue were five.
> **ETHEL:** What happened?
> **DAUGHTER:** You decorated the cakes wrong.
> **ETHEL:** Yes, I did. I put a frog on the chocolate cake and a kitten on the white cake.
> **DAUGHTER:** When did you remember that the chocolate cake was for Sue, and she wanted the kitten?
> **ETHEL:** Sue told me after she finished watching me put the frog on her cake.

The script was developed with the help of Ethel's daughter, because it was a story that Ethel had enjoyed talking about with family members and friends over the years. Ethel's daughter watched Ethel's reactions to what was being said about the birthday cake mix-up that had occurred 45 years earlier to see whether Ethel agreed with the messages that would be her part of the dialogue. Line drawings were selected to represent the messages. Some of the messages, such as "I put a frog on the chocolate cake and a kitten on the white cake," are specific to the story. Some of the utterances such as "What happened?" and "Yes, I did," however, can be used in many dialogues.

In addition to creating scripts that Ethel can use to retell old stories to her friends and relatives, the AAC team created a pool of vocabulary to meet Ethel's communication needs in her new environment at the extended care facility. They used a daily routine diary to document events and activities to guide them in selecting vocabulary. Table 12.4 shows two of Ethel's typical activities and the selected vocabulary to support participation.

TABLE 12.4   Daily Routines and Selected Vocabulary for Ethel

GETTING UP IN THE MORNING

Can I get up now (later)?*
I'm (not) getting up now.
What day is it?
Will you get my glasses (watch)?
I want to wear the blue (brown) dress.
Where is my sweater (jacket)?
I want my face (hair) washed.
Do I get a shower (bath) today?
I can do it myself.
Will you help me with this?
Thanks for helping me.

EATING LUNCH

What is this?
I (don't) like this stuff.
I (don't) want more.
I need a fork (spoon).
This is too hot (cold).
Where is my food (drink)?
Will you help me?
I can do it myself.
Where is Edith (Elsie)?
Who are you?
I dropped my spoon (napkin).
I want to go to my room (watch television).

*Words in parentheses are examples of additional or alternative words.

EVALUATING SELECTED VOCABULARY

Selecting vocabulary for an initial lexicon requires familiarity with language development and communicative competence, symbol systems and their constraints, and the communication needs of the individuals for whom the vocabulary is being selected (Blau, 1983). Vocabulary must be individualized, but it must also be dynamic to meet the changing communication needs of users over time. Vocabulary selection is not a one-time task; it is an ongoing process.

Selected vocabulary should be evaluated and revised so that it meets the changing needs of AAC users. Updating vocabulary involves determining how frequently and under what circumstances vocabulary is being used. This can be accomplished through observation and data collection. Determination of the adequacy of vocabulary can also be guided by answering key questions. Several possibilities are listed below.

1. Can the AAC user communicate needs and wants effectively? Does the vocabulary provide opportunity for the AAC user to go beyond expressing helplessness to expressing helpfulness? Is the user able to find out about the needs and wants of communication partners?

2. Can the AAC user convey feelings, attitudes, and opinions to others? Can the AAC user elicit the same information from communication partners?

3. Can the AAC user share enough personal information to promote the development of social closeness and the formation of relationships?

4. Can the AAC user speak about a variety of topics that go beyond the here and now? That is, does the vocabulary allow for the indication and elaboration of events of the past, present, and future?

5. Can the AAC user discuss a topic in some depth? Does the vocabulary allow the user to take at least three turns during discourse on a topic? Does the vocabulary allow the AAC user to express intelligence?

6. Can the AAC user repair communication breakdowns without frustration? For example, does the vocabulary include utterances such as "I need the other board to say what I want to say" or "You misunderstood me; listen again"?

7. Can the AAC user take more than a passive role in the interaction? Can the AAC user initiate, question, and direct?

8. In summary, does the AAC user have the vocabulary to be an equal communication partner?

Haney (1995) suggested putting selected vocabulary to a test. Clearly, vocabulary designed to meet the communication needs of one individual is not expected to meet the needs of another individual even under similar circumstances, but some insight can be gained as to its potential effectiveness. If the AAC user is an adult, one of the adults involved in vocabulary selection could use the selected vocabulary to communicate with a typically speaking individual. This person could also communicate with the AAC user for whom the vocabulary was selected. Similarly, if the vocabulary was selected for a child, a child who participated in the selection process could use it to communicate with a typically speaking peer and additionally with the child for whom the vocabulary was selected. This exercise may help answer the questions: How much communication can this vocabulary support? Does it meet my needs as I engage in conversation with the AAC user? Will it meet the needs of the AAC user?

SUMMARY

The goal of ongoing vocabulary selection is to provide AAC users with vocabulary that allows communication to the greatest extent possible currently and in the future. Carefully selected vocabulary should provide AAC users with the means to create and convey messages and engage in communicative interaction with a variety of partners across a variety of contexts. Recent developments in technology have affected some of the considerations involved in vocabulary selection. Expanded computing capacity and organizational options made possible by dynamic displays, for example, have reduced some of the need for prioritization and decision making as to which vocabulary to include and which to exclude. Much of the technology today allows for the storage and retrieval of ample vocabulary to meet the communication needs of AAC users, even as they become more integrated into schools and communities (Beukelman, 1995). For the many AAC users who do not have high-technology communication devices and for those contexts in which these devices are not the devices of choice, however, prioritization and careful selection continue to be important if individuals are to have vocabulary that supports effective communication.

CHAPTER 13

SYMBOL SELECTION

DONALD R. FULLER AND LYLE L. LLOYD

The development, organization, construction, and implementation of an effective **augmentative and alternative communication (AAC)** system for individuals with severe cognitive and/or physical impairments is a complex task. First, individuals with severe communication disabilities must be thoroughly assessed for strengths and weaknesses to determine whether they can benefit from an AAC system (see Chapter 11). Second, a systematic and thorough evaluation of vocabulary needs must be determined (see Chapter 12). Third, a determination must be made as to whether AAC users' needs will be met by using aided AAC, unaided AAC, or a combination of both. In addition, clinicians/educators must decide whether the AAC system will serve as an augmentation or alternative to natural speech and/or writing. Finally, the means to represent, the means to select, and the means to transmit must be determined (see Table 3.1).

This chapter takes a closer look at the **means to represent** and discusses symbol selection for use in AAC devices for individuals with little or no functional speech. The following discussion assumes that the abilities of a hypothetical user have been thoroughly assessed and that a starter set of vocabulary items has been determined. The question then is this: What symbols should be chosen to represent the vocabulary items? Chapters 6 and 7 described literally dozens of aided and unaided symbols that represent concrete and abstract referents. To design a truly effective AAC system, clinicians/educators must first know what symbols are available and then know the strengths and limitations of those symbols. Too often, practicing clinicians/educators have limited knowledge of symbols or simply rely on whatever symbols are available. In either case, users may not be pro-

vided with the most effective symbols for their communication needs.

This chapter describes a two-phase process for symbol selection. The first phase involves the selection of AAC symbols based on general issues and/or principles. The second phase is more specific to certain types of symbols and includes guidelines on how to choose and arrange them to maximize potential for learning and retention.

PHASE I: GENERAL AAC SYMBOL SELECTION CONSIDERATIONS

Armed with the knowledge of available symbols, clinicians/educators turn their attention to the selection process. An overriding principle that should be kept in mind is that *not all symbols are created equal*. What may be an excellent choice of symbols for one individual in one situation may be a poor choice for a second individual in the same situation. Additionally, what may be an excellent choice of symbols for one individual in one situation may be a poor choice for the same individual in a different situation. Therefore, symbol selection should always focus their attention on users and their situations.

Over the past few decades, several other guiding principles have been suggested to assist clinicians/educators in choosing AAC symbols for potential users. These guiding principles have come primarily from practicing clinicians and educators, with a smaller number of principles coming from empirical research. Collectively, these principles have been referred to as **selection considerations**, and they govern the choice of assistive technology as well as the choice of symbols. Selection considerations for assistive technology are addressed in Chapter 14. This chapter discusses the selection of *symbols*.

A large number of symbol selection considerations have been presented over the past several years (Goodenough-Trepagnier, 1981; Jones & Cregan, 1986; Kiernan, Reid, & Jones, 1982; Lloyd & Karlan, 1983, 1984; Musselwhite, 1982; Musselwhite & St. Louis, 1988; Nietupski & Hamre-Nietupski, 1979; Silverman, 1995; Vanderheiden & Harris-Vanderheiden, 1976; Vanderheiden & Lloyd, 1986; Yoder, 1980). Some of these considerations have focused on the characteristics of users, whereas others have concerned themselves with characteristics of symbols. Still other considerations are relevant to the clinical and/or educational environments. To facilitate discussion, symbol selection considerations have been grouped into 10 major categories: (1) user variables, (2) acceptability variables, (3) use variables, (4) vocabulary variables, (5) intelligibility variables, (6) linguistic variables, (7) interaction variables, (8) efficiency variables, (9) audience variable, and (10) teaching variables. These categories and their pertinent selection considerations are listed in Table 13.1.

In the following section, the individual symbol selection considerations are defined and discussed. Then, suggestions for rating symbols is discussed and a few aided and unaided AAC symbol types are compared. The final section discusses phase II of the symbol selection process, selecting specific symbols and teaching considerations.

User Variables

Clinicians/educators should consider user variables relative to the cognitive and physical abilities of the potential AAC user. The type and severity of *impairment(s)* are important considerations in selecting AAC symbols. The demands that different symbols place on the individual's *auditory, cognitive, memory, motor, receptive language, tactile*, and *visual skills* vary widely and must be matched with individual abilities.

Clinicians/educators should also consider individual *preferences* for modality and/or symbols to the extent possible. No matter how wonderful clinicians/educators think a symbol is, or how well the symbol may meet the user's needs, if the user does not like or want the symbol, it may be useless. Clinicians/educators must also get to know potential users well enough to learn about their *experiential background* and *cultural background* so that appropriate symbols will be selected. A symbol depicting a cow being milked, for example, may be an inappropriate symbol for milk if the user's only reference to milk is a carton or glass of white liquid. Cultural background is also important. Nigam and Karlan (1994) conducted a cross-cultural validation study of Picture Communication Symbols (PCS) with Asian Indians. They found a number of PCS that were inappropriate for referents in that culture. Although presently this is the only known cultural validation study of aided symbols, further studies might indicate additional aided (and unaided) symbols that are inappropriate in different cultures. Clinicians/educators must understand the culture of potential users to select appropriate symbols.

The wide range and extent of disability conditions preclude providing a rating of aided and unaided AAC symbols according to the above considerations. The selection of symbols based on these variables depends on the user's abilities, which must be thoroughly assessed. Service providers must be careful not to overgeneralize the limitations of a condition and rule out specific symbols prematurely just because it first appears that they may not be the best choice. Blischak & Lloyd (1996), for example, described a young woman with hearing impairment who, despite physical impairments, developed some competency using manual signs as part of her multimodal communication system.

Acceptability Variables

Clinicians/educators need to determine the acceptability of the symbols to the potential user, individuals close to the user (e.g., caregivers, peers), and other communication partners in the general community. Spoken language is commonly accepted and rewarded in the general community and is therefore the standard by which other symbols are compared. Individuals who do not have functional speech to communicate rely on AAC systems that may or may not be accepted when

TABLE 13.1   AAC Symbol Selection Considerations

SELECTION CATEGORIES	SELECTION CONSIDERATIONS
User variables	1. Impairment (type and severity) 2. Auditory skills 3. Cognitive skills 4. Memory skills 5. Motor skills 6. Receptive language skills 7. Tactile skills 8. Visual skills 9. Preference 10. Experiential background 11. Cultural background
Acceptability variables	12. Cosmesis 13. Perceived difficulty or complexity 14. Prior intervention outcomes 15. Correspondence to community language
Use variables	16. Accessibility 17. Display permanence 18. Durability 19. Portability 20. Reproducibility
Vocabulary variables	21. Vocabulary size 22. Logic 23. Expansion capability 24. Representational range
Intelligibility variables	25. Iconicity to user 26. Iconicity to communication partners
Linguistic variables	27. Degree of inherent linguistic structure 28. Correspondence to spoken language 29. Correspondence to written language 30. Development of literacy
Interaction variables	31. Potential for assertiveness 32. Opportunity for active participation 33. Face-to-face interaction 34. Projectability 35. Facilitation of independence
Efficiency variables	36. Overall set/system efficiency 37. Rate of communication
Audience variable	38. Potential communication partners
Teaching variables	39. Adaptability to educational setting 40. Ease of learning 41. Ease of teaching

compared to the benchmark of spoken communication.

Cosmesis (aesthetic quality) usually relates more to the acceptability of the aid or device being used to transmit messages (e.g., a communication board, ETRAN, or voice output communication aid [VOCA]) than to symbols themselves. Symbols do, however, have some degree of aesthetic appeal. Some symbols may be more visually or psychologically appealing than others due to such factors as design, use of color, use of detail, and figure-ground differential. Cosmesis—like beauty—is in the eye of the beholder. What is aesthetically appealing to one individual may not be to another. Therefore, it is important that the symbols chosen be aesthetically appealing to the user. Less important (but important nonetheless), is that they be aesthetically appealing to communication partners.

Variables other than cosmesis may also influence acceptability. One is the *perceived difficulty* or *complexity* of the symbols. For example, McNaughton and Kates (1980) have stated that the initial acceptability of Blissymbols is generally low because most people who are introduced to the system perceive it as being complicated. However, once the system is understood, it may become more acceptable. Another variable that may influence acceptability is the experience of the AAC user and/or caregivers with *prior intervention outcomes*. Previously failed attempts at using AAC may adversely affect acceptability of a newly introduced symbol set/system. In an anecdotal report, Reuss (1991) commented that the parents of her student with physical disabilities viewed the introduction of Blissymbols as just another approach that would probably be unsuccessful in improving their daughter's life. Finally, acceptability may be influenced by the degree of *correspondence to community language*. As more and more AAC users move to less restrictive environments, the acceptability of symbols by general education classroom teachers, employers, and the community at large becomes increasingly important. Symbols closely related to the community language (e.g., Braille, fingerspelling, synthetic speech) or symbols that can be readily adapted to the community language (e.g., Blissymbols, manually coded English) may be more acceptable than symbols that

are not as related to the community language (e.g., objects, Amer-Ind, Gestuno). Graphic (aided) symbols, however, typically provide a **gloss** in traditional orthography (TO), which corresponds to the words used in the community.

Use Variables

Use variables describe the basic characteristics of symbols, including **accessibility**, **display permanence**, **durability**, **portability**, and **reproducibility**. Accessibility refers to how easy it is to access the symbols for message transmission. This variable may not be as relevant to the symbols as it is to the aids or devices that are used to transmit messages. In general, though, aided symbols are less readily accessible than unaided symbols, because the user of aided symbols must access them through an aid or device external to the user's body. Unaided symbols, on the other hand, require only parts of the user's body for transmission.

Display permanence and reproducibility are more specifically related to AAC symbols. Display permanence refers to whether a symbol is visually permanent and enduring or dynamic and temporary. Reproducibility is defined as the ease with which a symbol can be copied or drawn in the immediate clinical/educational environment. These two variables are related to each other in that permanent and enduring symbols are easier to reproduce. Most aided symbol sets/systems are graphic, and therefore, are permanent. Generally speaking, symbols with display permanence place fewer demands on the user's recall memory. Unaided symbols are predominantly dynamic, and therefore, are nonpermanent and more difficult to reproduce.

Durability and portability are more relevant to devices, but can apply to symbols as well. Because aided symbols are used with communication aids, their durability and portability are affected by the devices that house them. Unaided symbols, however, are readily durable and portable.

Vocabulary Variables

Vocabulary variables include vocabulary size, **logic**, **expansion capability**, and **representational range**. The aided and unaided symbol sets and systems listed in Table 5.1 differ considerably in their numbers of symbols. Smaller sets have only a few symbols, whereas some of the more sophisticated systems have literally thousands. Obviously, the larger the vocabulary, the larger the vocabulary from which to choose. Larger vocabularies contain a wide range of concepts, from objects to feelings to action words and, in some cases, function words (e.g., conjunctions, articles). As a general rule, symbol systems have a larger vocabulary size than symbol sets. An exception to this is PCS, which contains approximately 3,000 symbols.

By definition, a symbol *system* is a collection of symbols that has a logic and rules that provide expansion capability. A symbol *set*, by comparison, does not have a logic or rules for expansion beyond the original set. Within the domains of aided and unaided symbol systems, one can witness varying degrees of success in logic and expansion capability. Systems with expansion capability tend to have a good representational range and depict not only concrete concepts, but also abstract concepts. These systems allow the user to express ideas beyond the here and now.

Sometimes an AAC user's vocabulary is limited not by the number of symbols in a set/system, but rather by the AAC display. At this point in the selection process, symbols that represent concentrated message pools (i.e., those having high frequency of use) should be selected first, with symbols that represent special messages being added as needed (Goossens', Crain, & Elder, 1992).

Intelligibility Variables

The term *intelligibility* originally was used to describe the ability of people to understand synthesized speech. Because of the technological limitations at the time, the earliest VOCAs used a microcomputer chip to produce synthetic speech that sounded characteristically unnatural and robotic. Several comparative studies were conducted to compare the intelligibility of speech output produced by the early microcomputer chips (e.g., J. E. Clark, 1983; Hoover, Reichle, Van Tasell, & Cole, 1987; Huntress, Lee, Creaghead, Wheeler, &

Braverman, 1990; Nye & Gaitenby, 1974; Pisoni & Koen, 1982). Intelligibility research is still being conducted today, although speech output has improved dramatically over the past several years. Now, speech output may be digitized, synthesized, or a combination of both. A more thorough discussion about speech output technology can be found in Chapter 10.

More recently, the term *intelligibility* has taken on a similar but slightly different meaning. This second definition refers to the ease with which symbols are understood by users and their communication partners. A more commonly used term for this is **iconicity**, which refers to the degree to which an individual perceives the relationship between a symbol and its referent (Bellugi & Klima, 1976; Brown, 1977, 1978). Symbol iconicity includes transparency and translucency, and the absence of iconicity is referred to as opaqueness. **Transparent** symbols are those in which the observer can readily see the relationship between the symbol and its referent in the absence of the referent. The referent is guessable. For example, most individuals would guess that Symbol 1 in Figure 13.1 depicts a house, and indeed it does. Some symbols, on the other hand, are so arbitrary that the relationship between the symbol and its referent is generally not understood even when the symbol and referent appear together. These symbols are classified as **opaque**. Symbol 2 in Figure 13.1 is an example of an opaque symbol that represents "the." Most symbols, however, are neither transparent nor opaque, but are classified as translucent. **Translucent** symbols may not be readily guessable, but the relationship between symbols and referents is generally understood once the two appear together. Symbol 3 in Figure 13.1 is an example of a translucent symbol. Some individuals may guess that this symbol represents "lollipop,"

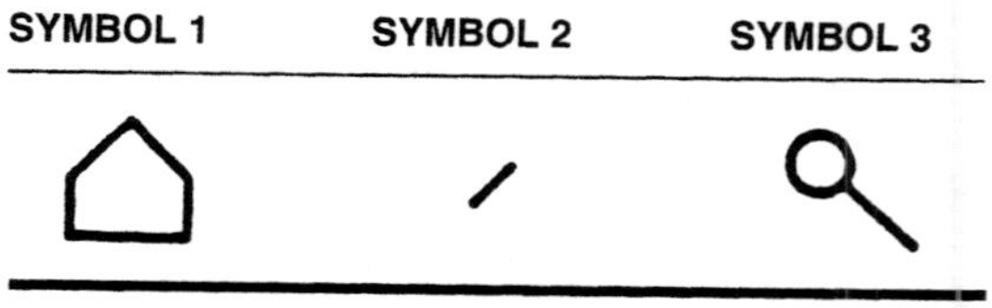

SYMBOL 1	SYMBOL 2	SYMBOL 3

FIGURE 13.1 Illustrations of Iconicity and Opaqueness in Blissymbols

some may think it represents "tennis racket," and still others may believe it represents "balloon." This symbol is not readily guessable. However, once its true meaning ("spoon") is provided, most people can understand the relationship. Iconicity then, refers to the degree to which symbols represent their referents. Intelligibility, as defined by iconicity, is relevant to all aided and unaided symbols, including speech. For example, natural speech is by and large opaque. For the most part, the acoustic signal that is produced when a person says a word bears little relationship to the referent symbolized by that word. A small number of English words, however, do sound like their referents (e.g., cuckoo, buzz, hiss). These onomatopoetic words are iconic. Other aided and unaided symbol sets/systems have varying proportions of iconic and opaque symbols.

The symbol intelligibility category refers to the symbol *iconicity to the users* and their *communication partners* (e.g., caregivers, peers, and the general community). Of all the symbol selection considerations, the variable of iconicity has received the most empirical attention. Fristoe and Lloyd (1979a) postulated what is commonly referred to as the *iconicity hypothesis*, which states that the visual representation (i.e., iconicity) afforded by some AAC symbols may facilitate the learning and memory of symbol–referent associations. In other words, ". . . symbols having a strong resemblance to their referents would be easier to learn and remember than those symbols having a weak visual relationship" (Fuller & Stratton, 1991, p. 52). Subsequently, a vast body of research has predominately supported the iconicity hypothesis for graphic symbols (C. R. Clark, 1984; Fuller, 1987/1988; Goossens', 1983/1984; Hern, Lammers, & Fuller, 1994; Luftig & Bersani, 1985; Mizuko, 1987; Nail-Chiwetalu, 1991/1992; Yovetich & Paivio, 1980) and for unaided symbols (Brown, 1977, 1978; Doherty, 1985/1986; Goossens', 1983/1984; Griffith, 1979; Griffith & Robinson, 1980; Konstantareas, Oxman, & Webster, 1978; Luftig & Lloyd, 1981; Mandel, 1977; Polzer, Wankoff, & Wollner, 1979; Snyder-McLean, 1978). This finding is consistent for children and adults having typical cognitive and physical abilities as well as for individuals with autism and cognitive impairments (except in persons with cognitive impairments, the iconicity hypothesis is supported only when comprehension tasks instead of production tasks are considered). Nevertheless, if other factors are equal, iconic symbols should be used, especially by individuals with cognitive impairments (Mirenda & Locke, 1989; Mizuko & Reichle, 1989). Iconicity, however, is also in the eye of the beholder. What may be a strong visual relationship between symbol and referent for one individual may not be strong for another. Consequently, for iconicity to be used to its best advantage, it must be in relation to the user and communication partners. For partners who can read, a gloss will assist intelligibility.

Linguistic Variables

Linguistic variables include the *degree of inherent linguistic structure* of the set/system, the level of *correspondence to the spoken and written language* of the community at large, and how well the symbols provide for the *development of literacy*. All of these variables are related to a large degree. For example, if a symbol system has a great degree of inherent linguistic structure and corresponds well to the spoken and written language of the community, it will maximize the development of literacy.

Some aided and unaided symbol systems have their own unique linguistic structures, although their structure may not be used as part of the AAC system. For example, Blissymbolics uses its own syntactic structure, which is not the same as in English. ASL also has its own unique linguistic structure. Typically, when these systems are used in an AAC system (for a person who is not a member of the Deaf community), the symbols are simply borrowed and placed in English syntactical order. In ASL, adaptations of this nature have resulted in a number of pedagogical sign systems such as Seeing Essential English (SEE-I), Signing Exact English (SEE-II), and Signed English. Although systems with their own unique linguistic structures may not correspond well to the spoken and written language of the larger community, they are still useful and powerful in other environments. Who would question the efficacy of ASL within the Deaf community?

As a whole, symbols that are an analog of the community language correspond quite well with the spoken and written language of that community and assist in the development of literacy. TO, fingerspelling, Morse code, and Braille are all analogs of the English language because they use letters or codes for letters that can be combined into English words. These are probably the most highly rated symbol systems in this category of selection considerations. Objects, simple pictures, pointing, yes/no gestures, and other simple gestures (when used as the primary means of communication) have virtually no linguistic structure and therefore do not have a high correspondence to the spoken and written language of the general community due to their limited nature. As such, they tend not to facilitate the development of literacy.

Approximation to the spoken and/or written language of the community can be achieved through symbols representing function words or through other strategies. For example, the use of Blissymbolics has been suggested as a means to facilitate the development of literacy because some of the processes involved in the reading of written language are similar to those used in the linguistic processing of Blissymbols. Schulte-Sasse (1991) hypothesized that users of Blissymbolics may have the potential to develop a level of visual perception that is a crucial skill in the reading process. Because of the parallels of Blissymbols and written language, the use of Blissymbolics may have further facilitated the development of the following skill clusters: understanding of pictographs and word pictures; insight into the utility of language; differentiation of word and object; formulation of concepts and word finding; utilization of segmentation in reading (semantic elements in Blissymbolics may facilitate segmentation); and sentence finding according to grammatical rules. Any aided or unaided symbol system that has a large proportion of function words or that approximates the skills necessary for literacy may be easily adaptable to the community language and therefore may be beneficial to the development of literacy. A more thorough discussion of literacy issues is presented in Chapter 23.

Interaction Variables

Interaction variables describe the ease with which a user can communicate with others. Although the variables included in this category may relate more to the transmission technique being used, they pertain at least to some degree to AAC symbols as well. These variables include *potential for assertiveness*, *opportunity for active participation*, *face-to-face interaction*, *projectability*, and *facilitation of independence*.

The potential for assertiveness refers to the capability of the user to interrupt a communication partner, to protest about something, or to ward off interruptions from others. Although some may consider these behaviors as rude, many individuals use them in the course of typical conversations. The AAC user should be afforded the opportunity to engage in these behaviors as well by being given access to symbols conducive to these behaviors (e.g., synthesized speech).

Opportunity for active participation refers to both the AAC user and the communication partners. As a general rule, aided symbols allow for active participation because the aid or device displaying the symbols becomes the focal point of the conversation. Both user and communication partner must attend to the symbols on the aid or device for effective exchanges to take place. Ideally, conversational input from the communication partner should also occur via the aided symbols. This has been referred to as augmented input (Romski & Sevcik, 1988a). When several AAC users who have the opportunity to communicate with each other use the same symbols, interaction is promoted (Mizuko & Reichle, 1989).

Face-to-face interaction is detrimentally affected with aided symbols as a whole because the user and communication partner must attend to the aid or device during message transmission. Unaided symbols, conversely, allow for better face-to-face interaction between the AAC user and communication partner.

Projectability is defined as the ability for communication to take place over a distance. Aided symbols (except synthetic speech) rate poorly on this variable. Typically, the communication partner must be within at least 3 feet of the

AAC user for effective communication to take place. On the other hand, many of the unaided symbol sets and systems can be projected over fairly long distances. This is especially true of unaided symbols that use a fairly large sign space (e.g., Amer-Ind, manual signs, and pantomime). Unaided symbols that are more restricted in their production space (e.g., fingerspelling, hand-cued speech) are not as easily projected.

Facilitation of independence only partially depends on the specific symbols being used. It is more related to the type of aid or device that houses aided symbols, the method of access, and the motor abilities of the potential user. Generally speaking, aided or unaided symbols that are idiosyncratic or arbitrary will require an assistant or aide to decipher the user's messages. This, in turn, inhibits independence.

Efficiency Variables

The efficiency of AAC symbols in communicating a message is determined by the *overall set/system efficiency* and *rate of communication*. Overall set/system efficiency is evaluated by the relationship between symbols and the messages they convey. Blissymbols, PICSYMS, Sigsymbols, manual signs in ASL, and pedagogical sign systems tend to have high overall efficiency. These systems have a one-to-one relationship between symbols and concepts. Aided and unaided symbol sets and systems that have a less than one-to-one relationship are less efficient. For example, all systems based on TO (e.g., Braille, fingerspelling, Morse code) require that the user combine letters to form words. If words must be spelled individually, the user must engage in many activations to produce single words (e.g., Y-E-S-T-E-R-D-A-Y involves nine symbols in fingerspelling to convey a single concept).

Rate of communication refers to the speed in which a message can be transmitted. Because natural speech is the standard by which all other symbols are compared, having a rate of communication that approximates that of spoken communication is desirable. Examples of AAC symbols that can accomplish this are ASL, manually coded English (MCE), Tadoma, and hand-cued speech. A high degree of proficiency is required to approximate the rate of natural speech. Digitized and synthesized speech are capable of approximating the rate of natural speech, but a user may only be able to produce about two to five words per minute due to the constraints of assistive device access and input. Although producing manual signs takes more time than producing the acoustic symbols of natural speech, ASL has much less redundancy than spoken English. An expression in ASL can convey the same amount of information more quickly than a spoken phrase. The net effect is that identical messages in ASL and natural speech tend to be transmitted at a comparable rate. Proficient users of MCE, Tadoma, and hand-cued speech, which make natural speech more visual and/or tactile, can communicate at a rate that approaches natural speech. Not all unaided symbols, however, allow such efficiency. Aided symbols are typically more slowly transmitted than unaided symbols because a selection technique must be used (e.g., direct selection, scanning). When feasible, it can be advantageous to use the same symbol type across low- and high-technology applications. AAC users should have access to the most flexible and efficient symbol types that meet their needs (Silverman, 1995).

Audience Variables

Audience refers to the number of *potential communication partners* available to a person using AAC. Symbols that are equivalent to (e.g., TO) or closely approximate the community language allow for a large number of potential communication partners. As a whole, aided symbols provide for a relatively large potential audience because the gloss is typically displayed with the symbol. Most aided symbols also tend to be fairly iconic so that even if potential partners cannot read, they may still be able to understand the symbols' meanings. Unaided symbols, on the other hand, are generally limiting because most have to be learned by communication partners. The potential audience is affected by the knowledge members of the community have of different symbol sets/systems. A person who knows ASL may have a relatively small potential audience in the community at large, but a relatively large potential audience within the Deaf community.

Teaching Variables

Teaching variables relate to whether the symbols are *adaptable to the educational setting*, the *ease of learning*, and the *ease of teaching*. The adaptability to the educational environment depends on several factors: (1) the degree to which the symbols approximate the language being used in the educational setting, (2) the capability of the user to convey abstract as well as concrete ideas through the use of symbols, (3) the opportunity the symbols afford the user for independence, and (4) the ease with which the symbols can be reproduced or generated.

Symbols that are analogs of the English alphabet may be the most easily adaptable to the educational setting. These include Braille, Morse code, expanded rebus symbols (to a certain extent), digitized speech, synthesized speech, electrolaryngeal speech, and fingerspelling. Other symbol sets and systems that can be readily adapted to the community language (e.g., Blissymbols, PICSYMS, Sigsymbols, pedagogical sign systems, and hand-cued speech) may also be adaptable to the educational setting. Symbols that are easily reproducible on the spot (e.g., PICSYMS, Sigsymbols) also have an advantage over those that are not. The more powerful aided and unaided symbol systems will also allow the individual to express a wide range of ideas, thereby enhancing independence. Independence is also enhanced when symbols are easily understood and do not require an aide or interpreter.

Ease of learning and of teaching are interdependent variables (Hooper & Lloyd, 1986; Hurlbut, Iwata, & Green, 1982; Raghavendra & Fristoe, 1990; Schlosser & Lloyd, 1993b; Schlosser, Lloyd, & Quist, 1991). Because iconic symbols that have strong visual relationships to their referents are easier to acquire and retain, one could argue that these symbols should be taught. However, the *manner* in which symbols are taught may be just as important (Hooper & Lloyd, 1986; Hurlbut, Iwata, & Green, 1982; McNaughton & Warrick, 1984; Quist & Lloyd, 1990; Raghavendra

& Fristoe, 1990; Schlosser, 1994/1995; Schlosser & Lloyd, 1993b; Schlosser, Lloyd, & Quist, 1991). At present, there is not a solid research base from which to draw conclusions regarding the manner and ease of teaching.

Several cross-set/system comparisons have been made on the ease of learning of various aided symbols. In order of most to least difficult to learn, the general trend appears to be TO, lexigrams, Premack symbols, Blissymbols, rebus symbols, Pictogram Ideogram Communication (PIC) symbols, PICSYMS, and PCS (Briggs, 1983; Burroughs, Albritton, Eaton, & Montague, 1990; Clark, 1977, 1981; Clark, Davies, & Woodcock, 1974; Ecklund & Reichle, 1987; Goossens', 1983/1984; Hughes, 1979; Hurlbut, Iwata, & Green, 1982; Kuntz, 1974/1975; Leonhart & Maharaj, 1979; Mizuko, 1987; Romski, Sevcik, Pate, & Rumbaugh, 1985; Woodcock, 1968). This observation should be viewed with caution, however, because it is based on studies that predominantly explored short-term learning and recall of aided symbols. Retention and generalization of symbols were not addressed. Intersystem comparisons of the ease of learning unaided symbols have not been conducted.

Comparing Aided and Unaided AAC Symbols

Symbol selection is a task that requires clinicians/educators to know about available aided and unaided symbols. Through the use of the selection considerations just described, clinicians/educators can systematically evaluate a wide range of aided and unaided symbols to determine which ones are most appropriate for inclusion in an AAC system for a specific user. General comparisons can be made between and among symbol types, with more in-depth analysis being conducted according to the characteristics of the user.

Clinicians/educators can use a rating system based on research, clinical judgment, and intuition to evaluate different symbol types. For example, a simple three-point rating scale (e.g., poor, fair, good) or a more elaborate five-point scale can be used to describe the degree to which each symbol type meets the selection considerations. User variables and acceptability variables that relate more to users' abilities and personal preferences than to symbol characteristics are critical considerations for making in-depth analyses and judgments regarding symbols for specific AAC users. Ratings of the other selection considerations are helpful in making general comparisons.

Natural speech is the standard by which all other symbols are compared. The only shortcomings of natural speech, for example, are its display permanence, reproducibility, and iconicity. Synthetic speech closely approximates natural speech except that accessibility, durability, and portability would not be rated as highly. These variables depend to a large extent on the aid or device that houses the synthetic speech. TO, which would rate high in representational range, has no iconicity. Conversely, pictures that would rate low in representational range would rate high in iconicity. As a final example, Blissymbols would be rated as having some degree of both representational range and iconicity, but not the highest.

Rating symbol sets and systems allows clinicians/educators to make gross judgments about particular AAC symbols based on how they compare with one another and how closely they compare with the standard of natural speech. Fine judgments can only be made when the user is placed in the center of the decision-making process. By taking user characteristics and acceptability variables into consideration, clinicians/educators will be able to refine their gross judgments concerning symbols, thereby narrowing down the type of symbols that would be appropriate. Once a decision has been made as to which symbols (aided and/or unaided) are best for inclusion in an AAC system, clinicians/educators are ready to enter phase II of the symbol selection process.

PHASE II: SELECTING SPECIFIC SYMBOLS AND TEACHING CONSIDERATIONS

One of the first decisions to be made with an individual who is being provided with symbols for the first time relates to the purpose of AAC, because the purpose to some extent governs the symbols that will be used. Will AAC serve only as a means of here and now communication, or should it also provide powerful language that can serve as a

bridge to literacy? Should the AAC symbols include an eclectic blend of several symbol sets and/or systems (e.g., will manual signs be used in conjunction with graphic symbols)? If the purpose is to provide a means of immediate communication (without regard to language or literacy), a more eclectic approach to symbol selection may be desirable. That is, it is often advantageous to select symbols from a variety of aided and/or unaided sets and systems. However, if the user has the capability to learn language and/or become literate, symbols from a single set or system may be preferred for consistency and for the capacity to generate sentences. Selecting symbols from specific aided and unaided sets and/or systems (e.g., exclusively Sigsymbols and Signed English) may be more appropriate than selecting symbols from several sets or systems. If the user is already using symbols in the school and/or other environments, the symbols should be retained whenever possible. When updating or expanding vocabulary, the decision becomes whether to continue using symbols from the established set/system or to select symbols from other sets/systems. Once again, knowing the purpose for AAC can guide clinicians/educators in determining what symbols may be most appropriate.

The remainder of this chapter describes a process by which symbols can be selected for specific vocabulary and how they can be arranged to maximize the possibility for immediately successful communication. This section assumes that AAC will serve only as a means of communication without regard to language learning (see Chapter 15) or literacy (see Chapter 23). This purpose points to using symbols drawn from several symbol sets and systems. The following exercise shows the appropriateness of taking an eclectic approach and using symbols from more than one set/system.

Refer back to Figures 6.1 and 6.2, which illustrate how various aided symbol sets and systems depict concrete (Figure 6.1) and more abstract (Figure 6.2) concepts. Take the next several minutes to study these figures. Observe how each aided symbol set/system (PCS, Oakland, Rebus, Sigsymbols, PICSYMS, PIC, and Blissymbols) depicts the concepts in Figure 6.1 (ball, bed, book, candy, car, cookie, and door) and the concepts in Figure 6.2 (big, cold, dirty, fall, little, make, and want). Then, for each concept, select the symbol that does the best job of depiction. Look closely at the responses. Chances are good that the same symbol set/system was not selected for every concept (e.g., PCS were probably selected for some but not every concept). Instead, symbols were probably chosen from several different sets/systems. If several people were asked to perform this task, it is doubtful that the entire group would agree on which symbols were the best depictions of the various concepts. This exercise is intended to show that *no one symbol set/system has all the best symbols.* This is one reason clinicians/educators must know what is available, must have access to all possible symbols, and must work with the user to learn the user's preferences. Although this exercise used aided symbols, the same could be said about unaided symbols. No one unaided symbol set/system has all the best symbols.

The guiding principle in choosing symbols, whether they be aided or unaided, is that *the user is at the center of the selection process.* Any choice of symbol for a particular concept must consider the preferences of the user. There are, however, other considerations that relate directly to the user. One of the earliest determinations that must be made when selecting aided symbols is the conceptual development of the user. Visual/graphic symbolic representation has several levels of conceptual development. From simplest to most complex, these are (1) identical object to object associations (where an object is used to represent itself); (2) nonidentical object to object associations (where a nonidentical object such as a miniature is used to represent the real object); (3) picture to object associations (where the individual must understand that a two-dimensional picture is being used to represent the three-dimensional real object); (4) part to whole associations (where the individual must recognize a concept although only part of it is being depicted); (5) ideographic symbol to picture or object associations (where the symbols become less realistic and more schematic); and (6) abstract symbol to picture or object associations (where the relationship between symbol and referent is arbitrarily assigned). Generally

speaking, one's choice of symbols will be governed to some extent by the user's level of conceptual development. As an extreme example, selecting TO or fingerspelling (which requires abstract symbol to picture or object associations at the sixth conceptual level) would be inappropriate if the user is functioning at the first or second conceptual level. Determination of conceptual development should take place during a thorough AAC assessment (see Chapter 11).

Functionality is an important consideration in selecting symbols. Individuals must have certain abilities to use certain symbols. Symbols should be as functional as possible. Selecting TO for a blind individual, for example, would not be a functional choice. Braille, on the other hand, could be.

Beyond preference and functionality, iconicity should be considered as a factor in symbol selection for both aided and unaided symbols. Research has shown that iconicity is a powerful variable in the acquisition and retention of both aided and unaided symbols. Selecting symbols that are more representative of their referents maximizes the possibility for immediate success. Remember, however, that iconicity should be in reference to the user. Although determining iconicity for the user is difficult, it is somewhat generalizable to different populations. What may be highly iconic for clinicians/educators may also be somewhat iconic for the user. Until further research is conducted on iconicity, however, this statement should be viewed with caution.

For aided symbols, complexity is also a variable to consider (Fuller, 1987/1988; Hern, Lammers, & Fuller, 1994; Luftig & Bersani, 1985; Nail-Chiwetalu, 1991/1992). However, at present this variable is not well defined, and empirical research has given only mixed results. Until complexity can be more thoroughly investigated, clinicians/educators must rely on a user's opinion and their own professional intuition in determining what constitutes complexity for aided symbols.

For unaided symbols, several characteristics (discussed in Chapter 7) must be considered during selection to maximize success. These include touch vs. nontouch (touch signs are easier to learn than nontouch), symmetrical vs. asymmetrical (symmetrical signs are easier to learn), one-handed vs. two-handed (one-handed signs are simpler to produce), complexity of handshape and/or movement (some handshapes and movements are simpler than others), visible vs. invisible (some signs are more readily seen as they are not obscured by another aspect of the same sign), and one movement vs. two or more movements (one movement signs are simpler to produce). When choosing unaided symbols, clinicians/educators should select manual signs and/or gestures that match the user's cognitive and physical abilities.

Once symbols have been chosen for the user's vocabulary, clinicians/educators should set up the teaching environment to heighten the opportunity for success. As a final strategy, clinicians/educators may want to consider grouping vocabulary so that the easiest symbols are taught first. With a large vocabulary (e.g., 100 or more functional concepts), teaching all symbols at once would be difficult, if not impossible. Therefore, clinicians/educators may want to teach the symbols in sets. For example, 100 symbols could be taught in several sets of five to ten. Symbols appearing in the first few sets should be those that are (1) highly preferred by the user, (2) transparent or highly translucent, (3) easy to produce (unaided symbols), (4) as dissimilar as possible, and (5) likely to have communicative impact. Minimal pairs exist in many of the aided symbol sets and systems (e.g., the Blissymbols for "happy" and "sad" are identical except for the orientation of the arrow). Similarly, many manual signs share handshapes, locations, and/or movements. This is referred to as topographical similarity. Minimal pairs should be avoided when teaching initial sets of both aided and unaided symbols. Immediate success in communication is virtually ensured if clinicians/educators begin the training process with symbols that are highly motivating to the user, highly iconic, easy to produce, and visually distinct.

SUMMARY

Symbol selection is not a process that clinicians/educators can rush through. With the almost overwhelming number of aided and unaided symbols sets/systems available, one must make a systematic attempt to determine which are most appropriate for a specific user. In other words, which symbol sets and/or systems best match the user's purposes, abilities, and needs, with different communication partners across environments? The first phase in this process is to evaluate all possible symbols to determine which are the most appropriate. By using the selection considerations discussed in this chapter, clinicians/educators will be able to eliminate the inappropriate symbols, thereby paring the possibilities down to a more manageable number. Once this is accomplished, clinicians/educators will be ready to match symbols with referents in such a manner as to maximize the opportunity for successful communication. Several variables have been discussed to assist clinicians/educators in matching process, and suggestions have been offered for maximizing the potential for immediate success in communication.

CHAPTER 14

TECHNOLOGY SELECTION

CHARLOTTE A. WASSON, HELEN H. ARVIDSON, AND LYLE L. LLOYD

Matching the strengths and needs of AAC users to the features of low-technology and high-technology **augmentative and alternative communication (AAC)** devices is the purpose of technology selection (Costello & Shane, 1994; Demasco, 1994; McNairn & Smith, 1996). Because of the myriad of AAC devices that now exist, choosing just the right one or ones can seem, at first consideration, like an overwhelming challenge. Errors can not only cost time, energy, and money, but also waste communication opportunities. Throughout this text, the need to identify and provide for the current and future communication needs of individuals with little or no functional speech and/or writing in an effective and efficient manner has been stressed. Meeting AAC users' diverse communication needs for today, tomorrow, and the future in a broad range of life activities frequently calls for **assistive technology (AT)** and always calls for collaborative teams. Professional and nonprofessional members of AAC

service delivery teams must conjointly participate in selecting technology and determining goodness of fit (Beukelman & Mirenda, 1992; Fried-Oken, 1992). This process of matching the features of technologies to the strengths and needs of users has come to be known as **feature matching**.

As indicated in Chapter 11, the assessment process involves consideration of the AAC user, partners, environments, and AAC system. Table 14.1 provides a sequence of the steps involved in selecting AAC devices. Steps 1 through 4 were previously discussed in Chapters 11, 12, and 13. Step 10 will be discussed later, in Chapter 21. This chapter will focus on steps 5 through 9. This chapter discusses (1) the roles and responsibilities of the AAC service delivery teams in selecting technology, (2) technology selection variables to be considered, (3) the process of feature matching, (4) the purpose and process of evaluating trial use during the selection process.

TABLE 14.1 Steps Involved in Selecting AAC Devices

1. Assess AAC user.
2. Assess partners.
3. Assess current and future communication environments.
4. Assess the AAC user's vocabulary needs and the symbols to represent the vocabulary/messages.
5. Determine the relevant features needed to meet the AAC user's needs, considering partners and environments.
6. Identify devices that have most of the desired features.
7. Narrow list to two or three devices that represent a goodness of fit.
8. Conduct trials with selected devices, modifying devices and clinical approaches as necessary.
9. Select most appropriate device.
10. Assist in procuring device and appropriate further training in its effective use.

ROLES AND RESPONSIBILITIES IN SELECTING TECHNOLOGY

Just as no single member of the AAC service delivery team will be able to identify the current and projected communication needs of individuals with little or no functional speech, no single team member will be capable of selecting the most appropriate AAC technology. Feature matching, then, should be the joint endeavor of several, if not all, team members. AAC users and their family members hold key roles in that they will have personal information regarding current and projected communication needs. Their input is also essential in determining the acceptability of recommended and implemented technology.

The roles and responsibilities of professional members of assistive technology service delivery teams in guiding technology selection have been discussed by numerous authors (e.g., Golinker, 1992; Parette et al., 1993; Uslan, 1992). Several AT selection themes have emerged that have direct applicability to the selection of AAC technology. Parette and colleagues (1993), for example, noted that the professional members of service delivery teams must (1) identify specific characteristics of individuals needing AT, (2) identify characteristics of available technology, and (3) arrange a best fit between individuals and technology. These broad feature-matching roles and responsibilities take on greater specificity as they are put into action; therefore, one or more members of the AAC service delivery team must possess low- and high-technology expertise to meet AAC technology selection challenges. A number of technology selection responsibilities that continue well beyond the initial process of technology selection during intervention are listed below (Golinker, 1992; Parette et al., 1993; Uslan, 1992, Yaida & Rubin, 1992).

1. Establish, conduct, and monitor trial use with AAC and other AT.
2. Select appropriate AAC and other AT.
3. Conduct administrative activities related to acquisition and use of AAC and other AT.
4. Train user for appropriate use of AAC and other AT.
5. Maintain AAC and other AT.
6. Assist in partner acceptance of AAC and other AT.
7. Modify environment to support the use of AAC and other AT.
8. Evaluate the suitability of selected AAC and other AT.
9. Assist in the development, modification, and/or upgrade of AAC and other AT.

TECHNOLOGY SELECTION VARIABLES

Making technology selection decisions as part of AAC service delivery is a challenging process. In addition to making general decisions about how low- and/or high-technology devices might effectively and efficiently blend with unaided systems to meet current and projected communication needs, specific decisions must be made about selecting specific low- and/or high-technology. Decisions are complex because they are shaped by multiple interrelated user, partner, environmental, and device variables that influence the appropriateness of one group of devices or specific piece of technology over another (Beukelman, Yorkston, & Dowden, 1985; Fried-Oken, 1992).

In general, AAC technology selection is based on selecting devices that (1) provide the desired symbol set or system, (2) support ease of access, (3) have the necessary output(s), and (4) meet special needs or considerations. For example, for one individual, technology may be needed to provide a symbol system that would allow construction of infinite communication messages, support the use of an expanded keyboard switching mechanism as an interface between the user and a computer, allow for both speech and print output, and support upgrades to accommodate for changing needs.

As part of their work on a symbol taxonomy, Fuller, Lloyd, and Schlosser (1991) determined that nearly 50 discrete AAC selection variables exist in the AAC literature. These variables may be grouped into areas of (1) functionality/ability to meet needs, (2) availability/useability, and (3) acceptability/compatibility, as they were by Vanderheiden and Lloyd (1986) (see Appendix A-5, Functional Dimensions of Individual System Components). Several others (e.g., Cress & French,

1994; Cress & Goltz, 1989; Demasco, 1994; Goodenough-Trepagnier, 1994; Koester & Levine, 1994; Light, 1989; Light & Lindsay, 1991) have suggested design goals or variables to be considered in selecting AAC technology. Devices that (1) support learnability, (2) promote consistency, (3) provide immediate utility, (4) promote spontaneity, (5) minimize motor demands, (6) minimize cognitive/memory demands, (7) minimize attention shifting, and (8) support updates/upgrades should receive high consideration when selecting devices for trial use. Each of these eight variables is briefly discussed below relative to the abilities and needs of the user.

Learnability

Device mastery is a critical issue in the selection of AT. Learning basic competence and developing proficient and sophisticated use of a communication device should be within the abilities of the user (Goodenough-Trepagnier, 1994). When learning to use a device is too complex, users may be tempted to discard the technology. As devices are considered and selected for trial use, ease of learning should be heavily weighed.

Consistency

AAC service providers should ensure that skills learned in device training are generalizable to later-learned aspects of the device's operation (Goodenough-Trepagnier, 1994), and that a communication device is compatible (or consistent) with other products that the AAC user may have mastered. For instance, if an AAC user has had experience with standard keyboards, considering systems that have QWERTY arrangements seems appropriate.

Immediate Utility

Although service providers generally agree that the use of technology should lead to immediate improvement in communication, achieving instant benefits with either low or high technology is often difficult (Goodenough-Trepagnier, 1994).

With multiple device characteristics interrelating with multiple user, partner, and environmental variables, an extended period of practice with the AAC device(s) selected may temporarily interrupt communication growth (Smith-Lewis, 1994). Although achieving a "best fit" on all features may be difficult, some immediate, positive change in communication will help maintain enthusiasm for further use and learning.

Spontaneity

The production of speech and/or print output via AAC devices is much slower than the production of natural speech. Therefore, for many AAC users, communication rate or spontaneity is an important judge of technology success (Vanderheiden & Kelso, 1987). Various rate enhancers have become an almost standard part of several current AAC devices. Word prediction and abbreviation expansion, for example, have been found to enhance rate for many AAC users but not all (e.g., individuals who have difficulty shifting gaze from the main part of a computer screen to a corner inset with word choices). Other less obvious device features that promote rate and spontaneity include on-line systems and screen organizers. If these features are new to the AAC user, a part of the trial process may be to teach their use so that overall proficient use of the device is possible.

Motor Demands

Successful use of AT will be influenced by physical performance capabilities (Beukelman & Mirenda, 1992; Demasco, 1994; Ratcliff, 1994). Motor skills required of technology, in and of themselves, are important because extensive motor demands fatigue technology users. Additionally, when motor demands are high, cognitive demands are also high. Goodenough-Trepagnier (1994) noted that "the more difficult the motor task, the more we concentrate, to the exclusion of whatever else is going on, even if we are not visually guiding our actions" (p. 5). Recent work by Ratcliff (1994) further addressed motor demands, specifically as they apply to AAC devices using scanning as an access mode. Ratcliff noted that several factors should be evaluated conjointly with motor functioning such as memory and cognitive loads and visual and visual-perceptual loads when scanning is being considered.

Goodness of fit has been achieved when a device minimally taxes the motor system. Information regarding such motor demands, however, can frequently be ascertained only after a period of device use, because consistency, speed, and economy of motor activity typically improve with device use (Treviranus, 1994). In fact, in addition to developing a cognitive awareness of the elements and locations of device features, most users develop a motor patterning impression that facilitates efficient and effective use. For most individuals, such automaticity emerges only after extensive practice (Koester & Levine, 1994). Therefore, a period of use with any device is necessary prior to procurement.

Cognitive/Memory Demands

Considerable attention has recently been focused on the cognitive load that is inherent in achieving operational competence with many AAC devices (e.g., Cress & French, 1994; Cress & Goltz, 1989; Demasco, 1994; Koester & Levine, 1994; Light, 1989; Light & Lindsay, 1991). Multiple interrelated elements of a device (e.g., access mode, symbols and symbol arrangement, and output) are noted to concomitantly influence cognitive load. Recent attempts to add more and more desirable features to devices has brought with it increased cognitive complexity. For example, when certain features (e.g., abbreviation expansion) are available in a device, but are not readily visible, the cognitive load required to recall and access them is sometimes so heavy that the AAC user may actually avoid their use (Demasco, 1994). When so much mental energy is invested in achieving the means to an end (i.e., message constructions), then too little may be left to achieve the end itself (i.e., functional communication) (Treviranus, 1994). As with motor demands, cognitive demands may be truly assessed only after trials with devices, because experience facilitates fine-tuning and automatic, effortless use (Goodenough-Trepagnier, 1994).

Attention Shifting

In general, AAC users should be provided with devices that require minimal attention shifting (Goodenough-Trepagnier, 1994). This may involve shifting from one visual focus to another (e.g., from the location of the switch to the location of the communication display in a scanning system), from one type of sensory information to another (e.g., auditory to visual), or even from an AAC device to a communication partner. Devices should be chosen that require minimal monitoring of auditory or visual features, so that energies can be conserved for the actual process of communication. Although everyone expends some energy monitoring the sensory demands of the communication process, speaking individuals do so using minimal mental energy. AAC service delivery teams should seek those devices that minimize the energy required to monitor device features and shift from one sensory modality to another (Demasco, 1994).

The auditory scanning option of high-technology AAC devices that was developed primarily as a feature to assist individuals who needed an alternative to visual scanning (e.g., those with visual impairments) (Piché & Reichle, 1991) may be considered as a means of reducing attention-shifting demands for a broader population of AAC users. With auditory scanning, AAC users may be more fully supported in their attempts to maintain communication as a primarily auditory event.

Updates/Upgrades

Advancements in AAC technology are likely to continue at the present or an even faster rate, as inventors and modifiers of technology provide updates/upgrades for AAC users. Additionally, AAC user needs will change whereby device features that were once not essential become so. One goal of technology selection should be to acquire devices that easily and inexpensively support updates/upgrades, while minimizing the need for new learning (Smith-Lewis, 1994; Treviranus, 1994). AAC service delivery teams should select technology that can grow and evolve with the user and the advances of the field without forcing the abandonment of previously mastered skills. The team must predict skill acquisition and device modifications in its attempt to achieve current and projected goodness of fit.

Although update/upgrade variables apply most often to high-technology devices, they must also be considered when selecting low-technology devices. Adding new vocabulary, shifting from one symbol type to another, or rearranging an existing display may all disrupt the current level of low-technology device functioning. Therefore, teams must engage in forward thinking in anticipation of the effects of updates/upgrades.

Decisions to update/upgrade both low technology and high technology must not only be well justified, but also appropriately timed. When a current device is providing appropriate communication support, but an upgrade is available, service providers may want to gradually introduce the change or postpone its introduction to some other time. For example, if a school-aged child is being provided with a high-technology upgrade to facilitate fuller educational inclusion, the summer months may be a more appropriate time to introduce and practice the upgraded device than the school months, when demands for effective and efficient use are higher (Beukelman & Mirenda, 1992).

FEATURE MATCHING

After considering user, partner, environmental, and device variables, clinicians/educators begin the feature-matching process (steps 5 and 6 in Table 14.1). Feature matching must be considered against the backdrop of both current and future communication needs. AAC teams typically develop a set of device features to match to an individual's needs. For example, the transdisciplinary Purdue-GLASS (Greater Lafayette Area Special Services) AAC Assessment Team has a basic list of more than 30 features it considers when devices are evaluated, including the following:

1. Direct selection
2. Auditory scanning
3. Visual scanning
4. Switch capability (switch type)
5. Activation feedback (auditory, tactile, visual)
6. Flexible grid size (variable size cells)
7. Voice output (digitized, synthesized)
8. Text-to-speech capability
9. Visual display (static, dynamic, color)
10. Monitor glareguard
11. Visual clarity
12. Print output
13. Accessories
14. Mounting capability
15. Portability (size, weight, carrying case)
16. Durability
17. Moisture resistance
18. Keyguard (availability)
19. Ease of programming
20. Technical support
21. Computer interface
22. Environmental control
23. Memory: multiple levels
24. Vocabulary size
25. Symbols available
26. Symbol sequencing potential
27. Expanded keyboard
28. Adjustable activation delay
29. No repeat function
30. Cost
31. Other

Figure 14.1 is an example of a feature matching worksheet developed by the Purdue-GLASS AAC Assessment Team for John. The left column lists 18 features that would meet his needs. Three devices that have been identified as having most of these features appear across the top. Notations in the individual cells indicate presence and/or specific information about the features that enable the team to determine the most appropriate devices for trial use. John, a 5-year-old with good cognitive abilities but severe physical impairments, was enrolled in a self-contained kindergarten program. He required a voice output communication aid (VOCA) that could accommodate both traditional orthography (TO) and other graphic symbols, which he could access with his right index finger. Because of the tendency to drag his hand and his fluctuating range of motion, John needed a keyboard with flexible cell sizes and a keyguard. He had questionable visual difficulties and required auditory feedback for cell activations and a static visual display. Special features he needed included a computer interface so he could print out his

NAME: JOHN	DATE:		
NEEDS/FEATURES	**DEVICE A**	**DEVICE B**	**DEVICE C**
Direct selection	√	√	√
Auditory activation feedback	√	√	√
Flexible grid size (variable size cells)	√	√	√
Voice output	Digitized and synthesized	Synthesized	Digitized and synthesized
Text-to-speech	√	√	√
Static visual display	√	√	
Visual clarity	√	√	
Mounting capability	√	√	√
Durability	√	√	√
Keyguard	√	√	√
Technical support	√	√	√
Computer interface	√	√	√
Environmental control	√	√	√
Extended memory	√	√	√
Symbol types	Any	Any	Manufacturer's only
Symbol sequencing potential	√	√	
Adjustable activation delay	√	√	√
No-Repeat function	√	√	√

FIGURE 14.1 Sample Feature-Matching Worksheet

drawings and written work, adjustable activation delays so the length of time a cell must be activated could be adjusted based upon his fatigue level, and a no-repeat function so if his hand or finger rested on a key, it would only produce a single character or command.

Three devices were identified by the team to be procured for trial use. Low-technology communication displays were developed that matched the device displays as well. It was recommended that John use these displays when device use was not feasible (e.g., in the bathtub, riding the bus).

Recently, several individuals have developed software to facilitate the feature-matching process (Garrett et al., 1990; McNairn & Smith, 1996). McNairn & Smith (1996) developed a tool for matching an individual's strengths and needs with device features. The *AAC Feature Match Software* contains a device database with information on more than 120 devices from more than 20 manufacturers. There are nine main categories of features related to (1) language organization/encoding methods, (2) speech output, (3) direct selection and scanning/switch input, (4) keyboards, (5) switch types, (6) display types, (7) mounting options, (8) power sources, and (9) support options and additional features. Appendix A-6 provides a copy of the Feature Checklist form indicating all the features in the device database. The most critical aspects of developing a feature-matching worksheet or using feature-matching software is the team's clinical judgment in determining the features that will be of most importance to the AAC user. If the features are not accurately identified and entered into the computer, for example, the devices that will be recommended will not be the most appropriate.

AAC teams must consider several options when selecting technology. No one piece of AAC technology is likely to have all the features that are desired to meet an individual's current and projected communication needs. Rather, several devices will have some of the desired features. Consider Jill, a young adult with severe physical and speech impairments and a progressive visual impairment whose AAC team is now assisting her with technology selection. The team's consensus is that Jill will be successful in pairing a simple, low-technology device (a general-use message recorder) with her existing unaided gesturing and limited natural speech to achieve functional communication in brief community interactions (e.g., describing a desired hair style to her stylist). The team has agreed that Jill will, however, require an advanced computer system with an expanded QWERTY keyboard and multiple outputs as a viable communication and employment tool for use at her workstation in a telecommunications office. Once Jill's needs have been noted, several potentially useful communication devices are identified and two to three of these are recommended for trial use. Because Jill and her team anticipate that her visual impairment will progress, all of the high-technology devices are chosen for their capacity to be upgraded to include auditory scanning, a screen enlarger, or both. After a period of trial use with two or three of the selected devices (set up through rental agreements with manufacturers of the devices), Jill, assisted by her service delivery team, selects the one that best fits her communication and work needs, and eventually purchases it.

Many AAC users, like Jill, achieve maximal benefit when both low- and high-technology devices meld with one another and with various unaided and natural communication options to yield multimodal communication (Iacono, Mirenda, & Beukelman, 1993; Murphy, Markova, Moodie, Scott, & Boa, 1995). A thorough overview of the basic components of low- and high-technology communication devices is provided in Chapters 9 and 10.

TRIAL USE OF AAC DEVICES

At the cornerstone of being able to procure the best fit AT for individual AAC users is acquiring data that a device will have a positive functional outcome on the user's communication abilities and overall quality of life. These data are essential to convincing AAC users, partners, potential financial supporters of the technology procurement, and even AAC teams that feature matching has indeed occurred and that optimal pieces of technology are about to be recommended.

Data regarding the potential positive utility of the devices being considered for eventual procurement should be gathered through trials and clinical documentation. These data may typically be gathered on several devices that have been selected. Trial use should involve best-case scenarios, wherein the AAC user is provided with an adequate amount of training (often in both clinical and nonclinical environments) under maximal levels of cueing with maximal levels of professional and nonprofessional partner and environmental support. The outcome of such trials should determine both the immediate and eventual success with the given pieces of communication technology. Both qualitative and quantitative data should be gathered about variables that have been established prior to data collection. Data can be obtained through multiple avenues (e.g., observation of frequency and effectiveness of use, interviews, or social validation measures).

No set time frame can be suggested for the trials, because each AAC user and device form a unique set of circumstances. In some cases, a particular device may show immediately a strong potential for being effective and efficient, whereas in other cases, the device's potential will take longer to determine.

Functional Outcome Measures

Feature matching works very well as a tool to determine appropriate devices, however, the field does not have a tool that gives valid, reliable, and sensitive measures that capture critical differences in levels of function that are attributable to use of the various AAC technology. Although not specifically devised for AAC, the American Speech-Language-Hearing Association's (ASHA, 1995) Functional Assessment of Communication Skills for Adults (FACS) was recently developed to address functional outcome measures in adult speech-language therapy. The FACS measures four domains—social communication; communication of basic needs; reading, writing, and number concepts; and daily planning—that are rated on a 7-point scale in dimensions of adequacy, appropriateness, promptness, and communication sharing. Because these four domains are so similar to the areas of AAC communicative competency suggested by Light (1989) several years ago, a scale similar to the FACS could easily be developed for use as an outcome-oriented measure of trial use of AAC devices.

Avoiding Common Pitfalls

This chapter has outlined steps in selecting appropriate AAC devices using a transdisciplinary team and the AAC model that considers the user, the partners, the environments, and the total AAC system. However, there are many pitfalls possible for individual professionals and/or users. The following list of common AAC device selection pitfalls was developed by Blischak (1993).

1. Selecting a device without team input (especially without the AAC user's input).
2. Trying to fit the device to the client rather than selecting a device based on a thorough assessment.
3. Believing that acquiring an assistive device is the goal in AAC intervention. In many ways, it is just the beginning.
4. Believing that acquiring an assistive device will solve all of the individual's problems.
5. Believing that an assistive device is the only means of communication; that is, failing to integrate use of an assistive device into an individual's total communication system.
6. Settling for preprogrammed vocabulary without considering individual needs.
7. Failing to consider time and funding for communication-partner training.
8. Failing to consider long-term communication needs in different contexts.
9. Overlooking the importance of environmental support.
10. Putting the user's life on hold until a device can be obtained.
11. Falling for a sales pitch.
12. Failing to follow up on funding denials.

SUMMARY

The sheer number and interrelationships of variables influencing the matching of the strengths and needs of AAC users to the features of low- and high-technology devices might seem to suggest that achieving any goodness of fit is overwhelming, if not virtually impossible. Teams that are most successful in technology selection are those that systematically proceed through the process. The process begins by identifying the current and projected communication needs of the AAC user, which forms the basis for determining the various device features needed. The team must then identify technology—either low technology, high technology, or both—that offers the maximal number of desirable feature matches.

Some of the most challenging issues of AAC service provision relate to selecting technology that will provide AAC users with maximal communication support with numerous communication partners in a variety of functional environments. Multiple, interrelated variables include the positive and negative attributes of any given device or group of devices. No consensus presently exists on the priorities of these variables, on how to choose or use them to maximize systems design, or on how to resolve conflicts when mismatches occur (Goodenough-Trepagnier, 1994). Consequently, technology selection will continue to be a major challenge for many years to come, as the cost and benefit of technology use is further investigated. The benchmark of successful technology selection will be when AAC users use several types of AAC technology naturally to meet multiple daily communication needs and bring about positive life changes.

CHAPTER 15

INTERVENTION PRINCIPLES
AND PROCEDURES

CAROLE ZANGARI AND KATHLEEN KANGAS

Some might argue that intervention issues in **augmentative and alternative communication (AAC)** are unnecessary to address. After all, AAC is about communication, and the same principles that are applied to any type of communication intervention would apply to AAC. In any intervention program, the treatment is developed based on careful assessment. The role of the clinician/educator is to assist an individual to become a more effective communicator. The clinician/educator must establish appropriate goals with the individual, build skills that either remediate or compensate for deficit areas, and evaluate and document the effectiveness of the intervention program. AAC practice should be viewed in the broader context of principles of speech and language intervention. However, because the communication process of AAC is distinctly different from natural speech, these principles are addressed somewhat differently. This chapter focuses on the application of AAC intervention principles and procedures.

APPROPRIATE CANDIDATES FOR AAC SERVICES

AAC intervention services have not always been available to individuals with severe communication disabilities. As the field of AAC emerged, many professionals were reluctant to shift their focus to include various aided/unaided AAC strategies and techniques, often fearing that the use of AAC would negatively affect future development of intelligible speech. Parents often resisted AAC intervention for their children thinking that professionals were giving up on improving spoken communication skills.

In general, AAC techniques were not used with individuals who would eventually develop or regain natural speech. Children with developmental apraxia, adults with aphasia, and individuals with traumatic brain injury (TBI) often did not have the opportunity to learn AAC strategies until it became apparent that natural speech was not progressing to a point where it would be functional. At times, intervention focusing on alternatives to speech was delayed months, or even years, often leading to excessive frustration, social isolation, depression, and reduced opportunities for typical life experiences.

Other individuals were denied access to formal AAC intervention because they were unable to demonstrate certain behaviors thought to be prerequisites to the development of symbolic communication. Despite a paucity of supporting data (Kangas & Lloyd, 1988; Reichle & Karlan, 1988), many clinicians/educators withheld AAC training from individuals who could not demonstrate certain cognitive skills, such as **means-ends relationships, imitation**, and **object permanence**. Other individuals were denied AAC services because they did not exhibit behavioral skills such as sitting quietly, making eye contact, and taking turns, thought to be necessary before more formal communication teaching would be successful. Intervention with these individuals focused on teaching the specific cognitive and/or behavioral skills that were lacking. The client was believed to be ready for communication intervention when these prerequisite skills were mastered.

Current thinking in AAC intervention holds that AAC strategies and techniques should be taught to any individual who exhibits a discrepancy between communication needs and abilities (Blackstone & Painter, 1985). It is now known that AAC does not inhibit the development of speech. In fact, in some individuals with a variety of disorders including **aphasia** (Beukelman & Garrett, 1988; Eagleson, Vaughn, & Knudson, 1970; Goldstein & Cameron, 1952; Schlanger, 1976; Sklar & Bennett, 1956), **apraxia** (Ellsworth & Kotkin, 1975; Skelly, Schinsky, Smith, & Fust, 1974), **dysarthria** (Gitlis, 1975; Kates & McNaughton, 1975; Kladde, 1974; Levett, 1971; Ontario Crippled Children's Centre, 1971), **autism** (Creedon, 1975; Ellsworth & Kotkin, 1975; Fulwiler & Fouts, 1976; Konstantareas, Oxman, Webster, Fischer, & Miller, 1975; Miller & Miller, 1973; Offir, 1976; Schaeffer, McDowell, Musil, & Kollinzas, 1976), and cognitive impairment (Balick, Spiegel, & Greene, 1976; Brookner & Murphy, 1975; Duncan & Silverman, 1977; Kimble, 1975; Leibeis & Leibeis, 1975; Linville, 1977; Prinz & Shaw, 1981; Schmidt, Carrier, & Parsons, 1971; Wills, 1981), AAC has been shown to actually facilitate the development of speech.

The current view of appropriate candidates for AAC intervention also considers future needs. If individuals are at risk for developing a discrepancy between their communication needs and abilities, AAC should be explored. For example, individuals with **amyotrophic lateral sclerosis (ALS)** may visit a speech-language pathologist when their speech skills are declining, but still effective. The treatment team may choose to pursue AAC options immediately, rather than wait until the speech deteriorates to the point where making decisions about communication options becomes more difficult. In other cases, a discrepancy develops not because potential AAC users' abilities change over time, but rather because their environments change. Consider the example of a woman with cognitive impairment who has lived at home all of her life, interacting primarily with individuals she has known since childhood. Although her speech is severely impaired, through the years her family and neighbors have learned to interpret her speech quite accurately. If this woman moved into a supported living apartment and/or got a job in the community, her new communication partners might not be able to decipher her spoken messages. In this case, a change in environment would create a discrepancy between communication needs and abilities and, thus, would make this woman a candidate for AAC intervention.

DEVELOPING AND IMPLEMENTING AAC INTERVENTION PROGRAMS

Communication involves an integrated system that may include speech, traditional orthography (TO), and aided and/or unaided AAC. Because communication is so essential in daily life, any resolution of communication disabilities should be measured in terms of real-life performance. Like other types of communication intervention, AAC intervention should facilitate meaningful and functional communication in real-life activities. Both the content of intervention and the form of AAC teaching should provide skills that make observable differences in the lives of individuals with AAC needs.

Effective AAC intervention programs include a strong link between assessment and intervention. An important aspect of the AAC assessment process is to identify potential AAC users' abilities in terms of both strengths and needs. Although assessment is critical in providing information for planning intervention, one often cannot afford to defer intervention until assessment is complete. A complete AAC assessment may take many months. If intervention is delayed accordingly, the potential AAC user is likely to be faced with unmet communication needs. Intervention programs should be built on the information gathered in the assessment process, building on the individual's strengths to address communication needs. AAC service providers must sometimes begin intervention based on minimal assessment data and include the results of such intervention as part of an ongoing assessment (Goossens', 1989). Thus, assessment and intervention are seen as parallel and interrelated processes rather than two discrete stages of AAC service delivery.

Both content (*what* is taught) and context (*where* and *how* something is taught) are important considerations in AAC intervention. Content, or the focus of intervention, sets the course for developing communication skills that can help overcome barriers to participation in life activities. Although most potential AAC users have many limitations in their skills and abilities (access barriers), some barriers to effective communication are functions of the environments in which they live, learn, work, and play (opportunity barriers). AAC intervention must address all barriers to successful communication, regardless of whether they are a function of the AAC user or of the environment. Intervention must also address each aspect of the individual's multicomponent AAC system, including residual speech, gestures, and aided techniques. Because each of these components contributes to an overall pattern of communication effectiveness, they each require systematic attention. Addressing only one component of the individual's AAC system may improve skills, yet do little to improve the overall success of daily communication. Consider the situation of Jim, a 14-year-old adolescent with moderate cognitive impairment. After a considerable amount of training, he was able to operate his voice output communication aid (VOCA) quite effectively in therapy sessions. However, because he did not have the pragmatic skills to initiate or maintain conversation, he rarely used it. Thus, his overall effectiveness as a communicator was only marginally improved.

A successful outcome depends not only on the content of intervention, but also on the context of an intervention program, including the setting in which it occurs, the format of the teaching situation, and specific instructional methods. As with any teaching situation, the details of how new skills are taught are important considerations in planning and implementing AAC intervention. The context of intervention may vary greatly depending not only on the content of what is being taught, but also on such factors as individuals' learning styles, ability to generalize information, stamina, and attention span. For example, one AAC user might begin to learn to use an alphabet board in one session, whereas a seriously ill patient in an acute care facility may require several brief intervention sessions to learn those same skills.

AAC GOALS

As in any area of clinical practice, appropriate goals must be established to guide AAC intervention. These goals should be established as part of a team assessment, with the AAC user and/or the family being an important part of the decision-making team. Setting appropriate goals requires the team to consider a number of factors in addition to the potential AAC user's strengths and weaknesses. For example, the team needs to consider the individual's cultural background and native language environment so that AAC skills being taught will be consistent with the individual's values, customs, traditions, and beliefs (see Chapter 22 for a discussion of multicultural issues).

General Guidelines

AAC intervention goals should have outcomes that are functional and beneficial to the AAC user. In most cases, regaining or developing typical communication is not a realistic goal. Eight criteria have been established to guide clinicians/educators in developing AAC goals (Mirenda, Iacono, & Williams, 1990; Rainforth, York, & Macdonald, 1992). Any goal of AAC intervention should meet one or more of the following criteria.

1. **Maintain health and vitality.** For some AAC users, communication relates directly to physical care and basic needs. Goals to meet this criterion would include indicating comfort or discomfort, requesting medications, and communicating symptoms to a physician.

2. **Enhance participation in current and future integrated environments.** Many AAC interventions are directed toward enhancing students' abilities to participate in general education classrooms or facilitating adults to communicate at job sites. Communicating critical messages about tasks in those environments enhances an individual's ability to remain in a particular setting and to expand to similar environments.

3. **Increase social integration (especially with peers).** Social communication is an important part of life and a critical purpose of communication. Social interaction skills help to establish close relationships with family members, develop a circle of friends with whom to share leisure time, and engage in exchanges with casual acquaintances or

strangers. AAC users have the same social communication needs as typically speaking individuals. Unfortunately, many individuals with disabilities find their social interactions restricted to close family members and to staff or service personnel who are paid to interact with them.

4. **Have frequent or multiple applications across environments and activities.** Communication skills and strategies that can be applied in many settings are more efficient for learning than idiosyncratic techniques that work in only one situation. For example, the use of graphic symbols with printed words that can be read even by relative strangers would be more efficient than the use of idiosyncratic gestures that can be understood only by someone familiar with these gestures.

5. **Be essential for further development.** Some skills may be chosen because they provide access to further development. Early academic skills are a good example of this. Recognition of letters and letter sounds may not be immediately functional, but learning these skills successfully may assist with keyboard access as well as with reading and writing skills.

6. **Be a priority for the client (interest/performance/talent).** Client-centered decision making requires the interests of the AAC user to be a major factor in selecting goals. If a teenager is especially interested in sports and wants to attend sporting events and hold conversations about a favorite team, sports vocabulary should be incorporated into the communication training. An adult who wants to return to participation in a social club or church circle would also need vocabulary and strategies designed specifically for those individual interests.

7. **Be a family priority.** The priorities of the family members are also important. Parents may want their child to take part in religious training or to communicate with grandparents over the telephone. Spouses may want their partners to be more effective in communicating feelings of sadness, illness, or fatigue, so that misunderstandings do not lead to frustration between couples. Family needs should be given high priority in the intervention program.

8. **Be a priority of significant people in the target environment.** Priorities of other people who function in the target environments should also be considered. For example, a teacher might feel that a student with disabilities should follow previously established classroom routines (e.g., asking permission before speaking, giving a spoken response to roll call). Co-workers might value courtesies such as saying "please" and "thank you" or acknowledging instructions when they are given.

These criteria ensure that the goals set for AAC users will have an important impact on their lives. People with severe communication disabilities often invest great amounts of time and energy to obtain and learn AAC strategies and techniques. These efforts must be directed toward goals that are realistic and important.

Integrated Goals and Objectives

The overall purpose of the AAC program is to provide a person with more effective communication. Clearly, the criteria discussed above require the clinician/educator to focus on the important life activities and environments of the AAC user. With this approach, goals and objectives are integrated into daily routines. When goals are integrated, they address the actual use of AAC in natural and realistic communication situations. Specific skills such as producing manual signs or accessing graphic symbols are effective only if they are used in actual communication situations.

Some might argue that following integrated goals and objectives is no different than teaching generalization which is included in any speech and language training program. AAC intervention, however, involves additional issues, and so the concern about using skills in natural environments is magnified. AAC users are often in situations where they are the only individuals using a particular communication strategy or technique. Because AAC is very different from natural speech and/or writing, AAC users may initially require significant assistance to communicate in realistic situations.

Many AAC users have had limited experience with successful communication. Consider, for example, Ryan, a 4-year-old who has good language comprehension, but unintelligible speech. If a communication device is provided, Ryan might be expected to use it effectively to communicate. At 4 years old, however, Ryan has had no experience asking questions, playing word games, or guessing at reading words. It should not be surprising, then, if Ryan learns to access the vocabulary of the device but still fails to use it to ask questions or tell stories. Appropriate and effective use of a device requires practice in natural settings where there are opportunities to communicate with family and friends.

Teaching the skills of operating a communication device in an isolated setting is sometimes appropriate. Some techniques do require significant learning time, and sometimes this is efficiently accomplished in a quiet and distraction-free setting where the AAC user can concentrate on operating the device. As quickly as possible, however, communication should be related to real-life needs in natural environments. Samples of isolated and integrated goals are presented in Table 15.1.

Ensuring Accountability

As in any area of intervention, appropriate measures of progress are required. Measures of the specific use of AAC approaches during intervention are widely used for documenting progress. Clinicians/educators record data on the number of symbols an individual can identify, the number of words and phrases expressed through AAC modes during specified activities, and the time required to transmit messages. Although these measures show how the client is responding to the training program in a therapy context, they are not sufficient to document the full effects of the intervention program.

For some individuals, it may be appropriate to modify the measures used for speech and language assessment of persons with milder speech and language impairments. For example, a conversational speech sample could be analyzed for length of response, diversity of vocabulary, appropriate pragmatic functions, use of syntactic structures, or any other parameter relevant to the conversation of the AAC user. Although developmental norms are not typically applicable to an individual who uses AAC, repeated measures would reflect changing abilities to produce more advanced and varied language. Some measures can be applied to any communication technique. For voice or print output, messages can be analyzed directly. For signs or gestures, the gloss can be transcribed and analyzed in a way similar to that of natural speech.

One limitation of this approach is that these measures encourage the comparison of communication samples of AAC users' communication with those of typically speaking peers. Some believe such comparisons are inappropriate. On the other hand, such comparisons are useful to determine discrepancies. At best, comparing the communication skill samples of AAC users with those of typically speaking peers is a limited approach that should not be a sole frame of reference.

TABLE 15.1   Sample Goals Contrasting Isolated and Integrated Goals

ISOLATED GOAL	INTEGRATED GOAL	COMMENTS
Child will match objects to pictures during a structured activity in a quiet setting.	Child will select a desired toy or food by pointing to the picture of the object during recess or lunch times.	Both goals focus on learning picture symbols, but embedding the skill in a choice-making structure helps the child establish communicative power in natural environments.
Adult will use a communication device to produce sentences with correct use of present progressive, past, and future tense verbs when describing sequenced pictures.	Adult will prepare a letter to a friend or relative with correct use of present progressive, past, and future tense verbs.	Both goals focus on learning different verb tenses, but working on this skill in the functional context of letter writing is more meaningful and serves to improve the quality of the letter.

If the main purpose of AAC intervention is to improve functional communication, assessment of progress must include assessment of communication in real-life activities. For example, Mitchell, a young adult with a head injury, works during therapy sessions to increase his vocabulary. He practices labeling pictures and answering questions by providing one or two words typed out on a computer keyboard, but his vocabulary access can be considered truly functional only when he can type out answers to real-life questions such as "What do you want for lunch today?" or "Do you need to buy anything at the grocery store?" Although Mitchell's answers might still be single words and short phrases, his ability to use vocabulary in more meaningful ways and in a greater number of settings would reflect progress.

INSTRUCTIONAL DELIVERY

How AAC skills are taught can be just as important as *what* skills are taught. If AAC users are to be successful in real-life communication, intervention methods must be effective and efficient. Although many questions about the most efficacious approaches to teach AAC skills remain unanswered, most professionals are guided by instructional methods and principles that have emerged from the fields of education and psychology.

General Strategies for Instruction

Structured versus Situational Teaching.   Structured teaching uses specific activities devised for teaching targeted skills. For example, a teacher might direct a child to complete a page in a workbook or to describe the actions of a pictured story. The main purpose of these activities is for the child to learn or practice communication skills, in particular, vocabulary development or sentence structure. Structured teaching often occurs during therapy sessions that are designated for intervention in a certain domain (e.g., a 30-minute period might be designated as speech and language time).

Situational teaching, in contrast, takes advantage of daily activities to teach skills. Kopchick and Lloyd (1976), for example, described a 24-hour approach to teaching manual signs. In this approach, staff members were expected to teach manual signs all day long—during dressing, at mealtime, and when going to and from school. Teaching greeting skills when a child first enters the school building and teaching requests for objects within a meal or snack time are examples of situational teaching. Many authors have advocated working with parents (Kaiser, 1993) or peers (Ostrosky, Kaiser, & Odom, 1993) to implement intervention programs with children. Because these people interact with the AAC user on a regular basis, they can take advantage of many situational teaching opportunities.

Teaching in meaningful and relevant contexts (e.g., milieu teaching) plays a central role in the AAC intervention process. Milieu teaching has been extensively researched and found to be effective in enhancing communication skills of children with communication disabilities (see Kaiser, 1994). Some individuals with learning problems, such as those with autism, brain injury, and cognitive impairment find it difficult to transfer skills learned in one set of conditions to other situations (Anderson & Spradlin, 1980; Warren & Rogers-Warren, 1985). For example, a boy with autism who has learned to indicate a picture symbol for "I want to leave" when an activity has ended in the speech therapy room may not be able to use that same symbol to indicate the same concept with his classroom teacher when computer time is over. Teaching in natural contexts allows the clinician/educator to take advantage of cues and consequences that are natural parts of the setting. If this boy learned to use his "I want to leave" symbol in a relevant setting, such as the classroom, he could take advantage of natural cues that typically signal the end of an activity period (e.g., other students cleaning up materials) and consequences (gaining acknowledgment and a response to his request).

Promoting Generalization.   Generalization, which refers to the transfer of learned behaviors from a training situation to an untrained situation, is a critical issue (Calculator, 1988b; Hegde, 1985; Reichle & Sigafoos, 1991). This includes generalization to (1) untrained stimuli (e.g., a person is taught to comment on a set of pictures, and is then provided with new pictures that call for similar vocabulary), (2) untrained environments (e.g., a child is taught to use picture symbols to request items at school, and is then expected to used the same symbols to make similar requests at home), and (3) untrained persons (e.g., an adult is taught to use a social greeting with familiar peers and staff members in a group home, and is then encouraged to greet additional co-workers in a job setting).

When structured teaching approaches are used, especially in isolated or clinical settings, generalization is usually considered to be a final phase of teaching for a particular skill. Generalization can be encouraged by using a wide variety of materials, cues, and prompts in the structured setting, as well as by completing structured activities in more than one setting and with more than one communication partner. Professionals often involve familiar members or paraprofessionals in generalization.

When naturalistic approaches are used, generalization is promoted throughout the training sequence. Opportunities to generalize newly trained skills may occur even while establishing a new skill. Because this type of teaching often occurs in natural environments, the need to specifically program for generalization may be reduced. For example, if greetings are trained in the natural situation of arriving at school, once the clinician/educator reduces prompts, the individual is already greeting people appropriately in the natural setting. However, even with naturalistic strategies and situational teaching, generalization is an important phase of the teaching sequence and should not be overlooked. Some individuals may have great difficulty in establishing the spontaneous use of new skills, so specific support for generalization may be needed.

Collaborative Approach to Service Delivery.
Contextual relevance is important, but not sufficient for the development of communication skills. Another component of how AAC skills are taught relates to who does the teaching. In transdisciplinary approaches, professionals engage in a great deal of **collaboration**, working across traditional discipline boundaries to better serve individuals with disabilities. The speech-language pathologist, for example, may be working with a child learning to use a VOCA to answer questions in music class. Although certainly attending to the communication objectives of this activity, the speech-language pathologist may also be facilitating the acquisition and practice of new motor, academic, and behavioral skills. In this example, the child may be refining hand control for pointing (motor domain) while using the AAC device to identify which percussion instrument was used in the last sonata (academic domain). This approach recognizes that people generally do not learn new skills in isolation. It encourages professionals to teach functionally interrelated clusters of skills. Successful integration of AAC intervention into existing activities requires collaboration among all members of the team and is appropriate regardless of what approach or setting is used.

Designing Integrated Instructional Strategies.
Good intervention, no matter what aspects of communication are being addressed, is well-grounded in theory and research and is structured by sound educational practices. Rainforth, York, and Macdonald (1992) describe a practice of designing comprehensive instructional programs that integrate several programmatic domains including communication. Although specifically designed for use in educational programs, the basic concepts can be applied to AAC users in a variety of settings.

In this approach, systematic instruction is used to teach a variety of skills within the context of a meaningful activity. The first step is to identify the context for instruction by determining what environments and activities have the highest priority for a specific individual at a given time. The second step is to examine these environments and activities to identify the specific skills needed for participation. These skills, sometimes called **embedded skills**, are then targeted for intervention. The third step is to determine the specifics of how the embedded skills are to be taught (e.g., What teaching methods will be used? When and where will the skills be taught? How will the program be implemented?). Only after careful observation, analysis, and planning does actual teaching begin. When the intervention program is implemented, the performance is carefully monitored so that difficulties can be identified and modifications can be made.

This systematic approach to instruction offers a number of advantages. First, it ensures that the teaching of communication skills occurs not in an isolated or arbitrary context, but as part of a high-priority, real-life activity. Second, it helps protect against loose threads and details that fall between the cracks in less systematic approaches.

The ultimate goal of AAC intervention is to improve communication skills to enhance participation in life experiences (Beukelman & Mirenda, 1992). In successful intervention programs, individuals show measurable gains in meeting the communication requirements of meaningful life activities, not in the achievement of arbitrary goals or scores on discipline-specific tests.

Instructional Procedures

Mand-model. Mand-model is an instructional procedure used by professionals and nonprofessionals that has been successful in teaching individuals with disabilities. Clinicians/educators ask questions or provide direct instructions to create instructional opportunities in natural environments (Reichle & Sigafoos, 1991). For example, the clinician/educator might "mand" (command/request) a response by saying "Where are you going?" or "Show me what you need." If the listener fails to respond after a pause, the speaker provides a model of the expected response.

Modeling for Imitation. **Modeling** for imitation (Hegde, 1985) is another teaching procedure used by both professionals and nonprofessionals. For example, a parent might look at a picture book with a young child and name the pictures, expecting the child to repeat the names.

In AAC intervention, clinicians/educators and other communication partners model the use of modes that the individual is expected to use. For example, if a child is using manual signs to communicate, a teacher might produce a new sign vocabulary and ask the child to repeat or imitate the signs. When assisting a child to use a communica-tion board, an adult might point to the symbols first, expecting the child to imitate. An instructional aide might model how to make a specific request, such as asking for help with an art project, by pointing to symbols for "Help me paint red." Immediately after modeling, the aide might coach the child to use that response to ask a peer for assistance.

Molding/Physical Guidance. One step further in providing assistance to the learner is to provide **molding** or **physical guidance**. This means providing a full physical prompt or whatever motor assistance is needed. For manual signs or gestures, this may involve physical movement of the learner's hands. For use of a device, it may include physical guidance to select a symbol, press a location, and/or activate a switch.

The ability to provide physical guidance is sometimes discussed as one of the potential benefits of AAC strategies (Fristoe & Lloyd, 1977a, 1977b, 1979a; Lloyd & Karlan, 1984). Although physically facilitating speech would be difficult, using physical guidance to facilitate aided and unaided communication is fairly simple. One could assist a person, for example, to touch a symbol for a simple request, then allow the person to experience the result of that request (e.g., help a young adult point to the symbol for "Listen to music" to get someone to turn on the radio). Molding/physical guidance is not as helpful in teaching someone to say "Listen to music," because the clinician/educator cannot physically guide the articulators into producing a spoken phrase.

In using this strategy, the clinician/educator must be sensitive to the individual's level of participation. In the early stages of intervention, considerable physical guidance may be required. As an individual demonstrates increased participation, the clinician/educator may reduce the amount of physical guidance to the point that the response can be produced independently. If the learner remained passive or if the individual physically resisted guidance, the clinician/educator should introduce a different strategy.

Using molding/physical guidance is a key area for collaboration with occupational and physical therapists. If a person experiences a motor impairment, AAC team members must understand what types of motor control are in the person's ability range, what reflexes might be present and how they are triggered, and what type of physical guidance is most conducive to appropriate motor control.

Time Delay.   **Time delay** (Spradlin, Karlan, & Wetherby, 1976) can be used to introduce new symbols to the individual. With this procedure, the clinician/educator first pairs two stimuli, one that already elicits a response from the individual, and one that is selected to be taught. A time delay is then introduced, in which the new stimulus is presented first. For example, Angela, a 4-year-old girl with autism, gets excited and signs WANT as soon as she sees her favorite kind of cookie. Her teacher could pair a picture symbol of a cookie with the real object, and present the two things to Angela simultaneously, expecting Angela to continue to respond excitedly to the cookie. Gradually, a time delay is introduced, and the picture symbol is shown before the cookie, with the time delay gradually extended. When Angela learns the meaning of the picture symbol, she will show her anticipation by signing WANT or pointing to the picture symbol as soon as the graphic symbol is presented.

Time delay also refers to the practice of waiting between presenting a natural cue and introducing an instructional prompt designed to elicit a response (Reichle & Sigafoos, 1991). Clinicians/educators use time delay when they introduce choices and allow an interval of time to pass before they provide a prompt (for example, a manual sign or pointing to a graphic symbol). Time delay, in this sense, has also been referred to as **pause time**. While the introduction of time delay/pause time cannot be used to teach new communicative behaviors, it provides learners the opportunity to develop competence in previously learned communication skills. Time delay/pause time is more than an instructional procedure, however. Because AAC users are often at a disadvantage during conversations because they simply need more time to communicate, the purposeful introduction of time delay/pause time can facilitate interaction.

Shaping.   **Shaping** refers to the initial acceptance of a response that may be quite different from the desired one, and then the gradual refinement of the response by requiring successively more accurate abilities (Hegde, 1985). In unaided communication, this would mean initially responding to gross gestures or rough approximations of new signs, and then gradually responding to only increasingly precise responses. In aided communication, it might mean initially accepting a single fist point toward a symbol, and later requiring the sequencing of two or three key presses to access the message. Gradually shifting from accepting large targets separated in space toward accepting smaller targets placed closer together might also be considered shaping a response. Throughout the shaping process, the AAC user should experience a high rate of success, because even very gross approximations of the desired response are accepted at first.

Enhancement.   **Enhancement** is an approach to teaching symbols that involves providing cues or embedding symbols in a meaningful visual context. Blissymbols may be enhanced by incorporating the actual Blissymbol into a drawing that relates to the meaning (Blissymbolics Communication Institute, 1984). For example, a graphic of the numeral 1 is a part of the first person pronoun "I" in Blissymbolics. In enhanced Blissymbols, the number 1 is still included, but it is enhanced to look like a stick figure pointing to itself. The recommended teaching approach is to gradually fade the use of enhancements so that the individual learns the meanings of the unenhanced Blissymbols. Refer back to Figure 6.5 for examples of embellished or enhanced Blissymbols. TO may also be enhanced so that the printed words look like their meanings (Clark, Davies, & Woodcock, 1974). For example, the word *big* might be printed in large bold type whereas the word *little* could be printed in small type. Thus, the physical appearance of the words are enhanced to provide a clue to the meaning. These enhancements may be faded until both words become the same size as all other words.

Fading.   **Fading**, which involves reducing the strength, frequency, and/or duration of prompts can be used within the context of instructional procedures to improve communication skills, but is especially critical to the first three procedures described. In molding/physical guidance, for example, the physical molding/guidance of placing an AAC user's hand on a communication board to select a symbol may be faded to simply touching the arm to prompt a selection. The rate at which one implements fading during the instructional process is key to positive clinical/educational outcomes.

Prompting.   In many forms of teaching, the service provider initially provides whatever **prompts** are needed to generate the desired communication. Verbal prompts (e.g., "Tell me what you want"), gestural prompts (e.g., a puzzled look, a vague sweep of the hand over the communication board), and physical prompts (e.g., forming the learner's hands into a manual sign) can all be used to elicit the desired behavior. If the AAC user visually attends to the clinician/educator carefully, the service provider might also deliver a visual prompt by looking at the needed symbol.

The mode in which prompts are presented and the level of assistance they provide to the learner vary. The clinician/educator must first select an appropriate type of prompt (e.g., verbal, gestural, physical) and then provide that prompt at an appropriate level of assistance. Table 15.2 gives examples of different types and levels (partial, full) of prompts. Optimally, the clinician/educator attempts to identify a prompt that is sufficient to elicit the desired communicative response but does not offer more help than the AAC user actually needs. For example, a young woman learning to turn on her communication device may initially need full physical assistance (e.g., placing her hand on the switch and pressing). Later, as her abilities increase, she may only need a partial physical prompt (e.g., moving her hand toward the switch). Later a partial gestural prompt (e.g., pointing to the on/off switch) may be all that is needed to turn on the device. Still later, the young woman may be able to turn on the device in response to being given pause time. Sometimes prompts are referred to as **cues**. In this text, however, cues are considered to be naturally occurring stimuli in the environment. If the young woman turns on her device in response to seeing it, she is responding to a naturally occurring visual cue. No prompt was needed.

Several authors have delineated hierarchies of prompts (e.g., Culp & Carlisle, 1988; Sigafoos, Mustonen, DePaepe, Reichle, & York, 1991). Clinicians/educators may follow a most-to-least prompt hierarchy as just described or a least-to-most prompt hierarchy, in which the level of prompts is increased until a response is elicited. Performance is considered to be improving if fewer prompts are needed or if the prompts used are at a lower level of assistance to the AAC user.

TABLE 15.2   Examples of Different Types and Levels of Prompts

TYPE OF PROMPT	PARTIAL PROMPT	FULL PROMPT
Verbal (spoken, signed, or written)	"What's next?"	"Tell me, 'Check schedule'."
Gestural	Shrug, look puzzled; pantomime opening communication book.	Open communication book to correct page and point to desired symbol.
Physical	Gently move learner's elbow so that the arm is extended in the direction of the communication book.	Use hand-over-hand assistance to help learner point to the correct symbol.
Visual	Gaze directly at communication book.	Not applicable.

Even if the actual response provided by the AAC user does not change significantly, the reduction in prompts is considered a sign of progress.

An Integrative Framework for Intervention

So far, this chapter has discussed a number of issues regarding how AAC skills are taught. In this section, the content of intervention is addressed by considering the importance of four areas of communication. Communication involves (1) information/messages to communicate, (2) reasons to communicate, (3) ways in which to communicate, and (4) partners with whom to communicate. Regardless of how much progress is made in any *one* of these areas, barriers in *any* of the remaining areas are likely to impede successful communication.

Information/Messages to Communicate. An important part of any communicative act is the thought or idea behind it. Like natural speakers, AAC users must have something to say; that is, information/messages to communicate. At least four things are needed to compose a message: sociolinguistic knowledge, means of representation, appropriate vocabulary, and experiential/world knowledge.

Sociolinguistic Knowledge. First, the communicator must have an idea of what to say. To do that, one must have sufficient sociolinguistic knowledge. A girl who wants to play with her father, for example, must have some understanding that she can use communication to inform him of her wishes. If a true language is used, such as American Sign Language (ASL), she must possess enough knowledge of that language's semantic, morphological, grammatical, and syntactical rules so that an intelligible message can be formed (e.g., MUSIC, DADDY!). The amount of sociolinguistic knowledge needed by the communicator depends both on the content of the message itself and the components of the specific AAC system being used.

Some potential AAC users lack basic sociocommunicative knowledge and must be taught that communication is a tool that can be used to get

one's needs and desires met. Five-year-old David, for example, is severely autistic. At lunch time, he is frequently unable to open the plastic containers that hold his sandwich and dessert. Although he is usually hungry, he does not know to request help from his teachers. Before they teach David specific vocabulary or symbols, his teachers must help David become aware of the power of communication. That is, he needs to learn that he can exert control over his environment through communication.

Other AAC users, particularly those with acquired disorders, understand the dynamics of human interaction, but are unable to participate as fully as they would like. Their intervention programs would probably include teaching the rule-based aspects of language, such as morphology, grammar, and syntax.

Means of Representation. Second, the communicator must have some means of representing the message. The representation can be symbolic or nonsymbolic. With symbolic representation, one thing (e.g., a picture of a cat, the manual sign CAT, or the word *cat*) is used to stand for something else (i.e., the actual cat). In most cases, the communicator must have some receptive understanding of the representation and be able to use it expressively. As its name implies, nonsymbolic communication does not use symbols to represent ideas. Instead, facial expressions, touch, and movement are the primary means of conveying information. Suppose the girl who wanted to play with her father communicated without the use of symbols, perhaps by picking up the music box, shaking it, and putting it in her father's lap. She is using nonsymbolic strategies (e.g., movement and manipulation of objects) to convey her wishes. A goal for her could be that in a year's time she would be able to point to picture-based symbols along with using nonsymbolic strategies to communicate an entire message (e.g., pick up a music box picture and put it in her father's lap).

Most AAC intervention addresses the means of representation at least once during the course of treatment. Symbol selection is an important part of the assessment process. For individuals learning a new symbol set/system, symbol teaching becomes a critical part of the intervention process. For example, Mrs. A has a communication book with single words and short phrases that she used frequently. After her third stroke, she was no longer able to read well. Her therapy plan addressed this by reteaching some basic reading skills and pairing picture symbols with many of the words in her communication book. She is gradually reacquiring her reading skills. In the meantime, however, she has learned to use the picture symbols (such as a map next to the word *where* and a blank face next to the word *who*) to communicate in everyday situations. Refer to Chapter 13 for a review of symbol selection.

Appropriate Vocabulary.   Third, the communicator must understand, have access to, and be able to retrieve appropriate vocabulary needed to convey a specific message. Selecting appropriate vocabulary that allows the AAC user to interact effectively is a constant challenge. A discrepancy often exists between the amount of vocabulary needed to function in a variety of environments and the number of messages that can be stored and accessed. Unless the AAC user can spell and create the vocabulary, clinicians/educators (with input from the user and others) assume responsibility for determining what vocabulary to provide. The exact wording of messages is important because it can set the tone of a conversation. Messages with the same content may be phrased very differently to carry various tones (e.g., casual/formal, complimentary/insulting). Clinicians/educators must address many important issues in the vocabulary selection process, including the following:

1. What communicative functions does the AAC user need to express?
2. What are the AAC user's needs and preferences for specific messages?
3. How long should each vocabulary unit be (e.g., a single letter, a word, a sentence)?
4. How should vocabulary/messages be organized and stored?

The vocabulary/message needs of most AAC users change greatly over time, requiring clinicians/educators to monitor and periodically modify available message sets. For example, children will need additional messages as their vocabular-

ies and syntactic abilities expand. Adolescents may need different ways of expressing the same content appropriate for various contexts (e.g., "I don't agree." vs. "No way!"). Adults may need vocabulary that accommodates life changes, such as a new job, a move to a different city, or a change in an intimate relationship. Refer to Chapter 12 for a review of vocabulary selection.

Experiential/World Knowledge.   Finally, the communicator wanting to express ideas outside the here and now must possess enough experiential/world knowledge to have some areas of content about which to communicate. Some individuals with AAC needs require a sophisticated degree of background knowledge to communicate effectively in school, at work, and during leisure activities. Other AAC users need lesser degrees of background knowledge to meet the communication demands of their current environments. A major consideration must be the background knowledge they will need to participate in both present and future environments.

In many cases, background knowledge is addressed along with AAC intervention. JJ's intervention is a case in point. As a preschool child with almost no intelligible speech, JJ was assumed to have severe to profound cognitive impairment similar to his speaking classmates. Because his school believed that individuals with this level of cognitive impairment required a specialized curriculum, he did not participate in a typical preschool curriculum. When JJ was provided with some basic AAC strategies, he showed that he probably did not have cognitive impairment and was slated to enter a regular kindergarten class in his neighborhood school. Because of his lack of exposure to certain kinds of educational experiences, however, JJ did not have the same background knowledge that his future classmates had, putting him at risk for failure. No combination of AAC strategies and techniques could help JJ be academically competitive without the background knowledge that teachers assume kindergartners have. Therefore, his AAC intervention program aggressively addressed areas such as basic concepts, letters, and numbers as contexts for learning and using new communication skills.

AAC intervention generally requires significant attention to the aspect of communication that deals with having something to say. Many AAC users require specific instruction in learning to use new symbols and vocabulary. Some must be taught specific grammatical and syntactical structures to enable them to communicate sophisticated, pragmatically appropriate messages. Still others will need experiences that allow them to learn about the world—its people, cultures, and environments.

Reasons to Communicate.   Individuals with AAC needs often have few reasons to communicate and few opportunities for meaningful expression. Some communication partners have little or no expectations that the AAC user can or will participate in interaction and, therefore, make no communication demands on the AAC user. Research has also shown that naturally speaking communication partners may dominate conversations and preempt communicative acts on the part of the AAC user (Light, Collier, & Parnes, 1985a). This unfortunate reality has two negative consequences that the clinician/educator must address. First, having few meaningful opportunities for interaction leaves the potential AAC user with very little motivation to develop more effective communication skills. If one has no reason to communicate, why work hard at communicating better? Second, the number of opportunities to practice emerging communication skills is often quite limited. AAC users must have not only a reasonable need or desire to communicate but also sufficient opportunities to learn new communication skills. In many cases, professionals must intervene before changes in communication abilities can be expected. Reasons or opportunities for communication arise out of three sets of conditions: internal states, environmental demands, and partner expectations.

Internal States.   Most people are motivated into action by their own internal states. Bodies signal hunger, thirst, and pain, and prompt individuals to act by getting something to eat, drink, or seek relief. Individuals with severe cognitive and/or physical impairments may be unable to independently resolve their own needs; they may have to rely on another person to assist them in getting food or drink, for example. Although many individuals are quite capable of communicating their needs to someone who could assist them, many others are not.

Some potential AAC users are not sufficiently aware of their own needs. Others may be aware of their internal states, such as hunger or thirst, but may not understand that communication can be used to help them get their needs met. These individuals may not realize that they can communicate their needs to another person who will then assist them. In these cases, the mere presence of internal states is not sufficient to elicit communication.

Environmental Demands.   Another source of motivation for communication is environmental demands; that is, situations in which communication is needed to satisfactorily complete an activity. A father, for example, discovers that his daughter left her toys at the bottom of his wheelchair ramp, and he needs to ask someone to move the toys before he can safely use the ramp. That communicative act comes not from any internal state, but from the situation. He cannot accomplish his objective to get down the ramp without the help of another person.

Individuals with little or no functional speech often participate in activities and situations in which few, if any, environmental demands for communication are made. Efforts to nurture and care for individuals with disabilities have resulted in a reduced number of opportunities in which they need or are even tempted to communicate. Consider the case of a young boy who is a beginning AAC user getting ready for bed. The boy's parents undress him, put on his pajamas, help him brush his teeth and wash his face, and tuck him into bed. Although the parents may be talking to him throughout this process, there may be no real need for *him* to communicate. Why should he bother communicating if all his needs are being attended to lovingly, without his having to ask for anything? By manipulating this situation somewhat, the bedtime routine can be used as an opportunity for teaching new communication skills. For example, the parents might create opportunities for developing choice-making skills by asking the boy which pajamas he wants to wear. Pausing expectantly before putting on the pajamas may encourage him to signal for continuation of the activity. These changes in the environment set the stage and tempt the child to communicate.

Adult AAC users may also be faced with fewer opportunities for communication. Mr. M, a successful businessman, was very outgoing and independent before a stroke left him with severe apraxia. Upon return from the rehabilitation facility, his wife of 32 years anticipated and responded immediately to his every need. Though motivated by the best intentions, Mrs. M was, in fact, hampering her husband's progress. With fewer reasons for communicating, Mr. M learned to be passive and only minimally communicative.

Partner Expectations.   A third source of reasons or opportunities for communication arise out of the expectations held by the AAC user's communication partner. One is more likely to contribute to an interaction if the communication partner expects it. This expectation, which begins with the belief that the AAC user is *capable* of initiating and responding, may influence how the interaction proceeds. Consider Charlie, a young boy whose presymbolic communication strategies are quite subtle and easily overlooked. Charlie's day care provider does not notice many of his presymbolic behaviors and does not consider those that she does notice to be meaningful communicative acts. Therefore, it does not occur to her to offer Charlie choices or other opportunities to communicate. Charlie's mother, on the other hand, clearly expects him to communicate, and she provides him with many opportunities for communication (e.g., by engaging him in social interaction and offering choices). The lack of opportunities to communicate may also be problematic for adult AAC users, such as Hank, a 55-year-old man who had a stroke. Like Mrs. M, Hank's wife now provides care for him in ways she did not before his stroke. In their daily routines, Mrs. M makes many decisions without any input from Hank. She selects his clothes, plans their meals, and turns the TV to his favorite sporting events, without expecting Hank to convey any opinions about these issues. In doing

these things, she may be discouraging Hank from using the communication skills that he is recovering or developing.

In some cases, rhetorical questions are used as a substitute for conversation that requires meaningful participation by the individual with communication disabilities. For example, Shauna, a teenager with cerebral palsy, occasionally sees her bus driver while she's working at the library. Because he is uncomfortable and afraid of not being able to understand her, the bus driver attempts only superficial conversation that does not really require Shauna to respond (e.g., "It's a nice day, isn't it?"). A certain amount of rhetorical questioning is typical; however, AAC users who are rarely engaged as true communication partners may begin to feel frustrated and isolated when there is too much.

In summary, opportunities for communication provided to AAC users relate to their partners' perceptions of their ability to respond appropriately. Intervention that fails to examine and address the role of communication partners' expectations has limited benefit for the AAC user. Individuals who have something to say and who know how to express their thoughts are communicatively limited if the people with whom they interact have no realization that they can make an interesting, informative, and valid contribution if given the opportunity. Intervention in this area may involve raising partners' levels of awareness and teaching them to expect their AAC-using friends, relatives, and colleagues to play active roles in conversation. The clinician/educator would probably also work with the AAC user directly, teaching specific proactive strategies for entering, maintaining, redirecting, and discontinuing discourse.

Opportunities for Communication.   As discussed in the previous sections, the extent to which individuals attempt to learn new communication skills is related to the need for communication as a tool and its effect on the environment. Kaiser notes, "an environment that contains few reinforcers, few objects of interest, or meets the students' needs without requiring language, is not a functional environment for language" (Kaiser, 1994, p. 357). In some situations, the first step in teaching AAC skills includes manipulating aspects of the environments in which the potential AAC user participates to make those settings more conducive to meaningful communication. Table 15.3 lists a number of strategies that have been used successfully to create opportunities for communication. Research using these strategies has demonstrated that these environmental arrangements are effective in enhancing communication skills within a teaching milieu (e.g., Alpert, Kaiser, Hemmeter, & Ostrosky, 1987; Haring, Neetz, Lovinger, Peck, &

Semmel, 1987). They are most effective in eliciting emerging communicative behaviors rather than teaching completely new behaviors. These strategies can be used both to demonstrate how communication can be used as a tool and to illustrate the natural consequences that follow effective communication.

The first strategy, interrupting routines, involves structuring familiar routines, such as washing one's hands, so that communication is an important part of the process. This strategy is help-

TABLE 15.3 Strategies for Creating Opportunities for Communication

STRATEGY	DESCRIPTION	EXAMPLE
Interrupting routines	Clinician/educator interrupts a familiar routine.	Clinician/educator prepares to serve juice to the AAC user, then pauses expectantly just before pouring, watching for a communicative response (e.g., request continuance).
Pretending/teasing	Clinician/educator responds to a situation in a silly or teasing fashion.	Clinician/educator pours juice in the AAC user's cup, pretends to drink it, then pauses expectantly, watching for a communicative response (e.g., comment, direct action to object).
Providing inappropriate amounts of materials	Clinician/educator gives too much or too little of the material needed for a given activity.	Clinician/educator pours a tiny amount of juice, gives it to the AAC user, then pauses expectantly, watching for a communicative response (e.g., request recurrence).
Providing tasks that require assistance	Clinician/educator provides materials that require assistance.	Clinician/educator gives AAC user a container of juice that is difficult to open, then pauses expectantly for a communicative response (e.g., request assistance).
Providing materials within view, but out of reach	Clinician/educator provides materials needed to complete an activity within view, but out of reach of the AAC user.	AAC user gets ready to pour own juice in cup that is visible, but out of reach. Clinician/educator pauses expectantly, watching for a communicative response (e.g., request object or assistance).
Giving a purposefully incorrect response	Clinician/educator purposely responds incorrectly to the AAC user's previous action.	AAC user looks intently at juice. Clinician/educator gives milk instead, then pauses expectantly, watching for a communicative response (e.g., clarification strategy).

ful in making the need for communication salient to the potential AAC user. In this strategy, a familiar routine is set up and implemented frequently and consistently so that the learner is able to anticipate the next steps in the sequence. A planned interruption is then inserted, giving the learner an opportunity to signal awareness of the interruption and request that the routine be allowed to continue. During this planned pause, the clinician/educator carefully observes the learner, watching for any behaviors that either are or can become communicative. This strategy is most commonly used with individuals at the earliest stages of expressive communication who may be using presymbolic or early symbolic forms of communication. Table 15.4 lists the steps involved in this strategy. A variation on this strategy is the **behavior chain interruption technique** (Goetz, Gee, & Sailor, 1985), which provides additional structure for determining the points within the routine that are best suited for interruption.

Without a reason to communicate, individuals with even the most advanced AAC skills are unlikely to spontaneously express their needs, thoughts, and feelings. Therefore, professionals must intervene at the level of creating opportunities in which AAC skills can be taught. Creating a reason to communicate is an important aspect in the communication teaching process. It is not, however, sufficient for the development of effective AAC skills. The clinician/educator must also work with AAC users to design and develop ways to communicate and with communication partners to improve opportunities for communicative interaction.

Ways in Which to Communicate. It is perhaps with the ways in which to communicate that AAC users' communication differs most obviously from that of peers who do not have disabilities. By definition, AAC users are using some strategy or technique that others do not use for expressing thoughts and ideas. The most appropriate ways to

TABLE 15.4   Using Familiar Routines to Teach AAC Skills

STEPS	EXAMPLES
Engage the learner in a familiar, somewhat enjoyable routine.	Washing hands.
Go through the routine and pause at some point for 15 seconds or so. Observe the learner's reaction. Does the learner seem to be aware that the activity has stopped?	Clinician/educator helps learner begin washing hands, pauses before dispensing soap, and watches for any reaction on the part of the learner.
If yes, call attention to the interruption. Then teach a signal for requesting continuance, verbally labeling the intent or function of the signal.	Learner looks up when the clinician/ educator pauses. Clinician/educator says "Yes, we stopped," and molds learner's hands into sign for WANT, saying, "Want soap."
If no, call attention to the interruption. Then model or prompt a response that the learner may eventually use to communicate.*	Learner does not seem aware of the pause in the routine. Clinician/educator says "Uh-oh, we stopped," and helps the learner reach toward the soap dispenser.
Continue with the routine.	Clinician/educator resumes routine with the learner, getting soap, rubbing hands under water, and so on.

*The learner who shows no awareness that the routine has stopped will probably need more experiences with routines structured in this manner before a communicative response can be taught successfully.

communicate should be selected based on the message, the desire to communicate, and communication partners. AAC users who used aided symbols and strategies require specific training with their communication devices. AAC intervention requires consideration of operational issues and the use of different communication modes for different settings.

Operational issues can be divided into two parts: (a) *means to select* and (b) *means to transmit* messages. These issues are discussed in more detail in Chapters 8, 9, and 10. The means to select relates to the way in which AAC users activate a device or otherwise produce a message. Determination of how the messages will be selected should be made in relation to the abilities of the AAC users and needs of the situation. For example, messages related to personal care may require quick, efficient communication. An AAC user who is in pain or needs help in the bathroom will have little tolerance for slow scanning or misunderstood messages. In this case, however, the selection set for personal assistance may contain relatively few messages, which might be selected via an eye-gaze communication board. A small set of gestures or manual signs that can be easily learned by the most familiar communication partners may also be effective. These means would provide quick access to a small set of messages.

When participating in academic classes or when discussing work-related tasks, however, AAC users must have access to a much larger vocabulary. The individual who can spell and has access to the alphabet has a virtually unlimited vocabulary, although letter-by-letter spelling may be extremely slow and impede communication. Other approaches, such as the use of abbreviation expansion, dynamic displays, and encoding, can be used to increase the size of available vocabulary while increasing speed of selection over letter-by-letter spelling (see Chapter 8).

Transmission of messages relates to the way in which the message is sent to a communication partner. The transmission mode must be appropriate to the situation and the communication needs. Consider Peter, for example, a 12-year-old who spends half his school day in a resource room for children with special needs and the other half with typical fifth graders. He has a communication device that has a liquid crystal display (LCD), synthetic speech output, and print output. When he is with typical fifth graders and the class is doing silent reading, he must be quiet. Therefore, if he needs to speak to his teacher, he uses the LCD and gestures for the teacher to read the screen. His friend Gary, whom he sees in the resource room, does not read well, and therefore, Peter uses the speech output to communicate with him. During the lunch hour, Peter uses the print output to pass a secret message to his best buddy, Lamar. As Peter's case illustrates, the mode of communication is matched to the demands of the situation.

Appropriate goals of intervention may include establishing or expanding operational skills (e.g., introducing and teaching a scanning system or an abbreviation technique) as well as the appropriate selection and use of a way to communicate. Quite different modes of communication may be effective in different situations, and a client may require specific training in how to choose the best mode for the particular setting. Consider the case of Greg, for example, who had learned several modes of communication. He understood and could produce approximately 300 manual signs, had an extensive vocabulary of graphic symbols arranged in a communication notebook, and produced speech that familiar people could understand with extensive contextual support. He required specific training, however, in how to apply these different communication modes. When entering an unfamiliar environment, he might begin speaking or might use manual signs to communicate with strangers. Initially he showed no ability to evaluate whether someone was understanding him, and he never voluntarily switched modes of communication. With education, he was able to recognize when someone was confused, and he learned to try all three of his modes of communication in succession until one mode was effective. AAC users often have different modes of communicating with familiar partners and with strangers. Some AAC users need training on how to differentiate these situations.

Partners with Whom to Communicate. A final, but no less important aspect of communication that requires intervention relates to communication partners. Natural speakers often interact with AAC users in ways that make it difficult for the AAC user to communicate effectively.

Intervention should include teaching strategies and techniques to an AAC user's communication partners to optimize effective communication and promote continued development of AAC skills. Communication partners can be taught to do three basic things to enhance interaction. The first thing communication partners need to do is recognize the AAC user's communicative acts. Individuals who are just learning to communicate or who use presymbolic communication may use signals that are very subtle or ambiguous. Stefani, a 3-year-old with Rett syndrome, paced frequently. To indicate that she wanted something, she would walk over to it and stand quietly for a few seconds. This behavior was so subtle that most untrained observers failed to recognize it as communicative. Other AAC users may use overt, but highly idiosyncratic means of expression. Doug, a 34-year-old man with cognitive impairment, learned manual signs when he was an adolescent. Over the years, his way of making the signs changed to the extent that they would probably not be recognized by a person who knew only the standard version of those signs. AAC intervention with this individual might include teaching the people with whom Doug communicates regularly to recognize his nonstandard, idiosyncratic signs.

The second thing communication partners need to do is to acknowledge communicative acts/messages. Often this acknowledgment comes as a verbal confirmation. Paige, a preschooler with developmental delays, learned to tug on her partner's sleeve when she wanted to play. To acknowledge this request, her teacher often responded by labeling what she thought was Paige's intent (e.g., "Oh, you want to *play*"). This told Paige that her request had been heard. It also gave Paige some important information. By hearing the verbal label "play," she was eventually able to link her presymbolic gesture with another symbolic means of representing that concept, setting the stage for future communicative growth. For an individual who understands the verbal label, acknowledging a message can serve an additional function. AAC users can compare the acknowledgment to their original

intent to determine whether their message was interpreted correctly by the communication partner. This gives the AAC user an opportunity to correct a misunderstanding if one has occurred. For example, if Paige had actually wanted a hug, she could have followed up with another presymbolic message (e.g., outstretched arms) to provide her teacher with additional information.

Finally, communication partners need to respond contingently to the content of communicative acts/messages. For individuals just learning AAC skills, this positively reinforces their efforts. Communication partners should use naturally occurring consequences whenever possible (e.g., giving someone the item they just requested or providing help that was requested). Communication partners must respond to the intent of an AAC user's message, rather than its form. For example, the wife of Norton, a man with severe aphasia, insisted that he use his communication book, rather than point to what he wanted. Although her intent was to give him additional practice in using his AAC skills, Norton felt demeaned and angry at her attempts to redirect him.

Communication partners may also need specific training in the operational aspects of an AAC user's communication device. A spouse or parent who is the primary caregiver may have responsibility for such things as charging the batteries of a communication device, setting it up for use throughout the day, programming vocabulary, and troubleshooting when it is not working properly.

AAC INTERVENTION PRINCIPLES

Fourteen AAC intervention principles, some of which were also introduced as assessment principles (Chapter 11), emerge from the discussion in this and previous chapters.

> **Principle 1.** AAC intervention is based on the premise that everyone can and does communicate.
>
> **Principle 2.** AAC intervention must keep the AAC user as the central focus.
>
> **Principle 3.** AAC intervention should not be delayed or denied because individuals are unable to demonstrate certain behaviors.

Principle 4.   AAC intervention should focus not only on current, but also future, communication needs.

Principle 5.   AAC intervention should not focus on replacing communication behaviors that are functional and socially acceptable.

Principle 6.   AAC intervention often occurs in conjunction with the ongoing process of assessment.

Principle 7.   AAC intervention requires a team approach that promotes collaboration.

Principle 8.   AAC intervention should be guided by carefully constructed, appropriate, long-term and short-term goals.

Principle 9.   AAC intervention should occur primarily within functional contexts in natural environments.

Principle 10.   AAC intervention should include procedures to minimize or eliminate barriers to communication.

Principle 11.   AAC intervention should focus not only on what skills should be taught, but also on how they should be taught.

Principle 12.   AAC intervention must include ongoing appropriate evaluation of the progress of AAC users so that modifications in intervention strategies can be made.

Principle 13.   AAC intervention should result in positive change.

Principle 14.   AAC intervention must adhere to the law of parsimony.

These principles apply to AAC intervention in general and are not dependent on specific characteristics of AAC users. They are valid for users, partners, environments, and systems. There is, however, a principle that *does* depend upon specific characteristics that must not be overlooked. Many AAC users have some natural speech as well as the potential to improve and make it more functional. Many individuals with little or no functional speech benefit not only from AAC, but also from intervention to improve natural speech. ***When appropriate, AAC intervention should not dismiss, but rather include ways to optimize the use of natural speech.***

SUMMARY

According to current thinking, AAC users should not be denied access to AAC intervention because they have not demonstrated certain cognitive or behavioral skills. Intervention should be initiated whenever a discrepancy exists between communication needs and abilities, regardless of the type or severity of an individual's disabilities. Integrated goals and objectives should guide clinicians/educators as they use a variety of instructional procedures to minimize this discrepancy. Intervention should be directed toward four important aspects of communication: (1) information/messages to communicate, (2) reasons to communicate, (3) ways in which to communicate, and (4) partners with whom to communicate. Fourteen general principles should guide service delivery.

CHAPTER 16

SENSORY IMPAIRMENTS

DOREEN M. BLISCHAK AND CHARLOTTE A. WASSON

Many **augmentative and alternative communication (AAC)** users experience temporary, fluctuating, progressive, or permanent hearing and/or visual impairments. Too often, sensory impairments are undetected and undermanaged in individuals with multiple disabilities because their impact is masked by the effects of other disabilities. Additionally, multiple disabilities often produce a synergistic effect, whereby existing disabilities are magnified because other abilities are not available to compensate (Arkell, 1982). When speech is severely impaired, even a mild sensory impairment can greatly affect communication functioning and limit AAC options. The presence of sensory impairments should always be ruled in or ruled out as contributing factors in cases of communication disability. Thus, identification of and adaptations for sensory impairments should become a routine component of a comprehensive AAC service delivery program throughout an individual's life span. Contributions of hearing and vision specialists must be considered integral parts of AAC service delivery.

This chapter provides an overview of assessment and intervention geared toward overcoming or minimizing the effects of hearing, visual, and **dual sensory impairment (DSI)** for individuals with severe speech impairments. Brief introductory portions on hearing impairment may be a review for some service providers but have been included for others involved in AAC service delivery who may not be as familiar with hearing impairment terminology and issues.

HEARING IMPAIRMENT

Hearing impairment is the most frequently occurring impairment affecting communication, occurring in more than 21 million Americans. As many as 2 of every 100 children have a permanent hearing loss significant enough to affect speech and language development. Many more experience fluctuating hearing loss as a result of middle-ear dysfunction. Adult onset hearing loss is estimated to affect 25% to 35% of Americans over age 65 (Alpiner & McCarthy, 1993; Bess & Humes, 1990).

Individuals with hearing impairments represent a highly diverse group. Most who are members of a Deaf community and communicatively competent in **American Sign Language (ASL)**, their native language, experience few limitations within the Deaf community. Many have little or no functional speech, but they are not typically candidates for AAC intervention (for additional information regarding communication in American Deaf culture, see Padden & Humphries, 1988).

Many of the estimated 2 million individuals in the United States who have little or no functional speech, not as a direct result of hearing impairments, do experience some temporary or permanent hearing impairments (American Speech-Language-Hearing Association [ASHA], 1992). For instance, Lafontaine and DeRuyter (1987) reported that nearly 25% of individuals with cerebral palsy and little or no functional speech have hearing impairments, and Allaire, Gressard, Blackman, and Hostler (1991) reported a hearing impairment rate of 15% in children with severe speech impairments. Reports of hearing impairments in individuals with cognitive impairments vary widely, with an average of 15% (ranging from 6% to 68%) reported by D'Zamko and Hampton (1985). Although not all individuals with cognitive impairments may require AAC intervention, the presence of even a mild hearing loss can significantly interfere with speech and language development, increasing the potential need for AAC intervention.

Individuals with hearing impairments may also experience accidents, disease, or the effects of aging that may diminish their ability to use established communication methods. For example, consider the devastating effect of a spinal cord injury and resulting arm and hand paralysis on a deaf individual who communicated via ASL (Fried-Oken, 1992). Further, as AAC users age, many may acquire hearing impairments, requiring modifications in existing AAC methods. Aging Americans, with their high prevalence of hearing impairments, must also be considered potential candidates for AAC intervention (Hirdes, Ellis-Hale, & Hirdes, 1993).

Impact of Hearing Impairment

Hearing impairment may have far-reaching consequences, affecting opportunities for linguistic, social, educational, and vocational independence (Downs, 1994). Hearing is one of the two "distance" senses (along with vision) that enables individuals to monitor what occurs beyond the immediate environment. Hearing uniquely allows reception of information from all directions simultaneously. It enables individuals to maintain contact with the environment at all times. Hearing can be muffled, but not eliminated, even in sleep. It is through hearing that individuals are socialized, gaining knowledge of others and how they perceive their world (Spensley, 1989). A developing child with normal hearing, in typical circumstances, is immersed in spoken language and learns it rather effortlessly. The adverse effects of severe to profound **bilateral** hearing impairment on spoken language development are well documented, and evidence is mounting that even a mild to moderate loss may cause significant language delay (Davis, Elfenbein, Schum, & Bentler, 1986; Friel-Patti, 1990). Even a **unilateral** hearing loss may create difficulty in understanding speech in noise, putting school-aged individuals at risk for academic failure (Alpiner & McCarthy, 1993; Osberger, 1990). Further, the earlier the onset of the hearing impairment, the greater the impact on linguistic development.

Although an adult who already knows the language can comprehend speech even with a considerable hearing loss, part of that achievement is due to the redundancy of language as a system. This enables the experienced language user to decode the message "from the top down" even though the listener has relatively impoverished information from the auditory input. On the other hand, when one is acquiring the system, such impoverished or degraded information may simply be insufficient to support the comprehension of the message. (Jenkins, 1986, pp. 216–217)

Individuals with hearing and cognitive and/or motor speech impairments are at increased risk for difficulty in developing functional speech because the presence of a hearing impairment may interfere with feedback and self-monitoring. Visual communication **modes** such as manual signs, graphic symbols, or print may aid receptive and expressive communication, yet are no substitute for immersion in auditory language.

Causes of Hearing Impairment

Many prenatal, developmental, and acquired conditions may cause hearing and other serious impairments. Prenatally, the group of infections referred to as TORCH (toxoplasmosis, other infections, rubella, cytomegalovirus, herpes) are known to cause hearing and vision impairments and brain damage (Holvoet & Helmstetter, 1989). Other risk factors are listed in Table 16.1.

Acquired hearing loss may occur in isolation as a result of noise or drug exposure, diseases of the ear, or aging. Individuals who develop a hearing loss after acquiring language generally will not require AAC intervention. When hearing loss occurs in conjunction with other impairments as a result of head trauma, stroke, or in combination with failing motor or visual skills, however, the need for AAC intervention may increase.

Audiologic Assessment

The auditory status of all AAC users should be monitored throughout the life span, even if a prior hearing loss has not been documented. Identification of hearing loss in individuals with little or no

TABLE 16.1 Risk Factors for Hearing Impairment

- Autism
- Cerebral palsy
- Craniofacial anomalies (including cleft palate)
- Exposure to cytomegalovirus, diuretics, heavy metals (e.g., mercury), herpes, ototoxic drugs (e.g., streptomycin), rubella, toxoplasmosis, and/or untreated maternal syphilis in utero
- Exposure to ototoxic drugs after birth
- Head trauma
- HIV infection
- Jaundice (hyperbilirubinemia)
- Low birth weight
- Meningitis
- Mental retardation
- Parents or grandparents with hearing loss
- Perinatal anoxia (lack of oxygen during birth) or problems breathing shortly after birth
- Syndromes involving chromosomal abnormalities (e.g., Down, Hurler, Treacher Collins, Turner, Waardenburg)

Compiled from D. A. Clark (1980); Holvoet & Helmstetter (1989); Northern & Downs (1991).

TABLE 16.2 Indicators of Hearing Impairment

PRIMARY PHYSIOLOGICAL INDICATORS

- Crying
- Discharge from ears
- Frequent colds or upper respiratory infections
- Frequent wax buildup
- Mouth breathing
- Tinnitus (ringing in the ears)
- Tugging at ears

PRIMARY BEHAVIORAL INDICATORS

- Aggressive or withdrawn behavior
- Difficulty following spoken instructions
- Difficulty localizing source of sound
- Failure to respond to name or other speech
- Intolerance of loud and/or sudden sounds
- Puzzled facial expression
- Speech or vocalizations that are too loud or too soft
- Straining toward sound source

Adapted from Alpiner & McCarthy (1993); DuBose (1983); McCormick (1990b).

functional speech, however, may be difficult. Overt behaviors that are typically thought to indicate hearing impairment may be the same as those displayed by individuals with impairments not related to hearing. These behaviors and other indicators are provided in Table 16.2. Indicators are listed as primary physiological or primary behavioral, but there is overlap (e.g., crying may be physiological or a learned behavior).

A comprehensive auditory assessment involves **evaluation** of the outer ear, middle ear functioning, hearing sensitivity, and responses to speech audiometry. Every effort should be made to complete the full assessment battery, beyond a simple hearing **screening**. Although pinpointing exact hearing abilities may not always be possible in some individuals, AAC teams should try to "rule out moderate-profound, bilateral hearing impairments involving the speech frequencies (500–2000 Hz inclusive)" (Gans & Gans, 1993, p. 128).

General Considerations. To complete a reliable audiologic assessment, the AAC team often needs to make special adaptations to accommodate the communication, cognitive, physical, and behavioral needs of AAC users; no person is too young or too impaired for such assessment (Lloyd & Cox, 1972; Young, 1986). AAC users should prepare for and participate in the assessment process to the fullest extent possible. Preparation may involve creating and rehearsing vocabulary items for asking and answering questions, describing a problem, or responding to auditory stimuli. Contact should be made with the audiologist prior to the initial examination to determine what will be required of the AAC user. This initial contact also informs the audiologist of the unique communication needs and behaviors of the individual who will be assessed. Additional considerations are provided in Table 16.3.

Procedures. As with any assessment, an important first step is gathering a case history, including personal and family history and, when appropriate, a description of the onset and symptoms surrounding the hearing loss. The audiologist will

TABLE 16.3   Adaptations for Audiologic Assessment

GENERAL CONSIDERATIONS

- Be aware of attention span and physical stamina. Frequent breaks may be necessary or the assessment may need to be conducted over several sessions.
- Remember to establish eye contact, use gestures, simplify speech, repeat, and rephrase as necessary. Allow adequate pause time for all responses.
- Communicate with the AAC user and not with an accompanying caregiver exclusively. Actively involve the AAC user in the evaluation and counseling process by explaining procedures.

PLAN AHEAD

- Prepare the AAC user and accompanying caregiver by explaining, demonstrating, and role-playing what will happen during the audiologic assessment.
- Work with the AAC user and desensitize as needed to improve tolerance for otoscopic examination, insertion of probe tips, and headphone placement.
- Determine the AAC user's preferred mode of communicating for this situation. Preprogram and/or practice message items prior to the assessment session.
- Determine and practice an appropriate motor response and prepare adaptations (e.g., switches) as needed.
- Prepare materials such as objects, pictures, or written words for speech reception and identification testing. Practice the indicating response (eye gaze, pointing, switch).
- Ensure that all assessment locations are physically accessible and safe.
- Ensure that the AAC user can be positioned appropriately to maximize concentration and comfort and inhibit reflexive movement.
- Be aware that pure tones or sudden flashes of light may trigger seizures in some individuals. Find out whether an AAC user is at risk, what precautions to take, and how to manage a seizure.

Compiled from Bennet (1992); Byers & Bristow (1990); McEwen & Lloyd (1990a); Young (1986).

then examine the outer ear, ear canal, and eardrum for the presence of malformations, foreign objects, or impacted **cerumen** (wax). Elderly persons and individuals with mental retardation, particularly those with Down syndrome, are at risk for developing impacted wax. Many will require routine wax removal to maintain adequate hearing (Crandell & Roeser, 1993; Van Dyke, Lang, Heide, van Duyne, & Soucek, 1990).

Middle Ear.   The middle ear is a cavity containing the eardrum and three small bones (ossicles): the malleus (hammer), incus (anvil), and stapes (stirrup). These vibrate in response to sound and conduct the vibrations to the inner ear. A hearing loss caused by impairment of outer or middle ear structures is called a conductive hearing loss. The eustachian tube, which equalizes middle ear pressure, leads from the middle ear to the nasopharynx (see Figure 16.1).

Immittance audiometry is used to evaluate middle ear functioning. Each of three immittance tests contributes unique information, yet they are best interpreted as part of the total audiologic battery to confirm or rule out a conductive hearing loss (Bess & Humes, 1990; Ginsberg & White, 1985). Tympanometry involves introducing air into the ear canal via an inserted probe to provide an indirect measure of the mobility of the eardrum and ossicles. A **tympanogram** shows relative air pressure in decaPascals. A peak at 0 daPa indicates that middle ear pressure is the same as ambient air pressure (Kaplan, Gladstone, & Lloyd, 1993). The tympanogram shown in Figure 16.2 illustrates normal middle ear pressure.

Static acoustic immittance measures energy flow through the middle ear under varying degrees of air pressure and is recorded in cubic centimeters (cm^3). Values from 0.25 to 2.0 are considered within normal limits. Acoustic reflex testing measures the movement of the stapedius muscle, which contracts in response to loud sound. Reflexes should occur when tones are presented between 65 and 90 decibels (dB) (Bess & Humes, 1990).

Immittance testing is quick, relatively noninvasive, and useful for any individual who does

Outer ear   Middle ear   Inner ear   VIIIth cranial nerve

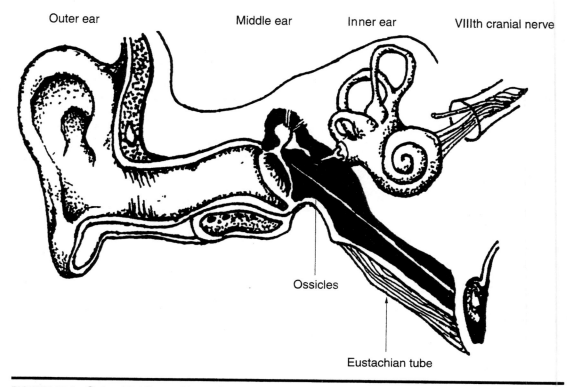

Ossicles

Eustachian tube

FIGURE 16.1   Outer, Middle, and Inner Ear.
Courtesy of Jacob Wasson.

not respond consistently on measures of hearing sensitivity. However, the individual must remain still without vocalizing or moving the head and tolerate insertion of the probe tip into the ear canal.

Pure Tone Testing.   Pure tone testing determines hearing threshold, the lowest level at which the presence of a tone is detected 50% of the time, across a range of frequencies (typically 250 to 8000 Hz). In normal adults, threshold is 0 to 20dB. Testing requires production of a voluntary motor response (e.g., hand raise). Children with a developmental age of 2 to 3 years may be taught to respond via **play audiometry**, where, for example, they are taught to drop a block in a box in response to a tone (Hodgson, 1985; Northern & Downs, 1991). For AAC users with physical impairments, any consistent voluntary motor response that is observable, repeatable, and resistant to fatigue, while not promoting abnormal posture or move-

ments, may be used. Use of adapted switches that activate a light or buzzer may also be appropriate.

Results of pure tone testing are plotted on an **audiogram** in dB, a unit of sound intensity (Figure 16.3). A pure tone average (PTA) of the frequencies 500, 1000, and 2000 Hz is also reported as an estimated response to speech stimuli.

Special Procedures.   Pure tones are ideally presented through headphones to isolate each ear, which is particularly important in cases of suspected unilateral loss or when sensitivity differs significantly between ears. However, sound field testing may be conducted to estimate general hearing sensitivity for individuals who do not tolerate headphones. Special procedures such as **visual reinforcement audiometry (VRA)** may be used with young children or individuals with cognitive impairments. Generally, the individual is positioned in a sound-treated booth where the audiologist can carefully observe responses. A loud tone

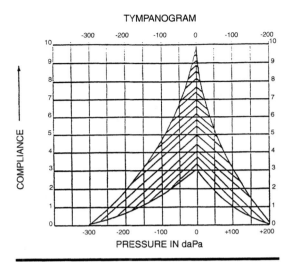

FIGURE 16.2 Normal (Type A) Tympanogram.
From Kaplan, Gladstone, & Lloyd (1993).

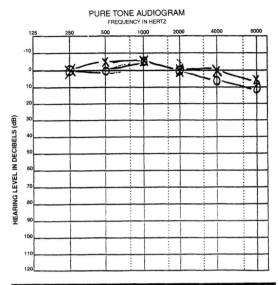

FIGURE 16.3 Normal Audiogram.
From Kaplan, Gladstone, & Lloyd (1993).

is presented, followed by the activation of a light, video display, and/or movement of a mechanical toy. As presentation of additional tones of varying frequencies and intensities occurs, the audiologist notes the individual's gaze in the direction of the toy in anticipation that it will be activated. Although VRA has the potential for use with older individuals by using more age-appropriate visual reinforcements (e.g., video), it may not be appropriate for everyone. Some individuals may be frightened by the toy or object, or may manifest seizure activity in response to the flash of light (Bennet, 1992; Gans & Gans, 1993; Goetz, Gee, & Sailor, 1983; Young, 1986).

Tangible reinforcement operant conditioning audiometry (TROCA) may also be used for pure tone testing. Here, an edible reinforcer is provided each time the individual responds appropriately to presentation of a tone (Lloyd, Spradlin, & Reid, 1968).

Speech Audiometry. Individuals who do not respond consistently to pure tones may respond to speech, as it is more meaningful. Evaluation of speech awareness (detection) may be obtained without production of a voluntary motor response, via observation of automatic responses such as cessation of movement, blink, or startle in re-

sponse to hearing one's own name. Adaptations are generally not necessary, as the individual need not interpret the spoken word but only respond to speech as sound.

Assessment of **speech reception thresholds (SRTs)** generally requires production of a spoken response, as the individual is required to repeat spondees (two-syllable words with equal syllabic stress, e.g., baseball, ice cream) presented at varying loudness levels. Threshold, here, is the level at which 50% of the words are correctly identified. Production of natural speech responses may be appropriate for some AAC users, given the high predictability of the spondees. An AAC user may also indicate common objects, line drawings, or written words via eye gaze, pointing, or adapted switches. Another option is to use familiar words that the AAC user can indicate via an established communication mode (e.g., manual signs). When adaptations are needed, the AAC service provider, in close collaboration with the audiologist, must determine the preferred response mode and prepare stimuli prior to the assessment.

Speech identification testing is a critical part of the assessment battery, because pure tone and speech reception thresholds are not always predictive of the ability to understand speech. Here, the individual is required to repeat 50 monosyllabic words presented above threshold. This typical speech identification testing is problematic for many AAC users, even with interpreting by a familiar partner. Although most speech identification tasks use open-set material, one commercially available closed-set adaptation, the *Word Intelligibility by Picture Identification (WIPI)* (Ross & Lerman, 1970), may be appropriate. Here, the individual may point or use eye gaze to indicate from a set of pictures. For further information regarding adaptations for AAC users, see Bess and Humes (1990), Byers and Bristow (1990), Penrod (1985), and Wasson, Tynan, and Gardiner (1981).

Auditory Brainstem Response. For individuals who do not respond consistently to behavioral audiometry or when results are questionable, **auditory brainstem response (ABR)*** evaluation is indicated, along with continued attempts to use behavioral methods (Allen, Rapin, & Wiznitzer, 1988). ABR is a noninvasive procedure that measures electrical responses along the auditory pathway at the level of the brainstem. It does not require production of a voluntary response. Surface electrodes attached to the head record responses to repeated "clicks" delivered via headphones. For this procedure, which takes approximately 45 minutes, some individuals require mild sedation.

ABR is best used in conjunction with the results of other tests in the audiologic assessment battery (Gans & Gans, 1993). However, results may serve as a point of departure for including or ruling out hearing loss as a contributing factor in speech-language delay for some individuals. For additional information regarding ABR testing, see Jacobson and Hyde (1985), Niswander (1987), or Northern and Downs (1991).

Classification of Hearing Impairment

Hearing impairment may be classified according to ear(s) affected (unilateral or bilateral) and age of onset (e.g., prelingual—before development of mature speech and spoken language). It may also be described according to degree of loss—reported in dB—and structures involved (conductive, sensorineural, mixed). Table 16.4 provides a general description of degree of hearing loss and resultant effect on communication. For some individuals, a mild hearing loss may interfere with communication, whereas others with a moderate loss may function with few adaptations. In general, (1) the age of onset, (2) the severity of the loss, (3) the frequencies involved, and (4) the presence of additional impairments will influence the impact of the hearing loss on communication.

Conductive.   **Conductive hearing impairment** occurs when problems affecting the outer and/or middle ear reduce conduction of sound, usually resulting in a mild to moderate degree of hearing impairment. Causes include foreign bodies or wax accumulation, middle ear fluid, and disease processes. Most conductive impairments are medically manageable, although many become permanent if left untreated. A common cause of conductive loss, particularly in children, is **otitis media (OM)**—inflammation of the middle ear. Antibiotics are generally used to treat cases of acute, purulent (infected) OM to prevent development of eardrum perforations, meningitis, or permanent hearing loss. A common, yet still controversial treatment for chronic OM involves insertion of pressure equalizing (PE) tubes into the eardrum (Alpiner & McCarthy, 1993; Ginsberg & White, 1985; Northern & Downs, 1991).

For AAC users, detection and treatment of OM may be hampered by difficulties in communicating pain or discomfort. Caregivers must remain alert to signs of possible OM (e.g., discharge from the ear, tugging at the ear, fever, irritability, restlessness). Routine audiologic and medical care are important for detecting and monitoring middle ear functioning.

Sensorineural.   Damage to the inner ear (cochlea and/or auditory nerve) may be present at birth or may result from infection, noise exposure,

---

*Auditory brainstem response may also be referred to as brainstem auditory evoked response (BSAER or BAER), auditory evoked response (AER), or brainstem response (BSR) audiometry.

TABLE 16.4 Classification of Hearing Impairment

CLASSIFICATION	HEARING LEVEL	IMPACT
Normal hearing	0–15 dB	No disability
Slight hearing loss	16–25 dB	Understands speech face to face, but may have some difficulty following conversation
Mild hearing loss	26–40 dB	
Moderate hearing loss	41–55 dB	Difficulty following conversation, particularly in noise, but can understand amplified speech
Moderately severe hearing loss	56–70 dB	Difficulty understanding amplified speech
Severe hearing loss	71–90 dB	
Profound hearing loss	> 90 dB	Little if any ability to hear speech, even with amplification

Based on Bess & Humes (1990); Kaplan, Gladstone, & Lloyd (1993); Thurman & Widerstrom (1990).

ototoxic medications, and/or age-related changes that can cause a generally irreversible, **sensorineural hearing impairment**. Degree of hearing loss related to inner ear damage ranges from mild to profound. Speech perception abilities are frequently more affected than responses to pure tones may indicate (Ginsberg & White, 1985; Hardick & Davis, 1986).

Mixed. In some individuals, factors may combine to produce **mixed hearing impairment** with both conductive and sensorineural components. For example, some individuals with Down syndrome may have a congenital sensorineural loss and experience recurrent OM or impacted wax. Another common combination is the occurrence of a conductive loss due to impacted wax in an elderly person who has a sensorineural loss. Mixed hearing impairment requires prompt medical management of the conductive component and ongoing audiologic management.

Management of Hearing Impairment

Amplification. Hearing is a background sense. It enables individuals to maintain contact with the environment while visual attention and concentration are devoted to other tasks. Even a mild loss

may compromise safety, independence, learning, and communication. Every effort should be made to secure appropriate amplification for AAC users with hearing impairments to maximize use of residual hearing. Although individuals differ in their ability to benefit from amplification, every person with hearing impairment should be given the opportunity to use some type of amplification (Ling, 1984; Northern & Downs, 1991; Osberger, 1990).

Hearing Aids. Four styles of hearing aids are most often fitted, depending on factors such as severity of loss, age, manual dexterity, and personal preference: behind-the-ear (BTE), in-the-canal (ITC), in-the-ear (ITE), and body-worn hearing aids. Body-worn hearing aids are occasionally prescribed for elderly individuals or individuals with physical disabilities who have difficulty manipulating the controls of smaller hearing aids (Figure 16.4) (Sobsey & Wolf-Schein, 1991).

Some AAC users may be independent in ongoing hearing aid management and in reporting hearing aid problems. For those who are not independent, caregivers should assume responsibility for daily and weekly hearing aid checks and maintenance. The hearing aid should also be checked by an audiologist any time that the aid is malfunctioning, or at least yearly for routine maintenance.

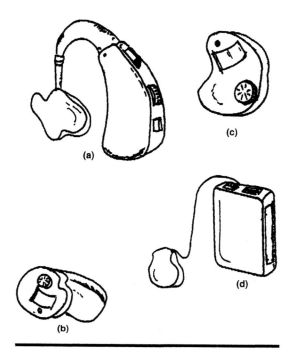

FIGURE 16.4 Hearing Aids. (a) Behind-the-ear (BTE) hearing aid. (b) In-the-canal (ITC) hearing aid. (c) In-the-ear (ITE) hearing aid. (d) Body-worn hearing aid.

Courtesy of Jacob Wasson.

As Smedley and Plapinger (1988) reported, a malfunctioning hearing aid may be worse than none, because wearing a "dead" hearing aid may create an additional loss of 25 to 40 dB (see Wayner (1990) for an excellent resource on hearing aid care and maintenance).

Assistive Listening Devices. **Assistive listening devices (ALDs)** are different from hearing aids in that they are designed to overcome the reduction in signal intensity resulting from background noise, distance, and reverberation. Because a hearing aid, by its very nature, amplifies all sound, it may have limited effectiveness when the wearer is in certain public areas, using the telephone, watching TV, or riding in a car. An ALD microphone is positioned close to the targeted sound source (e.g., another's voice, telephone receiver, or TV speaker), permit-

ting little or no amplification of extraneous sounds (Beaulac, Pehringer, & Shough, 1989). Many types of ALDs are used in conjunction with or in place of hearing aids. Audiologic consultation is strongly recommended in ALD selection.

Several types of ALDs may be appropriate for AAC users, two of which will be described. For further information, see Compton (1989). A hardwire system consists of a wire directly linking the sound source to a hearing aid or headphones (Figure 16.5a). Hardwire technology may allow for amplified or private listening to a TV, radio, or **voice output communication aid (VOCA)**. Another hardwire system that may be useful for individuals with physical impairments is a **personal amplification system (PAS)**, a body-worn amplifier with headphones. As with a body-worn hearing aid, the wearer must be independent in operating the device (Beaulac et al., 1989).

An alternative to hardwire is an FM system (Figure 16.5b), the ALD most frequently used in classrooms for students with hearing impairments (Bess & Sinclair, 1985). Here, the sound source, such as a teacher's voice, is transmitted via a wireless microphone to a body-worn receiver, which is attached to a hearing aid or headphones. FM (or similar) amplification systems have also improved classroom and therapy performance for hearing students with learning and/or communication disabilities (Blake, Field, Foster, Platt, & Wertz, 1991; Sudler & Flexer, 1986). Mild amplification may also increase auditory attention for some individuals with cerebral palsy who show deficits in auditory selective attention (Laraway, 1985).

Amplification should always be considered as a potential contributor to the development, participation, and independence of individuals with hearing impairments. Yet, individuals with multiple impairments, including many AAC users, may not always receive appropriate amplification. Sobsey and Wolf-Schein (1991) suggested several obstacles that may interfere with successful hearing aid use:

- Individuals at the ends of the hearing impairment continuum (i.e., mild or profound loss) may not receive amplification or may not receive it early in the course of the hearing loss, because it is believed that it would not be beneficial.

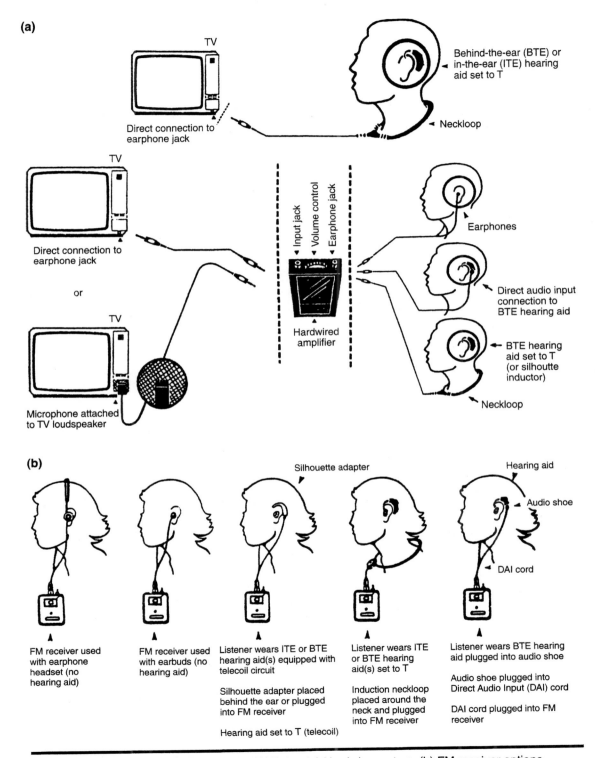

(a)

TV

Behind-the-ear (BTE) or
in-the-ear (ITE) hearing
aid set to T

Direct connection to
earphone jack

Neckloop

TV

Input jack
Volume control
Earphone jack

Direct connection to
earphone jack

or

Earphones

Hardwired
amplifier

Direct audio input
connection to
BTE hearing aid

TV

BTE hearing
aid set to T
(or silhoutte
inductor)

Microphone attached
to TV loudspeaker

Neckloop

(b)

Silhouette adapter

Hearing aid

Audio shoe

DAI cord

FM receiver used
with earphone
headset (no
hearing aid)

FM receiver used
with earbuds (no
hearing aid)

Listener wears ITE or BTE
hearing aid(s) equipped with
telecoil circuit

Silhouette adapter placed
behind the ear or plugged
into FM receiver

Hearing aid set to T (telecoil)

Listener wears ITE
or BTE hearing
aid(s) set to T

Induction neckloop
placed around the
neck and plugged
into FM receiver

Listener wears BTE hearing
aid plugged into audio shoe

Audio shoe plugged into
Direct Audio Input (DAI)
cord

DAI cord plugged into FM
receiver

FIGURE 16.5   Assistive Listening Devices (ALDs).   (a) Hardwire system. (b) FM receiver options.

- Hearing aids may not be powerful enough.
- Hearing aid functioning may not be consistently monitored.
- Hearing aid users may not receive appropriate orientation and training.

The key to overcoming these obstacles lies in appropriate audiologic management.

Other Sensory Aids. Other sensory aids to improve hearing include alerting devices, speech training aids, tactile aids, and cochlear implants. Little has been written regarding their use by AAC users. For additional, general information on sensory aids, see Boothroyd (1990) and Compton (1989).

VOCA Use. Although many studies have been done on synthetic speech intelligibility by persons without disabilities, only a few studies have involved persons with hearing impairments. Kangas and Allen (1990) found that adults with normal hearing and those with hearing impairments experienced more difficulty understanding high-quality synthetic speech than the speech of a natural male speaker, with the hearing-impaired adults understanding less accurately. Wasson and Binnie (1994) demonstrated that elderly adults with hearing impairments performed more poorly than elderly and young adults without hearing impairments on synthetic speech-recognition tasks and on tasks involving a natural female speaker in the presence of competing speech. Performance was poorer on the synthetic speech-recognition tasks. Of note in both studies is the broad performance variability by adults with hearing impairments, supporting the existence of a range of speech perception abilities.

Of concern for AAC users who may use VOCAs, then, regardless of their own hearing status, is the hearing abilities of their communication partners. AAC service providers should not assume that regular communication partners have adequate comprehension of synthetic speech. Audiologic assessment and/or consultation with regular communication partners is vital when selecting a VOCA.

Special Populations.

Autism. Audiologic evaluation is critical in differentiating **autism** from severe language impairment, profound hearing loss, and/or severe cognitive impairment (Wing, 1989). Further, children with autism tend to have a high rate of bilateral conductive hearing loss (Klin, 1993; Smith, Miller, Stewart, Walter, & McConnell, 1988). Some may demonstrate hypersensitivity to sound, yet others may seem impervious to loud noises. Still others may show bizarre or fluctuating responses to sound, for example, alternating underresponsiveness and overresponsiveness to a particular sound—such as a vacuum cleaner (Allen et al., 1988; Lovaas, Calori, & Jada, 1989). Thus, audiologic assessment and intervention for individuals with autism presents quite a challenge. ABR testing and frequent middle ear examinations may be of most benefit.

Little has been reported about the use of amplification for individuals with autism. One controversial treatment involves participation in several hours of auditory integration training (AIT) to overcome reported hyperacute hearing at certain frequencies (Rimland & Edelson, 1994; Veale, 1994). Little empirical evidence is available to support the efficacy of this approach. Given the difficulty in obtaining accurate, pure tone thresholds for many individuals with autism, use of such an approach is questionable (Friel-Patti, 1994; Gravel, 1994).

Cleft Palate. Individuals with **cleft palate** are at increased risk for sensorineural hearing loss, and invariably experience conductive hearing impairments (McWilliams, Morris, & Shelton, 1990). Although the presence of cleft palate alone rarely interferes with the development of functional speech to the degree that AAC intervention is needed, cleft palate occurs in a number of syndromes that affect physical and cognitive development (e.g., Klippel-Feil syndrome) (Northern & Downs, 1991). Thus, any AAC user with cleft palate must be considered at risk for hearing impairment.

Down Syndrome. Individuals with **Down syndrome** have a high incidence of hearing impairments. In addition to sensorineural loss, they are also vulnerable to middle ear problems such as impacted wax and recurrent OM (Van Dyke et al., 1990). Untreated hearing loss unnecessarily places individuals with Down syndrome at increased risk for communication difficulties. Audiologic assessment should be routine, even for individuals without prior history of hearing loss. Identification of hearing loss is especially critical to differentiate it from the behavioral, social, and communicative deterioration that signals the onset of dementia, a well-documented occurrence in some adults with Down syndrome (Burt, Loveland, & Lewis, 1992).

Acquired Impairments.   Like the general population, AAC users face the possibility of encountering illnesses or the effects of aging that may create additional impairments. Others who require AAC intervention as a result of head trauma or stroke may have a pre-existing hearing loss, lose additional hearing sensitivity as a result of the insult, or develop a hearing loss later on. Onset of each additional impairment affects the course of intervention—restricting communication options and potentially rendering previously used methods ineffective. Onset of hearing impairment may be mistaken for depression or dementia, with potentially disastrous results. Thorough audiologic management is critical for differential diagnosis, to maximize communication, and to reduce social isolation.

AAC Intervention.   Many aspects of AAC intervention with individuals with hearing impairments are similar to those for hearing individuals—to establish manual and/or visual means of communication to augment or replace spoken language—both receptively and expressively. Further, AAC intervention is consistent with the philosophy of **total communication (TC)** in deaf education (see Chapter 4) which promotes the acceptance and use of amplification; all visual, manual, and auditory modes of communication; as well as opportunities to communicate with individuals both with and without hearing impairments (Ling, 1984).

Each AAC user presents a unique combination of sensory, motor, cognitive, social, and commu-

nication abilities. Individuals with hearing impairments must receive intervention that takes into account their limitations in spoken language comprehension. Romski and Sevcik (1988a) stressed the role of receptive communication in individuals with cognitive impairments and the importance of addressing comprehension skills, suggesting that communication partners consistently augment their own speech production with AAC methods. The need for this augmentation becomes all the more critical for AAC users with hearing impairments who often miss communication that occurs during daily routines (e.g., meal preparation), because attention may be directed elsewhere. Even with amplification, many will have difficulty following conversation. Thus, communication partners need to take this into account by providing AAC "backup" to spoken utterances and by modeling functional communication during natural routines (Moeller, Osberger, & Morford, 1987). For example, gestures or manual signs may be easily modeled in many situations. Use of aided methods employing graphic symbols, by nature of their static presentation, can enhance comprehension as well.

Specific suggestions for auditory and communication intervention for AAC users with hearing impairments are listed in Table 16.5. Although these are intended primarily for children, age-appropriate adaptations may be made for older individuals. For a description of traditional aural rehabilitation techniques such as auditory training and speechreading (lipreading), see Alpiner & McCarthy (1993), English (1995), Hull (1992), and Schow & Nerbonne (1989).

Suggested intervention strategies may also be used when the auditory status of an AAC user is still undetermined. As mentioned throughout this chapter, pinpointing exact hearing abilities of some individuals with multiple disabilities is often difficult. As a rule, if an individual's behavior suggests difficulty in perceiving or comprehending speech, AAC service providers should proceed as if the person has a hearing impairment and provide communication adaptations, amplification, and auditory training, along with continued audiologic monitoring. A case study of a young AAC user by

TABLE 16.5   Intervention Suggestions for Working with AAC Users with Hearing Impairments

- Use appropriate assistive technology and monitor equipment functioning daily.
- Reduce background noise as much as possible in the home and classroom. Realize that hearing may not be optimal in noisy cafeterias, gymnasiums, or crowded public areas.
- Seat the child as close as possible to the speaker (e.g., teacher), away from distractions.
- Gain the child's attention before giving instructions or engaging in conversation.
- Encourage the child to respond to the sound of the child's own name.
- Look at the child when communicating and maintain eye contact as much as possible. Position child at eye level or move/bend to maintain eye contact. This is particularly important for children whose position is frequently varied from wheelchair to adapted stander to sidelyer.
- Speak in single words, phrases, and short sentences using natural pitch, rhythm, and intonation. Vary intonation naturally for conversation, reading aloud, expressing emotions. Use natural facial expression and body movements to supplement speech. Keep hands and papers away from face when speaking.
- Help the child notice environmental sounds (e.g., telephone, dog barking) by calling attention to them. Point out the direction from which the sound came to encourage localization skills. Provide toys, activities, and experiences that make noise and encourage auditory attention to them. Match the referent to a representation on the child's AAC device.
- Provide a variety of sensory experiences involving touch, taste, smell, sound, and other meaningful experiences within which language and communication can develop. Describe these using short meaningful sentences and model them with the child's own AAC device. Respond to what interests the child and provide appropriate spoken and AAC models.
- Associate a spoken word or phrase with the child's AAC representation and the actual referent. Use the word/phrase many times in varying contexts. Alternately speak, then indicate the referent to allow the child to shift visual attention between the two.
- Read aloud facing the child, giving the child the opportunity to alternately look at the pictures and the reader's face. As books become familiar, occasionally read from behind the child, and follow the print with an index finger.
- Give the child a chance to listen and then respond, to encourage turn-taking communication. Allow sufficient time for the child to process and respond.

Compiled from Bigge (1982); Gdowski, Sanger, & Decker (1986).

Hooper, Connell, and Flett (1987) illustrated the importance of repeated audiologic testing during ongoing AAC intervention. Although the child ultimately was found to have normal hearing acuity, she functioned as if she had a profound hearing loss, showing little to no response to most environmental sounds and speech. Her intervention program featured auditory training along with introduction of manual signs and Blissymbols to promote concurrent development of receptive and expressive communication.

VISUAL IMPAIRMENT

Visual impairment causes "suffering, disability, and loss of productivity for millions of people throughout the world" (Vision Research, 1983, p. 1). Among individuals most at risk for having or acquiring visual impairment are individuals with other disabilities (Tavernier, 1993), including those with little or no functional speech. AAC users with visual impairments, similar to those with hearing impairments, present special challenges to AAC team members.

Definition

As is true with many terms, the definition of visual impairment varies from source to source. According to the World Health Organization (WHO, 1980), blindness implies either no vision or no significant usable vision. An individual is considered legally blind if *corrected* acuity is less than 20/200 in the better eye, meaning that the individual distinguishes at 20 feet what someone with normal vision sees at 200 feet. Legal blindness involving peripheral field loss exists when the visual field is restricted to less than 20 degrees. The individual with normal vision has a bilateral visual field of 180 degrees (Karp, 1983; Nelson & Dimitrova, 1993; Robinson, Jan, & Kinnis, 1987). *Low vision* is a broader term, referring to a significant visual impairment with some usable vision and is a term that actually may be applied to many individuals who are classified with blindness (Hogg & Sebba, 1987; Lawrence, Lovie-Kitchin, & Brohier, 1992). Because many types and degrees of visual impairments are correctable, an individual should be classified as having a visual impairment only if the impairment remains once maximal correction is implemented.

Prevalence

Precise prevalence figures on visual impairment in AAC users are difficult to obtain, because a loss of vision may be unrecognized, unreported, or categorized secondary to a major classification or condition such as cerebral palsy or **traumatic brain injury (TBI)**. Worldwide as many as 35 million individuals are blind, and an equal number of persons have low vision (Lawrence et al., 1992). More than 10 million Americans have visual impairment beyond that which can be corrected by eye wear (Lawrence et al., 1992), and another 4.5 million have "severe" visual impairment—a figure that translates to "17 out of every 1,000 individuals in the civilian noninstitutionalized population" (Nelson & Dimitrova, 1993, p. 84). Determining more precise figures is difficult because no specific agency is charged with gathering such information (Lawrence et al., 1992).

In individuals with multiple impairments, visual impairment is more than 200 times that of the general population (Batshaw & Perret, 1992). This means that 75% to 85% of individuals with multiple impairments may have visual impairments (Tavernier, 1993). Many of these visual impairments occur early in life and affect males more than females (Hayes, 1985; Regenbogen & Coscas,

1985). Other visual impairments may emerge later in life. In fact, a group particularly at risk for visual impairment is elderly individuals, with nearly 10% reported to have severe visual impairments (Crew & Frey, 1993; Mann, Hurren, Karuza, & Bentley, 1993). Still further, as individuals with pre-existing congenital, acquired, or progressive impairments receive better medical care, their longevity increases, bringing additional risk of visual impairments related to the aging process (Aitchison, Easty, & Jancar, 1990). Table 16.6 summarizes visual abnormalities associated with selected syndromes and disorders.

Structure and Function of the Visual System

As illustrated in Figure 16.6, the visual system is a highly complex and well-organized body system, comprised of both peripheral and central components. Each ocular structure contributes to the receptive function of sight, the sense through which the brain receives as much as 75% of its information (Batshaw & Perret, 1992; Hayes, 1985; Vision Research, 1983). The actual processing of this sensory signal is called *vision*, which occurs as sensory information is sent through the visual pathway to the brain.

In normal binocular vision, individuals respond to objects by converging their eyes to position images on the two fovea centrali (maculae) in the retinal areas at the back of each eye, while increasing the accommodation of each lens to yield sharp retinal images. Vision is accomplished as the retina's rods and cones transform the physical energy of the visual image into nerve impulses. These electrosignals are processed at this level and are integrated with one another by a highly organized cellular system that is sensitive to different stimulus sizes, velocities, and locations in the field of vision. Neurosignals, through optic nerve impulses, are then routed to the brain. On their way, portions of each optic nerve cross one another before entering the occipital lobe. From there, some axons branch on into the midbrain to aid the body in orientation to visual stimuli. Additionally, neurons in the brainstem and their connections with the cerebellum assist in certain eye movements. The product of processing the visual signal is that

TABLE 16.6   Visual Abnormalities Associated with Selected Conditions and Syndromes

CONDITIONS/SYNDROMES	VISUAL ABNORMALITIES
Aging	Cataracts, macular degeneration
Brain damage	Amblyopia, cortical visual impairment, strabismus
Cerebral hypoxia	Cortical visual impairment
Cerebral palsy	Amblyopia, ocular motor dysfunctions, optic nerve atrophy, refractive errors, retinal abnormalities, strabismus
CHARGE syndrome	Coloboma, iris choroid, optic nerve atrophy
Diabetes mellitus	Cataracts, glaucoma, optic neuropathy, retinopathy
Fetal alcohol syndrome	Optic nerve hypoplasia, retinopathy, strabismus
HIV	Retinopathy
Hurler syndrome	Clouded cornea
Lowe syndrome	Cataracts, glaucoma
Marfan syndrome	Dislocated lens
Maternal rubella	Amblyopia, cataracts, nystagmus, pigmentary retinopathy, strabismus
Prematurity	Retinopathy
Prenatal or postnatal drug exposure	Strabismus
Tay-Sachs disease	Cherry red spot on macula, optic nerve atrophy
Trisomy 13, 18	Astigmatism, cataracts, coloboma, corneal opacities, hyperopia, microphthalmos, myopia, nystagmus, strabismus
Trisomy 21 (Down syndrome)	Astigmatism, cataracts, hypermetropia, myopia, nystagmus, strabismus
Turner syndrome	Cataracts, ptosis, strabismus
Zellweger syndrome	Cataracts, retinitis pigmentosa

Compiled from Alexander (1990); Batshaw & Perret (1992); Chalifoux (1991); Morse (1990); Nelson et al. (1987); Ponchillia (1993); Regenbogen & Coscas (1985); Trief et al. (1989); Trief & Morse (1988).

visual images are added to and coordinated with other sensory images (such as sound or smell) to yield a comprehensive sensory message (Batshaw & Perret, 1992; Erhardt, 1990).

Vision is described as the most "economic, flexible, expansive, and swift mode for processing information" (Erhardt, 1990, p. 35). Thus, an impairment of vision may immediately compromise an individual's overall well-being. Because visual impairment may be the expectation rather than the exception for persons with multiple impairments, AAC service providers must develop an awareness of common visual disorders and their general and medical management. Although core members of

the AAC team will more than likely not be directly involved in medical management, knowledge of such will promote effective collaboration between AAC service providers and vision specialists.

Types of Visual Impairment

Similar to hearing impairment, many different types and degrees of visual impairment exist (see Table 16.6). Loss of visual acuity may range from slight to profound. Visual field loss may also range from slight to profound and may be predominantly peripheral, central, or both (Jan & Groenveld, 1993; Morse, 1990; Vision Research, 1983). A

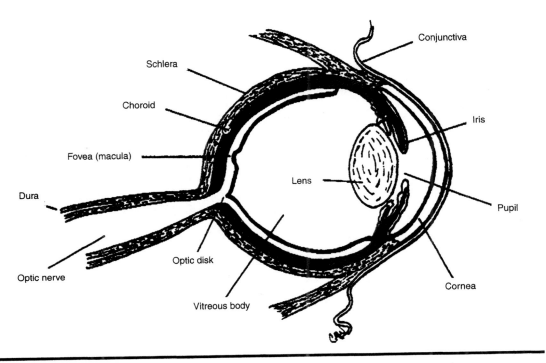

FIGURE 16.6 Schematic of the Visual System.
Courtesy of Jacob Wasson.

number of specific impairments of the peripheral and central visual system are associated with specific visual structures.

Eye Muscle Disorders. Strabismus, a general term referring to an abnormal ocular alignment due to disorders of any of six extraocular muscles, interferes with the eye's ability to fixate (Trief & Morse, 1988). Although not uncommon in children of the general population (3–4%), it occurs more frequently in preterm infants (15%) (Nelson, Ehrlick, Calhoun, Matteucci, & Finnegan, 1987) and in persons with cerebral palsy (40%) (Batshaw & Perret, 1992). Several conditions related to strabismus exist. **Esotropia** describes the turning in of one or both eyes, whereas **exotropia** refers to an outward turn. Treatment may involve eye patching, wearing of prescriptive lenses, surgical correction, and/or visual exercises. **Amblyopia,** characterized by a reduction in vision despite optimal visual management, is closely associated

with and directly caused by strabismus (Trief & Morse, 1988; Vision Research, 1983). Early management of strabismus is important in preventing the development of amblyopia.

Corneal Disorders. Corneal disorders result in blurred or reduced visual acuity. Causes include herpes simplex, swelling of the cornea, inherited and degenerative diseases, and toxic drug/chemical exposure (Batshaw & Perret, 1992; Erhardt, 1990; Hayes, 1985; Vision Research, 1983). The most common corneal disorder, refractive errors, affects more than 100 million Americans and is caused by misshaped corneas (Smith, 1982). Refractive errors range from mild to profound and include **myopia** (nearsightedness), **hyperopia** (farsightedness), and blurred vision due to **astigmatism.** Refractive errors are commonly corrected by prescriptive eyeglasses or contact lenses. Corneal clouding may occur as a consequence of glaucoma, metabolic disorders, trauma, or riboflavin deficiency (Batshaw & Perret, 1992; Hayes, 1985). In severe cases, corneal transplantation is performed to yield rapid correction (Hayes, 1985; Vision Research, 1983).

Glaucoma. **Glaucoma**, a collection of diseases resulting in increased pressure in the anterior chamber of the eye, can lead to optic nerve damage, vision loss, and blindness. Although vision loss is usually peripheral, glaucoma can also affect central vision. It is predominantly age related, yet it may occur at any time. Glaucoma is commonly associated with diabetes mellitus and with syndromes that include anatomic maldevelopment (Ponchillia, 1993; Rosenthal, 1993; Vision Research, 1983). It may also develop as a consequence of cataracts, congenital infections, retinopathy of prematurity (ROP), trauma, or chronic inflammation. Both drug and surgical management of glaucoma may be appropriate. Although no specific cause or cure is currently known, early detection and management can preserve remaining vision for many individuals (Batshaw & Perret, 1992; Rosenthal, 1993).

Impairments of the Lens. Two common disorders, presbyopia and cataracts, relate to a loss of lens clarity and flexibility. **Presbyopia**, which occurs in many persons as a part of the aging process, involves reduced flexibility and accommodation of the lens, resulting in blurred near vision. Prescriptive eyewear is often recommended. A **cataract** is any opacity or clouding of the lens. Although small, stable cataracts may not impede light transmission, dense ones severely impair vision. Cataracts can develop at any time (even prenatally) as an isolated disorder or as part of a syndrome (e.g., Down syndrome; diabetes mellitus) (Batshaw & Perret, 1992; Ponchillia, 1993; Rosenthal, 1993). Some estimates suggest that nearly 50% of individuals between 75 and 85 years of age develop cataracts (Vision Research, 1983). Successful surgical removal is often completed on an outpatient basis.

Retinal and Choroidal Impairments (Retinopathy). Most cases of visual impairment in the United States can be attributed to disorders of the retina and choroid, the underlying tissue layer containing blood vessels (Trief, Duckman, Morse,

& Silberman, 1989). One type of **retinopathy**, retinitis pigmentosa, is a progressive disease that may initially cause night blindness, eventually leading to severe vision loss. Another type of retinopathy, retinoblastoma (retinal tumor) is usually diagnosed early in life. Often, the affected eye is removed; however, a continued risk does exist for development of additional tumors in other areas of the body (Batshaw & Perret, 1992).

Retinopathy of prematurity (ROP) was once thought to be directly attributable to high levels of oxygen administered to preterm infants shortly after their birth. However, recent research indicates that birth weight and gestational age also factor into the occurrence and severity of ROP (Batshaw & Perret, 1992; Dekker & Koole, 1992; Trief et al., 1989; Vision Research, 1983). Given that preterm infants are at risk for multiple impairments, and that ROP is not curable, early detection and management of visual impairments in preterm infants are critical.

Diabetic retinopathy is a retinal disorder closely related in occurrence and severity to the duration of diabetes. Medical management includes drug therapy, laser procedures, and surgery. As with ROP, diabetic retinopathy is not curable and some individuals are nonresponsive to medical intervention (Rosenthal, 1993).

Other types of retinal disorders are associated with the **macula**. Because it is situated in the center of the retina, the macula provides the most acute vision and is particularly susceptible to damage. With macular damage, an individual experiences impaired ability to perform visual tasks requiring "close work" (Chalifoux, 1991). Early warning signs include mild blurring in one eye; later, a central vision field blind spot may develop. Rapidly progressing wet macular degeneration occurs when blood vessels beneath the macula hemorrhage. It is treated with laser therapy. Dry macular degeneration, which occurs without hemorrhage, progresses at a slower rate and may stabilize at a level that allows the retention of some functional vision. It is, however, generally unresponsive to treatment.

Anterior Visual Pathway Disorders. When the visual neural pathway, as opposed to the eye itself, is damaged anywhere from the lateral geniculate body up to and including the visual cortex, cortical visual impairment (CVI) will occur (Alexander, 1990; Jan & Groenveld, 1993). The damage may be localized within the brain's visual landmarks or generalized to various other cerebral areas (Morse, 1990). Individuals with CVI often present unique visual as well as general behavioral characteristics. To assist AAC team members in differential diagnosis, Table 16.7 compares these characteristics with those that may typically be displayed by individuals with ocular visual disorders.

Implications

The visual disorders summarized above, plus numerous others, exist in many AAC users. Sobsey and Wolf-Schein (1991) speculated that the high

correlation between visual and other impairments exist for a number of reasons (see Chapter 11 for a review). Failure to detect, manage, and monitor visual impairments in individuals with multiple impairments may seriously thwart social, communication, educational, and vocational opportunities. AAC service providers must become aware of the unique assessment and intervention issues relating to visual impairment, referring to and consulting with vision specialists on an ongoing basis.

Visual Assessment

Visual assessment should be completed any time that an AAC user is suspect for visual impairment, even when testing cannot be conducted through usual methods (Hall, Orel-Bixler, & Haegerstrom-Portnoy, 1991). Although the primary criteria for

TABLE 16.7 Characteristic Differences between Ocular and Cortical Visual Disorders

CHARACTERISTIC	OCULAR DISORDER	CORTICAL DISORDER
Appearance	Appears visually impaired	Usually appears normal
Close viewing	Common, used as a means of magnification	Common, used as a means of magnification, to reduce crowding, or both
Color perception	Dependent on particular eye disorder	Preserved
Compulsive light gazing	Rarely	Common
Eye examination	Usually abnormal	Normal
Eye pressing	Especially noted in congenital retinal disorders	Never
Light sensitivity	Dependent on particular eye disorder	In one-third of cases
Peripheral field loss	Occasionally	Nearly always
Poorly coordinated eye movements	Present when congenital and early onset	Usually normal
Presence of additional neurological impairments	Fairly common	Nearly always
Rapid horizontal head shaking	Occasionally	Never
Sensory nystagmus	Present when congenital and early onset	Not present
Visual attention span	Usually normal	Markedly short
Visual function	Consistent	Highly variable

Adapted from Batstone & Harris (1990); Erhardt (1990); Jan & Groenveld (1993).

determining visual impairment are visual acuity scores, additional standards are necessary because visual impairment is considerably more complex than any acuity scores or categories of scores might indicate (Sobsey & Wolf-Schein, 1991; Vision Research, 1983). Further, "the use of vision is not an isolated phenomenon. It is one behavior within a large constellation of behaviors, all of which are influenced by interactions with the environment" (Morse, 1992, p. 77).

Thus, no single test or approach is sufficient for examining the functional capacity of the visual system (Alexander, 1990; V. Bishop, 1988). Areas of both physiological functioning and functional visual use must be considered (Batstone & Harris, 1990; Erhardt, 1987; Sobsey & Wolf-Schein, 1991), and as is true in all areas of AAC service delivery, the efforts of a number of team members must be pooled to ensure appropriate identification and management. Just as the audiologist becomes a key member of the team serving the needs of AAC users with known or suspected hearing impairments, the vision specialist (e.g., optometrist and/or ophthalmologist) becomes a key member of teams working with AAC users with known or suspected visual impairments. Effective service delivery requires this collaborative effort because individuals who know the AAC user well may be unskilled in visual assessment, whereas vision specialists may not know the unique needs and behaviors of the AAC user.

Areas of Assessment. Several sources provide detailed discussions of the essential components of visual assessment for individuals with multiple impairments (e.g., Atkinson, 1989; Bane & Birch, 1992; V. Bishop, 1988; Hall et al., 1991; Macht, 1971; Morse, 1992; O'Dell, Harshaw, & Boothe, 1993; Sacks, Goren, & Burke, 1991; Sobsey & Wolf-Schein, 1991). Most of these procedures are specifically applicable to evaluating AAC users or can be effectively adapted.

Screening. A small number of formal and informal procedures are available to screen AAC users who are suspect for visual impairment (see, for example, Atkinson, 1989). The first step in any of these screening procedures involves visual inspection of the eye and its typical behaviors to detect obvious cosmetic and/or motor manifestations of visual impairment (e.g., esotropia, exotropia, or nystagmus). Trief and Morse (1988) recommend systematic repetition of this visual inspection, because many disorders of ocular alignment may change over time.

Although "subjective acuity tests are the single most effective tools available to screeners to determine the need for professional vision care" for individuals with multiple impairments (Cress et al., 1981, p. 43), several commercially available acuity tests have recently been criticized as being time consuming, unreliable, and difficult to administer (O'Dell et al., 1993). However, screening procedures can and should be adapted to fit particular individual abilities, as demonstrated by Sacks et al. (1991) in their screening of adults with moderate to profound cognitive impairments. Subjects were able to perform subjective acuity tasks using the conventional Snellen chart, "E" chart, Allen picture chart, finger counting, and/or perception of a handlight. O'Dell et al. (1993) also successfully screened individuals with severe to profound cognitive impairments using visual acuity cards (available through VisTech Consultants, Inc.) in a forced-choice preferential looking (FPL) task. Still further, Geruschat (1992) reported successful use of the Acuity Card Procedure (also available from VisTech) in screening children with multiple impairments. Such FPL tasks can be used for visual screening with many AAC users because FPL places few communication demands on the individual (Bane & Birch, 1992; Birch & Bane, 1991).

Assessment. When an individual has manifested behaviors during screening procedures or when general behavioral observations indicate that further diagnostic procedures are needed, more extensive evaluation should be carried out by the assessment team using both objective and subjective assessment tools (V. Bishop, 1988; Hall et al., 1991). Potential assessment tools (e.g., electrophysiological testing and more extensive FPL tasks) can be adapted by vision specialists or others under their guidance for use with AAC users. As part of the assessment, emphasis should be given to information gained from case histories, functional checklists, and behavioral observations (Atkinson, 1989; Hall et al., 1991; Jan & Groenveld, 1993; Sobsey & Wolf-Schein, 1991). Table 16.8 provides a summary of a visual assessment protocol, which includes both formal and informal assessments.

A vision specialist who works collaboratively with other core and tertiary team members may be a core member on the AAC assessment team for an individual with visual impairment. The speech-language pathologist may provide information regarding the visual demands of current and projected aided AAC methods, including information regarding the importance of illumination, size, space, contrast, color, and placement of graphic symbols. Team members may assist in preparing AAC users for assessment sessions by readying materials, adapting current AAC methods to facilitate responses, or role-playing the assessment scenario. Educational and/or vocational spe-

cialists can assess current skills and needs in educational and/or work environments and assist others in determining how unique visual and communication characteristics affect participation in functional activities (Dekker & Koole, 1992).

The **orientation and mobility (O & M)** specialist is often an underused member of assessment teams (Bailey & Head, 1993), including those serving AAC users with visual impairment. The O & M specialist can gather data regarding the individual's current travel skills and travel demands of the environment, and then assist in developing and monitoring O & M recommendations (Joffee & Rikhye, 1991; Kelley, Davidson, & Sanspree, 1993). In reality, O & M services for AAC users may be difficult to obtain. As noted by Chen and Smith (1992), "typically, a more capable student will receive orientation and mobility instruction more frequently than the child who is multihandicapped. The assumption is that the more capable student will attain the skills and will become an independent traveler" (p. 134).

TABLE 16.8   Summary of Vision Assessment Protocol

PROCEDURES/PROCESSES	TYPE OF INFORMATION PROVIDED
Caregiver interview	Preferred items or activities; current and preferred visual patterns; current travel and mobility skills; muscle balance; motivation for intake of visual information; current visual needs
Case history	Family history; possible etiology; current estimates regarding auditory, cognitive, motor, tactile, and visual abilities; current AAC system use
Elicited observation	Discrepancies in current and potential skills in cognitive, motor, and visual abilities
Environmental assessment	Sensory demands of materials and routines
Natural observation	Preferred items or activities; current and preferred visual patterns; current travel and mobility skills; muscle balance; motivation for intake of visual information
Seating and positioning	Relationship between motor functioning and visual functioning
Visual ability testing	Presence or absence of refractive errors; near and far acuity; central and peripheral visual field; visual localization, fixation, and tracking

Adapted from Alexander (1990); V. Bishop (1988); Hall, Orel-Bixler, & Haegerstrom-Portney (1991).

The ophthalmologist may conduct specialized assessment procedures to gather information about specific types of visual impairments, their potential etiology, and projected course. These procedures may include assessment of visual acuity, awareness, orientation and location, attention, fixation, and pursuit. Here, several forms of electrodiagnostic testing can augment subjective assessments (e.g., FLP tasks). These include electro-oculograms (EOG), electroencephalograms (EEG), visual evoked responses (VER), visual evoked potential mappings (VEPM), electroretinograms (ERG), and computed tomography (CT) scans (Alexander, 1990; Bane & Birch, 1992; Hall et al., 1991; Sacks et al., 1991).

Visual assessment may occur over an extended period and should be repeated, as necessary, throughout an AAC user's life span. Prior exchange of information between core AAC service providers and vision specialists who will be involved only on an intermittent basis will ensure optimal assessment. Various team members may assist with assessment adaptations, such as client and materials preparation, adapting seating/positioning, and acquiring and administering specialized tests similar to those described for AAC users with hearing impairments. Some of the adaptations AAC team members and vision specialists may consider in preparing for and conducting a functional visual assessment are listed in Table 16.9.

The necessity of ongoing visual assessment cannot be overemphasized. Too often, once a team has determined that no follow-up is possible or necessary, or that implemented management procedures (e.g., acquisition of prescriptive lenses) are adequate, an "abandoning attitude" develops (Hofstetter, 1991). Team members must observe an individual's functioning after management procedures are implemented or modified (Kelley et al., 1993). When no management has been initiated and there is still concern regarding visual functioning, the team should remain intact and continue to investigate other management strategies, as outlined in the next section.

TABLE 16.9 Adaptations for Visual Screening and Assessment

GENERAL CONSIDERATIONS

Be aware of attention span and physical stamina. Frequent breaks may be necessary.

Simplify procedures and materials to accommodate for the individual's level of functioning.

Talk to and involve the AAC user directly.

Talk to and involve the accompanying caregiver directly.

PLAN AHEAD

Inquire as to what specific information is desired from the assessment.

Schedule ample time to complete the assessment and be prepared to break up the assessment over several appointments.

Determine that all assessment sites are accessible and safe.

Prepare or adapt materials to fit the functional needs of the AAC user.

Involve caregivers in training necessary examination behaviors, such as sitting in particular positions (if possible), tolerating the shining of light into the eyes, and fixating on a distant target.

Determine the AAC user's preferred mode of communication and be prepared to allow responses in that mode.

Compiled from Atkinson (1989); Bane & Birch (1992); Batshaw & Perret (1992); Cress et al. (1981).

Functional Management of Visual Impairment

AAC users with visual impairments require special considerations to facilitate maximal development of functional communication. The service delivery team must bear in mind the AAC users' unique sensory, motor, concept development, social-emotional, academic, O & M, and vocational needs (Hazenkamp & Huebner, 1989). These needs, as related to receptive and expressive communication in general, and to AAC use in particular, will require careful and ongoing attention. Because most aided and unaided AAC modes have a heavy visual component, issues related to illumination, size, space, color, contrast, and placement must be addressed. The AAC user's physical positioning, position in relation to an AAC device or display, the visual demands entailed in using graphic symbols, and the potential adaptation of both low- and high-technology devices all become important issues in AAC intervention when vision loss is suspected or confirmed.

A Framework for Intervention. AAC users with visual impairment are not a homogeneous group. Each individual represents a unique blend of strengths and needs, successes and failures, and cultural-ethnic backgrounds. Although AAC intervention must be individualized, three guiding principles that frequently shape service delivery for individuals with visual impairments can be applied to AAC users as well. They include (1) optimizing residual visual abilities (Vision Research, 1983); (2) optimizing visual characteristics of stimuli (e.g., the AAC system) (Beevers & Hallinan, 1990; Boyd, Boyd, & Vanderheiden, 1990; Mann et al., 1993; Uslan, 1992); and (3) stimulating and/or training residual vision to maximal functional levels (Erhardt, 1987; Sobsey & Wolf-Schein, 1991; Sonksen, Petrie, & Drew, 1991; Tavernier, 1993).

Optimizing Visual Abilities. An individual may receive less than the maximal possible visual signal due to undercorrection. Although approximately 60% of the general population makes use of some sort of corrective eyewear (Vision Research, 1983), a much smaller proportion of indi-

viduals with multiple impairments seem to be fitted with corrective eyewear (O'Dell et al., 1993; Sacks et al., 1991). One possible reason for this may relate to the speculated inability of such individuals to independently manage their eyewear. Newer corrective lenses and procedures, such as extended wear contact lenses and radial keratonomy (RK), may hold merit for the management of certain visual impairments in AAC users, because they require one-time or infrequent care and maintenance. Members of the AAC team must be persistent advocates for the prescription of appropriate visual correction devices. Team members must also ensure the ongoing monitoring of existing eyewear and advocate that a proper replacement schedule be followed (Tavernier, 1993; Trief & Morse, 1988).

Optimizing Visual Characteristics of Stimuli. AAC service providers hold a key role in optimizing the visual characteristics of stimuli relevant to an AAC user. For AAC users who rely on unaided forms of communication, the obvious factor to consider is proximity to partners in environments relatively free of visual and auditory noise. For AAC users who rely on aided methods, a whole host of issues becomes relevant. Enormous amounts of cognitive and motor energy may be expended when materials are not optimally designed and placed in a supportive visual environment (Erhardt, 1987, 1990; Tavernier, 1993). Maximizing the salient features of graphic symbols may facilitate more efficient processing of visual input, allowing voluntary attention to be directed elsewhere (Erhardt, 1987). Design, size, spacing, and color/illumination of graphic symbols must be considered for each AAC user and must be addressed concurrently with issues of motor functioning, cognition, audition, and taction.

Assessment of trunk and neck position, head control, and range of motion should be conducted to determine symbol position(s) to optimize motor movements (see Batstone and Harris, 1990, as well as Chapter 17). Because many AAC users demonstrate motor fatigue over time, the assistive communication device itself, as well as the size and structure of its symbols, may need adjustment to accommodate coordination between motor and visual movements and most comfortable viewing distance. Although many service providers attend to issues of comfortable loudness level in regard to auditory stimuli, far too few are aware of the need to adjust for a similar component in the visual system (consider, for example, the natural adjustments individuals without disabilities make during reading or TV viewing). Thus an important part of AAC service delivery for individuals with visual impairments is to offer multiple symbol arrangements, distances, and positions.

An additional issue regarding position is worth noting. To achieve a steady visual gaze, some individuals (e.g., those with nystagmus or central vision deficits) may actually shift the head away from the viewed object. This is usually a functional, self-taught compensatory behavior and should not be discouraged (Batstone & Harris, 1990; Blischak, 1995; Vision Research, 1983).

AAC service providers working with individuals with documented or suspected visual impairments may learn critical skills from the efforts of individuals who work with the general population of individuals with low vision. For example, early Braille instruction can be optimized when the size and vertical and horizontal spacing of Braille symbols has been customized (Pester, Petrosko, & Poppe, 1994). Customizing the size, spacing, contrast color, and illumination of graphic symbols may similarly facilitate optimal use of residual vision in AAC users. Table 16.10 details several intervention suggestions.

Simple tactile enhancements such as texture may be provided to add a third dimension to graphic symbols. More sophisticated tactile enhancements such as the inclusion of Braille features as part of an overall symbol set/system or the use of Braille as the sole symbol system may also be considered. A Braille enlarger for individ-

TABLE 16.10 Intervention Suggestions for Working with AAC Users with Visual Impairments

VISUAL

Ensure maximal visual correction.

Train localization to symbol display.

Maximize ability to shift gaze from display to partner.

Adjust display as needed for most comfortable viewing distance.

DISPLAY

Use appropriate size, design, spacing, arrangement, color, contrast, and distance between symbols.

Minimize visual noise and glare.

MOTOR

Adjust trunk and head position to facilitate maximal intake of visual information.

Allow for frequent positional changes to accommodate for motor fatigue.

Ensure optimal distance between AAC user and display.

ENVIRONMENT

Ensure appropriate seating and positioning for trunk support and head control.

Provide sufficient illumination, without glare.

Present stimuli within the AAC user's field of vision, at an appropriate angle and distance.

Provide tactile and/or auditory supports.

Compiled from Batstone & Harris (1990); Downing & Eichinger (1990); van Hedel-van Grinsven (1989).

uals with both visual and tactile impairments is currently under development (Visser, 1994). An existing device, the Optacon, "produces a tactile image of printed material so that reading can be accomplished with a finger" (Vision Research, 1983, Vol. 2, p. 5). The Tactile Speech Indicator allows an individual with both visual and hearing impairments to use a telephone (Lynch, 1990).

Other sources of technology or technology features (e.g., the auditory scanning feature of several aided AAC devices) that may benefit AAC users with visual impairments are well reviewed (see, for example, Blischak, 1995; Boyd et al., 1990; Coleman & Meyers, 1991; Locke & Mirenda, 1988; Noyes & Frankish, 1992; Rowland, 1990). Although "assistive technology is recognized as key to independence for individuals with disabilities because it provides a means of access to the mainstream society" (Uslan, 1992, p. 402), acquiring such technology is a challenge for members of AAC teams working with AAC users with visual impairments (see Chapters 8 through 14). One example of AAC and other assistive technology (AT) used by a child with physical and visual impairments was described in a case study of Thomas by Blischak (1995). Thomas successfully used a switch-activated VOCA with auditory scanning, corrective lenses, and magnification in his elementary school classroom.

Stimulating and/or Training Residual Vision. Research has documented that typically developing children up to age 10 have the capacity to strengthen the neurological processes responsible for vision (Gellhaus & Olson, 1993). Because 90% of the population with visual impairments retain some degree of usable vision, the logic behind early and aggressive vision stimulation and training is obvious (Morse, 1990; Tavernier, 1993). A rich environment that includes varying sensory stimuli and experiences is critical if individuals with visual impairments are to reach maximal skill levels. Without visual stimulation, irreversible underdevelopment of the visual system may occur (Potenski, 1993; Sonksen et al., 1991).

Visual stimulation denotes presentation of visual stimuli to individuals who have little or no reaction to objects in the visual environment, whereas vision training refers to attempts to enhance the skills of individuals who demonstrate some involvement with objects (Tavernier, 1993). Typically, stimulation is implemented using operant conditioning strategies or by the presentation of highly contrasting visual stimuli (e.g., under "blacklight" conditions) (Sonksen et al., 1991). A gradated program involving scanning, recognition, and perception has been beneficial in vision training. Both procedures may hold merit for individual AAC users to stimulate interest in visual information, particularly when functional consequences are tied to the procedures (Batstone & Harris, 1990).

DUAL SENSORY IMPAIRMENT

Most individuals with DSI (formerly referred to as deaf-blind individuals) have some degree of residual hearing and vision, although for a small number (approximately 6%), neither sensory channel is functional for communication (Fredericks & Baldwin, 1987). Etiologies of DSI are much the same as those that cause hearing, visual, and other impairments, and include congenital, developmental, and acquired factors. Some individuals may have both sensory impairments at birth (e.g., maternal rubella), develop sensory impairments at differing rates (e.g., Usher's syndrome), or acquire one sensory loss in childhood, and another in adulthood (e.g., development of glaucoma in an elderly individual with pre-existing hearing impairment). Many of the same considerations regarding assessment and intervention for individuals with hearing or visual impairment apply to individuals with DSI. Often, tactile communication approaches are used to augment or serve as an alternative to information received through auditory and/or visual channels, along with previously described methods such as amplification and enlarged print.

Individuals with DSI have traditionally been identified and have received communication intervention, and as such, more information is readily available in texts (e.g., Goetz, Guess, & Stremel-Campbell, 1987; Kramer, Sullivan, & Hirsch, 1979; Orelove & Sobsey, 1996) and journal articles (e.g., Downing & Eichinger, 1990; Murray-Branch,

Udavari-Solner, & Bailey, 1991; Rowland, 1990; Rowland & Schweigert, 1989a). Further, many tactile communication approaches used with individuals with DSI such as touch cues, tangible symbols, and microswitch technology are broadly applicable for individuals with severe developmental disabilities and are described in detail in Chapter 18.

This chapter describes intervention approaches aimed at providing both receptive and expressive communication primarily for individuals with acquired DSI who have attained language and literacy skills but rely primarily on tactile means of communication. As such, these applications are limited to individuals with DSI who have intact motoric abilities. Intact motoric, language, and literacy abilities are also generally required of their communication partners.

Aided Communication

Low Technology.

Alphabet Glove/Glove Method. Use of the glove method requires that the individual with DSI wear a thin glove with alphabet letters and numbers printed across the fingers. The communication partner touches various areas of the hand to spell messages (Beukelman & Mirenda, 1992; Kramer et al., 1979). With memorization of letter/number locations by the communication partner, this method could also be used without the glove.

Braille Alphabet Card/Alphabet Plate. Cards containing a Braille and/or raised printed alphabet may also be used by individuals with DSI. For receptive use, the communication partner places the finger of the individual with DSI on each raised symbol to spell a message. For expressive communication, the individual with DSI touches the raised symbols and the partner reads the corresponding letters (Beukelman & Mirenda, 1992; Kramer et al., 1979).

High Technology.
Various assistive devices that translate between orthography and tactile methods are available for transmitting messages between communication partners and individuals with DSI. These have been previously described in this chapter and in Chapter 10. For information regarding adapting assistive communication devices for use by individuals with DSI, see Mathy-Laikko, Ratcliff, Villarruel, and Yoder (1988).

Unaided Communication

Tadoma.
In the **Tadoma method** of speech reception, an individual places a hand on the face of the speaker, with the thumb on the lips and fingers spread across the jaw and cheekbone. Few individuals with DSI actually are proficient in this technique, which is generally limited to use with communication partners with intelligible speech (Kramer et al., 1979).

Print-on-Palm/Palm Writing.
The palm writing method involves tracing alphabet letters or numbers one at a time on the palm of the individual with DSI (Beukelman & Mirenda, 1992; Kramer et al., 1979).

Manual Signs.

American One-Hand Manual Alphabet (Fingerspelling). Individuals with DSI may use fingerspelling, which is the same as that used by deaf individuals in the United States, for both receptive and expressive communication. Here, words are spelled by forming handshapes representing individual alphabet letters into the receiver's cupped hand(s) or in view of a sighted communication partner.

Sign Language. As with fingerspelling, sign language in both visual and tactile forms can continue to be used by deaf individuals who lose their vision. For those individuals with reduced linguistic abilities, simplified manual signs may be used instead. Like print-on-palm, use of manual signs also permits individuals with DSI to communicate with one another. (For additional information about unaided communication, see Chapter 7).

Coactive Signing. Used to teach signing to children with congenital DSI, coactive signing could also be used with older individuals who may have developed both vision and hearing loss concurrently. In coactive signing, the signer holds the learner's hands to actually form the signs. In time, the learner is expected to develop independent signing skill. For information regarding a standardized program of coactive signing developed at the SKI-HI Institute in Utah, see Watkins and Clark (1991).

Other Tactile Methods.

Morse Code. Messages may be transmitted via Morse code, though rather laboriously, by tapping on any part of the body. This method can be used both receptively and expressively by individuals with DSI (Beukelman & Mirenda, 1992).

Braille Hand Speech. The message receiver must know Braille to use Braille hand speech. It consists of positioning the fingers to represent configurations of Braille letters, which are then touched to the communication partner's arm or hand (Beukelman & Mirenda, 1992).

SUMMARY

AAC users with sensory impairments often require intensive assessment and intervention efforts along with lifelong monitoring of sensory status.

Team members should adopt a vigilant approach to assessing sensory status, providing intervention that takes advantage of the stronger sensory channel, and providing approaches and devices to augment or serve as an alternative for the impaired sensory channel(s). Of paramount importance is the preservation of current sensory abilities, which requires prompt medical management of conditions that can lead to additional sensory impairment and loss of successful communication skills.

The involvement of support staff such as hearing and vision specialists is vital to the functioning of a transdisciplinary team that can collaborate to provide intervention that occurs not in isolation, but in the context of meaningful, functional activities in the home, school, and community. Yet, assessment and intervention teams for children with DSI frequently lack hearing and vision support staff. This is also often the case for AAC users with hearing or vision impairments. Therefore, AAC team members must make every effort to enlist the involvement of essential professionals and work collaboratively in ongoing assessment and intervention to provide quality services to AAC users with sensory impairments.

CHAPTER 17

SEATING, OTHER POSITIONING, AND MOTOR CONTROL

IRENE R. McEWEN

Children and adults who have severe speech impairments also frequently have problems controlling their posture and extremities, which affect their ability to use **augmentative or alternative communication (AAC)**. Both aided and unaided AAC approaches require sufficiently skilled movement of a hand, the head, an eye, or other body part, which can be difficult for people who have cerebral palsy, amyotrophic lateral sclerosis (ALS), traumatic brain injury (TBI), and many other conditions. One factor that can affect motor performance is body position. Position may also influence other intrinsic and extrinsic aspects of a person's communication, such as cognitive performance, hearing, vision, attention, arousal, and opportunities for interaction.

As other chapters have emphasized, successful use of AAC nearly always depends on the quality of the team approach to assessment and intervention. When an AAC user or potential user has problems with motor control, an occupa-

tional or physical therapist can often provide valuable input. Some of the ways in which occupational and physical therapists can be helpful are listed in Table 17.1. Because occupational and physical therapists are usually not with people who use AAC throughout the day, other team members need to be able to recognize positioning and AAC access problems when they occur. Sometimes these team members can make necessary modifications themselves; other times they will need to consult with an occupational therapist, physical therapist, or other person with expertise.

This chapter begins with definitions of seating, positioning, and motor control; the terms are then applied in subsequent sections of the chapter. The definitions are followed by a discussion of common neuromusculoskeletal problems that users of AAC often have and that positioning can affect. Specific effects of positioning are then covered, followed by guidelines for the seated posi-

TABLE 17.1 Occupational and Physical Therapists' Contributions to AAC Assessment and Intervention

Occupational and physical therapists assist other team members to

1. Determine whether a person is likely to have the motor control necessary for unaided modes of communication, such as manual signs or gestures.

2. Identify body site(s) and movement(s) to control AAC devices.

3. Determine positioning and features of positioning devices to promote optimal neuromusculoskeletal benefits and use of devices.

4. Design an AAC system that best matches the motor abilities of the individual.

5. Design teaching strategies to promote development of motor control for all components of the AAC system.

tion. Then, means to identify control sites, promote motor control, and enhance motor learning are addressed. Finally, two case examples illustrate application of positioning principles.

DEFINITIONS OF SEATING, POSITIONING, AND MOTOR CONTROL

Seating refers to all of the seats and their components that assist people to maintain a sitting position. It includes ordinary seats that most people use everyday, such as couches and car seats, and the specialized seats designed to enhance the function of people with disabilities, such as adapted chairs and wheelchair seats.

Positioning means placing and maintaining a person in sitting, sidelying, standing, prone, or other postural alignment. A seat is one type of positioning device. Standers, sidelyers, and prone positioners are other types of positioning devices used by people with disabilities. The general goals of positioning people with disabilities are the same as all people have when they use such ordinary positioning devices as beds and desk chairs, including improved function, comfort, opportunities to participate in a variety of activities and environments, and prevention of musculoskeletal problems. When people have disabilities, additional goals of positioning are to (1) improve postural alignment and stability; (2) improve motor control; (3) prevent or minimize contractures and deformities; (4) improve sensory and bodily functions (e.g., vision and respiration); and (5) improve attention and arousal (Bergen, Presperin, & Tallman, 1990; Trefler, Hobson, Taylor, Monahan, & Shaw, 1993).

Motor control refers to initiation and execution of movement. Theories about how skilled movement is developed and produced have changed since the beginning of the twentieth century, from maturational-based theories to contemporary, dynamic systems-based theories (Bradley, 1994). As discussed later, positioning and other interventions designed to enhance the motor control of people with disabilities are currently changing as research supporting systems-based theories accumulates.

COMMON NEUROMUSCULOSKELETAL PROBLEMS

People who use AAC have many different medical diagnoses, most of which result from congenital or acquired central nervous system pathology. The brain is a common site of the pathology because brain damage or malformation can lead to lack of oral motor coordination as well as cognitive, perceptual, and sensory impairments that affect speech communication. Brain damage or malformation can also lead to problems in controlling muscles of the trunk, limbs, neck, and eyes, which also can affect communication. The type and severity of the motor problems depend on the location and the extent of the brain damage or malformation. For this reason, even people who have the same diagnosis, such as cerebral palsy, TBI, or stroke, may have much variation in their motor abilities.

Damage or malformation of the spinal cord and peripheral nerves can also affect communication, but written, rather than speech, communication is usually affected. People with a high spinal cord injury, for example, can usually speak but are unable to use their hands, so they may require alternative written communication. Speech production can be affected by cranial nerve damage. Specific intervention information related to various congenital and acquired impairments of AAC users is provided in Chapters 18 and 19.

When the neurological system does not appropriately innervate muscle, the resulting impairment is **neuromuscular**, a term that denotes the intimate relationship between the two systems. Similarly, the term **musculoskeletal** indicates the connection between the muscles of the body and the skeletal system, with the pull of muscles on the skeleton affecting both the alignment of the skeletal components and the shape of the bones. The term **neuromusculoskeletal** refers to the close linkages among the neurological system, the muscles of the body, and the skeletal system. The following sections discuss common neuromuscular, musculoskeletal, and associated problems of AAC users that can be modified or controlled through positioning.

Common Neuromuscular Problems

Muscle weakness may be either a primary or secondary impairment. Weakness as a primary impairment occurs when a muscle (or more typically a group of muscles) is not innervated or is inadequately innervated due to a brain, spinal cord, or peripheral nervous system disorder. It also results from muscle pathology, such as occurs in muscular dystrophy. The degree of weakness can range from mild to severe, with paralysis occurring when no activation of muscle is possible.

Weakness as a secondary impairment can occur from lack of exercise, which often results when people lack postural control, are unable to walk, and have poorly coordinated movement. Weakness can also occur secondary to muscle imbalance. If muscles on one side of a joint are stronger than the muscles on the other side, the muscles on the weaker side may be unable to overcome the power of the stronger side, thus becoming even weaker. Until recently, treatment philosophies cautioned against exercises to strengthen the weak muscles of people with cerebral palsy, stroke, and similar conditions resulting from upper motor neuron problems, fearing that the exercise would increase the neuromuscular dysfunction. Research, however, suggests that strengthening exercises may be valuable (Damiano, Kelly, & Vaughn, 1995; Horvat, 1987).

Muscle stiffness has a variety of causes, including spasticity, lack of muscle extensibility, and simultaneous contraction of muscles on both sides of a joint (reciprocal innervation) (Campbell, 1991; Olney & Wright, 1994). Muscle stiffness is sometimes referred to as high muscle tone or hypertonicity, although these terms are used less frequently than in the past because of their imprecision. Muscles may also lack sufficient stiffness, so they appear floppy (low tone or hypotonicity). Position, emotions, arousal, and health are some of the factors that can cause variation in a person's muscle stiffness.

Postural control regulates the body's position in space for stability and orientation. Stability (or balance) maintains or regains the position of the body over the base of support to prevent falling. Orientation aligns the body parts in relation to one another so they are appropriate for the task being accomplished (Shumway-Cook & Woollacott, 1993). When people have deficits that interfere with normal control of posture, they lack both the necessary stability and alignment for optimal function. Motor performance problems can be both related to and independent of other neuromuscular problems. People with cerebral palsy and similar conditions often have difficulty with several components of motor performance, such as (1) abnormal timing and force of muscle activation; (2) difficulty with initiation, maintenance, and/or termination of movement; (3) decreased speed of movement; and (4) use of abnormal compensatory patterns of movement as a person attempts to accomplish motor goals (Campbell, 1991; Olney & Wright, 1994). People with severe neuromotor problems often have few movement options available to them, so they must approach different tasks with **stereotypic movement** or paucity of movement. Position, practice, and other therapeutic interventions attempt to improve motor control and increase the variety and specificity of movement options.

Common Musculoskeletal Problems

Joint contractures and other skeletal deformities can be present at birth, but they usually develop over time, secondary to neuromuscular impairments. When a joint is contracted, it cannot be moved passively through its full range of motion. Other common skeletal deformities include **scoliosis** (sideways bending of the spine, which is usually combined with rotation of the vertebrae), **kyphosis** (forward bending of the spine), and hip dislocation (the hip joint separates, with the ball on the top of the femur coming out of the socket in the pelvis).

The primary causes of contractures and other deformities are position and muscle imbalance. Positional deformities occur when muscles and other soft tissue around a joint become tightened due to lack of joint movement. Anyone who has had a cast following an injury knows how quickly a joint can become stiff when it is not moved. The same thing occurs when people who are unable to move their joints fully are placed in one position for long periods of time. A person who sits all day, for example, and whose hips and knees are not in **extension** for a sufficiently long period will develop hip and knee **flexion** contractures. Although there is little evidence to indicate how long is enough, research suggests that joints must be at their maximum range for at least 6 to 7 hours each day (Tardieu, Lespargot, Tabary, & Bret, 1988). Thus, the value of periodic passive range-of-motion exercises to prevent contractures is questionable, and contracture prevention through selective positioning to provide a prolonged stretch is more likely to be of benefit.

Muscle imbalance can also contribute to joint contractures and is usually compounded by position. If the muscles that pull the thigh inward (adductor muscles) are more active than the muscles that move the thigh outward (abductor muscles), for example, then the thigh will be pulled inward and an adduction contracture will result if it is allowed to remain in this position. One way to prevent this and other contractures caused by muscle imbalance is through positioning that maintains the body in alignment opposite the pull of the more active muscles.

Associated Problems

In addition to neuromusculoskeletal problems, many people who use AAC have other impairments that can influence their use of AAC systems and may also be affected by position.

Sensory functions are important for effective use of AAC systems, particularly hearing and vision. Because hearing, vision, and dual sensory impairments (DSI) are common among people with central nervous system deficits, they must be carefully evaluated and considered when selecting AAC systems and training for their use, as described in Chapters 11 and 16. Hearing may be affected by positioning because involuntary body movements, which can be reduced by good positioning, generate as much as 30 to 40 dB of extraneous noise (Young, 1986). Vision can be enhanced or diminished by the position of both the individual and AAC devices. The sidelying position, for example, dictates a skewed view of the world, so that placing a communication display

board flat on a tray may not allow an AAC user to see all of the symbols.

Cognitive and communication functions are closely linked, not only through language but also through attention, memory, motivation, problem solving, and other functions (Cook & Hussey, 1995). Several studies suggest that cognitive functioning may be enhanced through positioning, particularly a well-seated position that provides the necessary supports (Sents & Marks, 1988).

Attention and **arousal** problems may be related to severe cognitive deficits or other associated central nervous system dysfunction (Rainforth, 1982; Thompson & Guess, 1989). Obviously, adequate attention to communication tasks and sufficient arousal is important for effective communication and use of AAC systems. Research generally supports the upright position as promoting greater attention and arousal than sidelying, prone, and other recumbent positions (Guess et al., 1993; Landesman-Dwyer & Sackett, 1978).

EFFECTS OF POSITIONING

Positioning can cause both immediate and delayed effects. Regardless of the positioning being used, service providers must understand when to expect effects to occur and to evaluate whether they are occurring as anticipated. If they are not, modifications must be made promptly.

Immediate Effects

Immediate effects occur as soon as a person is positioned, or relatively soon thereafter. Positioning in an adapted chair, for example, can have immediate effects if it provides the postural stability and alignment necessary to use a head-mounted light pointer more precisely or more rapidly. Similarly, immediate effects can be seen if a stander provides the support and alignment necessary for a person to touch symbols more effectively on a communication display. Immediate effects of a sidelying position can be seen in the muscle activity of some individuals who need a recumbent resting position but who become excessively flexed or extended when lying in **supine** (on the back) or **prone** (on the stomach) positions.

Many of the immediate effects of positioning are believed to result from improved postural stability and alignment that permits greater control of the arms and head (Myhr & von Wendt, 1991; Nwaobi, 1987). Other immediate effects include improved respiration (Nwaobi & Smith, 1986), improved performance on IQ tests (Sents & Marks, 1988), and enhanced opportunity for communicative interactions (McEwen, 1992). Position can also have an immediate effect on speed of switch activation. One study found that the activations of two preschool boys with cerebral palsy were slower when they were in a sidelying position than when they were sitting, standing, or lying prone on a wedge (McEwen & Karlan, 1989). Comfort is another important immediate effect of positioning.

Delayed Effects

Two types of positioning effects take place over time: developmental effects and musculoskeletal effects. Developmental effects are based primarily on neuromaturational theories of development and intervention, which presume that intervention for people with disabilities should approximate the sequence of motor development typically observed in infants and young children without disabilities (Atwater, 1991; Heriza, 1991). Most 4- to 5-month-old infants, for example, can raise their heads and prop themselves up on their elbows or hands when in a prone position. Observers of infant development have proposed that this activity is an important prerequisite for subsequent motor development, including development of head control, shoulder stability, and hand control (Alexander, Boehme, & Cupps, 1993). Similarly, a typically developing 6-month-old can assume and maintain a sidelying position, which may be important for developing hand function and for developing controlled balance of flexion and extension throughout the body (Bergen et al., 1990).

To promote the motor development of children with cerebral palsy and other neuromotor deficits, occupational and physical therapists have often recommended prone positioners, sidelyers, and other devices to support children in the developmental positions of typically developing infants. Recent research, however, has largely failed to support the neuromaturational theories of development. It suggests that intervention based on emulation of a normal developmental sequence is unlikely to be successful, particularly for people who are beyond the infant stage of development or have severe neuromotor disabilities (Atwater, 1991). Prone positioners and sidelyers may be used for resting; however, the presumed developmental effects should not prompt their use, especially if they interfere with access to AAC systems, opportunities for interaction, or ability to perform other functional tasks (Campbell, 1989; McEwen & Karlan, 1989; McEwen & Lloyd, 1990a).

Long-term positioning effects can also be seen on the musculoskeletal system. As mentioned above, people with neuromotor problems are at risk for contractures and deformities due to a lack of normal movement and muscle imbalances. Positioning is believed to prevent contractures and deformities, or reduce their severity, by maintaining muscles and joints in positions opposite the deforming forces (Bergen et al., 1990). A person who is typically seated in a chair, for example, should be positioned with the hips and knees extended (e.g., upright in a stander or resting prone) during times that these positions do not interfere with desirable activity. A splint can also provide positioning to one or more joints, such as a foot splint to maintain the ankle in a neutral position or an elbow splint to manage unopposed elbow flexion. Although research has not yet demonstrated that positioning influences the development or progression of spinal deformities, positioning that provides a well-aligned posture is likely to be an important preventive measure (Trefler et al., 1993).

SEATING AS THE PRIMARY POSITION

A seated position is usually the most appropriate and effective position for a variety of functional activities for AAC users, including social communicative interactions (Campbell, 1989; McEwen, 1994; McEwen & Lloyd, 1990a). Mital, Belkin, and Sullivan (1976) propose that with good upright positioning the "consistently presented visual, tactile, kinesthetic and proprioceptive cues may become integrated to the best advantage for full development of the (person's) abilities" (p. 198).

Opportunities for social interaction also are enhanced when children use assistive seating. McEwen (1992) observed the classroom interactions between children with multiple disabilities and adults when the children were positioned in wheelchairs, in sidelyers, and supine on mats. The study revealed that adults initiated interactions at higher rates when students were in their wheelchairs, perhaps because they were nearer the normal interaction height of the adults or because the adults expected the students to be more communicative when they were upright. This last hypothesis was supported by another study in which two of three groups of adults rated students to have greater communication skills when they were pictured sitting in wheelchairs than when pictured in sidelying or supine positions (Collins, 1994). Assistive seating has also been shown to increase the amount of time people with multiple disabilities spend with others and the number of places they visit in the community (Hulme, Poor, Schulein, & Pezzino, 1983).

An exception to the findings that the seated position is optimal was found in a study of students who have profound multiple disabilities and who scored less than a 24-month developmental level on a test of social interaction. When given an attentive communication partner, these students communicated more when they were lying on their backs than when seated in wheelchairs (McEwen, 1992). Adults, however, initiated interactions more often when the students were seated. The differences in the findings highlight the importance of individually evaluating optimal positioning to both enhance opportunities for interaction and promote communication by individual AAC users (MacNeela, 1987a, b).

Guidelines for Seating

A wide variety of adapted chairs are available that provide the alignment and postural support needed by people with severe neuromotor disorders. The type of chair (or chairs) needed by an individual depends on the person's age and neuromusculoskeletal status and on the activities for which the seating will be used. Rarely will standard, unadapted chairs (even wheelchairs) serve individual needs. For infants and young children, strollers and high chairs are commonly adapted with inserts to provide postural alignment and support. Various special chairs, many with modifiable components, that promote optimal alignment and motor control of young children are also available (Bergen et al., 1990; Finnie, 1977).

As children grow older and are more difficult to position and transport, an adapted wheelchair often becomes the primary chair. For some children, a manual or electric wheelchair may be their only means of functional independent mobility, making early access to a chair critical for their overall development. Independent mobility is believed to have such a powerful influence on social-communicative, cognitive, and emotional development that easy, independent movement from place to place should be provided at an early age, even if a child is expected to walk eventually (Butler, 1991; Campos & Bertenthal, 1987; Jaffe, 1987).

Some universal seating guidelines apply to all of the many types of seats. They are discussed below and then summarized in Table 17.2.

Positioning Hips and Pelvis Well: Key to Good Seating. In the seated position, the hips and pelvis provide a critical foundation for the rest of the body (Bergen et al., 1990; McEwen & Lloyd, 1990a; Trefler et al., 1993). If the hips and pelvis are not well-positioned on an appropriate seat, the goals of assistive seating cannot be accomplished, regardless of adaptations that might be made to a chair.

Seat Surface.   Seats (and chair backs) can be generally classified as planar, contoured, and custom contoured or molded (Bergen et al., 1990; Cook & Hussey, 1995). **Planar seats** are flat, which means that they support only those parts of the body that protrude. As such, planar seats not only concentrate pressure over protuberances, which can be uncomfortable and may result in pressure ulcers, but also provide insufficient support for people who lack good postural control

TABLE 17.2 General Guidelines for Wheelchair Seating*

HIPS AND PELVIS

_____ Seat has a comfortable, supportive surface
_____ Pelvis is level and centered on the seat
_____ Buttocks are all the way back in the seat
_____ Hips are flexed 90 degrees
_____ Thighs are apart with neutral hip rotation (lateral hip or thigh pads, or thigh separator are used, if needed)
_____ Pelvis restraint is easily fastened and snug

KNEES AND FEET

_____ Knees are flexed 90 degrees (footrests are straight down, seat depth leaves about a two-finger-width space behind the knees)
_____ Footrests are neither too high nor too low (thighs are supported by the seat)
_____ Feet are flat on the footrests (ankles dorsiflexed to 90 degrees, if possible)
_____ Feet are strapped down only if needed for stability or safety

TRUNK

_____ Trunk is maintained as symmetrical and erect as possible
_____ Chair back is reclined no more than an ordinary chair
_____ Chair back is contoured to accommodate the shape of the trunk, including fixed spinal deformities and spinal orthoses
_____ Lateral trunk supports are properly positioned
    _____ Provide needed support, but are not too tight
    _____ Do not interfere with arm use
    _____ Provide counterpressure when needed
_____ Trunk/shoulder restraints are properly positioned and secure
    _____ Shoulder straps go through or over the chair back just below shoulder height
    _____ Restraints are not too close to the neck, too high, too low, too tight, or too loose, and are angled correctly

HEAD

_____ Head is in a normally upright position
_____ Only the amount of head support necessary is provided (be sure that the chair does not have an unnecessarily high back and that hips/pelvis and trunk/shoulder positions are optimal before adding head supports)
_____ Head supports do not interfere with vision or movement

ARMS

_____ Arms are usually forward and can be brought forward easily
_____ Tray is at an optimal height and angle for function

OVERALL

_____ The person looks as symmetrical and normally aligned as possible, with the head up and the arms forward

*People who need assistive seating have many individual differences, and these guidelines are not intended to be fully appropriate for everyone. They can, however, serve as a starting point when evaluating the appropriateness of a seating system and exploring modifications to improve function.

(Bergen et al., 1990; Cook & Hussey, 1995). Planar seats are common in wheelchairs and other adapted chairs, so replacement is usually a necessary first step to improve overall seated positioning of people with moderate and severe postural problems. Sling seats, which are standard on many strollers for children and some wheelchairs, should always be replaced because they contribute to postural malalignment and deformities, and they are uncomfortable.

Contoured seats have curved surfaces that approximate the shape of the body. Several manufacturers make wheelchair seats of contoured foam and other materials in a variety of sizes. Individualized foam seats can also be constructed for wheelchairs, strollers, high chairs, and other seating devices. Contoured seats can provide adequate support for people who have mild to moderate postural problems, symmetrical posture, and few, if any, deformities (Cook & Hussey, 1995). Most of the seats that people without disabilities use everyday, such as seats in cars and desk chairs, have gently contoured surfaces.

Custom contoured/molded seats are usually needed by people with poor postural control, asymmetrical posture, and/or skeletal deformities. These seats are contoured or molded so that they conform precisely to the contours of the individual. The intimate contact of the contours provides the greatest amount of support and control (Bergen et al., 1990; Cook & Hussey, 1995). These seats can be expensive, and the expertise needed to make them is not readily available in many communities.

They are worth pursuing, however, when they can make an important difference in an AAC user's posture, function, and comfort.

Whatever the type of seat, it should not only provide the required support, but also be comfortable for hours of sitting. A good test is to imagine sitting in the seat all day. If a seat is uncomfortable, it will be difficult for the person to attend to much of anything except the desire to get out of the chair.

Hips. For most people, a hip flexion angle of approximately 90 degrees (the thigh at a right angle to the trunk) provides the greatest stability and promotes the best voluntary motor control (Bergen et al., 1990; Cook & Hussey, 1995). When the angle between the thigh and trunk is greater than 90 degrees, many people tend to extend their hips and backs, or slide forward on their seats so the pelvis tilts backward and the trunk and head are not well-aligned over the body. Good alignment, with a neutral or anterior pelvic tilt, is necessary for optimal postural control and control of voluntary motor activities (Figure 17.1).

Even when the seat-to-back angle of a chair is 90 degrees, the hip flexion angle should be checked. Less than 90 degrees of flexion and a posterior pelvic tilt are common, particularly when a person is not placed in the chair with the buttocks all the way to the back of the seat and the pelvic belt is not snug. This may occur because the footrests are misplaced (see the section on footrests) or because the seat depth is too long. When the buttocks are positioned against the back

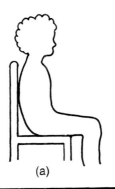 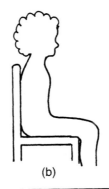 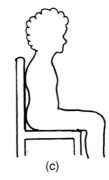

(a)   (b)   (c)

FIGURE 17.1   Pelvic Tilt.   (a) Posterior pelvic tilt. (b) Neutral pelvic tilt. (c) Anterior pelvic tilt.
Courtesy of Judy McEwen Richardson.

of the chair, a two-finger-width space should be between the back of the knees and the edge of the seat. If this much space is not found, the seat depth is probably too long.

Pelvis. Sometimes people have deformities that cause one side of the pelvis to be higher than the other (Bergen et al., 1990; Cook & Hussey, 1995). Unless the seat is modified to correct a flexible deformity or to accommodate a fixed deformity, the person's trunk will tilt sideways, causing poor postural alignment and instability. To check whether the pelvis is level, first make sure the person is all the way back in the chair and centered on the seat (not sitting toward one side or the other). Stand in front of the person, extend your elbows, and put your thumbs, with the thumb tips facing each other, on the person's **anterior superior iliac spines (ASIS)** (hip bones) (Figure 17.2). If the thumbs are correctly placed and level, the person's pelvis is level. If the thumbs are not level, try repositioning the person and check again. If they are still not level, seek the advice of someone with expertise in seating who can evaluate the need for seating modifications.

Thighs. The thighs provide important stability in the sitting position. If they are too close together or turned in, the base of support will be narrow and unstable. If the thighs are excessively separated or turned out, the pelvis and trunk can tilt too far forward, making it difficult to sit upright. Muscle imbalance and/or stiffness often cause thighs to be pulled together, whereas low muscle activity can

cause them to turn out. Sometimes a contoured seat with depressions for the thighs is all that is needed to maintain good alignment. In other cases, a wedge or block between the knees or thighs is needed to keep the thighs apart, or pads along the outside of the thighs or knees are needed to keep the thighs from turning out. Blocks or wedges between the legs are meant only to keep the thighs apart; they should *not* be used against the groin to keep a person from sliding down in a chair (Cook & Hussey, 1995). If a person is sliding down, check the hip angle, pelvis alignment, and pelvis restraint.

Pelvis Restraint. Some type of restraint is nearly always needed to keep the pelvis in place. The most common restraint is a belt that crosses the pelvis at a 45-degree angle (Figure 17.3). The belt must be snug enough to hold the pelvis in position, but not so snug that it is uncomfortable. If the hips and pelvis are positioned well on an appropriate seat surface, a tight belt should not be needed to maintain good alignment. Pelvic belts are most effective when they can be tightened with one hand while holding the person in position with the other hand. This is especially important when seating children (and some adults) who extend when they are placed in their wheelchairs. Belts that cannot be tightened with one hand, such as those with simply overlapping Velcro and no D-ring, should be replaced.

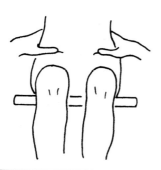

FIGURE 17.2 Correct Pelvis Level
Courtesy of Judy McEwen Richardson.

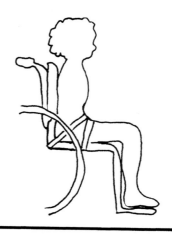

FIGURE 17.3 Pelvis Restraints (45- and 90-degree belts)
Courtesy of Judy McEwen Richardson.

If the person extends the hips excessively or if a 45-degree belt limits desired trunk or pelvis motion, then a 90-degree belt may be more appropriate (see Figure 17.3). Only one belt, however, is usually used at one time. In some cases, a rigid padded metal bar, called a **subASIS** (under the anterior superior iliac spines) **bar**, is used for people who require a great deal of control to maintain the position of the pelvis (Cook & Hussey, 1995). Knee blocks can also be used to keep the pelvis from sliding forward (Carlson & Ramsey, 1994).

Knees and Footrests.   If attempts to place the hips at a 90-degree angle with a neutral or anterior pelvic tilt have been unsuccessful, check the knees and footrests. Knee flexion tightness or contractures are common among people who use wheelchairs as a result of muscle imbalance and/or spending too much time with the knees flexed. The primary knee flexors are the hamstring muscles, which also extend the hip. Because the hamstring muscles cross both joints, tightness will cause the hip to extend as the knee is extended. Imagine a person sitting on a chair with one end of a rubber band attached to the lower leg, just below the back of knee, and the other end attached to the back of the pelvis, just above the hip joint. If the rubber band is flexible and long, straightening the knee will have no effect on the hip. If the rubber band is stiff or short, however, as with tight hamstring muscles, straightening the knee will cause the hip to extend and the pelvis to rotate posteriorly (Figure 17.4).

An easy way to check whether hamstring tightness is preventing good positioning of the hips and pelvis is to seat the person on a bench or chair with nothing under the feet or behind the legs. Permitting the knees to flex more often allows good positioning of the hips and pelvis. Footrests that are too far forward and straps behind the legs to keep the feet from slipping behind the footrests are common, but they demand more knee extension than many people can achieve without losing good hip and pelvis alignment (Hundertmark, 1985). Because the hardware often needs to be replaced to reposition the footrest, such footrest problems should be referred to a seating specialist.

Raising or lowering footrests that are not the correct height, however, usually does not require special expertise. Footrests should be at a height that supports the whole foot and allows the thighs to be supported on the seat surface. Footrests that are too high do not permit the thighs to broaden the base of support or distribute sitting pressure, leading to instability, discomfort, and localized pres-

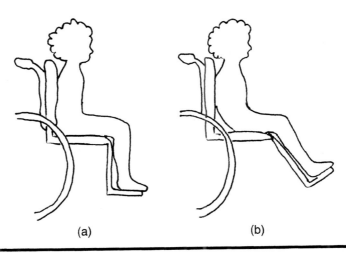

(a)   (b)

FIGURE 17.4   Person with Tight Hamstring Muscles.   (a) Positioning with the knees flexed 90 degrees permits a neutral or anterior pelvic tilt. (b) Positioning with the knees extended results in a posterior pelvic tilt. Courtesy of Judy McEwen Richardson.

sure. Footrests that are too low can leave the feet unsupported, which can cause pressure behind the thighs, contribute to ankle contractures, and encourage an individual to slide down in the chair in an attempt to reach the footrests.

The feet should be flat on the footrests with the ankles in a neutral position (a 90-degree angle between the foot and leg), if possible. Sometimes people have foot and ankle contractures that require specialized footrests to accommodate the limitations. To permit as much freedom of movement as possible, most people should not have their feet strapped down. Sometimes, however, it is necessary for stability or safety, especially for people who have excessive movement, such as **athetosis**.

Trunk. Once a good base of support is provided by the lower body, several chair features can further enhance trunk alignment and control, if necessary. A basic rule when attempting to improve trunk function through wheelchair positioning is to add or modify chair **posterior** (behind the body) elements first, then **lateral** (side) elements, and finally **anterior** (in front of the body) elements, if they are needed. One exception, however, is when an anteriorly tilted seat is used to promote a forward and extended trunk.

Posterior Elements. An important posterior element is the contour of the chair back. As with seats, chair backs can be planar, contoured, or custom contoured or molded. Planar backs are common, but do not provide the trunk contact typically found in the ordinary seats used by most people everyday, which is necessary for basic support and comfort. Contoured backs approximate the shape of the trunk and, depending on the depth of the contours and their similarity to the body shape, can provide the support and comfort needed by people with mild to moderate trunk instability and minimal, if any, spinal deformity.

Custom contoured or molded backs are usually needed by people with severe trunk instability and with moderate or severe spinal deformities, such as scoliosis or kyphosis. The intimate contact not only provides the support needed to maintain a well-aligned position and is the only surface that

can adequately accommodate spinal deformities. Before adding side supports, chest straps, or other restraints to a chair to improve trunk alignment, be sure the chair back is appropriately contoured.

Some chairs are fitted with mechanisms that permit the chair back to be reclined or the whole chair to be tilted in space (Figure 17.5). **Recline** refers to lowering (or raising) the back of the chair without altering the position of the seat and its relationship to the floor; the seat-to-back angle becomes larger when the back is lowered and smaller when the back is moved forward. **Tilt-in-space** refers to tilting the seat and back as a unit; the seat-to-back angle does not change. The primary reasons for using recline are (1) to redistribute pressure; (2) to accommodate the person who lacks 90 degrees of hip flexion; and (3) to provide a resting position without the need to transfer from the chair (Cook & Hussey, 1995). Tilt-in-space is also used for pressure redistribution and rest, as well as for fine-tuning postural control.

Although recline and tilt have benefits, they also may have negative effects; therefore, their use must be evaluated carefully. Reclining the back of a chair changes the seat-to-back angle, which changes the hip flexion angle, which often results in poor positioning of the hips and pelvis. Reclining the back more than a few degrees can also alter the line of vision to such an extent that a person's vision is directed toward the ceiling. This interferes with eye contact with communication partners and with vision needed to access a communication device. Moving the back of the chair also causes sheer forces on the trunk and buttocks, which can be dangerous for people who are at risk for skin breakdown (Cook & Hussey, 1995). A few degrees of permanent posterior recline, like that of most ordinary chairs, however, can be helpful. Because of the shape of the trunk and lower back, sitting in a chair with a perfectly vertical back actually forces one to lean forward a bit, especially if the chair back is planar and the buttocks are all the way back. A few degrees of recline can prevent this problem and help the person maintain an upright position more easily.

Chairs that tilt in space are increasingly common and can be helpful, but they can also be misused. This is especially true when chairs are tilted

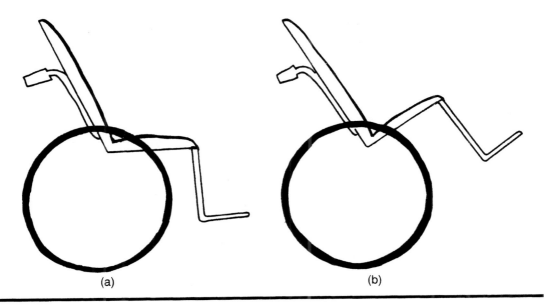

FIGURE 17.5   Wheelchairs.   (a) Recline. (b) Tilt-in-space.
Courtesy of Judy McEwen Richardson.

far back to keep a person's head from falling forward. Identifying and correcting the underlying cause of the problem, such as inadequate positioning or boredom, is a more appropriate course of action.

Just as a few degrees of recline can assist in maintaining an upright posture, a few degrees of anterior tilt may also be helpful, particularly for functional activities. Some researchers have suggested that an anteriorly tilted seat promotes a more upright posture in people who have the postural responses necessary to extend their backs when tilted forward (Miedaner, 1990; Myhr & von Wendt, 1991). Myhr and von Wendt found that seating children with cerebral palsy on an anteriorly tilted seat, combined with a cut out table to lean on, resulted in improved head control and hand function. Such improvement could positively influence an AAC user's ability to communicate. The effects of anteriorly tilted seats on long-term performance and fatigue, however, are unclear (Carlson & Ramsey, 1994).

Lateral Elements.   Lateral trunk supports can be placed along the sides of the trunk to prevent falling sideways. This is especially important to

consider when positioning a person in a seat with a planar back. A seat with a contoured back may provide enough support so that lateral trunk supports are not needed. If lateral supports are needed, they should be snug enough to be supportive, but not so snug that they interfere with arm use. Lateral supports should be prescribed by a seating specialist and mounted on the chair. Pillows, rolled towels, foam blocks, and other "fillers" can be used to roughly approximate the effect of lateral trunk supports, but they are too unstable to be used permanently.

Anterior Elements.   Types of anterior trunk supports, made by a number of manufacturers, include H- and V-straps, butterfly-type harnesses, rigid torso supports, rigid shoulder stabilizers, and vests (Bergen et al., 1990). Any anterior support should be used only if necessary because all are restrictive and limit forward trunk motion, which is important for arm and hand use.

One common problem with anterior supports is improper insertion of the straps over or through the back of the chair. Straps should be inserted just below the shoulders, so they provide slight downward pressure on the shoulders when they are fastened. Straps that are too high or too low tend to cause people to lean forward or slump. Another common problem, particularly with H-straps and butterfly-type harnesses, is that if they are not anchored firmly at the base, they will slide up under a person's neck and can interfere with breathing (Bergen et al., 1990).

Head.   After carefully attending to the alignment of the hips, pelvis, and trunk, a person's head will often be in a functional, upright position and require no further intervention. Poor positioning of the body, however, results in poor positioning of the head. No amount or type of support will be as effective in positioning the head as improving the overall positioning of the body. As with trunk support, if head support is needed, posterior support should be provided first, followed by lateral support. Anterior support should be provided only as a last resort.

Many types of head supports are available, and some of the newer types that permit some active movement while providing good control are more helpful than others. To the extent possible, any head support should not interfere with vision or movement. The Automotive Safety for Children Program at Riley Hospital for Children (1993) cautions against strapping a child's head to the chair while on a school bus because of the risk of a neck injury during a crash.

Bergen et al. (1990) describe five general types of head supports: (1) flat and gently curved posterior head rests; (2) contoured head rests that provide both posterior and lateral support; (3) lateral head supports, which are typically padded, planar supports; (4) anterior forehead supports; and (5) chin supports, such as soft foam neck rings or rigid supports. A seating specialist can help to select the head support that is likely to be the most effective for a given individual.

Arms.   Positioning of the arms is critical because hands can only function where the arms place them. Some people need slings or other supports to assist in overcoming gravity to move their hands. Simply ensuring that the arms are forward, however, is usually enough to place the hands in a functional position. Many people with cerebral palsy, in particular, have patterns of movement that cause their shoulders and arms to pull back. The hands cannot do much in this position, which makes it important to prevent the pattern to improve hand use.

In positioning the arms forward, place folded towels behind the shoulders and scapulae. If the pattern of pulling the shoulders and arms back is not too strong, sometimes this is enough. If this is successful, then wedges can be permanently mounted on the back of the chair (Bergen et al., 1990). However, blocks made of padded plastic, metal, or wood may be necessary to prevent the upper arms from pulling back. Clinicians/educators can easily see whether blocks will help by standing behind the person's chair and placing their palms in a position to hold the person's elbows forward when they are at rest on the wheelchair tray. Clinicians/educators should not hold the person's arms, but rather block them to keep them from pulling back. Different locations can be tried to find a spot that not only blocks the movement, but also results in better hand function. Blocks can then be constructed and mounted permanently on the chair back or tray.

The height and angle of the tray are also important to evaluate. Sometimes raising a tray will raise the arms enough to promote a more upright sitting posture. Raising the tray too much, however, can make it difficult to use the hands and to see things on the tray. Communication boards and other symbol displays are often placed on wheelchair trays, so their optimal height and angle is a critical component of a positioning evaluation. From a positioning perspective, no one best height or angle exists for a tray or for a communication display. An occupational or physical therapist can often provide initial suggestions, but fine-tuning is usually necessary as the person has opportunities to practice and motor control is observed over time.

In the final analysis, the seated AAC user should look as symmetrical and normally aligned as possible, with the head up and the arms forward. If not, first make sure the person has been placed in the chair correctly, because the best chair will not be effective if a person is positioned in it poorly. If a good position is still not achieved, more work probably needs to be done. Most seating, especially for people with severe disabilities, is never finished for long. Seats almost always require ongoing revision to accommodate growth, changes in motor control, and changes in musculoskeletal status. Revisions may also be indicated as more effective components and adaptations become available.

SELECTING BODY SITES AND METHODS TO CONTROL AAC DEVICES

Motor access to an AAC device can be considered after a person is positioned well. Determining the most effective method for a person to operate a device is an art rather than a science, so it usually takes time and much trial and error, particularly when a person has severe motor control problems. An occupational or physical therapist can often assist in making decisions, but a team effort is important, with input from the individual, the family, and everyone else who has observed the person's motor functioning under a variety of conditions. Two basic questions need to be answered when deciding how a person will control a device: Which body part will be used? Is direct or indirect selection likely to be most effective?

Body Site Considerations

To promote the most effective communication, the motor aspects of communication should be as effortless as possible. Many people with severe disabilities have better control of their eyes than other body sites, so eye-gaze techniques (Goossens' & Crain, 1987) can be a good means to develop communication skills, sometimes while control of other body sites is being developed through other activities (Cook & Hussey, 1995).

The hands are the preferred site for access because of the fine control that may be possible. Many people also prefer to use their hands, and hand use tends to be more socially acceptable. If hand function is not adequate, the head may be the control site of choice. The head can be used either to directly select symbols with a pointer or indirectly select with a switch, if direct selection is not possible (Cook & Hussey, 1995). Some people,

particularly those with athetosis, have the best control of their legs and feet. Although these sites are generally less desirable than the head or hands, they may be the most effective option. Some people can use more than one site, which can improve the efficiency of AAC use or may permit one site to be used for AAC and another to control other assistive technology such as a power wheelchair (Cook & Hussey, 1995). Speech-recognition technology is also becoming another possibility for access. With potential body sites in mind, the next decision is whether direct selection is possible.

Direct Selection Considerations

Direct selection is usually faster and cognitively easier than indirect selection. With direct selection, the person chooses from among an array of symbols by pointing with a hand, finger, eye, or other body part. Pointing can be done without a device or with a device such as a mouth wand or head pointer. Direct selection without a device is preferable, if possible, because there is one less component to break, lose, and manage.

Six elements of motor control are evaluated to determine whether a person is able to use direct selection and, if so, what the features should be. These elements are resolution of motion, range of motion, strength, endurance, versatility (Cook & Hussey, 1995), and speed.

Resolution of motion refers to a person's degree of fine motor control, as reflected by the smallest target, with the smallest separation between targets, that a person can accurately select. Some people are able to select small targets that are close together, such as keys on a computer keyboard, whereas others require larger and more widely spaced targets, such as a four- or six-location voice output communication aid (VOCA) or an expanded keyboard.

Range of motion is the distance that a person can move a body part. People without motor control problems, for example, can move the hand and fingers over a wide range in conjunction with trunk, shoulder, and elbow movement. The hand and fingers, separate from the trunk, shoulder, and elbow, have much smaller ranges. When a person has motor control problems, AAC service providers must determine not only the range of motion of the specific body site that may operate the device, but also the other parts that are responsible for placing that body part so it can do its work. This is especially important when evaluating use of distal body parts, such as hands and feet. Service providers should also determine the range of active motion that the person has when attempting to use a communication device, rather than just examining the passive range, or range when attempting other tasks.

Another important consideration when evaluating range is the placement of the communication display. Many people with motor control problems have difficulty reaching symbols on a display depending on its location. Move the display around to see whether location makes a difference. Try it on the right, the left, or in the middle (middle is usually best). Move it closer to or away from the person, change the angle, gradually move it from flat on the table or the tray to vertical, then hold it up in the air. People who are skilled at observing people with motor problems can often predict where the best placement might be, but anyone can experiment to see what works. Remember that even people with experience rarely get it right the first time.

Strength can also affect a person's ability to operate an AAC device. More strength is needed to press keys, for example, than to point; more strength is needed to raise an arm against the force of gravity to reach a display than to move a hand across a horizontal display. Sometimes people with motor control problems move too forcefully, so a device that is not sturdy enough can break. As with range of motion, strength should be evaluated when attempting to use the communication device in various locations. Many children with cerebral palsy, for example, are able to generate more force when a display is elevated than when it is flat on a table or a tray.

Endurance is necessary to sustain communication. If the movement required to operate a device is too tiring, the person will not be able to communicate at will. Sometimes endurance will increase as the person gains strength through the "exercise" of using a communication device. However, a communication device is not an exercise machine, so if endurance does not improve

quickly, a less tiring method of selection needs to be identified.

Versatility is another element that Cook and Hussey (1995) recommend evaluating. The most versatile body part is a finger and more than one usable finger increases versatility. One or more fingers can press keys, point to symbols, operate a joy stick, or press a switch. In contrast, the eye is limited to gazing and blinking, and without a sophisticated recognition system, a partner must be present who can interpret the symbols.

Speed is important because most AAC systems are slow and increasing the rate of communication will usually enhance both communication and opportunities for communication. Speed can be affected by the location and the type of display as well as the body part being used.

Evaluations of range, strength, endurance, versatility, and speed are generally more useful for determining which body part will operate the AAC device, and the features of the device, than for determining whether direct selection or indirect selection should be used. These elements can often be accommodated by the size, location, and type of communication display. Versatility usually comes into play when deciding which body part will give the most options.

Resolution (often in combination with speed) is the element that normally indicates whether a person can use direct selection. If a person does not have the motor control necessary to accurately select from among a number of symbols that is sufficiently large to meet communication needs within a reasonable amount of time, then indirect selection should be considered. Occasionally, the only body site with the necessary resolution for direct selection has such limited versatility that indirect selection is necessary (e.g., when eye gaze is the only direct selection option).

Indirect Selection Considerations

Indirect selection requires use of one or more switches to control scanning. As with direct selection, the body part, hardware, and location combination that enables the most accurate, consistent, and rapid operation must be determined. Resolution, range, strength, endurance, versatility, and speed all need to be considered. As with direct selection, no magic formula is available to determine the best configuration of body movement, type of switch, and switch location. Gaining knowledge of the person's voluntary movement during other activities is usually the best place to start. Potentially, any movement can be used to activate a switch, including eyebrow elevation, eye blinks, sipping and puffing air, as well as more common head, hand, and foot movements. As discussed above, hand movements are usually preferable if they are a viable option. In addition to potential advantages in resolution, range, and versatility, hand motions are visible to the person and more types of reliable switches are available for hand movements than for other types (see Chapter 9 for examples of switches).

Once a tentative body site has been identified, try switches that vary in size and are activated by differing pressures and types of movements. Try each switch in different locations until the best combination has been determined. Often many trials over time must be made to decide which body part, switch, and location enable the most effective switch operation. Unless a combination is clearly not working, however, be sure to give a person enough time to learn to use a switch without constant modification.

Regardless of the type of switch, it must be reliable so the person using it does not have to face the frustration of a switch that does not work or is not where it is supposed to be. For this reason, manufactured switches are usually preferable to homemade ones, and they must be mounted on the wheelchair tray or other selected location by someone who has the tools, hardware, and expertise to make them stay in place while in use.

MOTOR CONTROL, MOTOR LEARNING, AND MOTOR TEACHING

Acquiring the motor control necessary for the most effective use of an AAC device requires motor learning on the part of the AAC user. This motor learning can be greatly influenced by the motor teaching strategies used by speech-language pathologists, teachers, parents, and other caregivers and service providers.

From a systems perspective, motor behavior is the outcome of many dynamic and interacting components within a task-specific context (Heriza, 1991). The neuromusculoskeletal system is important, but it is only one element of the total picture that must be considered in motor control of AAC devices. Even if the neuromusculoskeletal system is adequate for the AAC task, motor behaviors will appear to be inadequate if the other systems are insufficiently developed. If motivation to communicate, for example, is inadequate, motor behaviors will appear to be deficient. Similarly, cognition, arousal, position, the communication display, opportunities for interaction, and a nearly limitless array of other environmental and personal factors can influence motor output. The team must evaluate as many of the components that contribute to motor behavior as possible and not just attribute observed behaviors to neuromusculoskeletal deficits.

Teaching motor control for the effective operation of AAC devices is much like teaching any other skill. Practice is essential for learning, and the way in which practice is organized affects not only a skill's acquisition and perfection, but also its maintenance and generalization. If the required motor activity is not yet in the person's repertoire (e.g., a child may never have pressed a switch), the teacher may need to prompt the behavior initially. From the least intrusive to the most intrusive, prompts include expectant pauses, comments (e.g., "I wonder what happens when the switch is pressed"), instructions (e.g., "touch the switch"), models (e.g., demonstrating pressing the switch and the outcome), cues (e.g., tapping the switch on the table), and physical guidance (e.g., moving the child's hand to the switch and pressing it) (Snell & Zirpoli, 1987). Remember to give the person *time* to respond to any prompt—count to 10 or 20, if necessary. People with motor impairments may need a long time to organize and produce a motor response, especially if they have sensory and cognitive limitations as well.

For optimal learning, the least intrusive effective prompt should be used. As learning occurs, the level of prompt should be reduced until only a natural cue, such as the presence of the switch, prompts the motor behavior (McEwen, 1994).

Physical guidance, in particular, should be used judiciously and only in the initial stages of learning. If hand-over-hand guidance or other physical prompts are needed for more than a short time when the person is given appropriate learning opportunities, then motivation, arousal, task complexity, or some other factor, rather than the neuromuscular aspects of motor control, may be influencing the motor behavior and require attention.

Practice to enhance motor control can be organized several ways (Larin, 1994). Drill-type or repeated practice within a relatively short time (called blocked or massed practice) can facilitate initial acquisition, but does not promote retention or generalization of a skill. To promote retention and generalization, short periods of practice throughout the day, in a variety of settings, with a variety of people (random or dispersed practice) is needed. For this reason, an important step in intervention should be to teach all communication partners or potential partners to provide appropriate practice.

Sufficient opportunity to practice is another critical factor for improving a motor behavior (Larin, 1994). Think about the number of times a tennis player hits a ball to improve a serve or a pianist plays a piece to improve a performance, then think about the number of opportunities people with severe neuromotor deficits typically have to practice using their AAC systems. A system may have been left at home or at school, be too much bother to place on a wheelchair, or have an unstable switch that is in a different location every time the person attempts to press it. A communication partner who does not take the time to interact with the AAC user also may limit opportunities for practice. Reasons for insufficient practice opportunities are endless. All interfere with improvement of motor control needed to acquire operational competence in using AAC devices.

Feedback is another essential component of motor teaching and learning. Extrinsic contingent feedback from communication partners is important for both accuracy of communication symbol selection and communication development. Intrinsic feedback, provided by the sensory system, is also important for error detection and correction.

Particularly when the sensory system is not intact, as with many AAC users, extrinsic feedback can augment or enhance learning (Larin, 1994). "If you sit a little straighter it will be easier to touch the ball" or "you touched the ball, so here it is" are examples of extrinsic verbal feedback. Other related intervention issues and procedures that can promote use of AAC systems are discussed in Chapters 15, 16, 18, and 19.

CASE EXAMPLES

Ramon

Ramon is a 16-year-old with profound multiple disabilities. He has spastic quadriplegic-type cerebral palsy, a seizure disorder, and severe cognitive impairment. Secondary to the cerebral palsy, he has a dislocated hip, thoracic kyphosis, and severe flexion contractures of elbows, knees, and hips.

Ramon's wheelchair had a planar seat and back. Because of his kyphosis, Ramon leaned far forward in the chair, which required an H-strap to hold him upright, a thick cushion behind his head, and a strap around his forehead to keep his head up. Because positioning was difficult and Ramon was uncomfortable in his chair, he spent much of his day at school lying on his side on a wedge or in a beanbag chair.

A primary educational goal for Ramon has been to improve his basic nonlinguistic social-communicative interaction. One of the major factors limiting his progress was his exceptionally poor school attendance. Over the past 5 years, Ramon was in school for only the first few weeks of each year, then was home sick with various upper respiratory infections, which often led to pneumonia.

At the beginning of the last school year, Ramon received a new wheelchair that was designed to accommodate his severe trunk and limb deformities. The most critical feature of the chair is a custom contoured chair back, which was designed to accommodate his kyphosis while maintaining his head in an upright position. The chair also has a custom contoured seat to level his pelvis and accommodate his dislocated hip, and footrests are placed slightly under the seat to accommodate his knee flexion contractures. Because Ramon lacks postural control, a chest restraint and posterior head support are still needed, but he no longer leans heavily into the chest panel and straps, and he is able to hold his head up without the anterior strap.

In his new chair, Ramon has been able to sit comfortably for several hours at a time, his eating has improved, and he has learned to press a switch. He has also remained healthy, missing only 6 days of school the whole year. His team is convinced that his upright position has contributed to pulmonary hygiene and has reduced the risk of aspiration, thus preventing the illnesses that were so common when he spent most of his day lying down. Perhaps as a result of his increased school attendance, better health, and greater comfort, Ramon is learning basic dyadic interaction skills that have never been possible for him before.

Lisa

Lisa is a 6-year-old with spastic quadriplegic-type cerebral palsy. She is in a general first-grade class and has had a VOCA for 2 years. Her ability to use the device is limited, however, and she usually communicates through facial expressions and answering yes/no questions. A goal for Lisa this year is to use the communication device to meet defined communication needs.

As part of the overall evaluation to determine intervention, Lisa's positioning was evaluated. She was positioned in a stander for an hour in the morning and an hour in the afternoon, in a sidelyer for 30 minutes in the morning, and on a prone wedge for 30 minutes in the afternoon. She was usually out of her chair on a mat for the daily 30-minute adaptive physical education class. For the rest of the school day, including lunch, she was positioned in her power wheelchair. Thus, of the 6-hour school day, Lisa spent, at most, 2.5 hours in her wheelchair.

Lisa's wheelchair seating was evaluated and found to be basically good, with only relatively minor modifications needed. Because Lisa's arms tended to pull back, making it difficult for her to use her right hand to select symbols on her communication device, blocks were secured to her tray. Although this modification kept her arms forward and immediately improved rate and accuracy, symbol selection was still motorically difficult.

Because Lisa's wheelchair was appropriate and access to her communication device was best when she was seated (and she liked being in her chair), her need for the other positions was evaluated. The team determined that standing was important to prevent flexion contractures; also Lisa's hand function seemed to be better in the standing position. So, the stander continued to be used during the 1-hour art-science block in the late morning when manipulation of materials was a major part of the lessons. Because the communication device was difficult to secure and difficult for Lisa to use when she was standing, topic boards with vocabulary useful for the art and science projects were provided.

Lisa's parents agreed to stand Lisa when she watched television after returning home from school and again when she helped wash the dishes after dinner to eliminate the need to stand in the afternoon at school. Lisa disliked being placed in the sidelyer and prone wedge because the other students did not use them, and when the team determined that they appeared to serve no important purpose, their use was discontinued. Lisa continued to be on the mats during adaptive PE, with the other students. She did not have the stability needed to use a communication display during this activity, so she relied on vocalizations, body and facial expressions, and answering yes/no questions.

Finally, Lisa's opportunities to practice using her communication device were evaluated. The team found that Lisa had her device on her chair and a responsive and knowledgeable communication partner for an average of only about 15 minutes a day at school. These opportunities were expanded greatly by ensuring that the device was always present and by teaching the other children and as many adults as possible how to interact with Lisa and facilitate her communication development.

SUMMARY

In general, a well-seated position is the best position for communication. It can offer more opportunities for interaction than other positions, promote the greatest motor control, and provide mobility to where the action is. Other positioning devices are needed as alternatives, but they should usually be used only when AAC needs are minimal. A notable exception may be people with the most profound disabilities who have been found to engage in more communicative behaviors when supine, given a responsive communication partner.

A well-seated position requires attention to certain guidelines, which is the responsibility of all caregivers and service providers. An occupational therapist, physical therapist, or other seating specialist can provide valuable assistance with seating, but they need input from other team members who can monitor positioning and positioning needs on a day-to-day basis.

Motor control that allows effective access and use of AAC devices requires extensive practice, which may be enhanced by the use of prompts and feedback. Effective motor teaching to improve skill in the operation of AAC devices provides opportunities for practice communicating on a variety of topics, in a variety of settings, with a variety of communication partners. Seating, other types of positioning, and motor control are critical components of the successful implementation of AAC.

CHAPTER 18

INTERVENTION FOR PERSONS WITH DEVELOPMENTAL DISABILITIES

DOREEN M. BLISCHAK, FILIP LONCKE, AND AMY WALLER

Many individuals who use **augmentative and alternative communication (AAC)**, either temporarily or across the life span, require assistance in developing spoken and/or written language as a result of impairments that occur prior to adulthood, during the **developmental period**. Many of these impairments are present at birth (congenital), although a definitive diagnosis is often not made until after infancy. Other impairments are incurred later during the developmental period, resulting in loss of previously gained skills and serious developmental delay. In this chapter, the term **developmental disabilities** refers to conditions such as autism, cerebral palsy, cognitive impairment, severe speech and/or language impairment, and other physical impairments that interfere with typical development during the developmental period prior to adolescence.

Developmental disabilities are associated with a group of relatively static, chronic conditions that are the result of neurological injury or malfunctioning. Neurological injury that occurs during prenatal development or as a result of trauma, asphyxia, disease, or stroke may cause physical, cognitive, and/or speech-language impairments that result in communication disabilities. Likewise, differences in neurological functioning characteristic of metabolic disorders, genetic abnormalities, or progressive diseases may also cause communication disabilities. Finally, a small number of children experience severe communication disabilities as a result of **glossectomy** or **laryngectomy** (surgical removal of the tongue or larynx) or performance of a **tracheotomy** to reduce breathing difficulties (Adamson & Dunbar, 1991; Batshaw & Perret, 1986; Capute & Accardo,

1991; Mirenda & Mathy-Laikko, 1989; Vanderheiden & Yoder, 1986). See Table 18.1 for a list of contributing factors in developmental disabilities that may create the need for AAC intervention.

The AAC intervention methods described in this chapter are based on thorough and ongoing assessment of individual needs across the life span and may be appropriate for any or all AAC users to support communication, speech, language, and literacy development. Because of the importance of early intervention for individuals with developmental disabilities, much of the material presented is geared toward young children. However, developmental and age-appropriate modifications are suggested for older children and young adults. Discussion begins with intervention approaches that use nonlinguistic AAC methods and progresses to approaches that use linguistic communication in social, educational, and employment settings. The use of multiple AAC methods and modes is emphasized, with overlap across situations and life span. Development of communicative competence is considered throughout as an integral component of a comprehensive AAC intervention plan.

DEVELOPMENT OF COMMUNICATIVE COMPETENCE

Light (1989) described competent communicators as individuals whose communication is functional and adequate and "premised on sufficient knowledge, judgment, and skill to perform as required given the partner, the environment, and the intent" (p. 139). An important distinction is made between **communicative mastery** and **communica-**

TABLE 18.1   Contributing Factors in Developmental Disabilities

PRENATAL	PERINATAL	POSTNATAL
Autism	Asphyxia	Asphyxia (e.g., near drowning)
Genetic abnormalities—inherited (e.g., Duchenne muscular dystrophy); not inherited (e.g., Down syndrome)	Birth trauma	Cerebrovascular accident (stroke)
	Low birth weight/prematurity	Infectious diseases (e.g., encephalitis)
Infectious diseases (e.g., maternal rubella)		Lead ingestion
Maternal trauma		Progressive diseases (e.g., muscular dystrophy)
Metabolic disorders (e.g., phenylketonuria)		Surgical procedures (e.g., glossectomy)
Neural tube disorders (e.g., spina bifida)		Trauma (e.g., head/spinal cord injury; laryngeal trauma)
Radiation exposure		Tumors
Toxins (e.g., maternal drug use)		

From Adamson & Dunbar (1991); Batshaw & Perret (1986); Capute & Accardo (1991); Mirenda & Mathy-Laikko (1989); Vanderheiden & Yoder (1986).

competence. Few native speakers of a language achieve total communicative mastery. This discussion, therefore, focuses on communicative competence, because it is most relevant for the majority of communicators. Also, individuals may be competent communicators in some contexts but not in others. For example, university professors may be competent when lecturing in a classroom, but may be less competent when negotiating the price of a new car. Likewise, AAC users may not exhibit communicative competence in certain contexts and, therefore, may not participate fully in all communication exchanges. Refer to Chapter 1 for a review of Light's four communicative competencies: **linguistic competence**, **operational competence**, **social competence**, and **strategic competence**.

Development of communicative competence begins almost from the moment of birth. Typically developing children are considered competent communicators if their communication is appropriate for their age and developmental level. Thus, communicative competence depends on the developmental level of the individual (Dunst & Lowe, 1986). For example, although AAC users may not use expressive language fully, they may still be considered competent if they use AAC to communicate *functionally* and *adequately*. Expectations for expansion of existing communication skills are important, but this progression may be different for AAC users than for typically developing children. Many AAC users do not acquire communication and language as a progressive mastery of phonology, lexicon, syntax, and discourse. For example, their development of an internalized phonological system may be based more on the perception of others' speech and less on their own speech articulation. AAC users' lexical development may also be affected if they have to rely on preselected vocabulary. By nature of the constraints inherent in using AAC methods, users also differ in their abilities to engage in discourse as equal and active members of a communicative dyad (Buzolich & Wiemann, 1988; Light, Collier, & Parnes, 1985a, 1985b; Romski & Sevcik, 1988a). Thus, their performance should not be perceived as merely having less communication and language, but as a manifestation of a unique configuration of performance (Nelson, 1992) on which the development of communicative competence rests.

Rowland and Stremel-Campbell (1987) have

provided a useful initial framework from which to view the development of communicative competence from early infancy to the development of linguistic communication, where "language is the culmination of a communicative competence that begins early in a child's life" (Rowland & Stremel-Campbell, 1987, p. 50). Further, Dunst and Lowe (1986) have listed six criteria from which to classify the development of communicative behaviors, beginning in infancy.

1. The degree to which the infant is *aware* of environmental events
2. The infant's ability to attain a *goal* or goal state through sustained interactions with the environment
3. The degree to which the behavior is *culturally defined* and thus has social and conventional readability
4. The extent to which the child *intentionally uses objects* to operate on adult attention or *uses adults* as means to obtain desired objects
5. The extent to which the communicative behavior is *linguistic* in nature
6. The extent to which communicative behaviors are used as *signifiers* for something *signified* in the absence of reference-giving cues (p. 12)

Table 18.2 provides a modification and extension of the developmental models of Rowland and Stremel-Campbell (1987) and Dunst and Lowe (1986). AAC examples that parallel "natural" communication methods at each stage are included, using terminology according to guidelines established in Chapter 4. In addition, a proposed course of development for each of Light's (1989) four areas of communicative competence is also included. Table 18.2 shows that linguistic, operational, and social competence develop simultaneously. For example, an infant's cry can demonstrate emerging linguistic competence (i.e., she is producing sounds in the same manner that she may eventually produce the phonology of her spoken language), emerging operational competence (i.e., she is using her vocal tract appropriately), and emerging social competence (i.e., she is communicating in a manner appropriate for her age and situation). Strategic competence may develop later, depending on the child's need to avoid and repair communication breakdowns (i.e., a child whose needs are correctly

interpreted and/or anticipated probably has less need to develop strategic competence). However, this interpretation was selected in an effort to mark the developmental stages at which these areas are emphasized in AAC use.

A major distinction is made between linguistic and nonlinguistic communication. Linguistic communication involves using symbols and combination rules of a naturally developed language (e.g., manual signs, spoken words, and/or a representation such as traditional orthography [TO]). During the first year of life, communication is exclusively nonlinguistic. Linguistic communication emerges in the second year of life in typically developing children. However, competent communicators, including many AAC users, use a variety of linguistic and nonlinguistic modes of communication. These described "stages" represent somewhat arbitrary divisions because there may be considerable overlap among them. For instance, in many typically developing children, communication via "transparent symbols" may not emerge as a distinct stage, but instead overlaps with use of early gestures and beginning speech production. However, for children with disabilities, this stage can represent an important transition from using gestural communication exclusively to beginning use of arbitrary symbols, a stage that may not develop without intervention in individuals with severe developmental disabilities (Rowland & Stremel-Campbell, 1987). Each of these stages will be discussed, along with AAC intervention for developing communicative competence and guidelines for transitioning to the next stage.

Although early communicative behaviors shown in Table 18.2 are primarily unaided, two primary forms of linguistic communication, spoken and sign language, are also unaided. Further, aided communication modes (i.e., transparent symbols and arbitrary symbols) may be introduced to AAC users during stages that in typical development are characterized by unaided communication modes. For further discussion of aided and unaided approaches in AAC, see Chapters 5, 6, and 7.

Throughout this chapter, the importance of symbol acquisition and functional symbol use is emphasized. Although typically developing children often require little explicit intervention to

TABLE 18.2 Developmental Levels of Nonlinguistic and Linguistic Communication

LEVEL	SYMBOLS	BEHAVIOR	EXAMPLES (INCLUDING AAC)	COMPETENCE*	INTERVENTION†
Nonlinguistic					
Preintentional reflexive behavior	Gestures Vocalizations	Reflexive behavior indicating physical state, which is interpreted by the caregiver	Grimace; crying to indicate hunger, pain	Social (emerging)	Ensure engagement
Preintentional anticipatory behavior	Gestures Vocalizations	Anticipatory behavior that is not intentionally communicative. The caregiver infers intent	Eye gaze; whole body movement and vocalizations directed to desired object	Social	Focus attention
Intentional behavior	Gestures Vocalizations Cause-and-effect movements	Use of nonconventional and conventional gestures with the intent of affecting another's behavior	Pushing, tugging, and other body movements (e.g., extending arms for "Pick me up"); whining Switch-activated buzzer	Social Strategic (emerging) Operational (emerging)	Sustain interaction
	Transparent symbols	Use of symbols that share one or more perceptual features of the referent	Some gestures (e.g., patting floor for "Sit down") Some vocalizations (e.g., "m-m-m" for eat) Some manual signs (e.g., "drink") Miniature objects Pictographs, photographs, pictographic Sigsymbols, pictographic Blissymbols	Social Strategic Operational	Elaborate interaction Work toward conventionalization

LEVEL	SYMBOLS	BEHAVIOR	EXAMPLES (INCLUDING AAC)	COMPETENCE*	INTERVENTION†
Nonlinguistic (*continued*)					
Intentional behavior (*continued*)	Arbitrary symbols	Use of symbols whose relationship to the referent is arbitrary	Some gestures (e.g., yes/no headshake) First spoken words Some manual signs (e.g., mother) Textured symbols 3-dimensional arbitrary symbols (e.g., NON-SLIP) Lexigrams Some Blissymbols, Sigsymbols Written sight words	Social Strategic Operational Linguistic (emerging)	Sustain elaboration Continue conventionalization
Linguistic	Arbitrary (and some transparent) symbols	Use of language, a rule-bound symbol system	Natural languages (i.e., spoken language, sign language) Language codes (e.g., orthographies, manual signs, fingerspelling, Morse code, Sigsymbols)	Social Strategic Operational Linguistic	Elaborate conventionalization

*Relates to all four types of communicative competence as described by Light (1989).

†Recommended areas of intervention (Dunst & Lowe, 1986).

learn functional linguistic and nonlinguistic communication, children with developmental disabilities often require intense and systematic intervention. Especially for the acquisition of the first functional symbols, caregivers and professionals need to employ intervention techniques such as shaping, fading, prompting, and expectant time delay. Use of each of these techniques will be illustrated at different points in this chapter, in conjunction with case examples illustrating various AAC approaches.

NONLINGUISTIC COMMUNICATION

Humans produce nonlinguistic communication behaviors alone or in conjunction with language, such as spoken English. These behaviors generally consist of vocalizations and gestures. The term *vocalization* includes unintentional vocal utterances, such as expressions of discomfort or pleasure, as well as the use of vocal patterns that may be idiosyncratic but nevertheless recognizable in certain situations. The term *gesture* broadly refers to unaided, nonlinguistic communication including generalized body movement; facial expression; hand, limb, or eye movement; and pantomime. Other forms of aided and unaided communication that may be employed nonlinguistically by AAC users include microswitch technology, objects or three-dimensional symbols, graphic symbols, and manual signs.

Gestures and Vocalizations

Considerable overlap exists among the early, gestural stages of nonlinguistic communication. Thus, discussion of assessment and intervention in the first three levels listed in Table 18.2 (preintentional reflexive behavior, preintentional anticipatory behavior, and intentional behavior) will be combined. Assessment and intervention techniques emphasize (1) engaging and sustaining interactions; (2) focusing attention on objects, persons, and events; and (3) promoting consistent, readable gestural and vocal communication.

Preintentional Reflexive Behavior.   During typical development, beginning with the birth cry, in-

fants naturally produce preintentional reflexive communicative behaviors to which caregivers contingently respond. These behaviors are initially produced without intent and are reflexive reactions to biological states (e.g., fussing, crying to indicate hunger, discomfort, or pain). When caregivers respond by providing attention and engaging the infant in interaction, an important bond that lays the groundwork for emerging communicative competence is formed.

Preintentional Anticipatory Behavior.   Preintentional anticipatory communicative behaviors emerge as typically developing children begin to recognize, focus attention, and anticipate desired objects, persons, or events. For example, a child may produce arm motions, sucking movements of the mouth, and vocalizations in response to viewing a bottle. Contingent, consistent, predictable responses from the caregiver focus the child's attention and lead toward the development of intentionally communicative, social interactions (Dunst & Lowe, 1986).

Research indicates that infants who produce nonlinguistic behaviors that are more readable are more likely to elicit responses from caregivers than infants who produce nonlinguistic behaviors that are less readable. The more readable behaviors thus lead to more frequent and sustained interactions and further development of communicative competence (Dunst & Lowe, 1986). In children with severe developmental disabilities, these early behaviors may be weak, infrequent, or absent and thus may not elicit contingent, consistent caregiver responses. Thus, an early important link in the chain of events leading to communicative competence is missing, as caregivers' attention to and interactions with the infant are reduced. Dunst and Lowe (1986) described the effect of infants' responsiveness on interactions with caregivers.

> [I]n instances where the infant responds to adult interventions in an expected manner, the caregiver's sense of efficacy is enhanced and (s)he is more likely to sustain ongoing interactions and initiate other interactions. This in turn is likely to increase the probability of the infant's acquisition of communicative competencies. Conversely, where the infant is unresponsive, the caregiver's feelings of

efficacy are diminished; (s)he is less likely to initiate and/or respond to communicative bids by the infant; and there is a decrease in the probability of the infant acquiring communicative competencies. (p. 12)

Intentional Behavior. Intentional communicative behaviors develop parallel to physical development when the child acquires the ability to isolate limb movements and vocalizations from whole body movement. With the emergence of communicative intent, a child's early preintentional communication (e.g., cries, gestures, vocalizations) gradually becomes overlaid with more conventional behaviors. Identifiable gestures, often produced with the hands and arms, emerge. For example, many young children whine and extend their arms upward to indicate that they would like to be picked up. Here, the extension of the arms is one element in the chain of actions involved in communicating the desire to be picked up. Subsequently, the child may produce another element of the action chain by screaming and/or pointing downward to indicate the desire to be released. Emerging strategic competence is evident here, as the child may repeat, modify, or increase the intensity of communicative behaviors to affect caregiver behavior. Anyone who has tried to restrain a squirming, screaming toddler can attest to the child's strategic efforts to communicate a desire to be freed.

Assessment. Capitalizing on the natural inclination toward gesture use may be particularly expedient and effective for all AAC users, regardless of impairment type(s) and severity. These unaided, nonlinguistic forms of communication may be used to fulfill a variety of communication functions, including getting and maintaining attention, requesting, indicating physical state (e.g., pain, hunger), or rejecting/protesting. Thus, assessment of communication abilities should always involve careful recording and documentation of nonlinguistic communicative behaviors that an individual is using effectively. For some individuals, nonlinguistic forms of communication build a foundation for eventual use of linguistic AAC and should not necessarily be eliminated from an individual's communication repertoire. In some cases, an individual should work toward more consistent production of and responses to existing behaviors (Baumgart, Johnson, & Helmstetter, 1990; Lloyd & Kangas, 1988).

Gestures involve consistent, recognizable body movements. As described previously, some children produce gestures that elicit contingent responses from caregivers. Other children, particularly those with cognitive, physical, and/or sensory impairments, produce gestures that go unrecognized and elicit no responses. Gestures produced with interfering behaviors such as extraneous or reflexive body movement can be difficult to interpret. Poor motor coordination may make it difficult for children to produce movements consistently. Thus, one of the first tasks of an AAC assessment team is to determine behaviors that are recognized and potentially communicative that could be shaped to become communicative and functional for the child. Communication partners must also learn to recognize and respond to these behaviors.

Caregivers should be interviewed to determine the child's current level of gesture use. Chapter 11 discusses observations and the use of interview forms for documenting and describing communicative behaviors. This information can be used as the basis for subsequent observation and elicitation of gestural communication. Evaluators should assess the child's physical abilities and note movements or actions that tend to occur consistently during daily routines, such as eating, bathing, and play. This is best done in conjunction with a specialist in motor development such as an adapted physical education specialist or occupational or physical therapist who can provide assistance in seating, positioning, and observing subtle motor behaviors (see Chapter 17). Further assessment should be conducted by engaging the child in an activity that is known to be pleasurable, according to the following general sequence.

1. Before beginning the activity, pause to allow the child time to anticipate and produce a movement that may be interpreted as anticipatory.
2. Begin the activity and pause periodically to observe any changes in muscle tone, movement,

touch, vocalization, and/or eye contact that may be interpreted as indicating a desire to continue.

3. Acknowledge the child's responses by providing spoken feedback and eye contact, along with the natural consequence inherent in the activity. The evaluator may also model or gently physically prompt a gesture if none is noted, but again, should guard against attempting to replace a child's natural movements in the initial stages of assessment and intervention.

The activity should be continued for a given length of time, with periodic pauses and responses to the child's gestures. Further assessment should be conducted across multiple sessions, with a variety of communication partners, such as caregivers, family members, friends, teachers, and therapists.

Evaluators should also note the child's desire to discontinue an activity. Children may indicate rejecting/protesting in a variety of ways, from increased vocalization, tension, and activity to sudden withdrawal or passivity. Any of these behaviors may be a "stop" signal to indicate desire to discontinue. If ignored, children may resort to more oppositional, problem behaviors (e.g., hitting, crying). See Chapter 24 for additional information regarding communication-based approaches to problem behavior.

Intervention. Intervention at these early levels of communication development emphasizes what communication partners can do within the context of predictable functional routines with the general goals of (1) increasing their own and others' responses to the child's communicative attempts, (2) encouraging the child's use of gestures/vocalizations, (3) arranging the environment to increase the number of situations in which gestures can be used, (4) providing opportunities for interaction with more communication partners, and (5) expanding the child's repertoire of communicative behaviors. Specific communication functions such as greeting, requesting (e.g., indicating desire for recurrence, making a choice, seeking assistance), rejecting, and closing may be targeted within such predictable routines.

Siegel-Causey and Guess (1989) described five general areas for beginning intervention, which are summarized below. These areas are not intended to be addressed sequentially, but rather concurrently within functional tasks.

1. *Developing nurturance* refers to providing a supportive, caring atmosphere and includes such techniques as giving support, comfort, and affection; creating a positive setting for interaction; expanding on individual-initiated behavior; and focusing on the individual's interest.

2. *Enhancing sensitivity* refers to being aware of and receptive to the subtle cues of others and includes such techniques as recognizing nonsymbolic behaviors, responding contingently, recognizing an individual's readiness for interaction, and responding to an individual's level of communication.

3. *Sequencing experiences* refers to organizing a related series of activities into a sequential, predictable format and includes such techniques as establishing routines, using patterns in games, providing turn-taking opportunities, and encouraging participation.

4. *Utilizing movement* refers to engaging in reciprocal dialogues with social partners and includes such techniques as using movements matched to the level of the learner's actions, selecting movements that accommodate the learner's immediate ability to respond or interact within particular contexts/moments, and using movements as communicative behaviors.

5. *Increasing opportunities* refers to providing a favorable situation for communicative participation and includes such techniques as using time delay, providing choices, creating need for requests, and providing opportunities to interact.

For further information regarding methods for developing nurturance, enhancing sensitivity, sequencing experiences, utilizing movement, and increasing opportunities, see Siegel-Causey and Guess (1989) and Baumgart et al. (1990). Various techniques for implementing movement-based approaches to communication, as adapted from the original work of Van Dijk (1966), have also been described (e.g., Beukelman & Mirenda, 1992; Romski & Sevcik, 1988a) and are summarized below.

1. **Resonance.** The learner and the caregiver engage in rhythmic movement while in direct physical contact to focus the learner's attention externally on people and objects. The caregiver responds to sub-

tle signals (as if they were communicative) for the individual to learn that movement can affect another's behavior (e.g., providing hand-over-hand assistance in wiping a tabletop with periodic pausing by the caregiver to wait for the learner to signal desire to resume/discontinue the activity).

2. **Coactive movement.** The learner and the caregiver engage in activities to promote anticipatory behavior within predictable sequences, with increasing physical distance (e.g., side by side). Models are produced concurrently with behaviors and are thus separated by space, but not time (e.g., blowing soap bubbles with periodic pausing by the caregiver to wait for the learner to signal desire to resume/discontinue the activity).

3. **Nonrepresentational reference.** The learner is encouraged to identify three- and eventually two-dimensional representations of body parts to develop body image, pointing skills, and independence (e.g., touching each foot and its representation before putting on each sock and shoe).

4. **Deferred imitation.** The caregiver gradually fades physically prompting the learner to produce the target movement, so that the learner imitates the movement in response to a model that is separated by space and time (e.g., rolling a ball back to the caregiver).

5. **Natural gestures.** The caregiver responds to and encourages the learner's natural gestures, without imposing more conventional gestures in the early stages of intervention (e.g., interpreting and commenting when the child is reaching for or pointing to a toy).

A case example of an instructional sequence using a movement-based approach for 3-year-old Sue is provided in Table 18.3. The long-term goals for Sue include using intentional gestural communication to build on anticipatory behaviors of leaning and reaching toward desired objects.

Prompting. A common issue in AAC intervention is the AAC user's difficulty initiating communication spontaneously, where *spontaneously* refers to "the ability of the learner to identify the need for, locate, and indicate or produce the correct communication symbol in response to naturally occurring cues *only*" (Mirenda & Santogrossi, 1985, p. 143). AAC users often depend upon **prompts** to communicate. An intervention program that uses prompts must include a systematic plan for reducing them in an effort to encourage spontaneous initiation and generalization of communication across situations. Reducing prompt dependency has been the subject of research studies involving a prompt-free strategy (Mirenda & Santogrossi, 1985), a verbal prompt-free strategy (Mirenda & Datillo, 1987), and varying time-delay strategies (Glennen & Calculator, 1985; Kozleski, 1991). Across these studies, increases were noted in subjects' requesting behaviors, in most cases, using aided communication (i.e., pictorial communication displays). However, as pointed out by Glennen and Calculator (1985), "An ideal communication program for the severely handicapped [sic] nonspeaking child would begin at an early age by training the initiation of nonlinguistic communicative skills" (p. 140).

Several techniques for reducing prompt dependency are illustrated in Amy's case example (see Table 18.3) that are appropriate at all levels of AAC intervention. The expectant **time delay** procedure, as described by Kozleski (1991) and illustrated under Procedures, step 1 (see Table 18.3), eliminates any spoken or physical prompts at the outset of an activity. Instead, a long expectant time delay, sometimes referred to as **pause time**, is provided during which the AAC user is given the opportunity to experience and respond to natural cues (e.g., sight, smell, and sounds of food), while the caregiver observes communicative behaviors. In Kozleski's (1991) study, high-interest items (e.g., a miniature car race track or a doll) were presented to two learners with severe cognitive and physical impairments, followed by a 45-second pause during which the caregiver established eye contact using an expectant facial expression (i.e., raised eyebrows). A more complete description of Kozleski's procedures is provided in the section below on graphic symbol communication.

Fading. Another important intervention technique illustrated in Table 18.3 is **fading**, in which physical and spoken prompts are initially provided and gradually reduced in strength, frequency, and/or duration. The reverse of fading is the use of a least-to-most prompting system, where initially no prompt is given and increasingly more intrusive prompts are provided if the learner fails to respond appropriately.

TABLE 18.3 Case Example—Movement-Based Approach

BACKGROUND

Sue, age 3, physical and developmental disabilities; mild hearing impairment; responds to environmental cues in context (e.g., sight of lunch area and items); limited gestural communication (i.e., guides another's hand to request object or action).

PLAN	GOALS
1. Recognize nonsymbolic behaviors.	1. Amy will produce a gesture to indicate desire for a bite of food and a drink of milk.
2. Create need for requests.	
3. Use expectant time delay.	2. Amy will produce the manual sign FINISHED.
4. Respond contingently.	3. Amy will wipe her face independently.
5. Provide opportunities to interact.	4. Amy will respond to simple gestural/spoken commands.

PROCEDURES

1. Following presentation of food, pause and wait for Amy to anticipate.	5. Periodically say "Look, Amy" and point to spoon/food in bowl.
2. Following Amy's reaction (e.g., leaning and reaching toward bowl), say "Amy wants to eat," then fill the spoon and hold it out. Pause.	6. Repeat sequence with drink until Amy refuses more food and drink.
	7. Take food away, say "Finished" and physically prompt Amy to produce the manual sign FINISHED.
3. Respond to Amy's movement (e.g., reaching for spoon) by saying "Take a bite" and assisting her in placing the spoon in her mouth.	8. Provide washing materials, say "Wash up" and model face washing. Physically assist Amy to wash her face.
4. Repeat steps 1 through 3, fading physical assistance for feeding.	9. Repeat sequence with face drying.
	10. Fade physical assistance for steps 8 and 9.

Adapted from Siegel-Causey & Guess (1989).

Shaping. The technique in which the learner's successive approximations of the targeted responses are reinforced is referred to as **shaping**. These approximations are learner initiated, and, in the beginning, they may only remotely resemble the targeted response. As intervention continues, however, the responses must begin to more closely resemble the targeted response for them to be reinforced. Mirenda and Santogrossi (1985) described shaping as a prompt-free strategy. They investigated its effectiveness in reducing prompt dependency in 8-year-old Amy, a student who appeared to have a severe cognitive impairment. Amy was taught to point to line drawings to request drinks, foods, and other items. Initially, a can of Amy's favorite soft drink, a cup, and a colored picture of the cola beverage were placed on the table in front of Amy. When Amy touched the can itself, she was told that she could not have a drink at that time; when she touched the picture representing the soft drink, she was told, "Yes, Amy, when you touch the picture you get some cola" (p. 145). The interventionists incorporated fading into this prompt-free strategy by gradually removing the can and cup from Amy's view, while the picture remained on the table. Subsequently, the picture was covered so that Amy needed to deliberately seek it out, and then the colored picture was replaced with a $2 \times 2''$ black-and-white Picture Communication Symbol (PCS). Amy reportedly continued to make progress in using graphic symbols for communication and eventually she began to use a 120-item picture communication book. Anecdotal reports by Amy's family members and school staff members suggested that Amy spontaneously and appropriately used her communication book to make requests both at home and at school.

Mand-Model Procedure.   The **mand-model procedure** has also been used successfully with learners with disabilities. In this procedure, clinicians/educators gain the learner's attention, produce a mand (a request or command that does not require a yes/no response, such as "What do you want?" or "Show me what you want"), pause, and, if the learner does not respond as desired, provide a model of the response. Venn et al. (1993) instructed three typically developing preschoolers to use the mand-model procedure during snack time with three preschoolers with disabilities. The six preschoolers were paired in three dyads, each with a typically developing preschooler and a preschooler with disabilities. One of the preschoolers with disabilities was diagnosed as having autism, pervasive developmental disorder, and no functional speech. His communication was described as consisting of vocalizations, pointing to objects to make choices, challenging behaviors, and manual signs. Manual signs were used in the mand-model procedure with this student.

The typically developing peers were taught individually how to implement the mand-model procedure. They were trained to use five scripts, each of which consisted of the following steps:

1. Providing the mand, "(Child's name), which one?"
2. Waiting 3 to 5 seconds
3. Providing access and praise if the child with disabilities responded correctly to the mand
4. Modeling the appropriate language response if the child with disabilities did not respond
5. Waiting 3 to 5 seconds for a response
6. Providing access and praise if the model was imitated correctly
7. Withholding access to the snack if there was an error or if no response was forthcoming (pp. 41–42)

The typically developing peers then implemented the procedure with the preschoolers with disabilities during snacktime. When the mand-model procedure was first introduced, all three preschoolers with disabilities began to engage in inappropriate behaviors (e.g., withdrawal, non-compliance). These inappropriate behaviors subsequently decreased after implementation of the procedure. Two of the three children with disabilities, including the preschooler with little functional speech, ultimately demonstrated an increased number of unprompted requests. See Beukelman and Mirenda (1992); Romski and Sevcik (1988a); Sigafoos, Mustonen, DePaepe, Reichle, and York (1991); and Chapter 15 for further description of various intervention techniques for reducing prompt dependency.

Intervention and assessment overlap, with ongoing assessment conducted as new communication responses, partners, and situations are added. Throughout intervention, AAC service providers must note where communication breakdowns occur so that appropriate plans can be implemented. Some children, particularly those with severe cognitive and/or sensory impairments, may not interpret environmental cues sufficiently to anticipate the initiation or termination of an activity. In this case, existing environmental cues (e.g., the sights, sounds, and smells of meal preparation and clean-up) could be exaggerated and used with "touch cues" that provide additional **tactile** information specific to a particular activity, such as placing a cup in child's hand (Beukelman & Mirenda, 1992; Siegel-Causey & Guess, 1989).

In other cases, a child may not be producing a gesture consistently due to differences in physical positioning across situations resulting in communication breakdown. Here, a two-pronged approach may be employed to intervention in which (1) intervention initially occurs in situations with optimal seating and positioning, and (2) caregivers are instructed to respond to minor variations in gesture production across situations. Communication breakdown may also occur when caregivers inconsistently respond to signals, fail to allow adequate pause time, or attempt to prematurely impose a different gesture on a child's existing gesture. All of these latter points can be addressed in a carefully designed intervention plan that takes into account communication breakdown points across communication situations and partners.

Gesture Dictionary.   Those implementing the intervention should construct a gesture dictionary (Table 18.4) for record keeping and to ensure consistency across communication situations and partners. This dictionary is especially important for children who are in the initial stages of gesture development or whose gestures are highly idiosyncratic. A personalized dictionary should note all the elements in a person's behavior that are part of the gesture, including facial expression, eye gaze, and vocalizations. The gesture dictionary should be kept with the AAC user at all times and updated as needed.

Microswitch Technology.   Activating microswitches to produce meaningful consequences can provide a means of acting on the physical and

social environment by individuals with severe multiple impairments to develop contingency awareness—"the realization of the association between behavior and environmental outcomes" (Schweigert, 1989, p. 192). For individuals, who may otherwise remain rather passive and noninteractive, switches may be used to shape more conventional, consistent intentional behavior in order to develop initiating skills or to replace idiosyncratic gestural signals. In focusing the learners' attention on consequences that they themselves control, groundwork is laid for sustaining social interaction and, in some cases, further development of communication involving transparent symbols.

Much of the early work involving the introduction of microswitches focused on access and activation of physical items such as mechanical toys, lights, music, and vibrating objects. Although this application was considered to be important in providing AAC users with a means of control over the physical (nonsocial) environment

TABLE 18.4   Sample Gesture Dictionary

BEHAVIOR	FUNCTION	RESPONSE
Moves head forward and blinks	Greeting	Wave and say "Hello."
Leans forward	Wants more	Model the manual sign. Say "More" and continue activity.
Arches back and vocalizes	Wants to stop	Model and physically prompt the manual sign. Say "Stop" and discontinue activity.
Extends right arm	Chooses object	Say "You want the _____" and give object.
Taps ear and continuously vocalizes	Wants to listen to music	Say "Music," provide choice of cassettes, and apply headphones.
Makes continuous, melodic vocalizations while listening to headphones	Singing	Continue music.
Activates buzzer	Needs assistance	Approach, say "Do you need help?" and offer assistance.
Shakes fist (manual sign approximation for TOILET)	Needs to use the restroom	Say "We'll go to the restroom" and proceed.

Based on Beukelman & Mirenda (1992), p. 189.

and opportunities for independent play, awareness of the link between nonsocial and social contingency was often not realized. Thus, this type of switch use did not always result in increased intentional communication and social contingency—"the knowledge that one's own behavior can reliably affect the behavior of another person" (Schweigert & Rowland, 1992, p. 274). The efficacy of using microswitches for development of social contingency awareness was illustrated in a single-subject study described by Mathy-Laikko et al. (1989). Here, an 8-year-old girl with severe motor, visual, cognitive, and hearing impairments learned to use a switch to request social interaction with caregivers via activation of an auditory message "J, please come and play with me" (p. 251). Schweigert (1989) also reported a case of a child who learned to activate a switch to request caregiver attention, yet did not activate a switch consistently to receive nonsocial consequences.

Expansion of switch use into an instructional sequence emphasizing development of a variety of communication functions was investigated by Schweigert and Rowland (1992) who described results of a 3-year study involving children with dual sensory and physical impairments. Their instructional sequence, termed the Early Communication Process (ECP), involves four levels of communication:

> Level I: Gaining attention
> Level II: Making requests or expressing interests
> Level III: Making choices or expressing preferences
> Level IV: Using symbols to make choices and express preferences (p. 276)

This program includes, as its final step, the introduction of communication via transparent (e.g., objects) and/or arbitrary (e.g., textured) symbols, an important transition in further development of communicative competence (described in more detail in subsequent sections). A case example, 5-year-old Jordan, is provided in Table 18.5.

Note the use of fading in level I of this instructional sequence, where the presentation of music as a consequence is paired with, faded, and gradually replaced by a tape-recorded voice requesting attention. Fading is also used at Level IV by gradually replacing one *stimulus* (i.e., real objects) with a new stimulus (i.e., tactile symbols representing those objects).

Prior to and throughout this instructional sequence, assessment must be conducted to determine appropriate switch type, placement, and activation method. This process may be quite time consuming, because it may be difficult to determine a consistent, voluntary movement for switch activation in the absence of a reinforcing consequence. This can be particularly problematic when low levels of switch activation occur as a result of unintentional, inconsistent motor movements. The services of a motor specialist such as an occupational or physical therapist are recommended to determine switch features that are most likely to be successful and to evaluate actual switch use. Other team members may provide additional help in observing subtle responses to social and nonsocial consequences of switch activation.

In addition to the obvious operational competence that may develop out of effective switch use, the AAC user also develops beginning linguistic, social, and strategic competence as switches are used to activate other aided communication displays, including symbol arrays and electronic assistive communication devices. Additional information regarding switches is provided in Chapter 9.

Nonlinguistic to Linguistic Transition Symbols

Transparent and arbitrary symbols may be used in both nonlinguistic and linguistic communication to serve as transition or bridging symbols. In typical development, linguistic communication appears after a child has used symbols in nonlinguistic ways. For example, single spoken words and manual signs are part of a linguistic system or language. However, this does not mean that they are being perceived and processed in a linguistic way (i.e., being combined according to syntactic rules). In these early stages, the child may process these symbols in routine activities, where one symbol refers to the next event. The transition from nonlinguistic to linguistic communication is apparent when a child begins to combine symbols. It may

TABLE 18.5   Case Example—Early Communication Process with Microswitch Technology

BACKGROUND

Jordan, age 5, profound physical and developmental disabilities; possible hearing impairment; severe visual impairment; occasional vocalizations, crying; no consistent anticipatory or intentional communication during daily routines.

PLAN	GOALS
1. Introduce contingent nonsocial and social consequences (communication partner attention) to microswitch activation.	1. Jordan will use a switch to activate a voice output communication aid (VOCA) to gain his communication partner's attention.
2. Determine preferred objects and provide opportunities to request.	2. Jordan will touch a tactile symbol to request a preferred object at school and at home.
3. Provide opportunities to make choices among preferred objects.	
4. Pair tactile symbols with objects for requesting.	

PROCEDURES

Level I: Gaining Attention

Determine preferences and appropriate motor behavior for switch activation.

Provide nonsocial consequence (music) to switch activation.

Pair social attention with music.

Gradually fade music as a consequence of switch activation, replacing it with tape loop recording for requesting attention.

Level II: Making Requests

After Jordan gains communication partner's attention, present a radio.

Assist Jordan in tactually scanning the radio, then remove his hand and wait for him to request the radio by touching it.

Level III: Making Choices

Identify additional preferred objects.

Present two preferred objects, assist Jordan in tactually scanning them, then remove his hand and wait for him to request an object by touching it.

Introduce across a variety of contexts and additional objects.

Level IV: Using Symbols

Attach tactile symbols to each object and assist Jordan in tactually scanning each as he scans the object, gradually fading presentation of objects with symbols.

Adapted from Schweigert & Rowland (1992).

even be this drive to combine that launches linguistic processing in the child.

Interestingly enough, single words and signs seem to have the potential of reinforcing this transition. Children have been observed to use the combination of a gesture and a spoken word prior to producing two-word utterances (e.g., pointing to a cookie and saying "More") (Acredolo & Goodwyn, 1990; Caprici, Iverson, Pizzuto, & Volterra, 1996). This is interpreted as an intermediate stage between using nonlinguistic and linguistic communication. Speaking the two-word utterance may still be too complex, so the child instead fills the empty slot of one of the words with a gesture. Linguistic communication, however, is not only a matter of using symbols that belong to linguistic systems (e.g., words in a spoken language or signs in a sign language). Linguistic communication involves perceiving and processing symbols as phonologic and syntactic combinations. Symbols that do not originate from a natural linguistic system, however, can also be processed in a linguistic way. That could be the case for graphic symbols such as Blissymbols. If users process these symbols as configurations of sublexical elements (the parts of the symbol) and as parts of a syntactic system, then they are communicating at a linguistic level. Sometimes when an individual uses one-symbol elements (e.g., one word, one manual sign, one graphic symbol), it is difficult to determine if the person is perceiving and producing the element as part of a linguistic system or just as a single signal.

It is important to bear in mind that individuals who have reached the linguistic level of communication continue to use symbols in a nonlinguistic way. Linguistic communication does not replace nonlinguistic communication, but rather adds a powerful way of organizing symbols. For most individuals, communication will always be a combination of nonlinguistic and linguistic means.

In the following sections, transparent and arbitrary symbols are discussed primarily as they are used in nonlinguistic communication. Later, some of the same symbols (e.g., Blissymbols and manual signs) will be discussed as they are used linguistically.

Transparent Symbols

The use of transparent symbols represents that stage at which AAC intervention first begins to depart, at least according to some features, from typical communication development. Here, a variety of symbols that bear perceptual resemblance to the referent may be used to encourage, supplement, or replace the use of gestures and vocalizations. Unlike these "natural" communication modes, AAC modes such as manual signs and object or pictographic communication displays must be devised

and introduced by intervention team members. With the introduction of these AAC modes comes the need to further develop operational competence; that is, the motor and sensory/perceptual skills necessary to form a manual sign or indicate a selection on a communication display (Light, 1989).

A major leap in communicative power may be realized with the introduction of transparent symbols. Previously described gestural communication methods, for the most part, are relegated to communicating in the here and now with familiar communication partners. With the introduction of more conventionalized transparent symbols such as manual signs and/or object or pictographic communication displays, AAC users can expand their number of communication partners and situations and begin to take an even more active role in the communication dyad. The AAC user is no longer as dependent on another person to set up opportunities to communicate and has much more potential to initiate the communication and expand the content of the message beyond items or referents that are immediately present.

Another important feature of transparent symbols is their potential for transitioning an AAC user into linguistic communication. As described below, manual signs, which are used linguistically by members of a Deaf community, may assist an AAC user in developing multiword utterances. Object and pictographic communication displays, like written language, are arranged in a visual-spatial format, which again share principles of ordering information. For example, in most forms of communication where symbols are sequentially combined, the same basic structures can be found, such as agent-action, or topic-comment.

In addition to expanding the expressive communication abilities of AAC users, receptive language development must also be considered. As Romski and Sevcik (1988a) pointed out, the development of receptive language and communication skills is frequently neglected. They suggested use of **augmented input**, in which the AAC user's communication partners provide communication models with the AAC user's system in addition to speech. This technique has also been referred to as **aided language stimulation** (Goossens' & Crain,

1986). Although research is needed to examine the effects of augmented input, Romski and Sevcik (1993a) suggested that the use of this technique may serve at least three purposes: (1) it provides the AAC user with a model of the AAC system in use, (2) it allows the AAC user to see the AAC symbols in use in everyday situations, and (3) it suggests to the AAC user that the AAC system is an acceptable means of communication. Romski and Sevcik (1993a) pointed out that digitized and synthesized voice output may play a special role in the development of receptive and expressive spoken language. In particular, they speculated that the consistency of a synthetic speech message may make it easier for some to process than natural speech. Again, however, further research is needed in this area to determine the effect of voice output in the language development of AAC users. Goossens', Crain, and Elder (1992) provided detailed instructions for implementing this technique.

Manual Signs.   As noted in Chapters 5 and 7, the term *manual signs* may be used to describe the use of natural sign language, such as American Sign Language (ASL) by members of a Deaf community, or the borrowing of these signs by AAC users for use as a code for spoken language. In

this chapter, discussion is primarily limited to use of manual signs as a mode of communication by individuals who are not deaf, although some may have impaired hearing. Further discussion of sensory impairments can be found in Chapter 16.

AAC users most often use manual signs in conjunction with spoken language and/or graphic symbols (Cregan, 1982; Cregan & Lloyd, 1984, 1990; Grove & Walker, 1990; Hooper, Connell, & Flett, 1987; Kopchik & Lloyd, 1976). Both input (communication directed to the AAC user) and output (communication produced by the AAC user) are therefore described as multimodal. Manual signs are used for some of the same reasons as other modes of AAC: to develop an organized, consistent mode of communication and/or to facilitate, supplement, or replace natural speech. Advantages and disadvantages of using manual signs are described in Table 18.6.

Manual signs may fill a variety of communication purposes. Some AAC users use a small number of single signs in limited situations, in much the same way as gestures. In fact, due to perceptual and/or motor difficulties, manual signs are sometimes interpreted as idiosyncratic gestures by unfamiliar communication partners. The manner in which signs and gestures are learned by the AAC user, however, can be used to distinguish the two.

TABLE 18.6   Advantages and Disadvantages of Using Manual Signs

ADVANTAGES	DISADVANTAGES
Quick, portable, accessible, flexible, inexpensive	Communication partners must learn sign
Motorically easier to produce than speech	Requires a fair degree of hand, finger control
May be multimodal, combining both visual and auditory input	Not always acceptable to parents and community
Transparency/translucency of many signs	May not be well suited for constructing multiword utterances
May be physically prompted	Does not allow for delayed message reception
Encourages face-to-face contact	Does not provide a permanent record
May be built on current natural gestures	
Longer duration than speech	
Allows for communication at a distance and in noise	

Compiled from Bryen & Joyce (1986); Fristoe & Lloyd (1977a, b); Musselwhite & St. Louis (1988).

Gestures generally develop naturally; manual signs are most often modeled or directly taught to provide consistency across communication partners and environments.

Because manual signs are conventionalized, they are recognized by individuals who know manual signs more readily than gestures. However, replacing natural gestures with manual signs is not always advisable if gestures are functional. This may be the case when an individual's capacity for lexical expansion is restricted. For instance, if an AAC user's total number of learnable manual symbols is limited, then switching to a sign vocabulary may add little communicative power. A second factor to take into consideration is the number of people with whom the AAC user interacts. If the number of communication partners is expected to remain limited, then little is to be gained by introducing manual signs, unless most communication partners know manual signs.

Some AAC users use manual signs to transition from nonlinguistic to linguistic communication (Blischak & Lloyd, 1996). Cathy, a young woman with severe physical and hearing impairments, was introduced to manual signs to expand her existing gestural communication. Over time, graphic symbols and TO were introduced, and eventually Cathy acquired a voice output communication aid (VOCA). Cathy became a competent multimodal communicator, appropriately switching communication modes to meet the needs of the communication situations and partners. For example, Cathy continued to use signs for face-to-face or urgent communication with familiar partners, but switched to graphic symbols and/or her VOCA in the community. Signing was functional for Cathy in limited situations, despite the limitations on arm, hand, and finger coordination imposed by athetoid cerebral palsy, but the other modes were more effective in less familiar situations. Cathy demonstrated strategic competence by her ability to switch among communication modes to avoid communication breakdowns.

Contrary to prior assumptions, use of manual signs has not been found to have a negative impact on the development of speech. Speech has often been observed to develop after a period of manual sign use (see Beukelman & Mirenda, 1992, p. 143;

Kopchik & Lloyd, 1976; and Silverman, 1995, Table 2.2, pp. 35–36 for overviews). The specific relationship between sign reception and production and speech reception and production is still unclear. However, there are several indications that signing and speech have common underlying cognitive and linguistic bases (Kimura, 1990; McNeill, 1985, 1993; Poizner, Klima, & Bellugi, 1990).

Motoric Aspects of Manual Signs.   Several authors (Dennis, Reichle, Williams, & Vogelsberg, 1982; Doherty, 1985; Fristoe & Lloyd, 1979b; Kohl, 1981) stressed that manual sign instruction should take into account the motoric complexity of signs, especially when an initial sign vocabulary is to be developed. Attempts to measure the motoric difficulty of signs have been based partly on distinguishing and determining the difficulties of the parameters of sign: location, movement, and handshape (Chapter 7; Doherty, 1985; Stokoe, 1960). In general, location is the easiest and typically first mastered parameter, followed by movement. Lloyd and Doherty (1983) also found that touch signs (signs that have physical contact with the signer's body) are easier to learn than nontouch signs, because touch signs provide a higher level of tactile feedback during performance. Handshape has generally proven to be the most difficult and last to be mastered by signers with and without physical impairments (Kantor, 1980; Wilbur & Jones, 1974). Additional discussion of sign parameters can be found in Chapter 7.

Bonvillian, Orlansky, Novack, Folven, and Holley-Wilcox (1985) and Folven and Bonvillian (1991) reported that early exposure to sign language can foster appearance of the "first sign" at a mean age of 8 months, 2 weeks, which is significantly earlier than the first word in typical spoken language acquisition (approximately 11 months). The authors attributed this phenomenon to the higher motor accessibility of signs compared to the relatively more difficult articulation processes required of speech production. However, this claim has been challenged and denied based on an overinterpretation of what is probably a form of manual babbling (Petitto, 1994; Petitto & Marentette, 1991). Typically developing children between the ages of 6 and 12 months generally have a much better command of the underlying receptive and motor skills for using manual signs than spoken words. Yet Petitto and colleagues (1983, 1991) purported that linguistic use of manual signs cannot be expected until a child has reached the developmental level of handling conventional and arbitrary linguistic forms. Nevertheless, it is these very characteristics of signs—greater receptive and motor accessibility, along with fewer linguistic constraints—that invite consideration of manual sign use by individuals with lower developmental levels. Signing makes use of the naturally developing visual-gestural modality, which forms the basis for early communication during this prelinguistic sensorimotor period.

Dunn (1982) developed a program for instruction in presigning motor skills, which attempts to follow general maturational lines in developing the motor skills important in sign production. This approach has three general principles, which are based on the underlying assumption that the motoric production of signs is directly and primarily related to the motor prerequisites of the three major sign parameters (location, movement, handshape).

1. Gross motor skills develop before finer skills
2. Maturation develops head-to-tail
3. First movements of the arms are toward the body (see also Grove, 1990)

Techniques for assessing movement, hand usage, and handshape are provided. If the individual demonstrates spontaneous use of critical motor patterns, assessment then focuses on elicitation and development of these skills. Intervention can then focus on the typical expected order, beginning with acquisition of hand and arm movements and progressing from unilateral to bilateral signs. In the final stage, signers learn to make the more complex asymmetrical signs with one dominant active hand performing the action while the other hand is passive.

This approach runs the risk of being overanalytical in the selection of manual signs while overlooking their basic communicative functions. Its implementation can easily lead to a situation in which manual signs are selected because of their supposedly more accessible physical characteristics rather than for their communicative potential. McEwen and Lloyd (1990b) thus challenged this view, stressing that there is little information available regarding the interaction of sign parameters and actual sign use. However, because intelligibility of sign production is related to motor skills, the question arises as to the point at which an individual's motoric difficulties are deemed too severe to consider signing as a viable AAC method. One approach is to analyze exactly which of the three major parameters (location, movement, handshape) may be affected by how accurate the manual sign attempts are. In many situations the motoric limitations do not have a significant effect on sign intelligibility. For example, Bornstein and Jordan (1984) studied the intelligibility of 330 signs most frequently used in sign programs (from Fristoe & Lloyd, 1977a, 1977b, 1979b) and found that accurate production of all three parameters was not generally necessary for comprehension.

Fawcet and Clibbens (1983) also proposed a technique to measure the intelligibility of a sample of an individual's sign lexicon by assessing the accuracy of the sign parameters of location, movement, and handshape. This technique can be used with individuals who have already acquired some functional sign vocabulary as well as with beginners. However, Grove (1990) cautioned AAC team members against focusing too explicitly on motor ability before any functional sign communication has been established. For more detailed discussion of motoric aspects of manual signs, see Chapter 7.

Assessment and Intervention. The decision to introduce manual signs should be based on the understanding that signing rarely suffices as a complete communication system. Learning signs should not be considered an end in and of itself: the goal should be increased communication. Because manual signs are not generally understood in the community at large, and because inclusion and independent communication and participation are considered to be desirable for AAC users, the combined use of signs with speech and aided AAC should be considered. As noted under advantages in Table 18.6, however, manual signs can be a viable early form of AAC. For many AAC users, particularly those with hearing impairments, manual signs may continue to function as part of a multimodal communication system throughout life.

During the assessment process, the AAC team must determine the individual's current modes of communication and the environment(s) in which they are functional. The environment(s) and the communication partners with whom manual signs are expected to be functional and the capacity of the environment(s) to support sign acquisition and use must also be evaluated. Assessment should also focus on the ability of the individual to produce signs bimodally (i.e., spontaneous speech attempts concomitant with sign production) and the ability to produce complex utterances. Although many individuals with severe cognitive impairments produce predominantly single-sign utterances, some produce two or more sign utterances. For example, Grove and Dockrell (1994) found that some individuals with cognitive impairments produced sign utterances resembling those produced by native signers.

The team must also carefully select the referents/messages, the signs that will represent them, and the source(s) from which signs will be selected. Signs, like spoken words, vary across geographic areas and social groups. Many different types of sign books and videos are commercially available. Teams should adopt a developmental approach regarding selection of the referents for which signs should be selected (Fristoe & Lloyd, 1980). Preference should be given to selecting meaningful vocabulary that is functional in daily living (Kopchik & Lloyd, 1976).

In principle, signs can be pulled from several sources. However, signs should be chosen predominantly from one single system for two reasons. If signs are selected from the same system, the user and others in the environment can profit from the internal logic of the system. For example, a particular sign system may have a specific way of combining elements into compound signs. GARAGE may be comprised of a combination of CAR and HOUSE. A similar internal logic may be found in other manual signs within the same system, such as KITCHEN as a compound sign that combines COOK and ROOM. A second reason why selection from one system may be preferable

is linked to the social function of communication itself: the more the lexicon is individualized, the less it will be understood by others.

One solution to the dilemma of sign selection has been developed by the originators of the Makaton approach to manual sign instruction, used predominantly in Great Britain (Grove & Walker, 1990). Manual signs used in the Makaton approach stem primarily from British Sign Language (BSL) and hence have naturally acquired linguistic strength. Makaton vocabulary is a collection of approximately 350 manual signs that have been selected to correspond with core vocabulary that is used by young children to cover a wide range of meanings.

Makaton vocabulary is classified into eight categories, which are presented as stages of approximately 35 items each. The notion of stages suggests that sign acquisition and use can reflect consecutive levels of functioning in daily life. For example, the first stage consists mainly of concepts that refer to physical needs (e.g., food, toileting) and to the immediate environment of a young child. To allow for personal adjustment of this scheme, the developers of Makaton proposed a ninth stage, in which additional concepts are added according to individual needs. Although the Makaton stages are purported to be developmentally sequenced, this aspect of the vocabulary is questionable. For example, MORE does not appear until stage 3 in the Makaton vocabulary. Some consider MORE to be a relatively early lexical item (Fried-Oken & More, 1992; Fristoe & Lloyd, 1980; Marvin, Beukelman, & Bilyeu, 1994). In fact, Fristoe and Lloyd (1980) considered MORE to be a critical word in an initial sign lexicon.

Developmental aspects should be one consideration in planning an initial sign lexicon. Other criteria to consider are iconicity and motor characteristics. Also important is the degree to which a motor approximation of a manual sign is still recognizable by others in the environment (Pennington, Karlan, & Lloyd, 1986). Excellent sources are available to assist AAC team members in introducing manual signs, including Bryen and Joyce (1986); Fristoe and Lloyd (1980); and Reichle, Williams, and Ryan (1981). Key points to consider are provided in Table 18.7.

TABLE 18.7   Considerations for Introducing Manual Signs

INITIAL STEPS	TECHNIQUES
Select objects, events, and communicative functions that are frequently occurring, motivating, meaningful, and age-appropriate.	Introduce signs in natural contexts with natural consequences, taking advantage of both planned and spontaneous opportunities.
Select signs that are relatively easy to produce.	Accompany sign production by speech.
Select signs that differ according to more than one parameter.	Use appropriate facial and vocal expression.
Select some signs that can be combined with others (e.g., MORE).	Accept sign approximations in the early stages.
	Eventually fade physical prompts and models.
Select signs that bear a high degree of visual similarity to the referent.	Combine signs with other bodily movements (e.g., headshake for no).
Do not necessarily select signs to replace natural gestures.	Model sign combinations.
	Gradually increase signing vocabulary and introduce aided AAC methods.

Compiled from Fristoe & Lloyd (1980); Pennington, Karlan, & Lloyd (1986); Reichle, Williams, & Ryan (1981).

After signs have been selected, team members should compile an individualized sign dictionary to promote consistency across communication partners. Signs relating to particular topics may be displayed in strategic areas (e.g., lunchbox, reading areas) to allow communication partners quick access.

Although signs often need to be taught within systematic training sessions using reinforcement techniques (Duker & Remington, 1991), signs should also be introduced and used in natural environments as much as possible to facilitate spontaneous discovery. In the 24-hour total communication or multimodal approach (Kopchik & Lloyd, 1976), the individual is exposed to signing models throughout the day in an effort to foster natural sign acquisition processes (Bryen & Joyce, 1986). One of the critical factors in the success of this approach is the signing proficiency of the communication partners. Sign instruction for parents, staff members, and other critical individuals is therefore recommended if manual signing is to become an effective mode of communication. Several systematic approaches to sign instruction have been developed, including a "working party" approach to public school staff inservice (Loeding, Zangari, & Lloyd, 1990), introducing "signs of the week" to group home staff (Spragale & Micucci,

1990), using videotaped lessons for student and staff instruction (Watkins, Sprafkin, & Krolikowski, 1993), and using any of the training courses offered by the Makaton Vocabulary Development Project (Grove & Walker, 1990).

McNaughton and Light (1989) described the introduction of signing to Linda, a 27-year-old woman with cognitive impairment. They emphasized the role of communication partners (referred to by McNaughton and Light as facilitators) in modeling and eliciting sign production in naturally occurring contexts at Linda's day program and group home. Other key points in this case study included (1) provision of general staff inservice; (2) participation of facilitators in assessment and goal setting; (3) individual sign instruction for two primary facilitators; and (4) follow-up general staff meetings to review communication goals and progress.

Two other important features of this intervention program also deserve special mention. First, facilitators were instructed to provide augmented input (as described by Romski & Sevcik, 1988a) by pairing speech production with facial expression, gestures, and presenting/pointing to objects to support Linda's spoken language comprehension. Second, as noted in Table 18.8, Linda's gestures and vocalizations for requesting objects continued

TABLE 18.8   Case Example—Introducing Manual Signs

BACKGROUND

Linda, age 27, severe cognitive impairment; physical disabilities; mild to moderate unilateral hearing loss; demonstrates functional use of objects and recognition of familiar persons, but does not respond to photographs or line drawings; occasionally aggressive (e.g., hitting, screaming) when required to complete a nonpreferred activity.

PLAN	GOALS
1. Model and prompt gestural and sign communication in these situations: • Selecting condiments at mealtime • Selecting free-time activities • Selecting clothing • Selecting physical activities • Selecting tasks during food preparation	1. Linda will request a preferred object by pointing to it and vocalizing. 2. Linda will produce the manual signs MORE and FINISHED at appropriate times during selected activities.

PROCEDURES

1. At the beginning of an activity, with objects in view, focus attention on Linda; pause.

2. If Linda vocalizes and points, provide the object. Also, provide a spoken and signed model of the object, if appropriate. If Linda does not request, go to step 3.

3. Question: Ask "What do you want?" accompanied by appropriate facial expression. If Linda requests, respond as in step 2. If Linda does not request, go to step 4.

4. Provide choices: Present two objects by pointing at and labeling them; pause. If Linda requests, respond as in step 2. If Linda does not request, provide choices again. If still no response, go to step 5.

5. Physical prompt: Touch Linda's arm; pause. If Linda does not request, model NO (spoken and headshake) and withdraw.

6. At appropriate times during selected activities, model the signs MORE and FINISHED.

Adapted from McNaughton & Light (1989).

to be accepted as communication attempts when signs MORE and FINISHED were introduced. In Table 18.8, a description of specific intervention procedures is provided.

Manual sign use should be oriented toward opening up more modalities, including speech and graphic symbol communication. The bimodal use of speech and manual signs is meant to strengthen the link between internal sign and word representation. This bimodal presentation can be simultaneous communication, where most spoken words of the sentences are represented in manual sign. Speech and sign are mirroring each other as two parallel channels. This technique has been used to teach and represent English (or another spoken language) to hearing-impaired children. Another form of bimodal use of speech and sign is key word-signing, where only the words that contain the highest content value are signed. For a discussion, see Chapter 7.

Another technique that is commonly used is the linking of signs to graphic symbols. This principle is particularly elaborated in the Sigsymbol system, devised in Great Britain by Cregan (1982) and adapted for the United States by Cregan and Lloyd (1990) (see also Chapter 6). Sigsymbols include a set of graphic representations of signs that may aid the user in establishing an internal multimodal (i.e., spoken, manual, graphic) representation. The use of Sigsymbols may also facilitate production of multiword utterances when used in combination with speech and manual signs, as de-

320   PART 5   AAC INTERVENTION

scribed in a case study by Cregan (1993). The basic principle is that throughout intervention the user is challenged to pair different types of symbols with each other to move toward use of more conventional, linguistic forms of communication (Romski & Sevcik, 1988a). Table 18.9 provides two case examples illustrating transition from manual signs to increased spoken and written communication.

Object Communication Displays. Object communication displays contain three-dimensional tangible symbols that bear varying degrees of physical relationship (i.e., iconicity) to the tactile or visual properties of a referent (Rowland & Schweigert, 1989a). At the transparent level are life-sized actual or artificial objects such as a cracker, a cup, or a piece of plastic fruit. Miniature objects such as a toy dish or spoon are also considered to be transparent or highly translucent to some AAC users. Referents may also be represented by attaching related objects to a communication display, such as a shoestring to represent "shoe," a straw to represent "drink," or a key to rep-

resent "car." These objects represent their referent by association.

Some objects may be represented by partial or miniature objects that share only one perceptual feature. For example, a piece of a basketball may represent the ball's texture or a ping-pong ball may represent its shape (Rowland & Stremel-Campbell, 1987). Last, the relationship between a tangible symbol and object or event may be strictly arbitrary, as in three-dimensional abstract shapes or **textured symbols** (see subsequent section on arbitrary symbol communication displays).

Object communication displays can be arranged and used in a variety of ways, depending on the particular abilities and needs of the AAC user. Objects can be placed in recessed wells on a wheelchair lapboard (Carlson, 1982) (Figure 18.1), attached to an apron worn by the communication partner (Goossens' & Crain, 1986) (Figure 18.2), or placed in schedule boxes (Baumgart et al., 1990; Beukelman & Mirenda, 1992).

Object communication displays are frequently used by individuals with visual impairments or dual sensory impairments (DSI), but may

TABLE 18.9 Two Case Examples of Use of Manual Signs

	DOMINIC, AGE 2.0*	CONRAD, AGE 8.0†
Syndrome	Down Syndrome	Fragile X Syndrome
Communication skills	Vocalizations Gestures	Developmental/receptive language disorder; a few one-word utterances
Sign system	Key word signing	Key word signing
Educational environment	Day-care center Home training program	Residential center Weekend parent counseling
Sign vocabulary	60 manual signs within 6 months	250 manual signs within 6 months
Effects on speech	Spontaneous speech production simultaneous with sign from 2 years, 6 months on	No observable effect on speech
Long-term effects	From 3 years on, speech becomes dominant modality; sign use fades	Signing will probably remain primary mode of direct communication; increase in importance of written language

*Based on a case reported by Hilde Lyssens (personal communication, August 1993)
†Based on a case reported by Loncke et al. (1993)

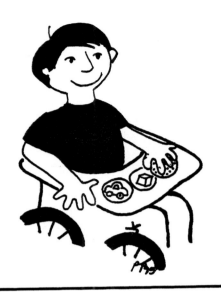

FIGURE 18.1 Wheelchair Tray Adaptation for Object Communication Display
Courtesy of G. S. Pennington.

also be used by individuals with severe cognitive impairments for whom two-dimensional symbols are not yet meaningful. Rowland and Schweigert (1989a) suggested that three major indicators suggest when tangible symbols may be appropriate for an AAC user. The individual must (1) demon-

strate some means of intentional communication, (2) have an intentional motor behavior that enables symbol selection, and (3) not already be using higher level symbols (e.g., manual signs).

Object communication displays are effective for functional routines. For example, a communication partner may present a child with an object communication board containing a cassette tape, a sand toy, and a building block to allow the child to choose a free-time activity. A child may benefit from use of an object display, such as the wheelchair tray adaptation that allows objects to be removed and given to the communication partner. This type of arrangement can be particularly beneficial as a transition communication display for individuals who have not engaged in the early communication behavior of requesting via extending an object (e.g., handing a cup to a communication partner to request more drink, as described by Rowland & Schweigert, 1989a). Another child with a severe physical impairment may use eye gaze during mealtime to indicate a food choice by gazing at a desired miniature food attached to a caregiver's communication vest. Here, use of a communication vest is particularly effective because its pockets or Velcro attachments allow objects to be changed as needed, and the caregiver's hands are free for feeding.

Table 18.10 provides a summary of a case study involving introducing a child to tangible symbols. For additional information regarding instructional strategies for use with tangible symbols, see Rowland and Schweigert (1989b).

One particular use of object communication displays involves providing a calendar or schedule box that can be used to promote both receptive and expressive communication. Here, a compartmented box holds objects representing activities that occur in sequence during the daily routine. As summarized by Beukelman and Mirenda (1992), a schedule box may serve several purposes:

1. Provide an overview of the sequence of activities
2. Provide information about what will happen next
3. Introduce the child to the concept of symbolization, which is the idea that one thing can stand for another
4. Make transitions from one activity to the next easier for the child (p. 194)

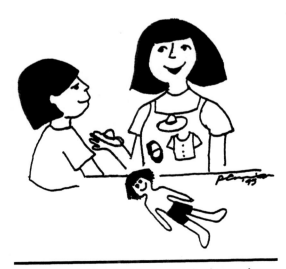

FIGURE 18.2 Small Objects Attached to an Apron
Courtesy of G. S. Pennington.

TABLE 18.10   Case Example—Object Communication Display

BACKGROUND

Sybil, age 6, dual sensory impairment (DSI); developmental disabilities; limited gestural communication (e.g., pushes away to protest; guides another's hand to request objects or action; extends object to request more).

PLAN	GOALS
1. Introduce symbols in school playroom. 2. Analyze Sybil's preference for playroom equipment. 3. Design three-dimensional symbols that are tactually similar to three pieces of equipment.	1. Sybil will touch a symbol to request or label desired objects. 2. Sybil will use existing gestures to maintain and terminate playground activities.

PROCEDURES	NOTE
1. Physically assist Sybil in tactually scanning each of three preferred objects. 2. Following Sybil's rejection (pushing away) of nonpreferred object or selection (physically orienting toward) of preferred object, present symbols, speak and sign WHAT, and physically prompt Sybil to tactually scan symbol array. 3. Remove Sybil's hand from display and wait for her to select the symbol and place it in instructor's hand. 4. When the correct symbol has been selected, provide activity. 5. Intermittently stop the activity and wait for Sybil to gesture her desire to continue or stop the activity.	Initially, only one meaningful symbol was presented along with a symbol for nothing (arbitrary shape). As Sybil reached criterion, the symbol for nothing was replaced by the second, and eventually the third three-dimensional symbol. **RESULTS** Sybil achieved mastery (80% criterion on three consecutive days for all three symbols). New staff and contexts were added to the instructional program. Sybil eventually used 22 symbols across a period of 2 school years.

Adapted from Rowland & Schweigert (1989a).

Rowland and Schweigert (1989a), however, emphasized that use of schedule boxes should extend beyond the typically described noninteractive use in which the child is required to retrieve the appropriate object prior to an activity, as a type of self-cueing procedure. Expressively, the child should be encouraged to retrieve an object in response to the teacher's question "What time is it?" or show the object to initiate a request for a particular activity. In Table 18.11, a least-to-most prompting intervention program for introducing a daily schedule system is provided.

Graphic Symbol Communication Displays. Although communication partners must acknowledge and respond to an AAC user's gestural, signed, and/or object-based communication, AAC users must have the option of accessing more conventional types of communication. Thus, graphic symbols are often introduced at some point during intervention to provide AAC users with another communication option. A wide variety of graphic symbols, as described in Chapter 6, has been employed by AAC users for both receptive and expressive communication. In this section, however,

TABLE 18.11   Case Example—Using a Daily Schedule System

BACKGROUND

Jodi, age 11, cognitive impairment; autism; Rett's syndrome; seizure disorder; inconsistent eye contact with people and objects; responds to simple spoken commands; requests desired items by whole body movement; produces manual signs only with physical prompting.

PLAN	**GOALS**
1. Place real objects to represent school activities in separate cardboard boxes.	1. Prior to each activity, Jodi will independently select the appropriate object from her communication display and proceed to the activity.
2. Use a least-to-most prompting system.	
3. Fade use of real objects and replace with more conventional, portable graphic symbols.	2. At the completion of each activity, Jodi will independently replace the object and select the appropriate object for the next activity.
4. Provide opportunities for Jodi to initiate communication.	
5. Use natural cues and consequences (e.g., retrieving and putting away materials; participating in the activity).	3. Jodi will initiate an activity by independently selecting an object and presenting it to a communication partner.

PROCEDURES

---

1. Prior to the beginning of an activity, provide no prompts. Observe Jodi's responses to natural cues (other students retrieving materials, movement toward an area of the classroom). If Jodi does not proceed to her schedule box, go to step 2.

2. Spoken prompt: Say, "Jodi, time for shopping. Get your purse." If Jodi does not respond appropriately, go to step 3.

3. Gestural prompt: Point to the appropriate object in Jodi's schedule box. If Jodi does not respond appropriately, go to step 4.

4. Physical orientation: Gently orient Jodi's head to the object in the schedule box. If Jodi does not respond appropriately, go to step 5.

5. Complete physical assistance: Place hand over Jodi's and assist her in retrieving the object.

6. Proceed to the activity. At its completion, begin at step 1 by providing no prompting and proceed from least-to-most prompts as described.

7. Continue steps 1 through 6 throughout the school day, documenting the level of assistance needed for each activity.

8. Be alert and respond to any attempt by Jodi to initiate communication using objects in her schedule box.

Adapted from Baumgart, Johnson, & Helmstetter (1990).

---

discussion will be limited to relatively transparent, pictographic symbols. Discussion of arbitrary graphic symbols (e.g., lexigrams) and linguistic graphic symbols (e.g., TO) is provided in subsequent sections.

Like gestures and manual signs, graphic symbols can be portable and relatively easy to access motorically, with the added advantage of being dis-played in a static format (i.e., graphic symbols typically do not depend on movement for their interpretation, as do speech and many manual signs). Additional advantages and disadvantages of using graphic symbols are described in Table 18.12.

Graphic symbol use has been described across a variety of individuals and situations. For example, Doss and Reichle (1991b) described use

TABLE 18.12   Advantages and Disadvantages of Using Graphic Symbols

ADVANTAGES	DISADVANTAGES
Are permanent, static	May not be immediately transparent to user and communication partners
May be accessed by limbs or eyes	
Have flexible display options (size, spacing, color)	Require communication partner to be close and at an appropriate viewing orientation
May be physically prompted	
Have longer duration than speech	May discourage face-to-face communication
May reduce memory demands	Have space and size limitations
Allow for delayed message reception	Can be damaged physically
May provide a permanent record	

Adapted from Lloyd & Kiernan (1984).

of graphic symbols in a similar manner to object-based schedule boxes. Here, graphic symbols are used to promote self-regulation and independence in the performance of daily living activities such as grooming, meal preparation, shopping, and household chores. Figure 18.3 provides an example of the use of graphic symbols to help individuals regulate and plan a weekly schedule.

McGregor, Young, Gerak, Thomas, and Vogelsberg (1992) described how an AAC user's intentional gestural communication was extended to include aided linguistic forms during an instructional program designed to increase functional VOCA use. Here, the communicative intent of the AAC user's gestures were noted and these messages were subsequently programmed into a VOCA. Kozleski's (1991) case studies show how the technique of expectant time delay can be used to teach individuals with severe cognitive and physical impairments to match objects with pictures on a communication board and how this can be a point of departure for initiating requests. One of the cases is summarized in Table 18.13.

Arbitrary Symbols

Most linguistic communication uses arbitrary symbols; however, arbitrary symbols can be used in both nonlinguistic and linguistic communication as discussed above.

Manual Signs.   Many manual signs are transparent symbols (as discussed above) or highly translucent, but the majority are arbitrary (either with low transparency or opaque). The arbitrary manual signs are used in nonlinguistic communication in the same way as transparent manual signs discussed above (e.g., one sign at a time).

Arbitrary Symbol Communication Displays.

Textured Symbols.   Three-dimensional textured symbols differ in one important way from the previously described three-dimensional transparent symbols in that their use involves forming a paired association between the texture and an object or activity. For example, a piece of corrugated cardboard may represent "soft drink," whereas a piece of a kitchen sponge may represent "milk." Such symbols may be perceived tactually (i.e., via passive stimulation of the skin) as opposed to partial or whole objects that require **haptic** perception (i.e., through active exploration). According to Murray-Branch, Udavari-Solner, and Bailey (1991), textured symbols may be easier to perceive and remember by individuals with severe cognitive impairments and/or DSI. Further, they may be perceived without correct spatial orientation, as the texture is uniform across the surface of the symbol.

Locke and Mirenda (1988) provided a case example whereby textured symbols were combined

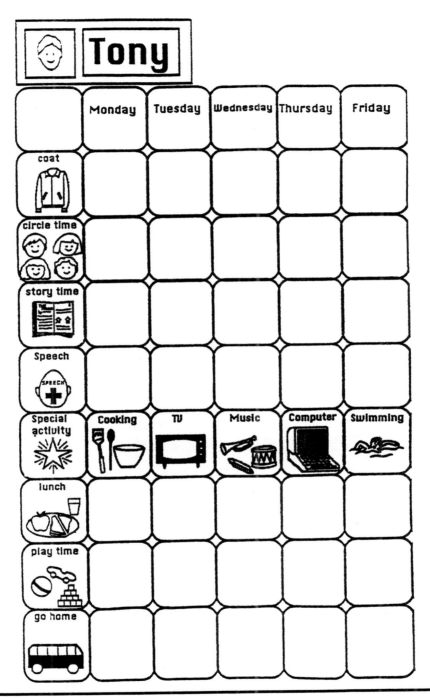

FIGURE 18.3   Chart with Graphic Symbols to Serve as a Weekly Schedule

TABLE 18.13 Case Example—Use of Expectant Time Delay

BACKGROUND

Oscar, age 15, severe athetoid quadriplegia with limited upper extremity range of motion; severe cognitive impairment; normal visual capacities; sensorimotor stage 4, indicating the ability to differentiate means from ends and to imitate movements observed in others; communicates via gestures, vocalizations, and smiles but communication attempts remain difficult to interpret.

PLAN	GOALS
1. Select high-interest objects (a miniature car race track, a battery-powered car).	1. Oscar will initiate requests for high-interest objects by using a communication board.
2. Determine optimal latency time.	2. Oscar will differentiate between three Polaroid pictures of three different high-interest objects.
3. Build a sequence of degrees in difficulty by using successively a board with only one Polaroid picture, then a board with two choices, and finally three.	3. Oscar will select the object of his choice by pushing the picture on the board.

PROCEDURES

1. Use a three-choice communication board with three photographs of high-preference items along with the objects. After he has touched an object, present the communication board to Oscar and wait 45 seconds (expectant time delay).

2. Use a three-choice communication board with only one photograph on a notebook switch. When he touches the switch with the photograph, give Oscar a 1-minute opportunity to interact with the object.

3. Repeat step 2 with two photographs.

4. Repeat step 2 with three photographs.

RESULTS

Oscar reached an 80% criterion level after 10 days in the one-choice training, after 15 days in the two-choice training, and after 15 days in the three-choice training step.

Adapted from Kozleski (1991).

with electronic voice output to increase requesting by an 11-year-old AAC user with cognitive and visual impairments. The addition of synthetic speech was a particularly critical component of this intervention, because it provided auditory feedback to the child in addition to tactile feedback.

Other Arbitrary Symbols. The most commonly used arbitrary symbols are the written orthography of alphabetic languages. TO is one of the most powerful **aided communication** symbol systems. Its use implies a developed level of linguistic skill and some mastery of spelling rules. TO is a form of linguistic communication, although word recognition and use of isolated printed words can be introduced at a developmental level where non-

linguistic symbols are the main carriers of communication. Printed words can also be used along with gestures, vocalizations, and graphic symbols such as Blissymbols and lexigrams.

One of the most well-known systems of graphic communication is Blissymbols. Since the system was introduced for children with physical disabilities in the early 1970s, it has received rapidly growing interest from parents, clinicians/educators, and researchers. Blissymbols are composed of meaning-based units (both pictographic and arbitrary), which differ in complexity according to the number of basic elements or strokes that are combined to form a symbol.

Lexigrams were originally designed to be used in research with nonhuman primates, but their use was extended to individuals with cognitive impairments. Each lexigram is composed of elements from a limited set of nine basic graphic forms. Because the symbols are arbitrary, their use requires an explicit learning process. Nevertheless, they are considered easier to learn than TO because (1) there are only nine different basic forms; (2) the basic forms are highly visually discriminable, even in superimposed positions; and (3) "spelling rules" (which elements can be combined to form symbols) are much less complicated. For more information about Blissymbols and lexigrams, see Chapter 6.

Most graphic symbols are not part of a linguistic communication system because they are not part of the lexicon of a naturally developed language. However, in some cases, graphic symbols may be processed as linguistic symbols. Some individuals may invest their linguistic capacity in these symbols, especially when graphic symbols are paired with spoken or written words. By using the graphic symbols in the word order of the spoken language, they may be processed as if they were actually the words. Individuals with severe expressive communication disabilities could also develop an idiosyncratic syntax that resembles a linguistic system (Goldin-Meadow & Morford, 1985).

LINGUISTIC COMMUNICATION

The development of **linguistic communication** should be an important consideration in AAC intervention for individuals with developmental disabilities. Although an impairment may affect linguistic abilities, the development of linguistic skills should not be abandoned too readily in the intervention plan for two reasons. The first reason is related to the unique characteristics of language that permit rapid processing of lexical items (words, signs) from a limited set of basic elements (sounds, handshapes) that are arranged in structured strings (sentences) (Levelt, 1993). This high degree of conventionalization makes language a superior means of expression in an infinite variety of communicative exchanges.

The second reason concerns the flexibility and apparent robustness of linguistic capacity,

even in individuals with limited access to language. For example, analysis of manual utterances in young deaf children who had almost no access to sign language models showed that they nevertheless had developed an idiosyncratic system that shared the basic characteristics of language. For example, their utterances showed phonological structure (Mylander & Goldin-Meadow, 1991) and consistency in the syntactic ordering of signs (Goldin-Meadow & Morford, 1985). Similar observations have been reported in children with cognitive impairments who were exposed to manual signing (Grove & Dockrell, 1994). For further discussion of the human capacity to develop language, see Pinker (1994) and Bishop and Mogford (1993).

The traditional approach to early language development assumes that the child does indeed have the ability to explore language rules, that is, the ability to freely modify and combine linguistic symbols. As Nelson (1992) pointed out, however, this is often not the case for many AAC users, who may be extremely limited in their ability to use language naturally and productively. Fortunately, the use of AAC methods, which originates from the need to develop overall communicative competence, may actually promote linguistic competence. Thus, the introduction of AAC should not be viewed as abandoning goals for developing speech and language, but rather as bringing a new impetus for their development. An interesting relationship between AAC use and linguistic competence is evident here. Access to and competence in using linguistic AAC (i.e., language and language codes) affords an AAC user unlimited capacity for expression. Moreover, introduction of linguistic AAC may contribute to further linguistic development.

Language

Theoretical Reference Model.   AAC service providers must understand typical language acquisition in order to evaluate an individual's linguistic competence. Although the developmental pattern of young AAC users may appear to be dramatically different from typically developing children, a developmental model of language acquisition can be useful in making decisions about the child's present linguistic competence and viable intervention strategies (Gerber & Kraat, 1992). However, a developmental model should not be considered as a descriptive and normative list of steps that are to be taken in a straightforward order. The model should be used as a guide to understand which language acquisition areas have been affected and to prioritize areas for intervention.

Crucial factors to consider in language development, as discussed by Rice and Schiefelbusch (1989), Snow and Ferguson (1977), and Wanner and Gleitman (1982) include the following:

1. **Language model(s) to which the child is exposed.** This includes the use of baby talk, monolingualism or bilingualism of the models, and consistency of the language.
2. **Accessibility of linguistic symbols.** A child uses symbols to explore the structure and the semantics of language. Hence, the child must be able to hear (spoken words) and/or see (manual signs, graphic symbols).
3. **Internal language capacity.** All humans are assumed to have a strong inclination toward acquiring language, and children play an active role in exploring the lexicon and rules of their language environment. During the first year of life, they develop the maturational (sensory, motor, cognitive, and articulatory) level that sets off an active search for language through interaction with the environment.
4. **Quality of linguistic interactions.** Interactions in which communication partners respond to the language learner by **recasting** (e.g., additions, deletions, expansions, reorderings, [Nelson, 1973]) have a particularly stimulating effect on language exploring behaviors. That is, during interactions involving recastings, the language learner is invited to explore both structural and lexical information as provided by the communication partner.

Language Assessment and Initiation of AAC. Development of linguistic competence is the internal force that drives the young learner to explore the underlying rules of language (Chomsky, 1965). However, assessing linguistic competence is a complicated issue for individuals with developmental disabilities, because performance can only be evaluated via overt behaviors. When dis-

abilities negatively affect speech perception and/or speech production, linguistic performance depends heavily on the introduction of AAC techniques. Hence, assessment of language skills can only be valid if it takes into account the amount and intensity of past intervention programs. In general, valid assessment of linguistic capacity is possible only if the individual has had the opportunity to experience multiple linguistic interactions across time.

A case study by Goossens' (1989) demonstrated how misleading initial assessment can be for individuals with severe communication disabilities who have not received AAC intervention. Prior to introduction of AAC, the described 6-year-old child was considered to have cognitive impairment. However, after 7 months of AAC intervention involving instruction in eye-gaze communication training and switch use, speech attempts emerged and the child appeared to function cognitively at a normal level.

Communication disabilities may disguise linguistic potential in other ways. As discussed previously, difficulties in speaking or reacting to spoken language may result in decreased quantity and quality of communication to which the child is exposed. This is particularly evident in cases of hearing impairment. For example, hearing parents appear to use more directive communication (i.e., more imperatives, fewer questions, shorter utterances) with children with hearing impairments than with children with normal hearing (Seyfried, Hutchinson, & Smith, 1989). This may be due to the fact that parents use language that matches their child's language level (Matey & Kretschmer, 1985). A similar phenomenon occurs with children with visual impairments who, because of their difficulty in responding to environmental cues, tend to receive more directives from adults than children without disabilities (Kekelis & Anderson, 1984). Such reduced language models may also occur for AAC users. If caregivers of AAC users attempt to match their child's expressive language and/or developmental level, AAC users probably also receive language input that is qualitatively different from that of typically developing children. Thus, AAC intervention often seeks to restore these interactions by providing symbols that are accessible according to the individual's sensory, motor, cognitive, and linguistic abilities and encouraging caregivers to communicate with AAC users in a more interactive manner.

However, introduction of AAC in and of itself does not guarantee full participation in communication. Many AAC users find themselves in situations where the speaker has predominant control over the conversation (Light, Collier, & Parnes, 1985a, 1985b). Upon initiating AAC systems, caregivers, peers, and other communication partners should be made aware of this unequal situation that restricts the AAC user. Jonker and Heim (1992) have proposed a training program for introducing interaction strategies to parents and caregivers such as allowing pauses and ensuring visual attention during the conversation. O'Keefe and Dattilo (1992) proposed a strategy that can be learned by AAC users to keep or to regain control over conversation. The response-recode (R-R) technique, which is easily learnable by individuals with cognitive impairments, consists of first responding to a communication partner and then immediately producing a recoding statement that requires the partner to reply. For example, in response to the question "Are you hungry?," the individual might respond by saying, "Yes" and then recode by saying, "What's for lunch?" This technique promotes active participation by the AAC user.

Buzolich, King, and Baroody (1991) described a study in which the expressive communicative repertoire of three AAC users was expanded to include commenting, a discourse function important in initiating and maintaining conversation. Using a least-to-most prompting hierarchy, all three subjects demonstrated appropriate commenting in group conversation situations. Two of the three generalized the commenting function to other classroom and community settings. Table 18.14 provides a case example illustrating goals and procedures.

Language Codes

Even if an individual has little or no access to primary linguistic expression, use of nonlinguistic symbols (e.g., pictographs) can pave the way toward linguistic communication. Nonlinguistic symbols can be used in ways that are similar to linguistic symbols. For example, pictographs or other graphic symbols can be used in the typical word order of spoken language. In this way, they are used as language codes, similar to use of manual signs as a code for a spoken language (see Chapter 7 for a discussion of manual codes). Moreover, by using linguistic and nonlinguistic symbols simultaneously, the more accessible nonlinguistic symbols may serve as a bridge to language use. When speech and nonlinguistic symbols are simultaneously presented to the user, all or part of the linguistic symbol will be processed by the receiver along with the nonlinguistic symbol. The principle here is that symbols that occur in earlier developmental stages (nonlinguistic) function as a basis for higher-level symbols (linguistic). Many forms of direct communication tend to be multimodal where different types of symbols are incorporated. For example, people tend to enhance speech with gestures when communication breaks down or when the message needs to be emphasized (McNeill, 1985). All modalities that are used in parallel tend to be redundant and complementary and have a mutually reinforcing effect on each other.

Because many AAC users rely solely on linguistic codes such as written language for expressive communication, acquisition of literacy skills is crucial. Chapter 23 discusses the development and use of written language by AAC users. One example of the use of written language by AAC users that warrants further discussion here, however, is the approach known as **facilitated communication (FC)**.

Facilitated Communication. This expressive communication approach was developed in Australia in the 1970s by Crossley (see Crossley, 1992) for use by a child with cerebral palsy. It was adopted in the 1990s by clinicians/educators in the United States for use with individuals with autism and other communication disabilities. With FC, an individual's arm or hand is supported by the facilitator during production of written communication, usually via an alphabet board, typewriter, or electronic communication device. This physical support, along with emotional support and belief in the person's competence, are the key elements of

TABLE 18.14　Case Example—Commenting with a Voice Output Communication Aid (VOCA)

BACKGROUND

Robin,* age 9, severe cerebral palsy; receptive language skills at age level; accesses a VOCA via an optical head pointer for expressive communication to greet, request, and ask and answer questions; reading, writing, spelling, and math at first- to second-grade level.

PLAN	GOALS
1. Program 10 comments into Robin's VOCA.	1. Robin will use her VOCA to spontaneously comment five times during daily 45-minute communication group sessions.
2. Have Robin practice activating the graphic symbols needed to produce the comment named by the clinician/educator.	
3. Provide opportunities to comment during group conversation time and cooking activities.	2. Robin will use her VOCA to spontaneously comment five times during weekly 45-minute cooking activities.

PROCEDURES

When an appropriate opportunity to produce a comment arises, prompt Robin to comment via her VOCA according to a least-to-most prompting hierarchy:

1. Expectant time delay: Establish eye contact with Robin and wait 10 seconds. If no or inappropriate response, go to step 2.
2. Indirect prompt: Provide an open-ended question, such as "What could you say?" If no or inappropriate response, go to step 3.
3. Direct prompt: Provide a spoken prompt and model of an appropriate response, such as "You could say 'Wow'." If no or inappropriate response, go to step 4.
4. Model: Activate Robin's VOCA to produce an appropriate comment.

Adapted from Buzolich, King, & Baroody (1991).

*Note: In the original case study, the child was referred to as "M"; a fictitious name has been assigned here to be consistent with other case examples in this chapter.

FC. It is purported to facilitate production of written language, and hence, communication, by linguistically competent individuals who were previously believed to have severe to profound disabilities (Biklin, 1990).

Several anecdotal reports and case studies (e.g., Biklin, Morton, Gold, Berrigan, & Swaminathan, 1992; Sabin & Donnellan, 1993) have supported the efficacy of facilitated communication as a breakthrough technology, yet controlled research studies using a variety of methodologies have failed to demonstrate that the individuals with communication disabilities actually authored the communications produced with facilitation (e.g., Eberlin, McConnachie, Ibel, & Volpe, 1993; Szempruch & Jacobson, 1993; Wheeler, Jacobson,

Paglieri, & Schwartz, 1993). At the same time, facilitators have denied that they were the authors or influenced the typed output.

Such extremely discrepant outcomes, along with the entry of FC issues into the popular media and the courtroom, have prompted organizations of professionals that serve individuals with disabilities to provide position statements regarding the appropriate use of FC. The position adopted by the American Speech-Language-Hearing Association (ASHA) on November 21, 1994, is as follows:

> Facilitated Communication is a technique by which a "facilitator" provides physical and other supports in an attempt to assist a person with a significant communication disability to point to pictures, objects, printed letters and words, or to a keyboard.

Personal accounts and qualitative descriptions suggest that messages produced using this technique may reveal previously undetected literacy and communication skills in people with autism and other disabilities. When information available to facilitators is controlled and objective evaluation methods are used, peer-reviewed studies and clinical assessment find no conclusive evidence that facilitated messages can be reliably attributed to people with disabilities. Rather, most messages originate with the facilitator. Moreover, Facilitated Communication may have negative consequences if it precludes the use of effective and appropriate treatment, supplants other forms of communication, and/or leads to false or unsubstantiated allegations of abuse or mistreatment.

It is the position of the American Speech-Language-Hearing Association (ASHA) that the scientific validity and reliability of Facilitated Communication have not been demonstrated to date. Information obtained through or based on Facilitated Communication should not form the sole basis for making any diagnostic or treatment decisions.

ASHA strongly supports continued research and clinical efforts to develop scientifically valid methods for developing or enhancing the independent communication and literacy skills of people with disabilities. Speech-language pathologists are autonomous professionals who are responsible for critically evaluating all treatment techniques in order to hold paramount the welfare of persons served in accordance with the ASHA Code of Ethics. Speech-language pathologists should inform prospective clients and their families or guardians that currently the scientific validity and reliability of Facilitated Communication have not been established, and should obtain their informed consent before using the technique. (ASHA, 1995, LC-94)

Thus, based on research to date, the decision to use FC to enhance the communication abilities of a given individual requires careful consideration of any and all other AAC options and should not, in any case, be used as the sole means of expressive communication. When combined with other AAC approaches, intervention should be planned toward the goal of increasing communication independence while decreasing physical, gestural, and spoken prompts and supports. As described in Chapter 23, a broad range of literacy experiences to enhance both reading and writing skills should

be provided for all AAC users. For an extensive review of published research regarding FC, see Green (1994) and Shane (1994).

EDUCATIONAL ISSUES

Educational services aim at providing the best options for the challenges posed by young AAC users. However, issues of which services are to be delivered, how, where, when, and by whom have been matters of ongoing discussion and debate. Children with disabilities will be best served if interventions are based on a collaborative team approach and systematic planning to increase functional skills, while tapping into the developmental tendencies of the child. Further, education of children with disabilities in integrated settings with typically developing peers holds great potential for optimal learning and development for all children (Rainforth, York, & Macdonald, 1992).

Community-Based Instruction

Individuals with severe disabilities, including many AAC users, have traditionally received education in special segregated settings, with little or no opportunity to interact with typical peers. Skills were generally taught according to a developmental sequence, where the introduction of higher-level skills were withheld until students demonstrated acquisition of various prerequisites (e.g., preacademic, prereading, prevocational). Further, skills were often taught out of the context of meaningful interactions and natural routines that could provide natural cues and consequences. For example, students practiced money skills by completing worksheets or games that used play money, rather than handling money during actual buying and selling transactions. In the late 1970s and early 1980s, however, this approach to special education met with opposition by those advocating a community-based (e.g., Falvey, 1986) or community-referenced (e.g., Ford, Schnorr, Meyer, Davern, Black, & Dempsey, 1989) curriculum. **Community-based instruction** emphasizes the following themes:

1. Content of learning—Students should learn to perform meaningful activities in areas that are impor-

tant to their daily lives and apply skills they learn in math, science, language, and other areas.

2. Process of learning—The most effective method of learning activities and basic skills involves practicing them in real-life activities. (Peterson, LeRoy, Field, & Wood, 1992, p. 210)

Inherent in this model for students with disabilities is the abandonment of a strictly developmental approach, particularly during the middle school and high school years. For some students, this may mean abandoning some goals altogether (e.g., color naming) in favor of more functional, meaningful, age-appropriate goals (e.g., recognizing different areas on a color-coded communication display; matching/sorting clothing items by color).

For other students, skills may be developed in meaningful contexts prior to attainment of previously required prerequisite skills. For example, a student may use a set of graphic symbol cards to prepare for and select groceries, rather than delaying shopping experiences until the student can write and read a list independently. Such a de-emphasis on prerequisites has been echoed in the field of AAC by Kangas and Lloyd (1988), who stressed the importance of not waiting for the development of certain cognitive prerequisites (e.g., cause-effect, means-ends) before introducing AAC, but rather using AAC as a means of realizing these cognitive skills.

Such a community-referenced approach to special education, by its nature, implies that students spend significant portions of the school day outside of the actual physical classroom. That is, the community *becomes* the classroom. With the advent of the full-inclusion model (described below) in the early 1990s, many clinicians/educators grappled with the obvious question: "How do we teach functional skills in community settings while at the same time provide maximum inclusive experiences for our students?" (Beck, Broers, Hogue, Shipstead, & Knowleton, 1994, p. 44).

Various options for resolving the conflict presented by these seemingly opposing educational trends have been proposed (e.g., Beck et al., 1994; Stainback & Stainback, 1992, 1996). Most center around providing integrated, heterogeneous classrooms in which community participation and preparation for adult life is emphasized for *all* students, in essence, a merging of the two approaches. This involves curricular modifications to include functional applications of basic skills along with elements that form the cornerstone of an inclusive approach to education (i.e., collaborative teaching, heterogeneous grouping, peer support).

Inclusion

Inclusion is at the same time a principle of educational organization and an educational goal in itself. It is based on the idea that the best educational opportunities are provided if all students can participate in the same learning environment (Stainback & Stainback, 1992). The presence of students with disabilities increases classroom heterogeneity, and many opportunities to enhance learning can emerge. Traditional educational thinking that homogeneous grouping is a necessary condition for maximal learning has been a fallacy. Homogeneous grouping itself is a relative phenomenon: even within a group of highly gifted students, dramatic differences may be apparent in intelligence, as well as in emotional, motivational, and social aspects of learning.

Heterogeneous grouping and the diversity of cognitive, linguistic, and social skills that it affords can be challenging and a beginning point of departure for clinicians and educators. Thousand, Villa, and Nevin (1994) have described cooperative learning or **collaborative learning** as an important technique for taking advantage of the learning opportunities inherent in heterogeneous grouping. In this technique, classrooms are divided into smaller groups within which children's abilities may differ considerably. The learning experience is fostered by the necessary exchange of information within each group as students tackle learning tasks. Group members are required to devise creative solutions to ensure participation of all members in the group task. Working together on such a project can increase the mutual acceptance and identification of group members, along with triggering willingness and creativity in exploring the unique contributions of each group member. Discovering options can lead to a high degree of appreciation of AAC users by other group members when it is shown that their contributions can improve the quality of group work. For example, graphic symbols may be used by all students during categorization or note-taking tasks.

This type of classroom arrangement requires both organizational and curricular adaptations, as well as involvement by a variety of support staff. The role of the transdisciplinary team is pivotal in the success of an inclusion approach, where identified specialists work collaboratively with the entire educational team to help identify problem areas related to their given areas of expertise as they arise during meaningful activities throughout the day. "Intervention is not provided in isolation but is incorporated into functional activities for the student that occur in the classroom, school environment, and community" (Downing & Eichinger, 1990, pp. 99–100). See Chapter 21 for additional information on service delivery.

For inclusion to be successful for AAC users, team members first need to be aware of the cognitive, linguistic, social, and emotional parameters of AAC use. As inclusion requires intense and frequent participation in all activities, AAC users must have sufficient knowledge, skills, and social sensitivity to actively take part in information sharing and social interaction. However, lack of these skills does not constitute sufficient cause to withhold a child from inclusion. The most recommended strategy is to use inclusion as a challenging and triggering situation for AAC users to develop the skills that are necessary for participating as fully as possible. AAC use is not an objective in and of itself, but rather one method for reaching functional outcomes (Calculator & Jorgensen, 1991). Classroom activities are the most natural settings for students, and communication skills have the highest chance of becoming part of a student's arsenal of skills if they are taught and challenged in natural situations.

The development of AAC skills by the user comprises only one element of entering an integrated classroom. Clinicians, educators, and other team members must also be sufficiently knowledgeable about the ways to facilitate information sharing through AAC. Attention should be given to actively involving peers to ensure frequent contact and interaction with the AAC user. Through games, activities, and discussions, a welcoming attitude toward the AAC user can be promoted. For example, Mirenda (1993) described the fascination of an AAC user's peers when they discovered that it was possible to store all kinds of interesting words and sounds in an electronic communication device.

Typically developing peers may require direct instruction in ways to increase interaction with AAC users, a process that can begin as early as preschool. As described previously, three typically developing preschoolers were successfully instructed to use a mand-model procedure to elicit communication from peers, one of whom was learning to request by using manual signs (Venn et al., 1993). Hunt, Alwell, and Goetz (1991) reported improved interaction by elementary students with severe disabilities via graphic symbol communication books when peers received instruction in eliciting conversational turn taking.

Rao (1994) also described an approach for reducing AAC user overdependency on familiar communication partners that features peer instruction. A basic feature of this approach involves use of a graphic symbol communication board by a small group of individuals involved in the communication exchange. Here, appropriate use of selected vocabulary is modeled by adults and peers repeatedly throughout an activity (e.g., tea party, card game). Adults begin by modeling vocabulary use and directing peers' attention to graphic symbols as indicated by the AAC user. Gradually, the adults become less involved by prompting peers to assist each other in "translating" the indicated graphic symbol(s). Thus, the role of support staff (e.g., special educator, speech-language pathologist, teaching assistant) is gradually decreased as increased peer interaction is promoted.

Although inclusion in regular classrooms may be a particularly challenging undertaking, with provisions for careful assessment, appropriate goals and teaching methods, adequate supports, and adaptations of classroom curricula, inclusion can be a successful experience for many AAC users. Students with severe, multiple disabilities may be successfully included in age-level classrooms, as described in the case of Thomas, a child with severe speech, physical, and visual impairments (Blischak, 1995).

IEP Development

At the heart of AAC intervention is the student's **individualized education program (IEP)**, which is required for all students who receive special education services. IEPs are designed to maximize the benefits of intervention by determining educational goals that can be met effectively according to a reasonable time schedule. IEPs delineate a student's current level of functioning, goals (long-term), objectives (short-term), individuals responsible for implementing the education plan, and environments in which instruction is to occur. Although an IEP identifies well-defined and measurable goals and objectives, goals are not necessarily meant to be pursued in isolation. On the contrary, much evidence suggests that students learn and integrate skills and knowledge best if they are part of the challenges within a functional context (Calculator & Jorgensen, 1991; Rainforth et al., 1992).

Definition and implementation of goals and objectives requires careful planning. Van Balkom and Welle Donker-Gimbrere (1994) proposed four steps in IEP planning for AAC users: assessment, implementation, extension, and independence.

Assessment. Assessment of all skills (strengths and needs) is generally considered to be the first step in IEP development. These skills must be considered in a dynamic, rather than a static, way. That is, communication development highly depends on opportunities to communicate, which in some cases may be severely limited. Therefore, assessment and observation results should always be viewed as somewhat provisional and open to adjustment after a period of intervention. Communication assessment should include evaluation of communicative competence (linguistic, operational, social, strategic); an inventory of needs and required adaptations (including physical and staff support); curriculum priorities; and vocabulary decisions. If the assessment team has recommended a communication device, the features of a device that would meet the student's needs should be included. Naming specific devices, however, should be avoided.

Implementation. The implementation of AAC within the classroom learning situation requires a participation plan that will allow the user as well as teachers and peers to guarantee maximal participation in learning and social situations. The participation plan should include all regular classroom activities, both curricular and extracurricular. At this stage, vocabulary selection is crucial. Whenever a change or adaptation of the AAC system is made, teachers and peers should be informed and given appropriate instructions.

Extension. Once an AAC user begins to take part in the classroom and school routine, adaptations or additions to the existing AAC system may be needed. This extension may include, for example, additional vocabulary or technology to facilitate group discussion or text production. At regular intervals, evaluation probes should be conducted to identify needs or adaptations that must be made to ensure more active participation in learning and social situations.

Independence. The independence step concerns maximal autonomy for participating in school activities. A condition is that parents as well as teachers and peers are familiar with the AAC system. This should evolve as naturally as possible so that the user will never be isolated or be placed in such specific situations that could lead to stigmatization. Therefore, AAC service providers must observe carefully how social relationships develop within the group and which position the AAC user takes. The teacher may try to draw the attention to positive skills if the AAC user has initially a rather marginal role. For example, a teacher can help the peers to discover that an AAC user can do exciting things with the communication device (Mirenda, 1993).

Such a distinction of separate steps suggests a successive, linear planning process, which can be quite misleading. In reality, AAC team members should consider all steps from the very start. Educational planning is actually a dynamic process where outcomes of interventions necessitate a reexamination of earlier set goals. For example, school performance may sometimes be even higher than was expected by team members who designed the first version of the IEP. The reason may be that the environment challenges the young AAC user to the extent that enhanced attention and motivation lead to faster learning, or it may be that the situation in the regular classroom simply increases the amount of information that is given and exchanged. Furthermore, through use of an appropriate AAC system, the student may have better and more access to information. If such positive and unpredicted development occurs, the team must revise the IEP and set even higher goals. However, some of the problems an AAC user has may be underestimated in the IEP. This can make the proposed goals impossible to reach. For example, the limited reading skills of an AAC user may have been considered to be easy to overcome if an intensive literacy program was offered in parallel with regular classroom activities. If the outcome of such literacy instruction remains under the level of expectations, other goals in the academic realm may also become less realistic. Such a case would require the team to question whether the proposed goals and methods actually fit the individual's level of competence and then restructure the IEP accordingly.

Beukelman and Mirenda (1992) proposed an educational model for AAC users that is particularly useful in IEP development. They noted that the degree to which a student participates in a given setting depends on four variables, within which different levels of participation can be distinguished:

- Integration: full-selective-none
- Academic participation: competitive-active-involved-none
- Social participation: competitive-active-involved-none
- Independence: independent-setup-assisted (p. 206)

AAC users show different patterns of participation, which changes over time with progress and maturation. For example, a young child at kindergarten age may not have a sufficient level of development to take advantage of all the challenges of an enriched environment and thus may not be fully integrated with typical peers. However, at a later age, the same child may become more oriented toward the environment and learn much more through daily interactions and incidental learning, thereby increasing integration, and academic and social participation.

Although it is beyond the range of this chapter to extensively describe IEP development, case examples throughout have provided a sampling of goals and procedures that may be suitable for inclusion in IEPs. For additional information regarding IEP development, see Beukelman and Mirenda (1992) and Calculator and Jorgensen (1991).

Transitioning

Transitioning is another important element of educational planning that should also be included on a student's IEP. For AAC users, each transition within the school system (e.g., from preschool to kindergarten) should be prepared for carefully, especially with regard to opportunities and risks that arise from academic, social, and vocational participation. In this section, special attention will be given to transitioning from school to adult life.

Although focus on the transition from school to adult life and employment should be of concern for all students, it should be a special concern for AAC users for two reasons. First, at the time of graduation, many AAC users will not sufficiently possess all of the skills required of adult life. Second, the new environments in which AAC users live and work may be inadequately prepared to respond appropriately to their needs. Both factors can seriously interfere with the graduate's access to employment, community living, and social/recreation opportunities. Further, dramatic changes in the requirements of the job market often occur. During the 3 to 5 years of high school attendance, the gap between the skills that were targeted for and actual job and living requirements may widen considerably. For example, for many AAC users, computer literacy may have become a more important goal than math skills, although traditionally oriented school programs may have failed to keep up with the change and give it sufficient weight in the curriculum.

At one time, students received intervention geared toward transitioning only during the senior year of high school. Presently, there is a growing consensus that transitioning and preparation for adulthood should be a part of the general IEP much earlier (Conti & Jenkins-Odorisio, 1994; Gallivan-Fenlon, 1994). However, the learning potential of students with severe disabilities may be easily underestimated, even by experienced team members. Precious time may be spent on prevocational (e.g., sorting tasks) and academic skills that may in fact relate little to actual demands of adult life. Sufficient attention should also be paid to the emotional aspects of transition to adult life. Feelings of uncertainty about the future may unintentionally prevent the student, relatives, and team members from considering adult life issues until the year of graduation.

Gallivan-Fenlon (1994) described several models of transitioning that have been successfully implemented, including provision of community-based education, use of collaborative teams, implementation of individualized transition plans, family involvement, and development of interagency agreements geared toward providing integrated community employment. The role of a "transition coordinator" who can support and guide other team members and "accept the role of systems change agent to help create new and different employment or residential options in local communities" (p. 21) was considered pivotal in successful transitioning.

Goals that reflect preparation for transition to adult life should be incorporated into IEPs during the elementary school years, with these critical components: a longitudinal, functional curriculum; an integrated learning environment; and community-based service delivery, where

> . . . a longitudinal, functional curriculum implies that students begin developing vocational skills at an early age, with increasing involvement as they become older. Early training during the elementary years must emphasize general work-related behaviors, such as attending to task, following schedules, completing assignments; independent mobility; grooming skills; and appropriate social interactions. Secondary training must be based on specific skills required in actual local employment situations, and youth should receive training in several potential types of jobs. By the time a youth

is ready to graduate, a specific job for which he or she has been trained should be identified for full-time placement. (Wehman, Wood, Everson, Goodwyn, & Conley, 1988, p. 30)

Wehman et al. (1988) also advocated implementing a formal, written transition plan at least 4 years prior to graduation that targets these areas:

1. Advocacy/legal
2. Employment—or—post secondary education
3. Financial and income
4. Independent living
5. Medical/therapeutic
6. Recreation/leisure
7. Social/sexual
8. Transportation (p. 234)

Clearly, effective communication skills overlay each of these targeted areas, and AAC users will require additional consideration of communication needs and adaptations.

VOCATIONAL ISSUES

Meaningful employment is the goal of many AAC users, just as it is for most individuals, yet until recently, many individuals with disabilities faced extreme physical and attitudinal barriers in gaining employment outside of sheltered workshops. These barriers range from reduced expectations and inadequate preparation to difficulties accommodating the various communication, physical, and technological needs of individuals with disabilities. As reported by Blackstone (1993d), two of the most significant barriers to successful employment of AAC users are "lack of education about the capabilities of AAC users and lack of information about the possible job-matches that exist" (p. 5). Overcoming these barriers often requires persistent effort on the part of the AAC user and other team members to achieve consistent, gainful employment.

Unfortunately, professional preparation programs in special education and speech-language pathology often do not provide coursework and/or practicum experience related to employment (Lloyd & Belfiore, 1994). Many AAC service providers may not be knowledgeable regarding vocational issues and available resources. Further, little research regarding employment of AAC users has been conducted. Thus, we turn to current research regarding employment of individuals with disabilities who are not necessarily AAC users, beginning with a discussion of **supported employment**, a successful approach that has been used with individuals across a broad range of disabilities (e.g., Rusch, 1990).

Supported Employment

Supported employment is one option that provides an individual with disabilities the opportunity to engage in competitive, community-based work with the central goal of accomplishing real work for real pay with on-the-job supports, job coaches, accommodations in the work place, and flexible work schedules in integrated job settings (Suter, 1990). The AAC team must work to identify and eliminate structural barriers (e.g., a desk that does not accommodate a wheelchair). Often a job coach is hired initially to ensure that tasks are completed correctly and in a timely manner. As time goes on, the trainee assumes greater responsibility in performing job tasks, with the ultimate goal of independent, competent job performance. Increasingly, employers of individuals with disabilities have begun to use co-workers as natural supports who take on a consultative role over hired job coaches (Rogan, Hagner, & Murphy, 1993). Successful use of this model with an AAC user was described by Butterworth and Strauch (1994) where co-workers suggested appropriate VOCA messages for an adult with physical disabilities employed in a university law library.

The benefits of supported over sheltered employment are many, not the least of which include cost-effectiveness, earning power, job satisfaction, and quality of life (McCaughrin, Ellis, Rusch, & Heal, 1993; Test, Hinson, Solow, & Keul, 1993; Thompson, Powers, & Houchard, 1992). Barriers to successful implementation, however, include the belief that individuals must be ready for community employment (i.e., focus on prerequisites); lack of financial resources such as start-up and overhead costs; worker-job mismatch; co-worker dissatisfaction; lack of coordination among ser-

vice providers and/or agencies; and, inadequate staff training (Beare, Severson, Lynch, & Schneider, 1992). In discussing the use of co-workers rather than traditional job coaches, Rogan et al. (1993) listed the following strategies to facilitate employment of persons with disabilities and circumvent these barriers.

1. Use personal connections to enhance social support.
2. Match employee preferences and attributes to work-site social climates.
3. Collaborate with work-site personnel to develop adaptations and modifications.
4. Facilitate and support the involvement of co-workers and employers.
5. Provide general consultation focused on person-environment factors that promote the success of the supported employee and the overall business (p. 277).

Each of these strategies requires careful examination by the AAC team, considering the roles of receptive and expressive communication and how AAC use may help or hinder job performance. Successful employment requires more than the ability to perform specific tasks and often hinges on communicative competence. Job-related communication skills are often quite different than those required in social and educational settings. Workers generally need to be able to communicate quickly and clearly to deliver messages, ask questions, and engage in social conversations with co-workers. To that end, modifications may need to be made in existing AAC systems to include appropriate messages, additional communication modes, and the means to interface with adaptive equipment.

Social competence is a critical factor in maintaining employment (see Salzberg, Lignugaris/Kraft, & McCuller, 1988, for a review). For instance, Butterworth and Strauch (1994) reported that interactions of workers with disabilities may not differ substantially from workers without disabilities for task-related interactions. However, difficulties with non-task-related communications interfere with the development of friendships and social support in the work site. AAC users may be particularly vulnerable to difficulties with social competence for a number of possible reasons:

1. Different timing, pragmatics of AAC use
2. Co-worker unfamiliarity with AAC methods
3. Difficulties with nonverbal aspects of communication (e.g., eye contact, maintaining appropriate physical distance)
4. Preoccupation with technology

Application of intervention strategies designed to identify and overcome these communication difficulties is important for AAC users and should be part of an overall intervention plan that begins early in life, with emphasis on development of linguistic, operational, social, and strategic competence (see Light, 1989). Suggested ways to develop communicative competence and increase employment options for AAC users are summarized in Table 18.15.

Independent Employment

Although supported employment may be appropriate for many AAC users, some may be independently employed in a variety of work settings involving technology, advocacy, and communication. Prentice (1994), for example, described his professional role in the Nuclear Division of a large corporation. Additional discussion of issues sur-

rounding independent employment by AAC users can be found in Conti and Jenkins-Odorisio (1993, 1994).

SUMMARY

Individuals with developmental disabilities are at particular risk for experiencing communication disabilities. For this broadly diverse group, AAC use can positively affect communication as well as overall development. The outcome of AAC intervention for children and adolescents with developmental disabilities depends on a number of factors. To make appropriate decisions about the introduction and use of AAC, a frame of reference about how AAC symbols may increase communication at particular levels of development is needed. Understanding how communication evolves from reflexive to intentional behavior and from nonlinguistic to linguistic symbol use helps clinicians/educators to make decisions about which symbols may be used. Equally important as symbol selection are the techniques to help AAC users acquire communication within integrated functional environments. Many individuals with developmental disabilities will require an explicit instructional approach that includes use of techniques such as shaping, fading, prompting, and expectant time delay.

The introduction of transparent symbols often means a major leap in communication development and power. Contrary to what is typical of early communication, transparent symbols have the potential to communicate beyond the here and now. They also may serve as a bridge to linguistic communication for individuals who have normal language capacity but who lack the skills to acquire language exclusively through unaided communication.

Development is also optimized if the AAC user can actively participate in a well-organized educational setting along with typical peers. An important instrument is the IEP, which sets goals and objectives in a way that allows parents and team members to direct and evaluate progress. Another important factor to consider is the organization of the environment. A community-referenced approach along with inclusion in age-level class-

TABLE 18.15   Suggested Ways to Increase Employment Options for AAC Users

Increase awareness of family members, educators, employers, and the community at large about possible employment options.

Begin during the preschool years with ongoing planning for transition from school to employment.

Present successful role models.

Develop functional community-based skills involving literacy, money management, personal care, use of transportation, interviewing, and self-advocacy.

Use technology appropriately.

Develop appropriate employment options.

Ensure an adequate level of job support.

Partially based on Blackstone (1993d); Conti & Jenkins-Odorisio (1993, 1994).

rooms provide the most appropriate challenges for a growing AAC user.

Although early AAC intervention for individuals with developmental disabilities is aimed at enhancing learning and developing opportunities, one of the most important issues to consider is improvement in quality of life and equipping individuals with skills that will enable, as much as possible, autonomy and self-fulfillment. Transition to adult life, vocational issues, and employment hold many challenges for AAC users, but can be met appropriately if they are approached with long-term planning when individuals are at a young age.

CHAPTER 19

INTERVENTION FOR PERSONS WITH ACQUIRED DISORDERS

RAJINDER KOUL, HELEN H. ARVIDSON, AND G. S. PENNINGTON

Individuals with acquired communication disorders demonstrate relatively selective impairments in attention, language, memory, motor skills, sensory processing, and vision. Studying the cognitive impairments that follow brain injury provides insight into the functioning of the normal brain and aids in developing rehabilitative programs and procedures that provide opportunities for individuals with brain damage to function more optimally. One area of rehabilitation that is different from traditional therapeutic procedures for severe speech and language impairment is **augmentative and alternative communication (AAC)**. AAC strategies and techniques have been used increasingly during the past two decades to facilitate, enhance, and improve the communication abilities of individuals with the following conditions: severe/global aphasia and/or apraxia; progressive neurogenic diseases such as amyotrophic lateral sclerosis (ALS), Parkinson's disease, progressive supranuclear palsy (PSP), multiple sclerosis (MS), and Alzheimer's disease (AD); and acquired physical disabilities such as cervical spinal cord injury and traumatic brain injury (TBI) (Bertoni, Stoffel, & Weniger, 1991; Beukelman & Mirenda, 1992; Bourgeois, 1990; Coelho & Duffy, 1987; Funnell & Allport, 1989; Gardner, Zurif, Berry, & Baker, 1976; Garrett, Beukelman, & Low-Morrow, 1989; Glass, Gazzaniga, & Premack, 1973; Helm-Estabrooks, Fitzpatrick, & Barresi, 1982; Herrmann, Reichle, Lucius-Hoene, Wallesch, & Johannsen-Horbach, 1988; Johannsen-Horbach, Cegla, Mager, Schempp, & Wallesch, 1985; Kraat, 1990; Lane & Samples, 1981; Ross, 1979; Sawyer-Woods, 1987; Skelly, 1979; Trunzo-Rahbar, 1980;

Weinrich et al., 1989). This chapter describes AAC assessment and intervention approaches for individuals who have severe speech and language impairments as a result of an acquired neurological condition.

APHASIA

Aphasia is defined as a language disturbance resulting from damage to certain subsystems of the brain that are responsible for the interpretation and formulation of language. Every day, approximately 300 individuals are diagnosed with aphasia in the United States (LaPointe, 1994). The foremost cause of aphasia is a **cerebrovascular accident (CVA)**, commonly called a stroke. Every year approximately 180,000 individuals in the United States require nursing home care as a result of a stroke (National Stroke Association, 1991). Other relatively less frequent causes of aphasia are TBI, intracranial tumors, toxicities, and infections.

Recovery patterns in individuals with aphasia depend on the lesion size, the remote effects of the lesion on distant brain regions, and the role of the damaged locus in language function (Mountcastle, 1978). Many individuals with aphasia show some degree of spontaneous recovery within 3 to 6 months after the incurrence of brain lesion. Some individuals may recover natural language (i.e., spoken or sign language) capabilities with or without speech and language intervention. Others, however, fail to demonstrate significant recovery of natural language abilities despite long and intensive speech-language intervention. This chapter focuses primarily on individuals with severe and global aphasia whose natural language is considered to be permanently impaired.

Severe and Global Aphasia

Although the terms **severe aphasia** and **global aphasia** both refer to neurological impairments that result in extensive disturbance in language function, there is a distinction. An individual with severe aphasia typically demonstrates severe deficits in one or more language areas (i.e., auditory comprehension, speech, reading, writing). For example, one individual with severe aphasia may have deficits in the ability to comprehend, but retain the ability to speak while another individual with severe aphasia may retain the ability to comprehend but have deficits in the ability to speak. An individual with global aphasia, on the other hand, demonstrates deficits across all language areas.

Communication Characteristics.   Varying types of aphasia symptomatology have led to the proliferation of classification schemes (Goodglass & Kaplan, 1983; Kertesz, 1982; Porch, 1981; Schuell, 1965; Wepman & Jones, 1961). Most of these classification schemes have resulted in instruments and/or standardized tests that evaluate areas of natural language performance such as auditory comprehension, speech, reading, and writing. Individuals who use American Sign Language (ASL) as their primary language have demonstrated deficits in language similar to those of their peers who use spoken language (Bellugi, Poizner, & Klima, 1983; Poizner, Bellugi, & Iragui, 1984). Most of the contemporary standardized tests such as the Boston Diagnostic Aphasia Examination (BDAE) (Goodglass & Kaplan, 1983) do not evaluate the performance of individuals with aphasia on various augmentative symbol sets and/or systems. Some tests, however, such as the Porch Index of Communicative Abilities (PICA) (Porch, 1981), Communicative Abilities in Daily Living (CADL) (Holland, 1980), and the Functional Communication Profile (FCP) (Sarno, 1969) evaluate aspects of gestural communication, a form of unaided AAC. The Boston Assessment of Severe Aphasia (BASA) (Helm-Estabrooks, Ramsberger,

Morgan, & Nicholas, 1989) evaluates and gives full credit for gestural responses on all items.

AAC Intervention.   In recent years, attempts have been made to improve the communicative abilities of individuals with severe aphasia by teaching them AAC symbol sets and/or systems. Early studies of individuals with severe aphasia indicated superior performance on some tasks when AAC techniques involving manual signs, gestures (Rao & Horner, 1979; Skelly, 1979), and visual-graphic symbols (Gardner et al., 1976) were used compared to when natural spoken language forms were used. However, this superior performance did not generalize outside structured treatment contexts (Coelho & Duffy, 1987), because most of the AAC techniques were applied without considering the language deficits of these individuals (Kraat, 1990). Problems observed in the natural language behavior of individuals with aphasia were also reflected in their use of AAC symbol sets and/or systems. Many of these individuals showed semantic paraphasias (substitutions of motorically similar or visually similar gestures) and inability to acquire and retain particular word classes and subclasses (Funnell & Allport, 1989; Steele, Illes, Weinrich, & Lakin, 1985; Weinrich et al., 1989). Service providers in extended care facilities have suggested that lack of generalization may also be due to the lack of encouragement and support from communication partners.

Graphic Symbol-Based Intervention.   Studies involving AAC intervention using graphic symbols with individuals with severe and global aphasia and/or apraxia are relatively few in number. Table 19.1 presents a concise summary of relevant studies. Early intervention studies using graphic symbols were devoted to studying the cognitive operations that were preserved in individuals with severe and global aphasia. Alternative symbol systems such as the visual input communication (VIC) system or cut-out paper symbols were taught to individuals with severe and global aphasia with encouraging results (Gardner et al., 1976; Glass et al., 1973; Helm-Estabrooks et al., 1982). Individuals demonstrated success in learning visual symbols.

TABLE 19.1 Summary of Graphic Symbol Intervention Studies Conducted with Individuals with Severe and Global Aphasia and/or Apraxia

AUTHORS	APHASIA TYPE AND SEVERITY	NUMBER OF SUBJECTS AND AGE RANGES	SITE OF LESIONS	TYPE OF SYMBOLS	GOALS/RESEARCH QUESTIONS	FINDINGS
Goodenough-Trepagnier (1995)	Global aphasia (N = 2), Broca's aphasia (N = 2), severe nonfluent aphasia (N = 3)	N = 7; 49–74 yrs.	Left CVA[1] (all 7 subjects)	C-VIC[2]; visual ana-logue repre-sentations (VAR)	To compare receptive and expressive performance on prepositions trained through C-VIC, VAR, and text.	Subjects obtained significantly more correct responses in the VAR than in C-VIC and text conditions in both receptive and expressive tasks.
Weinrich, McCall, Weber, Thomas, & Thornburg (1995)	Chronic Broca's aphasia	N = 2; 44–53 yrs.	Left CVA (both subjects)	C-VIC	Can training in the production of subject-verb-object (S-V-O) sentences and locative prepositional phrases on C-VIC result in improved verbal production of these constructions?	Both subjects demonstrated marked improvement in the verbal production of S-V-O sentences and prepositional phrases after C-VIC training. However, no significant difference between pretest and post-test was observed in the phonological aspects of their verbal productions.
Koul (1994); Koul and Lloyd (1994a)	Global aphasia (N = 5) Moderate aphasia (N = 5)	N = 10; 60–83 yrs.	CVA in left middle cerebral artery (all 10 subjects)	Blissymbols	How do translucency and complexity affect the acquisition and retention of Blissymbols by individuals with aphasia?	Subjects with aphasia and neurologically normal control subjects did not differ signifi-cantly in guessing, learning, and retaining Blissymbols. Subjects with aphasia learned symbols with low iconicity and symbols with high iconicity. Complexity had no influence on learning Blissymbols.
Naeser, Plaumbo, Baker, & Nicholas (1994)	Chronic severe aphasia with no spontaneous output	N = 7; 43–60 yrs.	Left CVA (all 7 subjects)	C-VIC	Does any relationship exist between the site of the lesion and good vs. poor response to C-VIC?	No relationship was observed between the site of the lesion in a single neuroanatomic area and response pattern to C-VIC. However, individuals who

Study	Diagnosis	N; Age	Etiology	Technique	Research question	Results
Weinrich, McCall, Shoosmith, Thomas, Katzenberger, & Weber (1993)	Global aphasia (N = 3) Broca's aphasia (N = 3)	N = 6; 46–63 yrs.	Left CVA (all 6 subjects)	C-VIC	Can individuals with global aphasia interpret and produce locative prepositional phrases in the absence of verbal memory load and morphosyntactic demands?	performed poorly on C-VIC had large cortical and deep lesions in the supplementary motor/cingulate gyrus, Wernicke's, and subcortical temporal isthmus areas. All subjects except one who had a prior history of right CVA could comprehend and produce prepositions at better than 90% accuracy. Only one subject was able to produce scorable verbal prepositional phrases.
Bertoni, Stoffel, & Weniger (1991)	Global aphasia	N = 1; 58 yrs.	Middle cerebral artery infarction	Pictographs	Can an individual with global aphasia use pictographs to communicate?	Subject was able to understand and express information in six communication domains (e.g., daily needs, public service) using pictographs.
Funnell & Allport (1989)	Severe aphasia	N = 2; 1. 58 yrs.; 2. 54 yrs.	Middle cerebral artery infarction (both subjects)	Blissymbols	1. Can individuals with severe aphasia learn to use Blissymbols? 2. How closely is the ability to use Blissymbols related to residual natural language abilities of aphasic patients?	1. Blissymbols that were highly translucent or transparent were learned and used more meaningfully than low translucent or opaque Blissymbols. 2. The performance on Blissymbols was consistant with performance on written words, indicating that Blissymbol processing is not independent of natural language processing.

[1]CVA = Cerebrovascular accident

[2]C-VIC = Computerized visual input communication

TABLE 19.1 (*Continued*)

AUTHORS	APHASIA TYPE AND SEVERITY	NUMBER OF SUBJECTS AND AGE RANGES	SITE OF LESIONS	TYPE OF SYMBOLS	GOALS/RESEARCH QUESTIONS	FINDINGS
Steele, Weinrich, Wertz, Kleczewska, & Carlson (1989)	Global aphasia (1, 2, & 3) Broca's aphasia (4 & 5)	N = 5; 47–64 yrs.	1. Left frontal lobe resection (head trauma) 2. Left fronto-temporal-parietal infarction 3. Left thalamic hemorrhage 4. Left frontal infarction 5. Left fronto-parietal infarction	C-VIC	Can subjects access and use icons? Are subjects able to combine these icons based on taught rules of combination? Can subjects communicate correctly using the system during communicative interactions?	All subjects were able to master the operations of the computer needed to access the icons. All subjects were able to use icons for communicative interactions such as asking and answering questions, describing events. All subjects performed markedly better on C-VIC than on natural language tasks as measured through several subsets of PICA.[3] All subjects in general demonstrated better receptive and expressive performances on concrete object and person designators than on abstract representations.
Weinrich, Steele, Carlson, Kleczewska, Wertz, & Baker (1989)	Global aphasia	N = 1; 57 yrs.	Middle cerebral artery infarction	C-VIC	To compare the subject's ability to discriminate between reversible locative prepositional phrases using C-VIC.	Subject's ability to discriminate prepositional phrases using C-VIC was significantly better than his ability to discriminate the same phrases using printed English.

Study	Disorder	N; Age	Etiology	Symbol System	Purpose	Results
Sawyer-Woods (1987)	Severe aphasia	N = 1; 59 yrs.	Large left parietal infarction	Blissymbols	To determine whether an individual with severe aphasia could use Blissymbols to identify and label. To determine whether type of symbols (pictographic vs. compound) would affect the ease of learning.	Subject learned all 60 symbols taught to criterion. Transparent Blissymbols were identified with 100% accuracy. The superimposed compound symbols vs. sequenced compound symbols were learned with equal ease.
Johannsen-Horbach, Cegla, Mager, Schempp, & Wallesch (1985)	Global aphasia	N = 4; 41–57 yrs.	1. Ischemic infarction in the area supplied by the left anterior cerebral artery and anterior branches of the left middle cerebral artery 2. Massive left subcortical hemorrhage 3. Left middle cerebral artery infarction 4. Infarction of the complete area of supply of the left middle cerebral artery	Blissymbols	To determine whether subjects could acquire a basic lexicon of nouns, verbs, adjectives, and adverbs in Blissymbols. To determine whether subjects could produce and understand simple sentences in Blissymbols.	All subjects learned more noun and verb symbols than symbols for other types of words. Three subjects, while pointing to the symbols, were able to articulate corresponding words correctly. Two subjects showed improvement in spontaneous communication.
Lane & Samples (1981)	Severe aphasia and apraxia of speech	N = 4; 45–63 yrs.	1. Left posterior temporal and parietal infarction 2. Left CVA 3. Infarction in the area of the distribution of the left middle cerebral artery 4. Diffuse left-sided brain atrophy due to subarachnoid hemorrhage	Blissymbols	To determine whether Blissymbols can be used to facilitate spoken and written communication.	Subjects 1 and 2, who had the highest auditory comprehension scores on the Token Test, performed significantly better on Blissymbols compared with subjects 3 and 4, whose comprehension scores on the Token Test were low. The learning of Blissymbols did facilitate writing in subjects 1 and 4; however, its effect on facilitating spoken language was limited.

[3]PICA = Porch Index of Communicative Abilities

TABLE 19.1 *(Continued)*

AUTHORS	APHASIA TYPE AND SEVERITY	NUMBER OF SUBJECTS AND AGE RANGES	SITE OF LESIONS	TYPE OF SYMBOLS	GOALS/RESEARCH QUESTIONS	FINDINGS
Trunzo-Rahbar (1980)	Severe aphasia and apraxia of speech	N = 4; 59–68 yrs.	CVA (all 4 subjects)	Blissymbols	To determine whether individuals with severe aphasia and apraxia of speech can acquire Blissymbols. To determine whether acquisition of Blissymbols can provide an overall improvement in functional communication skills.	All subjects were able to learn and use Blissymbols to varying degrees. Those subjects who had better receptive language skills learned a greater number of symbols. Spoken responses increase in intelligibility when occurring in conjunction with the use of Blissymbols. There was a significant change in functional communication skills after 20 hours of exposure to Blissymbols.
Nishikawa (1980)	Expressive aphasia	N = 9; age range = NA	NA	Blissymbols	To determine whether Blissymbols augment the expressive communication of adults with severe aphasia. To determine whether there will be a statistically significant difference in the ability of subjects to respond to the graphic subtest of PICA, using Blissymbols vs. traditional orthography (TO).	Subjects demonstrated significantly improved ability in responding to the graphic subtest of PICA when aided by Blissymbols. Subjects demonstrated improved ability in speech production and word finding as measured by PICA after 3 months training with Blissymbols.

Study	Disorder	Subjects	Etiology	Symbol System	Purpose	Results
Ross (1979)	Brain damage due to trauma	N = 1; 14.3 yrs.	Traumatic brain injury (TBI)	Blissymbols	To teach the Blissymbol system as an additional means of communication.	Results indicated that Blissymbols extended the subject's ability to communicate with increased speed and less effort. Subject was also able to form sentences with correct word order using the symbols.
Gardner, Zurif, Berry, & Baker (1976)	Global aphasia (N = 6) Mixed aphasia (N = 1) Wernicke's aphasia (N = 1)	N = 8; all subjects over 50 yrs. of age except one who incurred lesion from trauma	CVA for all subjects except one who had trauma	VIC[4] (A set of index cards on which simple or arbitrary geometric forms or ideographs are drawn)	To teach communicative functions such as carrying out commands, answering questions, describing events, and expressing feelings and immediate needs via arbitrary or ideographic visual symbols.	All subjects were able to learn a simple set of visual symbols to carry out commands, answer questions, and describe actions. Two subjects, one of whom was left-handed and another who suffered a lesion due to trauma and was under 50 years of age, performed beyond a basic level and were able to use symbols for novel communication.
Glass, Gazzaniga, & Premack (1973)	Global aphasia	N = 7; 59–84 yrs.	CVA (all 7 subjects)	Graphic symbols varying in color, size, and shape	To determine whether individuals with global aphasia can learn graphic symbols.	All subjects were able to convey information through simple constructions using symbols. Two subjects were also able to express and comprehend simple declarative statements.

[4]VIC = Visual input communication

In fact, some of these individuals were able to carry out sophisticated rule-bound communication using visual symbols. These findings suggested that individuals with global aphasia may not have cognitive impairment to the same degree as they have language impairment.

Initial investigations into learning graphic symbols and manual signs by individuals with aphasia have suggested that pairing a graphic symbol or manual sign with a vocabulary item influences rate of learning and retention of the symbols or signs (Coelho, 1982; Hughes-Wheatland, 1989; Weinrich, Steele, Kleczewska, Carlson, & Baker, 1987). Graphic symbols such as line drawings, pictographs, and less transparent symbol systems such as Blissymbolics have often been used as an alternative mode of communication for individuals with severe aphasia (Funnell & Allport, 1989; Johannsen-Horbach et al., 1985; Lane & Samples, 1981; Nishikawa, 1980; Ross, 1979; Sawyer-Woods, 1987; Trunzo-Rahbar, 1980). In most of these studies, individuals with aphasia learned symbols to varying degrees. Funnell and Allport (1989) found that words and graphic symbols with high iconicity were acquired more frequently than words and symbols with low iconicity by two subjects with severe aphasia. In addition, they observed that the influence of word class on performance and learning of graphic symbols or manual signs is secondary to iconicity. Johannsen-Horbach et al. (1985) observed that their subjects learned more Blissymbols that depicted nouns than those that depicted function words or adjectives. Blissymbols for nouns tend to be iconic compared with those for function words and adjectives.

Kraat (1990) observed that for individuals with severe aphasia, transparent and translucent graphic symbols and manual signs are more easily learned and retained than opaque symbols. Transparent symbols have meanings that can be easily identified in the absence of cues such as verbal hints or written words. Translucent symbols have a semantic, conceptual, or linguistic relationship with their referents that may be perceived when the symbols and referents are paired. Opaque symbols have no conceptual or semantic relationship with their referents. Lloyd and Fuller (1990) provide an extensive review of symbol iconicity research. For a further discussion of aided symbols, see Chapter 6, and for unaided symbols, see Chapter 7.

Koul and Lloyd (1994a) investigated the effects of symbol translucency and complexity on the recognition and retention of graphic symbols by individuals with aphasia. A group of subjects with aphasia resulting from lesions in the left middle cerebral artery, a group of subjects with damage in the right hemisphere, and a control group of neurologically normal individuals participated. A total of 40 Blissymbols were selected as stimulus items. Each subject participated in two experimental sessions. During Session 1, a visual matching task was administered to ensure that all subjects were able to adequately discriminate between the experimental stimuli. Subjects who successfully completed the visual matching task were exposed to the experimental task for the remaining part of the first experimental session. Session 2, which examined retention of symbols, was held one week after the completion of the first experimental session. A paired-associate learning paradigm was used to teach the symbol–referent pairs to all three groups of subjects in the experimental tasks. Results indicated that individuals with aphasia learned pictographic, ideographic, and opaque Blissymbols. Although no significant difference was found between the individuals with aphasia and the individuals in the neurologically normal control group in learning the arbitrary or opaque Blissymbols, the superior performance of individuals with aphasia on both arbitrary and pictographic Blissymbols compared with individuals with right hemisphere brain damage was interesting, especially because five of the aphasic individuals had global aphasia and demonstrated minimal competence on standard aphasia tests.

Although individuals with moderate aphasia performed better than individuals with global aphasia in guessing and learning symbols, the difference in performance failed to reach significant levels. This suggests that performance on recognition of single graphic symbols may be independent of the severity and type of aphasia. Transparency and high translucency were found to be potent factors in the recognition of Blissymbols by subjects in all three experimental groups. Complexity, defined by the number of strokes comprising the symbol, did not, on the other hand, have any influence on the recognition of Blissymbols by individuals with aphasia, individuals with right hemisphere damage, and individuals in the neurologically normal control group. In fact, no correlation was found between a priori determined complexity values and the symbols correctly recognized by the subjects in the three groups. Also, no significant interaction was found between translucency and complexity.

Lane and Samples (1981) and Sawyer-Woods (1987) reported a significant positive correlation between receptive language ability and learning Blissymbols. They observed that individuals with aphasia who had higher scores on receptive language tests performed significantly better on the task of learning Blissymbols than individuals who demonstrated lower receptive language skills.

The finding that individuals with aphasia can learn and retain graphic symbols has significant clinical implications for aphasia therapy. Currently there are several approaches to aphasia rehabilitation. One of these is to compensate for or provide alternatives to bypass damaged language components. Another is to focus on using an individual's intact abilities. The study by Koul and Lloyd (1994a) suggests that the undamaged right hemisphere in individuals with aphasia can be used to facilitate communication through graphic symbols. This approach to aphasia therapy for individuals with severe and global aphasia capitalizes on untapped capabilities of undamaged areas of the brain. However, further research is needed to evaluate whether individuals with aphasia can learn and use graphic symbols in naturally occurring communication environments.

The finding that translucency has a facilitative effect on learning also has clinical implications. If the goal of aphasia therapy is to provide an immediate means of communication for individuals with severe and global aphasia, one should consider choosing initial lexical items that have a strong visual relationship between symbol and referent. Several previous studies have agreed that a role does exist for alternative imagery enhancing techniques in aphasia therapy (Altman, 1977; Cannezzio, 1977; Fitch-West, 1983). Cannezzio (1977)

investigated the effects of imagery on a word-matching task in 16 individuals with aphasia. Subjects were asked to decide whether the second word was the same or different from the first word. Results indicated that words of high imageability were more quickly matched than words of low imageability. Similar findings were observed by Altman (1977) in individuals with aphasia who demonstrated greater recognition for picture-picture pairs than for word-picture or word-word pairs. In summary, using concrete words and iconic graphic symbols may greatly enhance and facilitate communication in individuals with severe and/or global aphasia.

With the recent rapid proliferation of AAC technologies, a computerized visual input communication (C-VIC) system has been developed and used by several researchers to observe whether individuals with severe aphasia can access, manipulate, and combine visual icons by following several rules of communication specific to the C-VIC system (Weinrich, 1991). C-VIC is primarily a computerized version of the Gardner et al. (1976) VIC. C-VIC contains a lexicon of iconographic symbols that subjects access by using a mouse. Symbols are arranged in a linear sequence in accordance with the taught syntax. Of interest is the ability of the subjects to communicate correctly using the computer system (Steele, Weinrich, Wertz, Kleczewska, & Carlson, 1989; Weinrich et al., 1989). Results indicated that subjects not only accessed the icons but also performed markedly better on C-VIC than on natural language tasks as measured through several subtests of the PICA (Porch, 1981). In addition, individuals with both Broca's and global aphasia were able to comprehend and produce locative prepositional phrases more easily using the C-VIC. They had difficulties performing a similar task with the same phrases in English (Weinrich et al., 1989; Weinrich et al., 1993).

In summary, individuals with severe and global aphasia perform significantly better on a variety of communication tasks using graphic symbols than when using natural language. However, aphasia intervention needs to go beyond simple modality exchange. Individuals with severe and global aphasia should be given opportunities to use multiple modes (natural and taught) to bring about maximum functional changes in their communication (Kraat, 1990).

Aphasia Classification Scheme to Guide Intervention. Garrett and Beukelman (1992) were the first in the AAC scientific community to provide a comprehensive scheme of classification for individuals with aphasia that can be used to guide AAC intervention. They classified individuals with aphasia into five distinct categories, each requiring somewhat different types of AAC intervention.

According to this classification scheme, individuals who exhibit the characteristics of global aphasia are **basic-choice communicators**. These individuals have severe impairment in both comprehension and expression of natural language. Comprehension, however, is often reported to be somewhat better than expression (Love & Webb, 1992). Spoken expressive language is typically limited to automatic speech and/or repetitive vocalizations. Garrett and Beukelman (1992) recommend that the goal of AAC intervention with basic-choice communicators is to provide a system through which they can express basic needs and choices, especially regarding activities of daily living. These communicators often require cues, prompts, and assistance in indicating choices. Making choices incorporates the skills of scanning, pointing, and grasping. Real items or communication boards can be used (Figure 19.1). Garrett and Beukelman (1992) emphasize the importance of encouragement and training for communication partners and caregivers so that they can facilitate communication for individuals with global aphasia.

Controlled-situation communicators are individuals with aphasia who can indicate their needs by spontaneously pointing to items and objects (Garrett & Beukelman, 1992). An individual with severe chronic Broca's aphasia will probably fall into this category. These individuals do not typically initiate communication and need a great degree of assistance in routine conversational exchanges. AAC intervention for controlled-situa-

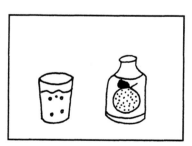

**Do you want your meds
with water or juice?**

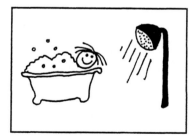

**Do you want a bath
or a shower today?**

FIGURE 19.1   Sample Boards for Basic-Choice Communicators

tion communicators typically includes the provision of picture symbols and/or words that can be used when individuals encounter difficulty initiating or sustaining conversation (Figure 19.2). Controlled-situation communicators can point to one of several topic choices on a communication board to indicate what they would like to talk about. After choosing a topic, they may be able to communicate more specific information. Garrett and Beukelman (1992) recommend providing controlled-situation communicators with notebooks containing words related to conversational topics that can be chosen to facilitate communication. Topic boards can also be used to direct and enhance communication exchanges.

Individuals who require graphic symbols or gestures to augment speech input from communication partners are categorized as **augmented-input communicators** (Garrett & Beukelman, 1992). These individuals demonstrate significant impairment in auditory comprehension, falling under the category of Wernicke's or transcortical sensory aphasia. The communication partners of augmented-input communicators typically require training to develop skill in providing augmented input. This training helps alleviate communication breakdowns. An augmented-input communicator can demonstrate comprehension of conversation by responding to written key words, gesturing, and indicating points on a rating scale. A communication board with a scale on it can be useful when communication partners want to express information and feelings about themselves and also when they seek information from the augmented-input communicator (Figure 19.3).

Comprehensive communicators include individuals with aphasia who typically have independent lifestyles and wish to participate in a variety of communication contexts. These individuals are typically able to point to symbols or words and can use gestures to augment their limited spoken language. AAC intervention for comprehensive communicators varies depending on participatory patterns and communication needs.

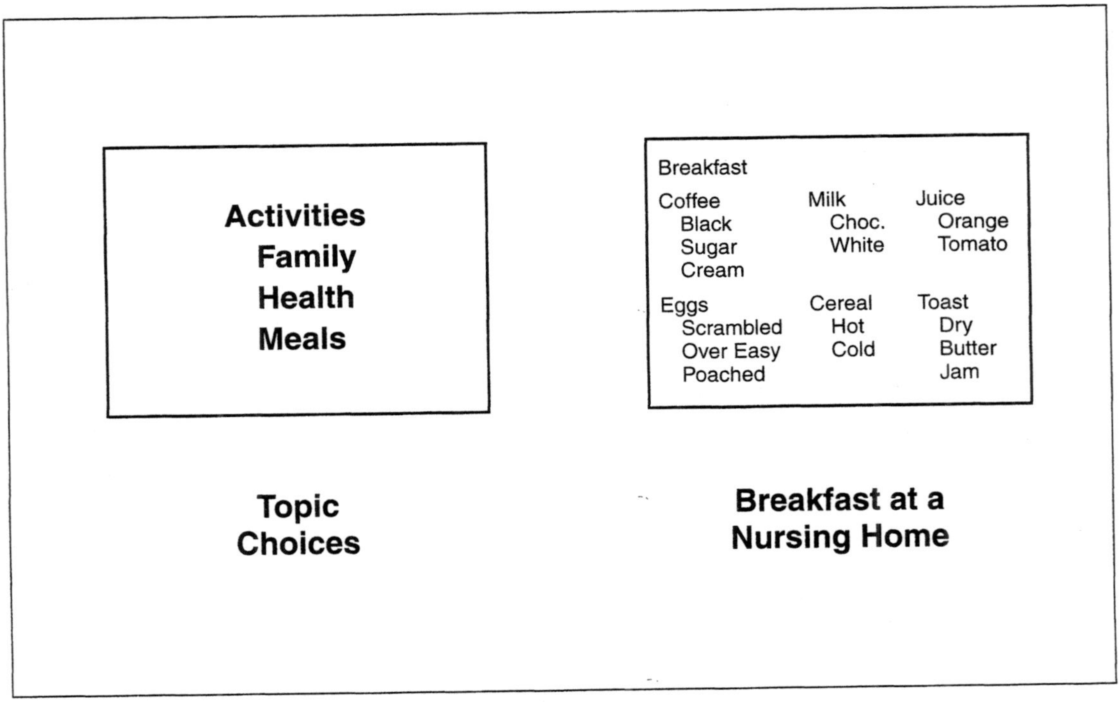

FIGURE 19.2   Sample Boards for Controlled-Situation Communicators

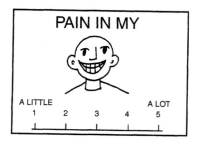

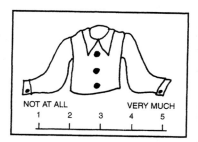

FIGURE 19.3   Sample Boards for Augmented-Input Communicators

Beukelman, Yorkston, and Dowden (1985) described an individual with Broca's aphasia who used a series of AAC techniques as he progressed through several stages of recovery. In the beginning, the individual communicated through simple photographs and line drawings mounted on a communication board. Later, he used a voice output communication aid (VOCA).

In many cases, individuals with aphasia develop reliable unaided yes/no responses. They may, for example, nod their heads or use eye-blink codes. They also may use aided approaches, however. Some clinicians have reported that a card with "yes" and "no" can still be useful. Garrett et al. (1989) listed alphabet cards, conversational control phrases, and breakdown resolution clues along with natural communication modes (e.g., gestures, writing) as possible components of an AAC system for comprehensive communicators (Figure 19.4). A comprehensive communicator may use both low technology and high technology (e.g., a letter board and/or a VOCA to communicate biographical information). An important aspect of successful AAC intervention with comprehensive communicators is the considerable training and practice required to become efficient with the various AAC techniques and devices (Garrett & Beukelman, 1992).

Individuals with mild to moderate aphasia who need communication support in specific situations may fall under the category of **specific-need communicators**. According to Garrett and Beukelman (1992), the scope of AAC intervention with specific-need communicators is limited because most of these individuals are able to communicate through simple syntactic constructions and gestures. In some instances, however, AAC strategies are helpful in facilitating accurate information efficiently.

An individual with aphasia who wants to communicate information during the leisure activity of playing bingo, for example, may use bingo paddles to aid in playing and for announcing that the game is over. A communication card with specific bank-

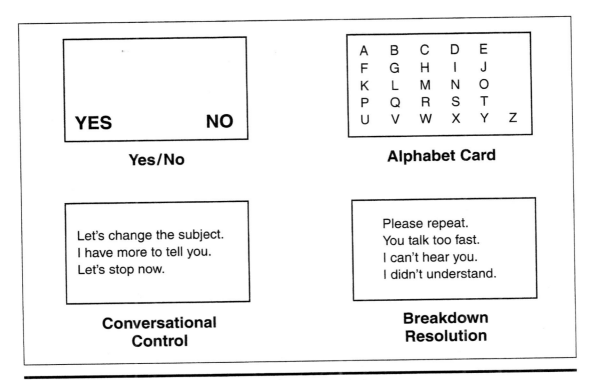

FIGURE 19.4   Sample Boards for Comprehensive Communicators

ing instructions and dollar amounts can facilitate specific information, which allows specific-need communicators more independence in controlling their finances (Figure 19.5).

Multiple Profile of Symbolic Capacities in Aphasia. Aphasiologists have debated frequently whether aphasia entails a central symbolic deficit in which a decrease in competence is seen across a range of symbol systems (i.e., from nonlinguistic pictures to purely linguistic symbols), or whether aphasia specifically impairs only the ability to process linguistic symbols. The theory that multiple profiles of symbolic capacities exist in aphasia is strongly supported by data obtained in research on disconnection syndromes, recognition and retention of graphic symbols, kanji/kana dissociation, pantomime interpretation, and sign and gesture dissociations (Corina, Poizner, Bellugi, Feinberg, Dowd, & O'Grady-Batch, 1992; Gainotti, Silveri, & Sena, 1989; Geschwind, 1965; Glass et al., 1973; Koul & Lloyd, 1994a; Sasanuma, 1986; Varney, 1978, 1982; Wang & Goodglass, 1992; Wap-

ner & Gardner, 1981). All of these data point to the fact that individuals with aphasia, although demonstrating deficits in both spoken linguistic competence and ASL, perform considerably better on tasks involving graphic or gestural symbolic systems. Wapner and Gardner (1981), for example, explored visual symbolic disturbances in individuals with aphasia, individuals with right hemisphere brain damage, and neurologically normal controls. Subjects were exposed to seven categories of visual symbols ranging from pictures to traffic signs to written phrases. Results indicated that individuals with aphasia and individuals from the control group performed similarly on tasks involving pictures, traffic signs, and trademarks. In contrast, a marked dissociation in performance was seen between individuals with aphasia and control subjects on purely linguistic stimuli. Linguistic stimuli posed special difficulties for individuals with aphasia. In addition, individuals with right hemisphere damage demonstrated poorer performance on pictures, traffic signs, and trademarks, but depicted profiles akin to controls on linguistic stimuli. These

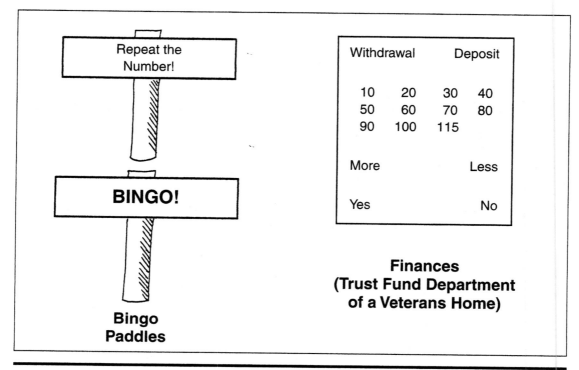

FIGURE 19.5   Sample Boards for Specific-Need Communicators

results are in accordance with results obtained by Koul and Lloyd (1994a), who observed that individuals with aphasia and control subjects did not demonstrate a significant difference on the learning and retaining of transparent, translucent, and opaque Blissymbols. However, individuals with right hemisphere damage learned significantly fewer low-translucent symbols as well as high-translucent symbols than individuals with aphasia and individuals in the neurologically normal control group.

The role of the right hemisphere in processing pictures was demonstrated by Gainotti et al. (1989) who observed that right hemisphere lesions lead to poorer visual recognition scores. Studies involving patients with focal brain lesions in the right hemisphere have established that the right hemisphere, particularly the right temporal lobe, plays a significant role in the learning, retention, and memory of representational drawings for concrete nouns and abstract geometric patterns, much as the left temporal lobe plays a critical role in processing verbal material (Cermak & Tarlow,

1978; De Renzi, 1968; Goldstein, Canavan, & Polkey, 1988; Jones-Gottman, 1979, 1986; Jones-Gottman & Milner, 1978). De Renzi and Lucchelli (1993) suggested that the right hemisphere may also be responsible for perception as well as meaningful recognition of visual symbols.

Several studies have reported that gestural/pantomime comprehension is strongly associated with language comprehension in individuals with aphasia (Duffy, Duffy, & Pearson, 1975; Gainotti & Lemmo, 1976). Duffy and Duffy (1981) observed that aphasia consists of dissolution of both linguistic and nonlinguistic behaviors and can be explained as a consequence of central symbolic deficit. However, data reported in several other studies suggested that impairment in pantomime comprehension is displayed by only a small percentage of patients with aphasia (Christopoulous & Bonvillian, 1985; Daniloff, Noll, Fristoe, & Lloyd, 1982; Varney, 1982) and that no correlation exists between pantomime comprehension and auditory comprehension (Varney & Benton, 1982). The absence of a correlation between pantomime comprehension and auditory comprehension may indicate that the reason for impaired pantomime comprehension may be more specific than a central symbolic disorder. Wang and Goodglass (1992) explained that impaired pantomime comprehension may be the result of **apraxia**. In their study on the performance of 30 patients with aphasia on several tests of pantomime production and comprehension, they observed that apraxia affects not only purposeful production of, but also comprehension of limb movements. Additionally, several studies have shown that individuals with severe aphasia can recognize manual signs and standardized gestures, such as Amer-Ind (Herrmann, Reichle, Lucius-Hoene, Wallesch, & Johannsen-Horbach, 1988; Kelsch, 1979; Rao & Horner, 1979; Skelly, 1979). The ability of individuals with severe aphasia to acquire manual signs, gestures, or graphic symbols and their inability to reacquire spoken language skills even after long and intensive speech therapy provides strong support for a theory of multiple symbolic capacities.

Further support for the multiple profile of symbolic capacities for individuals with aphasia comes from the dissociation of ideographic kanji and syllabic kana in Japanese individuals with aphasia. Case studies of Japanese individuals with brain damage show that the right hemisphere is more involved in the processing of ideographic kanji, and the left hemisphere is superior in the processing of syllabic kana (Paradis, Hagiwara, & Hildebrandt, 1985; Sugishita, Iwata, Toyokura, Yoshioka, & Yamada, 1978; Yamadori, Nagashima, & Tamaki, 1983; Yamadori, Osumi, Ikeda, & Kanazawa, 1980).

In summary, the multiple profile of symbolic capacities in aphasia has abundant support, which provides strong theoretical and empirical bases for using AAC symbol sets and/or systems with individuals with aphasia.

ACQUIRED PROGRESSIVE NEUROGENIC DISEASES

Several acquired progressive (also referred to as degenerative) neurogenic diseases present challenges to the provision of AAC services. AAC interventions that apply to specific progressive diseases are discussed in the following sections. Many of the same intervention principles that apply to individuals with aphasia also apply to those with acquired progressive neurogenic diseases. AAC service providers should focus on the following areas:

1. Recognize the need for transdisciplinary intervention involving professionals from disciplines such as nursing, occupational therapy, physical therapy, psychology, social services, and speech-language pathology.
2. Assess not only physical, sensory, cognitive, and linguistic impairments, but also comprehensively assess residual strengths and abilities.
3. Design AAC strategies and techniques that not only compensate for the loss of spoken language abilities, but also enhance and facilitate intact functional skills.
4. Recognize the need for ongoing support and follow-up.

Specific intervention strategies and techniques for individuals with acquired progressive neurogenic diseases, however, are quite different than those for individuals with aphasia. The chronic and degenerative nature of progressive neurogenic diseases brings additional issues to address.

Amyotrophic Lateral Sclerosis

Amyotrophic lateral sclerosis (ALS) is an insidious, progressive, degenerative disease of unknown etiology. The pathophysiology of ALS involves degeneration of both upper and lower motor neuron systems, which usually appears in midlife. The prevalence rate is 5 to 7 cases per 100,000 people (Rewcastle, 1991). The male-to-female ratio is 2:1 (Emery & Holloway, 1982). The general clinical picture of individuals with ALS at any particular point in the disease process depends on relative prominence of the upper motor neuron lesions, the lower motor neuron lesions, or the combined effects of both the upper and lower motor neuron lesions. When the disease process begins with the degeneration of the motor nuclei in the brain stem, the initial symptoms are usually **dysarthria** and **dysphagia**.

Communication Characteristics. Individuals with ALS usually do not exhibit language or sensory impairments as a result of the disease. Mixed dysarthria of the spastic-flaccid type and dysphagia, however, invariably occur at some point during the course of the disease (Darley, Aronson, & Brown, 1975). Tandan and Bradley (1985) reported that about 39% of individuals with ALS survive for about 5 years, about 10% survive 10 years, and a few may live up to 20 years after the onset of the disease. About 75% of individuals with ALS are unable to speak at the time of their death (Beukelman & Mirenda, 1992). The differential rates of mortality in individuals with ALS and increasing advances in medicine have led to an increase in the life span for individuals with degenerative diseases. To allow individuals with ALS to function optimally and be contributing members to society, AAC intervention is not only desirable, but necessary.

AAC Intervention. Assessment of motor control is the most important part of service delivery for individuals with ALS. Motor capabilities of persons with ALS depend on whether the disease process predominantly affects bulbar or spinal areas of the brain. Individuals with bulbar ALS are generally able to use their hands or fingers. They may be able to directly select a letter on an alphabet board or use a key alphabet or key-word encoding technique to produce sentences and phrases. However, individuals with spinal ALS have impairments predominantly related to limb control. Their main need is to obtain a supplement to enhance writing skills. These individuals can benefit from software writing programs with features such as word prediction and abbreviation expansion, which can improve writing efficiency by reducing the number of keystrokes required to convey messages.

Because ALS is progressive, an AAC system must be modified as individual abilities change. Initially, an individual with ALS may use natural speech or a direct selection device. As the disease progresses and impairment of upper extremities increases, the individual may require a device with single-switch scanning capabilities. Yorkston (1989) described early intervention using AAC

with a woman who had ALS, emphasizing the need for multiple AAC approaches as the patient's motor-speech disorders worsened. First, a portable speech amplifier was used to improve speech intelligibility due to compromised respiratory support. Later, this patient was taught to use a pocket-sized alphabet board. She either pointed to the first letter of each word she spoke or spelled out the entire word as necessary. Writing with pen and paper was used as a backup system for communicating longer messages. An adapted typewriter was given to her, but she preferred to use pen and paper (Yorkston, 1989). A VOCA and a message encoding technique that enhances the speed of communication may be an appropriate choice for individuals with ALS who have severe physical disabilities without cognitive impairments. Stephen Hawking, the British physicist, is an example of an individual with ALS who uses a sophisticated VOCA and power mobility to aid in maintaining an active lifestyle (Beukelman & Mirenda, 1992).

Parkinson's Disease

The clinical characteristics of **Parkinson's disease** typically include slowness in initiating and performing volitional motor movements, rigidity, flat affect (expressionless face), and a resting tremor of the pill-rolling type. The pathological basis for the syndrome lies in the degeneration of the substantia nigra due to deficiency of dopamine in the nigrostriatal pathway. However, recent research indicates that the locus of damage extends beyond the substantia nigra and includes locus ceruleus, a nucleus that generates the neurotransmitter norepinephrine, and raphe nuclei neurons that generate the neurotransmitters serotonin, noradrenaline, and dopamine (Hornykiewicz & Kish, 1986). Medical therapy for individuals with Parkinson's disease involves replacement of dopamine through the use of levodopa. This therapy is not totally effective, and, despite long-term use of levodopa, the disease progresses, possibly as a result of degeneration in the other neurotransmitter systems. The disease is usually sporadic with insidious onset occurring by the sixth decade (Rewcastle, 1991). Epidemiological data have shown a prevalence rate of 73 to 179 cases per 100,000 population worldwide (Schoenberg, 1987). Dementia is not commonly associated with individuals with Parkinson's disease; however, 15% of individuals with Parkinson's disease develop dementia, which is six times more than the percentage observed in an age-matched general population (Boller, Mitzutani, Roessmann, & Gambetti, 1980; Lees, 1985).

Communication Characteristics. The nature and type of speech disorders among individuals with Parkinson's disease vary depending on the stage of the disease as well as response to treatment (Love & Webb, 1992). Typical speech and voice characteristics of individuals with Parkinson's disease are imprecise articulation, excessively fast speaking rate, hoarseness, hypernasality, and reduced loudness (Darley et al., 1975; Logemann, Fisher, Boshes, & Blonsky, 1978). Logemann et al. (1978) observed 200 individuals with Parkinson's disease and found that 45% exhibited articulatory problems and 89% demonstrated laryngeally related problems.

Despite the rapid advances in medical treatment of Parkinson's disease, the long-term prognosis is still very bleak. As the disease progresses, most of the motor systems, including speech, rapidly deteriorate. AAC intervention provided at an appropriate stage may help these individuals communicate more effectively. To date, however, no data are available on the number of individuals with impaired speech due to Parkinson's disease who have benefited from AAC intervention.

AAC Intervention. Individuals with Parkinson's disease do not typically demonstrate cognitive and/or linguistic deficits unless dementia is associated with the disease process. In the absence of severe cognitive deficits, individuals with Parkinson's disease may be suitable candidates for high-technology AAC intervention. The primary motor control problems associated with Parkinson's disease need to be taken into account. Selection of an appropriate AAC device requires in-depth and individualized assessment of range and speed of movement, tremor, and rigidity. For example, if an individual with Parkinson's disease has a reduced range of movement of the upper limbs due to rigidity, the size of the selection display (e.g., on an alphabet keyboard) will need to be reduced (Beukelman & Mirenda, 1992). Beukelman and Mirenda (1992) recommend the use of a keyguard to dampen extensive tremor of the hands.

Very few studies document the effect of AAC intervention with individuals with Parkinson's disease. Yorkston, Beukelman, and Bell (1988) reported using an alphabet and/or word board to augment the communication of individuals with Parkinson's disease. The alphabet board technique requires the speaker to point to the first letter of each word as it is spoken. This technique not only provides additional information to communication partners but also forces speakers to reduce their speaking rates (Beukelman & Mirenda, 1992). Beukelman and Mirenda (1992) observe that for some individuals with Parkinson's disease, the reduction in speaking rate significantly contributes to improved intelligibility. A number of individuals with Parkinson's disease speak with reduced loudness. These individuals may also require some kind of speech amplification system to enhance and facilitate communication.

Progressive Supranuclear Palsy

Progressive supranuclear palsy (PSP) is a nonfamilial, degenerative disease. It is characterized by supranuclear opthalmoparesis (impaired vertical gaze in the upward direction, which progresses to involve the downward gaze), gait difficulty, falling, postural instability, and pseudobulbar palsy (Frasca, Blumbergs, Henschke, & Burns, 1991). The onset of PSP is gradual. The primary initial complaint is recurrent and/or unpredictable backward falls or gait disturbance characterized by slowness and hesitancy (Frasca et al., 1991). Patients tend to become progressively unable to ambulate independently. In later stages, patients require full care (Sosner, Wall, & Sznajder, 1993). PSP is difficult to diagnose and, as a result, is usually diagnosed in later stages. In its initial stages, symptoms are similar to Parkinson's disease. According to Sosner et al. (1993), 4% of individuals diagnosed with Parkinson's disease have PSP. Male-to-female ratio tends to be equal; age of onset can be 60 to 70 years (Frasca et al., 1991). In addition to the symptoms listed above, other (secondary) symptoms may include dysarthria, dementia, and in later stages, dysphagia. Initially the swallowing response is normal, but studies have shown that individuals with PSP develop a delayed swallow.

Communication Characteristics.   Initially, some individuals with PSP have reported word-finding difficulties (Sosner et al., 1993). For the most part, however, individuals with PSP have intact language. Language deficits are typically not present unless dementia is associated with the disease process. More common is mixed dysarthria with weak voice, which progresses in later stages to anarthria (Sosner et al., 1993). Behavioral characteristics may include distractibility and short attention span.

AAC Intervention.   An important factor to consider when designing an AAC system for these individuals is their visual impairment. The use of alphabet communication boards may not be appropriate unless carefully designed to accommodate vision. Symbol options must be carefully evaluated. There is currently little documentation on the effect of AAC intervention with individuals with PSP.

Multiple Sclerosis

Multiple sclerosis (MS) is a degenerative disease of the myelin sheath. The myelin in various areas of the central nervous system breaks down resulting in a variety of symptoms such as diplopia (double vision), loss or reduction of sensation, tingling in the extremities, dizziness, and dysarthria. This seemingly unrelated symptomatology provides an important clue in diagnosing the illness (Liebman & Tadmor, 1991). Multiple sclerosis primarily attacks young adults 20 to 40 years of age. The female-to-male ratio is approximately 1.5 : 1 (Arnason, 1982). One of the surprising characteristics of MS is the discrepancy in prevalence between warm and cold climates. Its prevalence rate in tropical areas is 1 per 100,000. In contrast, its prevalence rate in colder areas, such as

Canada, the Northern United States, and Northern Europe, is 30 to 80 per 100,000 (Liebman & Tadmor, 1991). The cause of MS is unknown, and at present there is no known cure.

The clinical course of MS presents itself in three main forms (Liebman & Tadmor, 1991; Poser, 1984). The first form accounts for approximately 20% of the individuals with MS. These individuals have few episodes and then recover completely. Individuals with the second form exhibit chronic, progressive symptoms. These individuals have a number of attacks and remissions that last for many years. The third form accounts for approximately 5 to 10% of the individuals with MS. This form predominantly affects young people. Attacks progress and spread rapidly over the entire nervous system resulting in death in a relatively short time.

Communication Characteristics.   Varying degrees of dysarthria ranging from mild to severe were reported in 41% of 168 patients diagnosed with MS in a Mayo Clinic study (Darley et al., 1975). Normal speech was observed in the remaining 59%. Beukelman and Mirenda (1992) reported that the prevalence of dysarthria in individuals with MS ranges from 19 to 41%, depending on the sampling procedure and the methodology involved in judging dysarthria. No single type of dysarthria is typical of MS; dysarthria is determined by site of lesion and not the disease process per se.

Beukelman, Kraft, and Freal (1985) conducted a survey of individuals with MS in which only 4% of 656 respondents indicated that their speech was severely unintelligible to the point that unfamiliar partners were unable to understand them. This suggests that most individuals with MS may not require an AAC system, at least in the initial stages of the disorder. However, temporary use of an AAC system may benefit individuals during relapses that occur in the early phases. Individuals with chronic MS may benefit from an AAC system that augments their communication skills as the disease progresses.

AAC Intervention.   Two major factors need to be taken into consideration in designing an AAC system for individuals with MS. One is the temporary nature of AAC intervention because of relapses and remissions in the early stages. The second is the impairment of sensory, perceptual, and/or motor skills that may constrain the use of AAC. Visual impairment, for example, is common in MS. About 16 to 30% of individuals with MS demonstrate subacute loss of central vision in one eye as the first symptom of the disease (Beukelman & Mirenda, 1992). Such visual limitations may constrain the use of AAC techniques. However, auditory scanning systems, large-print texts, and synthetic speech output of selected letters and words can help. Honsinger (1989) described an AAC device designed to meet the needs of a 30-year-old woman with visual impairment that consisted of an expanded keyboard with 1-inch square keys and synthetic speech output.

Assessment of motor abilities is an important aspect of AAC intervention with individuals with MS. The specific motor impairment depends on the site of lesion. Individuals with **pyramidal** lesions mainly demonstrate spasticity resulting in reduced range of movement. Intention tremor is a common motor control problem in individuals with **extrapyramidal** lesions. This tremor is often problematic for an individual when accessing a keyboard or a switch (Beukelman & Mirenda, 1992). Clinicians/educators must devise specific individualized strategies and techniques to reduce the interference of the tremor when accessing an AAC device.

A positive factor for AAC intervention is the noted absence of linguistic deficits in studies of MS patients (Olmos-Lau, Ginsberg, & Geller, 1977). However, Beukelman and Mirenda (1992) reported that earlier studies indicated that 1 to 3% of individuals with MS did have aphasia. The presence of aphasia in addition to severe motor and visual problems presents a challenge to successful AAC intervention.

Alzheimer's Disease

Alzheimer's disease (AD) is the most common cause of primary, degenerative dementia. Most epidemiological studies indicate the prevalence rate of AD over the age of 60 years ranges from 1,900 to 5,800 per 100,000 people (Rewcastle, 1991). According to one classification scheme, AD has been divided into three stages. Stage I is characterized by the onset of the deterioration of recent memory, disorientation, mood disturbances, and difficulty in dealing with day-to-day tasks. It lasts for approximately 7 years. Stage II involves rapid intellectual deterioration and symptoms resembling certain clinical aspects of aphasia, apraxia, and agnosia. It lasts approximately 3 years. During stage III, an individual is usually highly demented and bed bound. The individual is typically fed intravenously because the ability to chew food has been lost. Death occurs during this stage, most often due to bronchopneumonia because of stasis as well as aspiration (Nielsen, Homma, & Biorn-Henriksen, 1977; Rewcastle, 1991). Radiological investigations of the brains of individuals with AD indicate marked atrophy of the cerebral hemispheres and widening of the sulci and lateral ventricles (Liebman & Tadmor, 1991). Microscopically, neurofibrillary tangles and neuritic plaques are present in large numbers in frontal, parietal, and temporal regions of the brain (Rewcastle, 1991).

Communication Characteristics. Individuals with AD have communication disabilities that significantly reduce their ability to carry out satisfactory communicative interactions with friends and families (Bayles & Kaszniak, 1987; Fromm & Holland, 1989). During the initial stages of the disease, individuals demonstrate auditory comprehension deficits, word-finding difficulties, and pragmatic errors such as poor initiation and speaking for an unusually long time on a topic. Initially, there are no phonological errors. In the later stages, however, the ability to produce functional speech is progressively lost. Pragmatic and semantic deficits are replaced by confused and incoherent language. Some patients become mute, whereas others become echolalic (Nicholas, Obler, Albert, & Helm-Estabrooks, 1985).

Defining the role of the speech-language pathologist who works with individuals who have memory loss is a continuing challenge that is often not supported. This may be due to the progressive nature of the disease and the limited ability of individuals with AD to learn new information and maintain skills (Bourgeois, 1990). Many times, speech-language pathologists do not work with patients with AD because they have not had adequate training. Sometimes treatment is not initiated because of lack of third-party funding.

AAC Intervention. One important focus of intervention is to train communication partners, particularly caregivers and family members, how to interact with patients with AD (Ripich, 1994). Training should focus on teaching caregivers to understand the nature of language and cognitive losses as well as on teaching specific skills to facilitate communicative interactions. Environmental considerations to enhance the communication and well-being of patients are also important. Caregivers and family members should provide situations and facilitate interactions that minimize the effects of memory loss, use the patient's retained abilities, and eliminate the chance of failure. Communication partners should look for communication cues and listen for the message behind the words of patients with AD.

Interactions with patients who have AD should be direct and unambiguous. One should face patients, make eye contact, and use their names to gain their attention. Repeating utterances may be necessary to provide clarity. One should use short, simple sentences. One should not, however, talk down to patients. Individuals with AD are adults who merit respect and should not be spoken to as if they were children. Asking yes/no or choice questions is typically better than asking open-ended questions. Additionally, interactions are facilitated by using nondirective comments. Specific nouns should be used instead of pronouns or vague terms. Using the same spoken phrases to signal routine daily activities is helpful in communicating and establishing routines.

Patients with AD tend to focus on a communication partner's gestures, facial expressions, and body movements as well as a person's physical appearance. As the individual with AD becomes less able to speak and understand spoken language, these cues become more important. Gesturing and pointing to objects or persons can help

patients with AD to gain information. Appropriately touching patients to gain their attention (after gauging the individual's reaction to touch) can also be helpful (Bowlby, 1993). To avoid confusion, facial expression should match the message. Body movements can be used to supply additional information for individuals with memory loss. One clinician reported that she was not feeling well and was asked "What's the matter?" by a patient with middle-stage AD who had observed her sad face. In turn, communication partners gain information by paying attention to the gestures, facial expressions, and body movements of patients with AD (Bowlby, 1993; Tomoeda & Bayles, 1990). Because patients will often be embarrassed because they may not remember names, they sometimes focus on a person's physical appearance. Patients with middle-stage AD often comment on bright clothing and are very good at relating individuals to a description of their appearance (e.g., the patient may nod and look when the clinician says, "You know Lisa, the woman who wears earrings and smiles all the time."). Simply paying attention and allowing the patient the opportunity to communicate can be very helpful for the patient with middle-to-late stage AD. Social skills may remain intact for a long time, and patients may enjoy waving hello and using polite words such as "please" and "thank you." When an interaction is over, the communication partner should make it clear to the patient by using a departure signal or phrase (Bowlby, 1993; Clark & Witte, 1995; D. Clemens, personal communication, May 5, 1995; Ripich, 1994). Table 19.2 summarizes techniques to improve interactions with patients who have memory loss.

Very little empirical data exist on the effectiveness of AAC intervention with individuals with AD. AAC has, however, been found to aid the communication of some. Silverman (1994) found that only 4 out of 28 survey respondents (i.e., speech-language pathologists) who worked with individuals with AD tried AAC strategies and techniques. All four, however, reported that AAC intervention helped their patients to some degree. Bourgeois (1990, 1991, 1992, 1993) conducted a series of studies designed to remediate communi-

TABLE 19.2   Techniques To Improve Interactions with Patients with Memory Loss

1. Approach patients face-to-face, using names. "Hi, Mr. Smith. It's me, Sally, your nurse."

2. Use short, simple sentences. Ask one question or give one request at a time.

3. Talk about the here and now. Use gestures, point to objects or pictures to help illustrate the message.

4. Allow patients a chance to respond. Use pause time.

5. Use nouns rather than pronouns (which can be vague and confusing). "Where is Kathy?" is better than "Where is she?" "The book is over on the table" is better than "It's over there."

6. Speak in a calm manner. Speak slowly but not too slowly. Avoid speaking too loudly.

7. Facilitate communication with nondirective comments. "Let's go to the dining room" is more pleasant than "Come on to lunch."

8. Use the same spoken phrases for the same routine daily activities. "Your food is ready" can indicate mealtimes. "Let's go to bed" can indicate bedtime. "Put your coat on" can indicate going outside.

9. Realize that there is a capacity for understanding, but never assume a message has been received. Be prepared to repeat a message.

10. Communicate using a variety of modes (e.g., gestures, facial expressions, body movements). Use touch (which can both calm and excite) to reassure. Use calm and inviting facial expressions (e.g., smiles can be reassuring). Match facial expressions to messages to provide redundancy not dissonance (e.g., happy face for happy messages). Use direct eye contact. Use body movements to provide information.

11. Be responsive to patients' emotional states. "Oh, you look like you are having fun!" often elicits responses from patients.

12. Speak with all patients regardless of language abilities. Keep messages short, clear, and familiar (e.g., discuss caregiving activities, weather, how they look).

13. Listen attentively with an appropriate facial expression when patients want to communicate even if their vocalizations make no sense. Ask yes/no questions (which might help verify some of the information).

14. Say goodbye, wave, and/or give some departure signal so that patients know the interaction is over. "Goodbye, Mr. Brown."

Adapted from Bowlby (1993); Clark & Witte (1995); Ripich (1994).

cation deficits of individuals with AD. Her findings suggested using simple and easy retrieval strategies that involved recognition memory rather than recall memory. She observed that memory wallets containing picture symbols and written words were successful in enhancing the communication of individuals with moderate dementia (Bourgeois, 1990). She reported that individuals with AD were successful in maintaining the learned use of memory wallets at 3-week and 6-week follow-up sessions. In another study, Bourgeois (1992) reported that individuals with dementia who were provided with memory wallets and appropriate training were able to improve conversational content during conversations with their caregivers.

Bowlby (1993) reported that teaching compensatory memory techniques such as using sticky notes, signs, or lists is helpful for patients with AD. Clinicians have reported that photos, pictures, and maps are also helpful in facilitating interaction with individuals with memory loss.

Photos. Clinicians have used photographs and photograph albums to provide interesting, concrete material to facilitate conversation with patients with dementia during small-group activities or one-on-one interactions. Nurses, occupational therapists, and social workers use photographs to reminisce, alleviate depression, and promote a sense of well-being (Bowlby, 1993). Older individuals often enjoy sharing things about themselves. For individuals with memory loss, family photos can be excellent prompts that encourage and support interactions. Family members can prepare photo albums that chronologically highlight an individual's life. Clinicians have reported success placing one to four photos on a page, carefully arranged with regard to an individual's vision and ability to attend. Simple arrangements have been found to be the best. With some individuals, older photographs are more effective, because they are more recognizable. Short-term memory deficits common in individuals with dementia may preclude recognition of recent photos. Because of the possibility that old, irreplaceable photographs may be lost or damaged, however, photocopies should be used. Captions describing the photos provide information that can aid both individuals with AD and their communication partners. Some clinicians indicate that one short sentence for each photo is adequate. Others suggest that as memory loss becomes more severe, more sentences are useful to help the communication partner sustain interactions. A previously written one-sentence caption, such as "Aunt Mary in the rose garden in Shelbyville, 1949" does, however, provide communication partners with adequate information to include some content in the conversation. The communication partner can reinforce correct facts without putting the individual on the spot to recall certain information. Challenging the individual's memory by asking "Who is in the picture?" is typically not conducive to good conversation. Making comments about the affect of the person in the picture may be effective in establishing rapport and engaging an individual. The comments "She looks like she is having a good time in this picture," or "You look happy playing with your brothers," for example, may elicit appropriate responses and sustain the interaction (D. Clemens, personal communication, May 5, 1995).

Pictures. Magazines also provide concrete information for patients. Collections of pictures of various topics can be placed in notebooks (e.g., two pictures to a page). Topics such as cars, trucks, baseball, military affiliation, and farming are often of interest to males of the WWII generation. (The topic of baseball greats of the past has brightened the face of many older men with memory loss or aphasia!) Gardening, cooking, siblings, parents, and children are topics of interest to older women. Clearly, each generation has its own distinctive music, manners, tastes, and topics of interest. The clinician/educator must find out what is of interest to individuals and incorporate this knowledge when preparing therapy materials (Stuart, Vanderhoof, & Beukelman, 1993). Picture notebooks can help individuals with memory loss share their thoughts and past experiences and elicit conversations in small social groups.

Maps. For some patients with AD, state, county, and country maps can be used to reminisce about where they are now, places they have lived in the past, cities where they were stationed while serving in the military, and trips they have taken (D. Clemens, personal communication, May 5, 1995).

ACQUIRED PHYSICAL DISABILITIES

Cervical Spinal Cord Injury

The cervical spinal cord consists of eight spinal segments (C1 through C8) that include the pathway for neurons and fibers associated with the innervation of the upper limbs. Individuals with **cervical spinal cord injuries**, especially in the region of C5 to C8, frequently experience difficulties in writing because of the damage to the nerve cells that supply the upper limbs. The most frequent causes of spinal cord injuries are automobile accidents, falls, and gunshot wounds. Donovan (1981) reported the occurrence of 25 to 30 injuries per 1,000,000 people per year.

Communication Characteristics. Cervical spinal cord lesions usually cause impairment of writing skills due to paresis or paralysis of the upper limbs. However, if the spinal lesion occurs at the level of the first or second cervical vertebra, the individual will need a ventilator due to loss of nerve innervation to the diaphragm (Beukelman & Mirenda, 1992). Individuals who are ventilator dependent can speak by venting air past the tracheostomy tube and through the larynx (Beukelman & Garrett, 1988).

AAC Intervention. AAC intervention for individuals with cervical spinal cord injuries is primarily concerned with assistance in writing and keyboard control (Beukelman & Garrett, 1988; Beukelman & Mirenda, 1992). When the spinal cord injury is concomitant with severe head injury, different AAC strategies and techniques are needed to provide effective communication. A detailed discussion of AAC intervention for individuals with head injuries is provided in the section on TBI. Beukelman and Garrett (1988) noted that individuals with limited hand function may require an adaptive device to access and use a keyboard efficiently. A universal cuff for typing or an adaptive software program that supports multiple keystroke commands for individuals who are able to use only one hand are examples of assistive technology available to enhance written communication (Beukelman & Mirenda, 1992). Individuals who are literate prior to their injuries can use message-encoding strategies to enhance the speed of written communication. Voice recognition may be the technology of choice for rate enhancement of written language for individuals who are able to speak but are unable to write or access a computer keyboard. In the past, voice-recognition technology has been limited in its ability to accurately recognize a large number of messages (Coleman & Meyers, 1991). Currently available commercial voice-recognition systems, however, are much improved (Beukelman & Mirenda, 1992).

For individuals who have no functional arm or hand control but adequate control of neck and facial muscles, headsticks and mouthsticks may be the access devices of choice. Headsticks, however, obstruct the line of vision, and mouthsticks preclude voicing. Beukelman and Mirenda (1992) report that fatigue is commonly associated with headsticks and mouthsticks because of the precise positioning needed for keyboard activation. Fatigue can be reduced by employing light-based or sound-based head pointing options with standard desktop computer systems. Usually a sensor (light- or sound-based) is mounted on an individual's head. The individual is required to move the head and direct the sensor to the specific location on the screen-displayed keyboard to type or select a message.

Traumatic Brain Injury

Traumatic brain injury (TBI) is defined as a sudden injury to a neurologically normal brain that results in a cluster of neurobehavioral deficits. TBI can be categorized as penetrating and nonpenetrating or as open and closed head injuries. In a penetrating or open head injury, the skull is ruptured or broken. The most common causes of open head injury are bullet wounds, skull fractures from motor vehicle accidents, and sharp blows to the head. In nonpenetrating or closed head injury, the skull remains intact, but the brain is damaged by the ripping and tearing of the cellular structures, which causes bleeding inside the skull. Frequently both hemispheres are damaged in a closed head injury.

The overall occurrence of TBI in children and adults is estimated to be about 200 per 100,000 population per year in the United States. Of the 500,000 who acquire TBI in the United States each year, approximately 50,000 to 100,000 survive with severe behavioral and cognitive sequelae that affect independence and quality of life (Beukelman & Mirenda, 1992; Gualtieri, 1988; Kalsbeek, McLauren, Harris, & Miller, 1981). Motor vehicle accidents constitute a large proportion of closed head injuries (Sellars & Vegter, 1993). Head injuries are most prevalent among young adults between the ages of 15 and 24 (Adamovich, Henderson, & Auerbach, 1985). The National Institute on Disability and Rehabilitation Research (NIDRR) (1991) reports that closed head injury has been and continues to be the most frequent type of injury affecting children. The number of penetrating head injuries, however, has increased as a result of an increase in the number of gunshot wounds.

Extrapolations from epidemiological studies indicate that advances in medical sciences have led to the survival of a large number of individuals who sustain TBI. According to the NIDRR (1991), approximately 97% of the children who sustain TBI survive. Survivors, however, are frequently left with neurological deficits that may affect both cognitive and motor abilities. Individuals with TBI are particularly susceptible to speech and language disorders, sometimes to the extent that they are left with little or no functional speech. AAC intervention plays a major role in the rehabilitation of these individuals.

Communication Characteristics. Communication disorders associated with TBI depend on the size and type of the lesion and the resultant level of cognitive functioning. Diffuse brain lesions, for example, result in widespread cognitive deficits that include attentional disorders; reduced ability to comprehend or process information; deficits in long-term and short-term memory; impairment of reading, writing, and spoken language skills; and problems in planning, organizing, and engaging in goal-directed activities (Mitiguy, Thompson, & Wasco, 1990). In many cases, widespread brain lesions do not affect language per se but rather impair the cognitive operations necessary to facilitate effective communication. Focal brain lesions, on the other hand, most often associated with penetrating wounds, result in communication disorders typical of localized vascular lesions such as aphasia. Sarno, Buonaguro, and Levita (1986) studied 125 individuals with TBI and reported that 29% of their subjects exhibited symptoms associated with acquired aphasia, and 36% exhibited symptoms associated with subclinical aphasia. These authors defined subclinical aphasia as a subtle linguistic processing deficit in the absence of overt manifestation of linguistic impairment identified through testing. Still another type of speech impairment commonly associated with TBI is dysarthria. Rusk, Block, and Lowman (1969) reported that approximately one-third of a group of 96 individuals with TBI exhibited dysarthria during the acute stage of the trauma.

Several informal and formal scales such as the Ranchos Los Amigos Scale of Cognitive Functioning (Hagen & Malkmus, 1979) provide information to team members about the cognitive level and progressive stages of recovery in individuals

with TBI. The Ranchos Los Amigos scale, which outlines eight stages, has been extensively used in adult brain injury rehabilitation. The nature of AAC intervention in individuals with TBI primarily depends on the recovery stage and level of cognitive functioning (Beukelman & Mirenda, 1992; DeRuyter & Kennedy, 1991; Ladtkow & Culp, 1992).

AAC Intervention. Several published case studies describe AAC intervention in individuals with TBI (Beukelman & Yorkston, 1977; DeRuyter & Donoghue, 1989; Light, Beesly, & Collier, 1988). In most of these studies, several AAC systems were applied over time, depending on either the time post-trauma or the cognitive stage of recovery (DeRuyter & Donoghue, 1989; Light et al., 1988). Light et al., (1988) observed an individual with head injury for approximately 3½ years. Several AAC systems were provided, ranging from a simple communication board as a means to indicate basic needs and wants during phase 1 (6 to 9 months post-trauma) to a microcomputer to aid written communication during phase 3 (22 to 23 months post-trauma). A more traditional therapy designed to develop articulation skills, voicing, and the recognition of communication breakdowns was provided during the final phase (40 to 44 months post-trauma).

DeRuyter and Donoghue (1989) described several AAC approaches provided to an adult male with TBI over a period of more than 28 weeks. The first AAC intervention occurred 8 months post-trauma, when he demonstrated reliable yes/no head nods. During this phase, he also began to learn visuoperceptual and pointing skills necessary for using a communication board. By the 10th week of intervention, he was able to use a simple alphabet board with approximate 2-inch letters. He communicated effectively using the alphabet board by the 26th week of intervention. At this point in his rehabilitation program, a VOCA was introduced, and he was able to communicate with it at the rate of eight words per minute. At the time of discharge from the inpatient setting, the individual was able to communicate via limited speech, alphabet board, gestures, and an electronic AAC device.

This case study demonstrates that specific AAC intervention strategies must be devised and revised to meet the changing needs of individuals with TBI. Therefore, a multiple-phase AAC approach that spans cognitive stages of recovery is proposed to guide professionals in selecting appropriate AAC intervention strategies and techniques for individuals with TBI. This AAC approach is divided into five major phases.

Phase 1: Generalized Response to Sensory Stimulation. During phase 1, individuals with TBI may demonstrate a generalized response to specific stimulation. For example, an individual may demonstrate a startle response to loud sounds or an eye-blink response to an object coming rapidly toward the face. Because the therapeutic goal at this time is to heighten arousal and awareness of objects in the individual's immediate environment, the purpose of AAC intervention is to stimulate the individual to respond. Sellars and Vegter (1993) suggest using loud bike horns, recorded environmental sounds, assorted musical tapes, a feather duster, food extracts, and fluorescent sponge balls to stimulate the senses. Beukelman and Mirenda (1992) suggest collecting information from communication partners about interests and pre-trauma activities of individuals with TBI so that rehabilitation personnel can provide interesting and meaningful stimulation.

Phase 2: Localized Response to Sensory Stimulation. During phase 2, individuals with TBI are able to provide consistent and differential responses to various sensory stimuli. They can, for example, track visual stimuli and localize sounds. Severe motoric impairment, however, is invariably present during this phase. An adaptive switch that can provide an alternative access mode to a computer with voice output can be beneficial for an individual with a motor impairment who cannot direct select (Garrett, Schutz-Muehling, & Morrow, 1990). If individuals can achieve competence using adaptive switches, they can gain some control over their environments. For example, a switch that activates a VOCA can also be used as a remote control unit for electrical appliances such as lamps, televisions, radios, and fans. During this phase individuals with TBI may exhibit improved cognition and may begin to establish cause and ef-

fect relationships. Therapy should be designed to develop and strengthen these relationships (Beukelman & Mirenda, 1992). The important point to remember during this phase is that AAC techniques will vary considerably depending on an individual's cognitive and motoric impairments.

Phase 3: Increased Responsiveness and Purposeful Interaction with the Environment. Most of the individuals with TBI at this middle phase demonstrate impaired judgment, confusion, memory loss, and fatigue. Ladtkow and Culp (1992) report that individuals who do not have severe motor control impairments or cognitive-linguistic deficits begin to speak around this time, although their speech may be confused and contain pragmatically awkward constructions. A complete AAC assessment that includes evaluation of cognition, motor, and sensory capabilities must be carried out at this phase to determine the residual capabilities of individuals with TBI and to provide focus for future AAC intervention. Assessment of motor control capabilities should include determination of appropriate message selection techniques such as direct selection or scanning described in Chapter 8. Visuoperceptual and visual acuity disturbances, which are fairly common in individuals with TBI, must also be assessed (Beukelman & Mirenda, 1992).

AAC intervention for individuals with significant cognitive impairments should be designed to facilitate and maximize interactive communication. AAC strategies and techniques should be designed to accommodate reduced memory and attentional load. An individual at this phase may be provided with a nonelectronic AAC device such as a communication board. Putting a small number of highly iconic symbols on a board and using recognition memory instead of recall memory are strategies that may help facilitate communication for individuals in phase 3.

Individuals with TBI at this phase, however, should also be given the opportunity to try computers with adapted access. Clinicians/educators should gather information about the abilities of individuals with TBI before they consider recommending use of an electronic communication device. Because individuals with TBI are going through considerable changes in cognitive, communicative, and physical competence at this point in the recovery phase, however, a recommendation for the purchase of an electronic AAC device may not be appropriate at this time (Ylvisaker & Urbanczyk, 1994). Loan and lease options should be explored.

Phase 4: Impairments in Language and Speech. Individuals with TBI at this phase may exhibit symptoms of aphasia, apraxia, and/or dysarthria because of the diffuse nature of severe brain injuries. Baseline language measurements should be taken during this phase to determine specific skills and deficits that should guide the intervention plan. Individuals with severe aphasia or motor control deficits require a long-term AAC system to allow them to communicate effectively. DeRuyter and Kennedy (1991) and Ladtkow and Culp (1992) reported that identifying and assessing communication needs and matching specific capabilities and constraints to AAC intervention is an approach commonly used with persons in late-phase TBI.

Phase 5: Significant Transition. Individuals with TBI approach the return to pretrauma status during the last phase. Beukelman and Miranda (1992) observed that individuals in this stage have either regained almost all of their cognitive functions and become natural speakers or they remain unable to speak because of severe deficits in motor control. During this phase individuals are moved from acute care units to home and community, making a transition from dependent to independent living. However, although individuals with TBI at this stage have recovered some cognitive and communication skills, their recovery may still be far from complete. Creating communication opportunities and training individuals and communication partners to resolve communication breakdowns are important aspects of AAC intervention during this phase (Beukelman & Mirenda, 1992).

Individuals who fail to regain natural speech because of motor control disorders may desire commercially available AAC devices with synthetic speech capabilities. However, AAC service providers must work with the individuals and their families to determine exactly what features are needed. As individuals regain normal cognitive function, they may be provided with devices that allow for flexible vocabulary programming, innovative message encoding, and word prediction to enhance communication rate. Accessing a communication device may not be a major problem at this stage, as DeRuyter and Lafontaine (1987) report that 78% of the individuals with TBI who are unable to speak in the later stages of recovery use direct selection techniques, while 16% use scanning. Due to intact cognitive abilities of individuals with TBI at this stage, AAC intervention has great potential.

Ylvisaker and Urbanczyk (1994) suggest that AAC intervention for individuals with TBI should be designed to enhance success and reduce frustration and other emotional burdens as much as possible. Behavioral and emotional distress can be reduced by involving these individuals in decisions concerning the selection of the AAC device and providing extensive practice in using the device for functional interactive communication.

SUMMARY

In recent years, AAC strategies and techniques have been added to traditional therapy approaches designed to improve the functional communication skills of individuals who have lost them because of acquired neurogenic disorders. Individuals with aphasia have demonstrated the ability to learn and use graphic symbols. Individuals with acquired progressive neurogenic diseases and acquired physical disabilities have also learned to use AAC. AAC intervention for individuals with spinal cord injuries typically involves improving written communication. Individuals with TBI, on the other hand, typically need intervention to improve both spoken and written communication. Clinicians/educators working with individuals with TBI must be knowledgeable about the cognitive stages of recovery so that appropriate AAC strategies and techniques can be employed. AAC intervention is an especially dynamic process for individuals whose conditions are improving or declining.

CHAPTER 20

PROFESSIONAL CONCERNS AND ISSUES

RAYMOND W. QUIST, LYLE L. LLOYD, AND KEVIN C. McDOWELL

Individuals who provide **augmentative and alternative communication (AAC)** services should be practicing within the ethical guidelines as well as any legal requirements, for their respective professions. AAC remains a relatively new field; consequently, critical issues such as training and credentialing need to be addressed to ensure that individuals using AAC are receiving quality services. In this chapter, legal bases and ethics, as well as competencies, certification, and licensure concerns, will be discussed.

LEGAL BASES

The development of special education law in the United States is a tribute to society's concern with the needs and rights of individuals. However, the real changes in special education evolved as an extension of the U.S. civil rights movement. As a result, the delivery of special education services today has changed in many significant ways (e.g., increased accessibility, parental involvement, accountability, and legal repercussions).

History

Any discussion of the legal basis of AAC requires a brief review of the evolution of special education law within the United States. During the mid-1800s, society recognized a need to provide for individuals with disabilities by establishing institutions for their care (e.g., institutions for individuals who were mentally incompetent, blind, or deaf). Although some parents chose to have their child remain part of the family, if the impairment was particularly severe, the family physician often encouraged institutionalization. As a consequence, these individuals often were invisible to society.

Many individuals with physical disabilities were able to participate in a number of activities by using wheelchairs or customized artificial limbs. Viscardi (1952), prior to having artificial limbs, wrapped the stubs of his legs in padded material so that he could "walk" on them. He, like many other individuals with physical disabilities, insisted on participating in the mainstream throughout his education and later as he entered the workforce. However, these were the special individuals who persisted despite the good intentions of many, including professionals. Within the educational system persons judged by school officials to be unable to function in general education (e.g., they scored low on an IQ test, were confined to a wheelchair, or were unable to talk) were sent to special schools. Individuals who had very severe disabilities and were not institutionalized were likely to be kept at home. Obviously, in these cases, public education was not really an option. Many parents, as a result, provided their children with home instruction.

The return of World War I and II veterans with injuries/disabilities resulted in the development of vocational rehabilitation and public assistance programs. Assistance for individuals with disabilities included **Medicare** (Title XVIII) and **Medicaid** (Title XIX) of the 1965 **Social Security Act** (PL 89-97) programs, and Veterans Administration benefits. Since World War II, concern for individuals with disabilities has increased. More services became available because of a greater visibility of returning veterans, improved economics, increased public concern toward the public welfare, increased education and awareness, and more assertiveness on the part of individuals with disabilities and their families. As is often the case, individuals may be unaware of the needs of persons with disabilities until they are personally involved. Because many of these veterans were influential (or at least highly articulate) prior to acquiring their disabilities, they became effective advocates for appropriate services.

With the onset of the civil rights movement, increasing numbers of people within the United States began to think about the rights of individuals who belonged to minority groups. During this period, the central focus was on African Americans. *Brown v. Topeka Board of Education* (1954) was the first major legal step in the journey toward equal educational rights for all persons.

President John Kennedy and Vice President Hubert Humphrey (under President Lyndon Johnson) had family members with cognitive impairments. The Association for Retarded Citizens (ARC) of the United States, currently named the Arc, gained national prominence because of Kennedy's and Humphrey's encouragement for the development of a President's Committee on Mental Retardation (Turnbull, 1993).

The 1960s were marked by dramatic social changes that resulted in a number of laws designed to expand the rights of all individuals, including improvements in the education of all children. Major legislation that provided federal funding to states for the construction of mental retardation and mental health facilities (PL 88-164, 1963; PL 90-170, 1967; PL 91-517, 1970) addressed the needs of individuals with developmental disabilities. Subsequent legislation (PL 94-103, 1975) focused on services, including protection and advocacy programs for individuals with developmental disabilities. Education was seen as critical for all individuals to achieve meaningful, productive lives.

Table 20.1 depicts the chronology of the development of laws that have an impact on special education and AAC along with brief descriptions of each law or amendment. A more in-depth study of special education law can be found in Rothstein (1994), Turnbull (1993), and Wehman (1993).

School practices over the years clearly demonstrated a need for strong government direction in education. Schools were exclusionary—that is, many children with disabilities were never allowed to enroll with typically developing children. They often were placed in special schools.

For those children who did get into the school building (access), the result often was functional exclusion. For example, if a child were placed in a class without appropriate support, failure was ensured. Schools practiced partial exclusion by admitting some children with disabilities and not others. Schools often practiced discrimination (e.g., excluding individuals with behavioral problems or limiting enrollments on the basis of artificial quotas). Inadequate funding frequently resulted in limited resources, which resulted in waiting lists or placement in programs that were inappropriate. With the application of specified admission criteria, large numbers of children from racially underrepresented groups were inappropriately categorized due to the use of tests standardized on other populations. For children with severe communication disabilities, psychological testing frequently was flawed due to the many problems in obtaining and interpreting responses. Because language is so integral to the judgment of cognitive abilities, these children often were included in classrooms for students with cognitive impairments.

A number of other factors also contributed to inappropriate educational classification or placement: (1) architectural barriers that made a particular building inaccessible for individuals with disabilities; (2) reliance on private or special public schools to provide services for children with disabilities; (3) use of noncertified personnel to provide services or claiming inability to provide services due to unavailability of certified personnel; (4) lack of early intervention programs to prepare children with disabilities for entry into school; and (5) a tendency for children, once classified, to remain classified for the duration of their educational careers. Parents' lack of knowledge, both of services available and of their rights, allowed the schools to continue to avoid their responsibilities to children with disabilities for many years.

Education for All Handicapped Children Act

The Elementary and Secondary Education Act (PL 89-10) was passed in 1965 to ensure improved quality in the nation's education. Because this Act did not address the educational needs of children

TABLE 20.1 Chronology of Laws Impacting AAC

1963 **PL 88-164 Mental Retardation Facilities and Community Mental Health Centers Construction Act of 1963** provided major federal funding to support state and local programs.

1965 **PL 89-10 Elementary and Secondary Education Act** established the federal government's role in education.

1965 **PL 89-97 Social Security Act of 1965** established Medicare (Title XVIII) and Medicaid (Title XIX).

1965 **PL 89-313 Elementary and Secondary Education Amendments of 1965 for Children with Handicaps** extended the focus on education to children with disabilities.

1966 **PL 89-750 Elementary and Secondary Education Amendments of 1966** established the Bureau of the Education of the Handicapped (BEH); developed and monitored programs for individuals with disabilities; forerunner of EHA.

1967 **PL 90-170 Mental Retardation Amendments of 1967** authorized funding for additional construction and services.

1967 **PL 90-247 Elementary and Secondary Education Amendments of 1967** established discretionary programs to support development and expansion of special education services.

1969 **PL 91-230 Elementary, Secondary, and Other Education Amendments of 1969** consolidated a number of federal grant programs for the education of children with disabilities.

1970 **PL 91-517 Developmental Disabilities Services and Facilities Construction Amendments of 1970** was the first congressional effort to address needs of individuals with developmental disabilities; allocated funds for construction of facilities and services for persons with developmental disabilities.

1973 **PL 93-112 Rehabilitation Act** mandated civil rights protection for all individuals with disabilities.

1975 **PL 94-103 Developmentally Disabled Assistance and Bill of Rights Act Amendments of 1975** required establishment of protection and advocacy programs for states to be eligible for grants.

1975 **PL 94-142 Education for All Handicapped Children Act (EHA)** mandated a free, appropriate public education (FAPE) for all children with handicaps.

1983 **PL 98-199 Education for All Handicapped Children Act (EHA) Amendments of 1983** provided incentives to states to develop preschool and special education early intervention programs for children with disabilities; replaced BEH with the Office of Special Education Programs (OSEP).

1984 **PL 98-524 Carl D. Perkins Vocational Education Act** included requirements for vocational education to be provided for children with special needs.

1984 **PL 98-527 Developmental Disabilities Act** provided assistance to states to ensure that persons with developmental disabilities receive care, treatment, and services to achieve maximum potential.

1986 **PL 99-457 Education of the Handicapped Act (EHA) Amendments of 1986** amended the EHA to reauthorize the discretionary programs and to authorize early intervention programs for all handicapped infants and toddlers and their families.

1987 **PL 100-146 Developmental Disabilities Assistance and Bill of Rights Act Amendments of 1987** created grants to support services, including protection and advocacy, for individuals with developmental disabilities.

1988 **PL 100-407 Technology-Related Assistance for Individuals with Disabilities Act (Tech Act)** provided states with funds to develop statewide technology services.

1990 **PL 101-336 Americans with Disabilities Act (ADA)** mandated equal opportunities in employment and public accommodations for individuals with disabilities.

1990 **PL 101-392 Carl D. Perkins Vocational and Applied Technology Act Amendments of 1990** expanded provisions to ensure equal opportunities for vocational education to include all individuals with disabilities.

TABLE 20.1   *(Continued)*

1990 **PL 101-476 Individuals with Disabilities Education Act (IDEA)** expanded EHA to include transition and assistive technology.	1994 **PL 103-218 Technology-Related Assistance for Individuals with Disabilities Amendments of 1994** provided financial assistance to support system change and advocacy activities and to assist in developing and implementing a comprehensive statewide program of technology-related assistance for individuals of all ages.
1991 **PL 102-119 Individuals with Disabilities Education Act Amendments of 1991** documented rights to assistive technology for individuals with disabilities.	
1992 **PL 102-569 Rehabilitation Act Amendments of 1992** provided for increased consumer decision-making and control; was intended to increase access to technology devices and services by requiring them to be included in the Individualized Written Rehabilitation Program (IWRP).	1997 **PL 105-17 Individuals with Disabilities Education Act Amendments of 1997** reauthorized and increased support for the development of a range of assistive instructional technologies.

with disabilities, the Elementary and Secondary Education Amendments for Children with Handicaps (PL 89-313,1965) was passed. This Act established the foundation for all future legislation dealing with the education of individuals with disabilities. The Elementary and Secondary Education Amendments of 1966 (PL-89-750, 1966) established the Bureau of the Education of the Handicapped to monitor programs for individuals with disabilities. Subsequent passage of the Elementary and Secondary Education Amendments of 1967 (PL 90-247, 1967) established discretionary programs to develop and expand special education services. Passage of the Elementary, Secondary, and Other Education Amendments (PL 91-230, 1969) consolidated a number of federal grant programs for educating children with disabilities. Through these legislative acts, Congress attempted to encourage states to develop personnel and resources for special education. They were the forerunners of the **Education for All Handicapped Children Act (EHA)** (PL 94-142, 1975).

During this same period two court cases, *Pennsylvania Association for Retarded Citizens (PARC) v. Commonwealth of Pennsylvania* (1972) and *Mills v. Board of Education* (1972) resulted in decisions that all children with disabilities should be provided access to an education. It was after these cases that Congress passed the EHA which required all children with disabilities to have access to **free, appropriate public education**

(FAPE). This Act initiated procedures to ensure that each public school system identify all children with disabilities within its district and provide them with appropriate education. In addition to providing support monies to see that these processes were carried out, the federal government mandated each state to establish procedures for enforcement.

During the four-year period from 1983 to 1987, a number of amendments to the EHA expanded educational opportunities for students with disabilities. The Education for All Handicapped Children Act Amendments of 1983 (PL 98-199, 1983) provided incentives to develop preschool and early intervention programs for children with disabilities. The Education of the Handicapped Act Amendments of 1986 (PL 99-457, 1986) lowered the age of eligibility for educational services to 3 years. Other complementary legislation such as the Developmental Disabilities Act (PL-527, 1984) and the Developmental Disabilities Assistance and Bill of Rights Act Amendments of 1987 (PL 100-146, 1987) created grants to support services for individuals with developmental disabilities.

The implementation of the EHA represented a major step toward the provision of equality in education. Schools identified many children with disabilities within their districts who were not attending school. As more parents and professionals encouraged the inclusion of children with disabilities in the mainstream of education, specialized schools were dismantled and children were moved into public school buildings. School administrators were challenged to find ways to include these children in their schools. Initially schools tended to include children with disabilities in areas within their schools (e.g., specially designated rooms or a wing of a building). In this way children were part of the same school, but were still separate from many educational activities; they really were not participating with children who did not have disabilities. For some children who were perceived as higher functioning, attempts were made at integration by mixing students at lunch or during special activities or classes, such as music and art. Certainly these steps enabled many children with disabilities to develop some socialization skills; however, as parents became more aware of their rights under the law, they began to press for the integration of their children into more educational activities.

When the EHA was passed, most professionals and parents of children with disabilities had only a sketchy idea of how the law should be implemented. As specific problems arose, hearings were held to answer these questions. Some issues needed to be resolved through civil suits that ultimately resulted in decisions that could serve as guiding principles. Inasmuch as the EHA guaranteed FAPE for all children with disabilities, it provided the framework for evaluating the education provided each child. Initially, many hearings were focused on the child's identification and placement with questions such as the following:

1. Was the diagnosis/category appropriate?
2. Was the child placed with children having similar disabilities and was the teacher appropriately certified for that category?
3. Was the child entitled to paid transportation to and from related services?
4. If a school could not provide the appropriate services for the child, to what extent must it pay for those services in another setting?
5. What are the school's responsibilities for notifying parents regarding their rights under the law?
6. If a child is appropriately classified and placed, are the teaching materials/approaches appropriate?
7. Should aides be provided for children within the classroom to assist in their education?
8. If a child needs intensive education during the year and is likely to regress over the summer, what is the school's responsibility during the summer (e.g., extended school year)?
9. How accessible must a school building be for individuals with disabilities?
10. Should parents have the option to place their children in a specialized facility (e.g., a state school for the deaf, a school for the blind, or other specialized private residential facility) even when the school has an appropriate program available?
11. Must a child demonstrate ability to benefit from special education, or is there a zero reject principle?
12. To what extent do school officials have to provide special, medically related services in their delivery of educational services (e.g., catheterizations, cleaning/suctioning of tracheal tubes)?

The concept of FAPE was at the heart of the EHA, but it was not well defined. Does FAPE mean the best education possible? *Board of Education of Hendrick Hudson Central School District v. Rowley* (1982) was significant in that it set a standard for defining FAPE. It involved an appeal of a decision requiring the school to write into the IEP an in-class interpreter for a child who was deaf. This child was functioning in a general education classroom, demonstrating educational success similar to his peers, and progressing from class to class without the use of an interpreter. The U.S. Supreme Court determined the child had access to an appropriate education and was achieving success without the use of an interpreter. Although the Court admitted the child might do better with an interpreter, it maintained that the law did not require that the education ensure a better or the best education. Therefore, the Supreme Court ruled that the child was receiving FAPE.

Another case raised questions concerning criteria for determining eligibility for special education services. *Timothy W. v. Rochester, New Hampshire School District* (1989) involved a child who was multiply handicapped with profound cognitive impairment. Among his many conditions were spastic quadriplegia, cerebral palsy, seizures, hydrocephalus, and cortical blindness. Although a developmental pediatrician testified that Timothy W. could not benefit from education due to very limited responses to stimuli, a number of rehabilitation and special education experts testified that he could benefit. The Court ruled that Timothy W. could not be denied an education—that all persons with disabilities can benefit from special education and, therefore, no minimal criteria of potential benefit exist for determining eligibility for special education services. This interpretation has been called the **zero reject principle** and is particularly important because it supports the notion that all school-aged persons with severe disabilities are eligible for special education services. The question then becomes one of determining what supports are needed to enable a child to participate in the educational process.

Irving Independent School District v. Tatro (1984) involved a Texas child who needed intermittent catheterization while present in school. A major question in this case was whether catheterization constituted a medical service or a related service. In this case, the Supreme Court determined that a nurse or other person can be qualified to provide the service and that a physician is not required. The Court also determined that such services be considered "related services" and must be provided by the school. **Local education agencies (LEAs)**, however, do not have to provide medical services except when needed for diagnostic reasons.

Recently, more attention has focused on the following issues: (1) functional training in community and work activities for individuals with disabilities, (2) planning for activities to facilitate a smooth transition from high school to work, and (3) implementation of preschool programs for children with disabilities and including them in the general education classroom to the fullest extent possible. These questions center around the concept of **least restrictive environment (LRE)**. Some individuals interpret LRE to mean full participation of children with extremely severe disabilities in a general education classroom with typically developing children. Because of the LRE movement, educators now are focusing more efforts toward preparing classroom teachers to work with children who have special education needs.

When Congress passed the EHA mandating the delivery of special education services, the legislation did not indicate specific dollar amounts. Rather, as is often the case with legislation, monies for special education were provided through the annual federal budget. Initially, federal dollars represented significant but partial support to encourage states to develop services with the expectation that the states would pick up a greater portion of the cost over time. When monies are sent to the states earmarked for special education, the state is allowed to keep a percentage of the funds for carrying out its legislative mandates and other activities (e.g., mandated monitoring/enforcement and other selected special projects). The vast majority of funds, however, are passed through to the individual LEAs to implement special education services and related obligations (e.g., inservice programs, supplies and materials, and assistive technology) for individuals within their jurisdiction.

As the national budget has become more strained, federal dollars appropriated for special education have not increased to keep up with inflation or increased needs. As a consequence, many state officials and special educators now use the term **unfunded mandates** to show that the federal government continues to mandate services without providing adequate funds to carry them out. Inasmuch as state budgets also have been strained, many states have failed to increase their share of the cost. The result is an increasing disparity between special education needs and the funding to provide for them.

However, substantial changes may be occurring in the funding approaches for special education. The current attitude of many U.S. legislators is that, because state officials are closer to the problem, they have a better idea of the needs of their people and how to fund those needs. As a result, Congress is considering **block grants**, which are federal monies provided to states with no mandates that can be allocated as state officials deem appropriate. Although local control appears reasonable, it is no guarantee that the allocation of these funds will be any less subject to political influences than federal funds. In fact, local control may create a greater disparity among states in the amount and types of special education services, a condition that existed years ago when state officials did have more say in allocating funds and distributing services.

Technology-Related Assistance for Individuals with Disabilities Act

The development of computer technology captured the imagination of many legislators. Rehabilitation professionals had demonstrated the value of technology in retraining individuals with acquired disabilities to re-enter the workforce. Increasingly, legislators, employers, and educators came to realize that technology could play a significant role in returning individuals to productive and personally meaningful lives. As a result, the **Technology-Related Assistance for Individuals with Disabilities Act** (also known as the **Tech Act**) (PL 100-407, 1988) was passed. This legislation authorized funds for states to establish and implement a consumer-responsive, statewide program of technology-related assistance for individuals with disabilities. Included in this legislative charge were the identification of federal policies that impede payments and services for assistive technology and the development of approaches to overcome these barriers. Over a period of 3 years, all 50 states were funded, but not necessarily at the levels originally authorized.

The Tech Act defined an **assistive technology device** as "any item, piece of equipment, or product system, whether acquired commercially, off the shelf, modified, or customized, that is used to increase, maintain, or improve the functional capabilities of individuals with disabilities" [20 U.S.C.)1401(a)(25), Tech Act, 1988]. Legislators who wrote the Tech Act recognized that the availability of a technological device by itself would not be sufficient; consequently, they provided for accompanying services to ensure the integration of the technology into daily living functions. A technology service was defined as "any service that directly assists an individual with a disability in the selection, acquisition, or use of an assistive technology device" (20 U.S.C.) 2201, Tech Act, 1988). Included within the scope of such definitions were (1) evaluating the needs of individuals, including such variables as functioning within the environment; (2) selecting, customizing, maintaining, or replacing a device; (3) coordinating therapists and intervention services with devices in existing education and rehabilitation programs; and (4) providing technical assistance in the use of the device and techniques to individuals, their families and caregivers, professionals, and any other individuals having a role in the user's daily life functions.

The Technology-Related Assistance for Individuals with Disabilities Amendments of 1994 (PL 103-218, 1994) reauthorized the original Tech Act and delineated desired directions for the next 5 years. Among priorities for the continuation of Tech Act activities are the following:

1. The development and implementation of strategies (including coordination, outreach, and empowerment) to overcome barriers regarding access to, provision of, and funding for assistive technology devices and services.
2. The development and implementation of strategies to ensure timely acquisition and delivery of assistive technology devices and services, particularly for children.
3. The development and implementation of strategies for training regarding assistive technology within existing federal and state funded training initiatives to enhance assistive technology skills and competencies.
4. The development and implementation of strategies to empower individuals with disabilities, family members, guardians, advocates, and authorized representatives to advocate successfully for increased access to funding for, and provision of, assistive technology devices and services, and to increase participation, choice, and control in the selection and procurement of assistive technology devices and services.
5. The provision for outreach to underrepresented populations and rural populations, the provision of activities to increase accessibility of services and training for representatives of the populations to become service providers, and training staff of the consumer-responsive comprehensive statewide program of technology-related assistance to work with their populations.

These stated goals show that major concerns center on promoting more active involvement of consumers in decision-making processes, as well as on monitoring and influencing future legislation affecting assistive technology and on developing faster, more efficient ways to get devices to the consumer, including funding approaches through currently existing agencies. Although the Tech Act is concerned with identifying barriers for device acquisition and use, it does not mention any additional funds to facilitate it. However, the Act does mention implementing strategies for training within existing federal and state funded initiatives to upgrade skills and competencies of those providing the services, as well as consumers and their family members. Considerable emphasis now appears to be on strengthening consumers' advocacy roles and developing more comprehensive community networks on assistive technology.

Individuals with Disabilities Education Act

In 1990, a number of amendments to the EHA resulted in a change in its name to **Individuals with Disabilities Education Act (IDEA)** (PL 101-476, 1990). Significant changes resulting from these amendments included recognizing and serving children in underrepresented groups with conditions such as autism and brain trauma, as well as rural and minority children. In addition, the amendments called for the provision of transition/extensions of services for deaf-blind individuals from school to work, as well as special education services for preschool children with disabilities. IDEA also called for integrating the concepts of the Tech Act into the educational plans for children with disabilities. It included the same definitions as the Tech Act, except that it substituted "children" for "individuals" and applied everything to the educational environment. The definitions are broad enough to include the full range from low technology (e.g., communication boards) to high technology (e.g., computerized communication systems) that are deemed necessary by a duly constituted group of individuals, such as a rehabilitation evaluation team or an **Individualized Education Program (IEP)** team. The assistive technology activities originally mandated by the Tech Act and included in IDEA (with the substitution of child/children for individual/individuals) are discussed briefly in the following paragraphs (as identified by letters in the law):

(a)   **The evaluation of the needs of a child with a disability, including a functional evaluation of the child in the child's customary environment.** The authors of the Tech Act recognized that assistive technology evaluations typically involve the cooperative efforts of a variety of rehabilitation and educational personnel and should include observations of the individual's everyday performance across environments. The consideration of these factors is important to ensure an appropriate AAC evaluation. Also, such considerations help to ensure more focus on the specific needs of the individual with little or no functional speech so an appropriate communication device can be selected.

(b)   **Purchasing, leasing, or otherwise providing for the acquisition of assistive technology devices for children with disabilities.** In the past, an evaluation team often recommended a communication device only to discover that there was no way to fund it. An important part of this legislation is to mandate that appropriately recommended devices are made available through a variety of mechanisms (e.g., leasing, loaning, purchasing). In the school environment, the acquisition of assistive technology can only be ensured by specifying the need in the child's IEP.

(c)   **Selecting, designing, fitting, customizing, adapting, applying, refining, repairing, or replacing assistive technology devices.** Outfitting an individual with a communication device is important; however, providing for adaptations, maintenance, and repair is essential. There may be costs for adapting the device specifically to the needs of the individual, as well as for repairs over time. Individuals might be outfitted with a device, but they may not be able to afford the additional costs of modification or repair. In some cases, they may not wish to spend the extra time involved for the changes needed. As a result, the device may sit on a shelf unused, or it may be used without the modifications needed for the AAC user to realize maximum benefits. This Act provides for the initial cost, appropriate modifications, and needed repairs for recommended devices.

(d)   **Coordinating and using other therapies, interventions, or services with assistive technology devices, such as those associated with existing education and rehabilitation plans and programs.** Although acquisition of a device is critical, its value is determined by the extent to which an individual is able to use it effectively. This means that a great deal of time and effort will be needed not only to teach AAC participants to program the device and make simple repairs or adjustments, but also to teach and reinforce the integration of the device into communication across environments (e.g., home, educational, recreational).

(e) **Training or technical assistance for a child with a disability or, if appropriate, that child's family.**

(f) **Training or technological assistance for professionals (including individuals providing education or rehabilitation services), employers, or other individuals who provide services to, employ, or are otherwise substantially involved in the major life functions of children with disabilities.** Parts (e) and (f) of the definitions of services recognize the need for providing appropriate training for all concerned AAC participants, focusing primarily on family members and those professionals who play a role in the child's rehabilitation/education.

Assistive Technology Issues

Individuals with Disabilities Education Act Amendments of 1991 (PL 102-119), extended rights to assistive technology for individuals with disabilities. Julnes and Brown (1993) noted that, although IDEA was amended to include the definitions of assistive technology devices and services, there were no new accompanying statutory mandates requiring participating states to provide them. These mandates were implicit in the EHA and further assumed under the new rules in IDEA, which specified that "each public agency shall insure that assistive technology devices or assistive technology services, or both, as those terms are defined in (Section 300.5-300.6), are made available to a child with a disability if required as part of the child's (a) special education (Section 300.17); (b) related services (Section 300.18); or (c) supplementary aids and services [Section 300.550(b)(2)]." Julnes and Brown (1993) provide excellent legal analyses of the mandate for providing assistive technology under any of three approaches: special education (Section 300.17); related services (Section 300.18); or supplementary aids and services [Section 300.550(b)(2)]. Specifically, IDEA mandates FAPE and goes on to mandate ". . . to the maximum extent appropriate, children with disabilities are educated with children who are not disabled . . . and are to be educated in regular classrooms unless the nature or severity is such that education in regular classes

with the use of supplementary aids and services cannot be achieved satisfactorily . . ." [Section 300.550(b) (1) & (2)]. *Board of Education of Hendrick Hudson Central School District v. Rowley* (1982), *Timothy W. v. Rochester, New Hampshire School District* (1989), and *Irving Independent School District v. Tatro* (1984) were instrumental in establishing the legal bases for the requirement to provide assistive technology.

Julnes and Brown (1993) discuss the applications of these cases and specific parts of IDEA that determine whether technology for students with disabilities must be provided. The ruling in the *Board of Education of Hendrick Hudson Central School District v. Rowley* (special education) is interpreted to mean that the school is not obligated to provide assistive technology if it provides more than FAPE. The standard is that a child with disabilities will receive an education consistent with what is offered children who do not have disabilities. The ruling in *Irving Independent School District v. Tatro* (related services) is interpreted to mean that assistive technology must be provided if it is needed for the child to attend school and benefit from special education. Questions still exist as to whether computers would provide merely a personal benefit or would be of such a nature that the school must provide them as part of FAPE.

Currently, no legal standard specifies the limits of personal use. The judgment as to what is personal relates to whether providing a device at home in addition to its use in school makes it personal. No problems currently exist unless the parents refuse or are unable to provide a home computer when it would support the child's special education programming in school as specified in the IEP. Litigation is likely to occur in this area. The provision of assistive technology will also be influenced by LRE decisions in terms of how it benefits the student, influences curriculum adjustments, and facilitates interaction with others in the classroom. Assistive technology must *always* be a consideration when determining the child's potential to acquire FAPE within the LRE.

In an Office of Special Education Programs (OSEP) Letter to Anonymous (1994), the following questions were answered. First, if a school district needs a device to implement the IEP, should it assume the liability for a home-purchased device from the time the student gets on the school bus until returning home? Second, if the school is not liable, then should it purchase a device for use at school? OSEP's response included the consideration of the school's obligation under special education, related services, or supplementary aids and services. It stressed that the determination of such services was to be made on an individual basis by the IEP team. Although federal law does not specify such a liability for family-owned devices, OSEP believes that the school would otherwise be held responsible for supplying a device and, therefore, the liability for a family-owned device would be reasonable.

The **Rehabilitation Act** (PL 93-112, 1973) mandated civil rights protection for all individuals with disabilities. Although Section 504 of the Rehabilitation Act does not specifically require the provision of assistive technology, the issue becomes one of equal access under the law. Section 504 specifies "no otherwise qualified handicapped person . . . shall on the basis of handicap, be excluded from the participation in, be denied the benefits of, or otherwise be subjected to discrimination under any program or activity receiving federal financial assistance" [34 CFR 104.4(a)]. Section 504 also requires reasonable accommodations to be made for the individual. Two important investigations by the Office for Civil Rights (OCR) applying Section 504 include *Eldon (MO) v. R-1 School District* (1986) and *Cleveland (OH) v. Public School District* (1988). In the first investigation, the parents requested a hearing on behalf of their son who had disabilities and was enrolled in the school's computer course. They bought their son a computer and arranged for the purchase of an adaptive device so he could operate it. They claimed the school had failed to notify them that computers were provided for children enrolled in a computer course. According to the Letter of Finding, the school was in violation and its officials were ordered to arrange for either rental or purchase of a computer for the child's use in the course. The second investigation involved a child with a hearing impairment who was to be provided with a hearing amplification device. Because the school was a year late in providing the device, the

Letter of Finding ruled that it was in violation of Section 504.

Since the passage of the Rehabilitation Act, a number of amendments have been passed to expand services to individuals with disabilities. The Vocational Education Act (PL 98-524, 1984), commonly referred to as the Perkins Act, included requirements to provide vocational education for children with special needs. The Carl D. Perkins Vocational and Applied Technology Act Amendments of 1990 (PL 101-392, 1990) expanded these rights for all individuals with disabilities. The Rehabilitation Act Amendments of 1992 (PL 102-569, 1992) focused on increasing awareness and access to technology devices and services by requiring them to be included in the Individualized Written Rehabilitation Program (IWRP).

When considering the need for assistive technology, all of the legal analyses are important to consider in their proper perspectives. The appropriate use of assistive technology provides the student access to FAPE and allows for less interruption of the classroom and less adaptation of curriculum and techniques than when no assistive technology is used. It also encourages active rather than passive participation and facilitates interaction with peers without disabilities (something that is highly compatible with the goals of LRE). A number of OCR investigations, **state education agency (SEA)** administrative decisions, and OSEP responses to letters support this position and make it clear that the provision of assistive technology is the responsibility of the school as part of FAPE. The decision regarding the need for assistive technology is made on a case-by-case basis by the IEP team. Once a recommendation for assistive technology is written into the IEP, the school or state is obligated to provide it. The recommendation should include what features of assistive technology will meet the needs of the student. The names of specific devices should not be included.

In *San Francisco Unified School District*, 1985 (SEA), an 8-year-old student with cerebral palsy was determined to need a computer with a speech synthesizer. The parents had managed to obtain a system and have it operative within 3 weeks. One and one-half years later, the school's case conference IEP team wrote the use of an identical computer system into the IEP. Because the school took 5 months to acquire the system and have it operative, the student continued to receive private speech-language therapy in the interim. At a subsequent hearing, the school was ordered to provide one-to-one therapy with a person who could communicate with him through a computerized communication system and to reimburse the family for the speech-language therapy provided while waiting for the system.

In *Alexis B. v. Harwich Public Schools*, 1988 (SEA), the issue involved dual placement of a child in two school programs, Harwich preschool and a local nursery school. The school had purchased a computer system for the child so he could participate in a summer computer program. The **impartial hearing officer (IHO)** recognized that the school had shown good faith in supplying a computer for the child's use; she further ruled that the school had no obligation to provide this computer for the child at the other school (i.e., the nursery school).

Letter to Goodman (OSEP, 1990) dealt with a question as to (1) whether a school could presumptively deny assistive technology to a student with disabilities and (2) whether a need is determined on a case-by-case basis. OSEP's response indicated that assistive technology could be considered appropriate under either special education or related services and that, if specified in the IEP, the school is obligated to provide it. The determination is on a case-by-case basis.

Greenwood County (SC) School District #52, 1992 (SEA), involved the question of amending an IEP to provide a Liberator™ communication device for a 13-year-old girl with multiple disabilities and limited communication skills. The child had been using a Wolf™ communication device and an Apple IIGS® computer. Because the child had been functioning at a relatively low level, the school felt a lower-cost IntroTalker™ would fit her needs more appropriately. Because the Liberator was viewed as a device that allowed greater growth in language skills, the IHO ruled that the school purchase the Liberator. Although he recognized the Liberator to be more costly, he saw it as more cost efficient because of its potential for accommodating growth.

In *re Child with a Disability (CT)*, 1994 (SEA), the issue involved a student with cerebral palsy and cognitive impairment who was provided with a computer by the school to facilitate his communication. When the computer disappeared, the school replaced it with a letterboard; consequently, the parents requested a hearing for its replacement. The IHO ruled that either the computer or the letterboard fulfilled the requirements of the IEP and that the School Board was not a party to the disappearance of the computer and therefore not responsible to replace it. The letterboard was deemed acceptable because it was reasonably calculated to enable the student to achieve passing grades and to advance from grade to grade. This particular example reflects some differences in thinking among IHOs and interpretation of *what* constitutes FAPE. Although some IHOs would feel that the electronic communication device would be appropriate because of the extreme limitations of a letterboard, this IHO felt that either was sufficient.

In *Board of Education of the City School District of New York City*, 1994 (SEA), a 15-year-old student with a learning disability could not write without the assistance of a computer. The school offered to provide a computer for the child in the classroom to be used in conjunction with his home computer. The parents requested that the child be provided a laptop computer, and an IHO directed the school to provide a laptop on a 12-month basis until he reached the age of 21. In review, the State Hearing Officer found that the laptop was not required under either IDEA or Section 504 of the Rehabilitation Act for the student to benefit from his educational program. He also ruled that the availability of the computer at home did not conflict with the requirement that a computer be provided the child under special education and related services. The issue here was not whether the school should make a computer available to the child, but that a specific type of computer, a laptop, was not necessary to accomplish the educational goals. This case is interesting because it clearly supported the student's need for a computer, but it did not support a specific computer even though it might provide much more flexibility for the student.

In *Westminister School District (CA)*, 1994 (SEA), one of the issues concerned a 13-year-old male student with a genetic disorder resulting in a variety of problems, including communication. Although the need for AAC services was not specified in the IEP, the evidence substantiated that the IEP team had frequently mentioned the need for such services for the child to benefit from special education. The IHO concluded that AAC services were needed and ruled that the school provide the student with the SpeakEasy™ communication device and that the AAC specialist program the device and provide the needed training.

Julnes and Brown (1993) suggest that the IEP team consider the following operational questions in determining a student's need for assistive technology devices/services: (1) Is the assistive technology device/service needed for the student to receive FAPE? (2) Is the assistive technology device/service needed as a related service? (3) Is the assistive technology device/service needed for LRE? (4) Is the assistive technology device/service needed to enable the student to have meaningful access to a school-sponsored program/activity on a nondiscriminatory basis? If the answer to any of these questions is yes, then the assistive technology device/service must be provided. With the increasing recognition of the value of assistive technology, more demands will be made for it in IEPs. IEP teams may find it increasingly helpful to use consultants to help them in their decisions involving assistive technology.

If the IEP team determines that a student can benefit from assistive technology and it is specified in the student's IEP, the device or services may be obtained from either the LEA or the statewide system, if one exists. Also, IDEA mandates that transition services focus on independent living, full participation in community programs, and the use of assistive technology and services [see 20 U.S.C. Sec. 1425. (1990)].

This section on the legal basis concludes with the most recent extension of EHA and IDEA. In June 1997, the president signed the Individuals with Disabilities Education Act Amendments of 1997 (PL 105-17, 1997). Many of the basic functions and ideas represented in IDEA have remained the same, but some additions or changes pertaining to assistive technology were made. Generally, there is support for the development of a range of assistive instructional technologies that would enable students with disabilities to be more fully included in their respective school communities. Changes include defining the IEP team's responsibilities to include consideration of programs for all children with communication needs and children with sensory impairments as well as support for the development of captioned videos, captioned television programming, and adapted educational media technology as a means of enhancing the educational and cultural experiences of students and other individuals who are deaf or have hearing impairments and who are blind or have visual impairments. The law also makes provisions for subgrants to LEAs to encourage the adoption of promising practices, materials, and technology.

DUE PROCESS AND EXPERT TESTIMONY

Due process is a key element in ensuring that FAPE is provided to all children with disabilities. Although structures vary among states, a general procedure is outlined in federal law at 20 U.S.C. Sec. 1415 (1990) and 34 CFR Sections 300.506-300.515. Due process, although not specifically defined in IDEA, consists of a number of procedures to ensure that the student's legal rights are protected and appropriate services are being provided.

School Responsibilities

The school has a responsibility to provide information to parents/guardians on special education services and rights relative to obtaining these services. Parents/guardians have a right to examine their child's educational records. A school must provide prior notice of intent to evaluate that includes a statement, in the parents/guardians' native language, as to the reason and the nature of evaluation. If parents/guardians disagree with the evaluation completed by the public agency, they may have an independent educational evaluation at public expense. Procedural safeguards ensure meetings with parents/guardians and school personnel to facilitate the assessment process when needed, to see that the child is properly placed for services, and to ensure that an appropriate IEP is developed and implemented. Required participants include a representative of the agency who is qualified to provide or supervise special education services (and commit resources), the child's teacher of record, and individuals who conducted assessments and who can interpret the data. One or both parents/guardians (and the child, if appropriate), and other individuals at the discretion of the parent/guardian or agency may also participate. A member of the assessment team should be present, as well as someone from the agency who knows the evaluation procedures used with the child and can explain the results obtained. Parents/guardians must receive prior notice, which includes a statement of the purpose and nature of the meeting, and the meeting must be scheduled at a time and place convenient for them. Although parents/ guardians are considered to be important to the IEP process, if they decline to participate, the school may conduct the meeting without them. The school is responsible for making a record of the meeting. School personnel have the responsibility to use their best professional judgments in the design of the IEP and to use good-faith efforts throughout. The parents/guardians may refuse to sign the IEP. In this event, either party may file for a hearing (i.e., the school to implement the IEP or the parents/guardians to obtain what they consider to be appropriate services) [IDEA d 300.350 (1990)].

Hearings and Appeals

A parent/guardian who disagrees with the program being implemented by the school can request a hearing before an IHO. In some states (e.g., Indiana) voluntary mediation may be used to see whether the conflict can be resolved without a hearing. Disagreement can be about evaluation, identification, placement, or any aspect concerning FAPE. Either parents/guardians (on behalf of their child) or the school can initiate a hearing. The party requesting the hearing is called the "petitioner," whereas the party responding is called the "respondent." The child may be represented by a

parent/guardian, an advocate, or an attorney. The advocate can be a friend, teacher, professor, tutor, or representative from the state's protection and advocacy services. The advocate may have attended training sessions on IDEA, state regulations, and principles of advocacy. The school may be represented by an administrator, such as a special education director, or an attorney. When the IHO's hearing decision is rendered, either party has a specified period of time to file an appeal. In some states an appointed Appeals Board reviews the record of the hearing and determines whether the IHO's decision was consistent with the documentation and requirements of due process. In other states the review may be done by a single person, often an attorney. Appeals do not constitute a rehearing, although new evidence could be considered or sought by the reviewing officer, in which case all hearing rights would apply. The usual grounds for reversal of the IHO's decision include the following: (1) the IHO was arbitrary or capricious in the rendering of the decision; (2) the IHO's decision was not consistent with what a reasonable person would conclude based on reading the hearing documents and reviewing testimony; and (3) the decision was contrary to the law. All individuals have a right to proceed with judicial review in a civil court action if not satisfied with the decision of the state's reviewing agency. If the parent/guardian is found to have prevailed, attorney's fees may be recovered from the public agency.

All the laws that have an impact on education for individuals with disabilities are designed to help parents/guardians and professionals work together to develop appropriate programs, something that did not always happen prior to the legislation. In the past, parents/guardians either knew nothing of their rights or the problem festered so long that litigation seemed the only available or viable recourse. Administrative hearings were designed to provide a means for resolution of a problem before it developed to a level where judicial intervention was needed. Initially, hearings were held by IHOs who were appointed by the state or LEA. Parents/guardians usually represented their child and the special education director usually represented the school. Over time, however, these hearings have become much more legalistic (i.e., parents/guardians and schools often are represented by attorneys), with significantly more time being spent with attorneys objecting to procedures and introducing documents and other evidence. As a result, these proceedings have become increasingly more expensive. As Congress became more aware of court actions and the economic burdens placed on the parent/guardian in hearings, it passed a law to provide reimbursement for legal fees if the child/parent ultimately prevailed [20 U.S.C. Sec. 1415 (e)(4); 34 CFR Sec. 300.515 (1990)].

Serving as a Witness and/or Consultant

Although AAC was recognized by many educators as important in ensuring FAPE, there was no systematic way to ensure that either the services or communication devices would be provided (some administrators have discouraged writing assistive devices into the IEP because of the cost). The passage of the Tech Act (PL 100-407, 1988) and the **Americans with Disabilities Act (ADA)** (PL 101-336, 1990), increased incentives to provide assistive devices and appropriate services. As a result of this federal legislation and increased awareness by clinicians/educators and AAC users, increased litigation on AAC technology and service issues can be expected. Individuals providing AAC services are more likely to be called to testify in legal proceedings (e.g., hearings, civil court, criminal court).[1] Those individuals who are best prepared in AAC may be called as expert witnesses (for either the petitioner/plaintiff or the respondent/defendant). The following suggestions are intended to assist the AAC service provider in preparing to testify in hearings and court cases.

1. **Recognize the differences between administrative hearings and civil court cases (with and without jury).** An administrative hearing is a due process procedure in which all concerned parties present information to an IHO who evaluates all evidence and renders a decision based on the law and the record. Due process also allows for civil action. In a special education dispute, either party can file action in a civil court if not satisfied with the hearing decision or its subsequent appeal. In most cases, civil court cases involving special education are heard by a judge without jury. Many civil or criminal cases may involve the use of a jury to evaluate all evidence and render a verdict to a judge who has presided over the proceedings to ensure compliance to trial rules. Each of these situations pose different expectations for the witness.

   A hearing is the least formal of the three situations. It is also the least binding legally. In the past, special education hearings have involved representation of the individual by the parent or advocate and representation of the school by the special education director. Attorneys are used more frequently today, particularly if either party believes the case may go into civil court. The IHO serves to maintain order in proceedings and to ensure that both parties have opportunities to present their information. Because the IHO alone hears and judges all evidence, compliance with the usual strict rules of evidence and argument is not necessary. If the LEA does not implement the decision of the IHO, the SEA can withhold special education funds. Generally, no actions can be taken against a parent/guardian who chooses not to comply with the IHO's decision.[2]

---

[1]At the time this book was being prepared, fewer than 50% of the speech-language pathologist professional preparation programs and fewer than 30% of the special education professional preparation programs offered as much as a single course on AAC. In other professions related to AAC, even fewer programs offered coursework and practica in this area. Consequently, a large number of persons enter the workforce with minimal academic training and practica in AAC. This means that individuals with AAC academic and clinical experience are in great demand to provide direct and consultative services. Because one should only provide services for areas in which one is competent, professionals who have had some coursework and some practica in AAC may find it appropriate to refer to someone who is better qualified.

[2]Although it is true that parents cannot be compelled to comply with the IHO's decision, if the school is concerned that the child's welfare is in serious jeopardy, legal action could be initiated to place custody of the child with welfare or a foster parent so that the proper education can be implemented.

In civil cases, all parties are expected to adhere to a strict set of rules for conducting court procedures and handling evidence (testimony and exhibits). These procedures ensure that all parties receive a fair trial. These rules become very strict when juries are involved, because the judge must guarantee that any testimony or evidence presented does not bias the jury in its decision. For this reason, attorneys will object to the entry of any documents that are considered irrelevant or prejudicial. Civil court decisions are enforceable by the courts.

2. **Be direct and confident in all answers.** Appearance can have a significant influence. The witness should maintain good eye contact with the individual asking the question at all times. Answers should be delivered in a clear and confident voice, but any hint of arrogance should be avoided. At all times the witness must remain calm and avoid any hint of anger or frustration. A fundamental rule for all witnesses to remember is *never* be intimidated by the attorney and *pay respect* to the IHO/judge. A major job of the witness is to educate the participants (IHO/judge and/or jury). Although the attorney will ask the questions, the witness will increase the effectiveness of the testimony if all answers are framed to the understanding level of the jury. The use of visual aids and direct answers consisting of major points with supportive documentation can help the IHO/judge and/or jury better understand the material.

3. **Demonstrate a solid knowledge base of AAC.** Inasmuch as no current certification or specialty recognition exists in AAC, the only way to demonstrate appropriate training is through coursework, publications, conference presentations, workshops, experience, and memberships in professional associations. In addition, the witness should be able to demonstrate familiarity with current research literature. Knowledge and clinical competency must be established for the witness's testimony to be given appropriate consideration in the decision.

The attorney representing the opposing party will try to cast doubt on the credibility of the expert witness. The IHO/judge can determine the credibility of a witness (on the basis of credentials and answers); juries, on the other hand, are more subject to being influenced by biases. The opposing attorney's questioning will be directed toward finding any weaknesses in testimony that will cast doubt on credibility. For this reason, professional integrity plays a significant role in any testimony, as reflected in the witness's recognition of limita-

tions in knowledge and scope of practice and in honestly admitting to not knowing the answer to a question. A trial is no place to bluff! Often a trial verdict depends on which of two witnesses is believed by the IHO/judge and/or jury.

4. **Maintain good records.** No witness can remember all the details of evaluations or clinical services provided to individuals. In any hearing, accuracy and consistency in the testimony is critical for credibility; consequently, one must maintain good notes on evaluations (tests and procedures used, nature of responses, interpretations of results) and discussions with other important people in the individual's environment. Witnesses may use notes to assist their memories during testimony. The IHO/judge will be looking for data that support or refute the need for AAC services. For this reason, the witness must be careful that all statements are clearly substantiated by the facts presented in the records and testimony. Juries are often impressed by well-organized and well-documented testimony.

5. **Answer the question, but do not add information.** The representatives for the petitioner/plaintiff and the respondent/defendant know what they want to demonstrate by asking their questions. The witness should answer each question as succinctly as possible, stressing salient points and avoiding becoming immersed in minute details or irrelevant information. Elaboration of answers may provide a key word or idea that could trigger a whole new direction of questioning. Address all remarks only to the person asking the question. Sometimes representatives will get into dialogue involving the witness, especially if the hearing is emotional. Although this is more likely when the parent/guardian is representing the child, attorneys can become involved as well. The IHO/judge has the responsibility to see that this does not happen.

In jury trials, the witness must pay attention to the judge and attorneys, answer directly and succinctly, and avoid any additional comments. Because consistency in the presentation of testimony is critical in determining the credibility of the witness, enhancement of the truth or omission of important details can be detrimental to the case. If witnesses are determined to be resistive or prejudicial, they may be treated as hostile, allowing more aggressive questioning, including leading questions. Furthermore, witnesses may be cited for contempt of court if the judge perceives them to be uncooperative or disrespectful of the court.

Prior to court testimony, and frequently when a witness may not be able to appear at a hearing, testimony may be taken by means of a conference call during a scheduled part of the hearing or in the form of a deposition. A **deposition** is a formal procedure in which both attorneys prepare specific questions to be answered. The witness is asked these questions, and the answers are transcribed into the formal record. In a hearing, a drawback to this approach might be the lack of opportunity for the IHO to observe the demeanor and credibility of the witness. In court cases, a deposition plays an important role because it discloses what the testimony is likely to be and is subject to verification under examination during the trial. For expert witnesses, it is not unusual for the deposition to involve an entire day.

All witnesses should be aware of a legal requirement that, other than the confidential communication afforded between client and attorney, no private communications can occur between involved parties (e.g., attorney, representative, client, or witness) and the IHO/judge. This rule regarding **ex parte communication** ensures that the IHO/judge's decision cannot later be challenged on the basis of unfair sharing of information germane to the case. For this reason, attorneys routinely share copies of any correspondence with the IHO/judge and with the opposing representative. If telephone contact is considered, it will generally be a conference call involving all concerned parties.

Although the above suggestions have been given to aid the potential witness in the event of being called on to testify, witnesses should confer with the representative/attorney at all stages of the hearing/trial process. The attorney is in the best position to prepare witnesses for any possible surprises, as well as to help them avoid any unknowing violations of legal procedure.

ETHICS

Individuals operate according to personally established principles or values that guide how they conduct their lives. When people become a part of an organization, their individual values or **ethics** are generally codified into a set of guidelines under which the group conducts itself and expects individual members to conduct themselves (e.g., business ethics, professional ethics). In govern-

ment, these values or ethics often are translated into laws. Codes of ethics are guidelines for encouraging behaviors by which individuals are judged to be good and honorable. Laws specify behaviors that are deemed unacceptable—even damaging—and indicate what sanctions will be exacted by society. Often laws are enacted when society judges that ethics or values are not resulting in those behaviors necessary for the welfare of society's members. As discussed earlier, laws were necessary because schools were not providing appropriate services for children with disabilities, something that was inconsistent with the expressed values of Americans.

Codes of Ethics

Several professional organizations have been founded on the principle of providing quality services for individuals with disabilities. Associations such as the **Council for Exceptional Children (CEC)**, an organization comprised of individuals with disabilities, special educators, and others concerned with special education services; **RESNA** (Rehabilitation Engineering Society of North America, subsequently renamed the Rehabilitation Engineering and Assistive Technology Society of North America), an interdisciplinary association for the advancement of rehabilitation and assistive technology; the **United States Society for Augmentative and Alternative Communication (USSAAC)**; and the **American Speech-Language-Hearing Association (ASHA)**, an organization comprised of audiologists and speech-language pathologists, have established codes of ethics for their members. Each professional association strongly encourages all students in training programs to become familiar with stated ethical principles so they will be able to adhere to them. The codes of ethics for these organizations will be discussed with particular emphasis on their relation to the provision of AAC services. Because CEC's, RESNA's, and USSAAC's codes of ethics are more general, they are presented here for general informational purposes. ASHA's Code of Ethics serves as an outline for consideration of applications to AAC practice and is discussed in more detail.

Council for Exceptional Children. The Code of Ethics of CEC (1991) is reproduced below in its entirety.

We declare the following principles to be the Code of Ethics for educators of exceptional persons. Members of the special education profession are responsible for upholding and advancing these principles. Members of the Council for Exceptional Children agree to judge them in accordance with the spirit and provisions of this Code.

I. Special education professionals are committed to developing the highest education and quality of life potential of exceptional individuals.

II. Special education professionals promote and maintain a high level of competence and integrity in practicing their profession.

III. Special education professionals engage in professional activities which benefit exceptional individuals, their families, other colleagues, students, or research subjects.

IV. Special education professionals exercise objective professional judgment in the practice of their profession.

V. Special education professionals strive to advance their knowledge and skills regarding the education of exceptional individuals.

VI. Special education professionals work within the standards and policies of the profession.

VII. Special education professionals seek to uphold and improve where necessary the laws, regulations, and policies preserving the delivery of special education and related services and the practice of their profession.

VIII. Special education professionals do not condone or participate in unethical or illegal acts, nor violate professional standards adopted by the Delegate Assembly of CEC.

RESNA. RESNA is an interdisciplinary association for the advancement of rehabilitation and assistive technology. It promotes the highest standards of ethical conduct. The Code of Ethics for RESNA (1993) states that its members shall adhere to the following:

1. Hold paramount the welfare of persons served professionally.
2. Practice only in area(s) of competence and maintain high standards.
3. Maintain the confidentiality of privileged information.
4. Engage in no conduct that constitutes a conflict of interest or that adversely reflects on the association and, more broadly, on professional practice.
5. Seek deserved and reasonable remuneration for services.
6. Inform and educate the public on rehabilitation/assistive technology and its applications.
7. Issue public statements in an objective and truthful manner.
8. Comply with the laws and policies that guide professional practice.

United States Society for Augmentative and Alternative Communication. USSAAC adopted a code of ethics in September 1994. The stated intent of the code is to inspire and educate members so that they may responsibly maintain and promote ethical standards (Lytton, 1995). The principles of this code of ethics are as follows:

1. Individuals shall abide by their responsibility to give the highest priority to the welfare of persons served professionally. Individuals shall respect the rights and dignity of all persons.
2. Individuals shall maintain and promote high standards for AAC practice, education, and research.
3. Individuals shall abide by their responsibility to achieve and maintain the highest level of professional competence to insure that the needs of the consumer are paramount.
4. Individuals shall provide accurate and current information to the consumer about AAC and the services they provide. Individuals shall not engage in dishonesty, fraud, deceit, misrepresentation, or any form of conduct that adversely affects AAC's professional practice or any consumer.
5. Individuals shall abide by promoting understanding of AAC and supporting the development of services designed to meet the needs of the consumer.
6. Individuals shall abide by their responsibility to enhance relationships among their colleagues, other professionals, consumers, and students.

7. Individuals shall not discriminate in the delivery of professional services on the basis of race, gender, age, religion, national origin, sexual orientation, or disability.

8. Individuals shall utilize a service delivery approach that incorporates the goals, objectives, skills, and knowledge of various disciplines including that of the consumer and family members.

9. Individuals shall accept the responsibility to expand and improve professional knowledge and skills to insure that the consumer receives the most appropriate technology and services available.

All of these codes of ethics with their delineated principles, although stated differently, share common features with the ASHA Code of Ethics. All professionals are expected to maintain high standards and exercise good judgment in their practice, as well as to work toward the overall betterment of their clients. Professionals are also expected to neither condone nor participate in unethical practices.

American Speech-Language-Hearing Association. ASHA has established a comprehensive, well-defined code of ethics to assist its members in decision making as they engage in their professional activities (ASHA, 1994). This code of ethics covers ASHA members, nonmembers who have the Certificate of Clinical Competence (CCC), and those individuals completing their clinical fellowship year (CFY) for certification. Adhering to these principles of ethics should encourage audiologists and speech-language pathologists to maintain a high standard of conduct and earn the trust of the individuals whom they serve. ASHA sets out four principles of ethics. Each of the principles is further subdivided to include a number of rules. Rather than listing each of the many rules individually under each principle, discussion is based on the rules in general.

Principle 1. "Individuals shall honor their responsibility to hold paramount the welfare of the persons they serve professionally." A true professional considers the needs of the client paramount, serves as a strong advocate for re-

sources and services, and refers to another professional if needed. The professional providing services is expected to be competent in the area and not to provide stated or implied guarantees for cure. The clinician/educator is expected to be appropriately trained and updated in AAC. The service provider should work actively to see that the client being served receives appropriate devices and services. The AAC professional is responsible for seeing that proper evaluations are completed. When AAC services/devices are needed, specific recommendations should be included in the IEP. The clinician/educator is also responsible for seeing that the AAC portion of the IEP is implemented and that all services provided and progress in treatment are documented.

Principle 2. "Individuals shall honor their responsibility to achieve and maintain the highest level of professional competence." Individuals are expected to be appropriately trained and certified/licensed in the area in which they provide services. They must also continue their professional education throughout their careers. Because no special certification/license in AAC is required at present, determining professional competency and whether a professional is operating within these ethical standards is difficult. Often AAC clinicians/educators have had no formal training. Experience working with other professionals who have AAC knowledge and experience, and frequent consultation with them helps to build AAC expertise. Additionally, they must remain current by reading the professional literature in the area and attending workshops in AAC. Also, because the provision of AAC services is a highly intensive effort, any aide who provides AAC assistance must have appropriate training and supervision.

Principle 3. "Individuals shall honor their responsibility to the public by promoting public understanding of the professions, by supporting the development of services designed to fulfill the unmet needs of the public, and by providing accurate information in all communications involving any aspect of the professions." Misrepresenting credentials, training, knowledge, or expertise in the area for which one is providing services is unethical. The public in general, and clients in particular, should be fully cognizant of a service provider's professional competencies in AAC. In addition, because AAC is a relatively new field and not widely known about by the public, as well as many other professionals, the AAC clinician/educator has a responsibility to promote understanding of AAC and to do everything possible to ensure the development, expansion, and delivery of AAC services. Because many individuals have an unrealistic idea regarding the role of technology in AAC (e.g., an electronic speech device will solve all speech problems), it behooves the AAC professional to help educate the public and other professionals about the full spectrum of AAC approaches, including unaided communication (e.g., signing, gestures) and low technology (e.g., communication boards), as well as high-technology electronic devices.

Principle 4. *"Individuals shall honor their responsibilities to the professions and their relationships with colleagues, students, and all members of allied professions. Individuals shall uphold the dignity and autonomy of the professions, maintain harmonious interprofessional and intraprofessional relationships, and accept the professions' self-imposed standards."* All professionals need to maintain openly honest, working relationships with other professionals. This is particularly true when speech-language pathologists work as part of an AAC assessment/treatment team with occupational therapists, physical therapists, and rehabilitation engineers. The speech-language pathologist must be able to make independent, professional decisions. In AAC, however, the speech-language pathologist must also be able to weigh individual professional judgments with the inputs of team members to achieve a collective judgment of what is best for the AAC user.

Ethical Situations

Many AAC professionals will be confronted with new situations for which there are no clearly defined rules, therefore, common sense combined with a knowledge of both law and ethics as applied to AAC is essential. Examples of ethical situations that the AAC practitioner might face are discussed in this section. These situations include (1) provision of AAC services for individuals with degenerating conditions; (2) specification of the need for AAC technology in the IEP; (3) determining one's own competency to deliver AAC services; (4) programming personally offensive language into a communication device; and (5) determining the appropriateness of providing facilitated communication.

1. Your patient, a 65-year-old male, has amyotrophic lateral sclerosis (ALS), which has resulted in severe neurophysiological deterioration. Although the patient has resisted the use of AAC for some time, his request now appears to be for the purpose of communicating his wish to die and to make arrangements for settling his estate. What are the ethical options?

    Many speech-language pathologists who work in rehabilitation settings have faced ethical dilemmas. Increasingly, AAC providers are working with individuals with a variety of degenerating diseases such as ALS and Parkinson's disease. Many of these individuals are older and may cling to using natural functions, including unaided communication, as long as possible. Although a means for communication with family members as well as medical staff would be helpful, these individuals may resist using any form of assistive technology. AAC devices may be perceived as artificial, nonnatural, and inconvenient. In many cases the selection of an AAC device is an acknowledgment of physical/neurological degeneration and represents a surrendering of independence. For this reason, the assistance of an AAC service provider may not be welcomed at first. However, with deterioration to a point of helplessness, the individual may finally give in to the reality of his condition and be motivated to communicate with loved ones by using anything that is available. At this point, the individual may accept AAC services. The point at which an ethical dilemma may arise, however, is when so much deterioration has occurred that the person wishes to die. At this point, AAC technology may suddenly be welcomed as a means of providing the communication necessary for completing the necessary legal and personal arrangements, including processing of documents for transferring funds, writing wills, or making funeral arrangements which may be disconcerting to an AAC service provider. Even more disconcerting to some may be the individual's use of AAC to provide a means to communicate a wish to die in the presence of witnesses. The AAC service provider, then, must wrestle with a conflict between professional and personal ethics. Professionally, the AAC service provider has an obligation to provide the services needed for the individual to communicate and tend to arrangements. Personal ethics, however, may dictate withdrawing from the situation and not committing to what is perceived to be an immoral or unethical act. The speech-language pathologist, if not comfortable assisting with such an arrangement, has a professional ethic to refer to another service provider.

2. You are a special educator. Several individuals developing the IEP, including you, believe an AAC device is needed for one of your students. Your director of special education will not let you include the recommendation for an electronic communication device in the IEP because of the expense and possible ramifications to an already constrained budget. This special education director has let it be known that people who do not comply with the request could be laid off. What are your ethical options?

    You have a professional and ethical responsibility to consider the welfare of your client above all other issues. Actually, so does your director of special education. Individuals are often placed in situations where they perceive their jobs or welfare may be placed at risk for acting on a professional conviction. If the individuals developing the IEP believe a recommendation for a device should be included, the critical features/specifications must be written into it. They may indicate what device(s) have these features. In such cases, you have support from fellow professionals. If you are alone in your opinion, you at least can write an opinion expressing your professional concerns. You must exercise your professional judgments and vigorously support what you believe to be appropriate. The CEC Code of Ethics commits you to serve as an advocate for your student. Inasmuch as the director of special education's action is inappropriate and in direct violation of IDEA, you would have justification to file a complaint and/or grievance. A complaint will result in an investigation by the department of education. At the very least, if you are unable to follow through with a grievance or serve as an effective advocate for your client, you should consider resigning and working in a setting more consistent with ethical practices.

3. You are a speech-language pathologist in an agency located in a rural part of the state. You have been approached by parents to evaluate and provide AAC services for their child and to recommend a communication device. You have a CCC in speech-language pathology, a state license, and attended one workshop on AAC evaluation. What are your ethical options?

    This situation can be very difficult. In these cases, an argument often is made for providing services because the alternative for the child is no service at all. Because all of the codes of ethics mandate that an individual provide services only if professionally trained and competent, you have an ethical responsibility to consider other alternatives, including referrals. Certainly, you should refer the child for an appropriate team evaluation. Because you are appropriately certified and licensed, you can provide some speech and language services, perhaps including limited AAC. However, if you decide to provide AAC services, you should consult with individuals who are well trained in AAC who can provide advice and supervision or guidance, as appropriate.

4. You are a female occupational therapist who has taken on the primary role of programming an electronic communication device and training the AAC user and significant others to use it properly. The AAC user is a 17-year-old male who demonstrates some typical teenage characteristics (e.g., interest in sex and use of swearing or dirty words). He would like you to program some of these words so they are available to him when he uses his communication device. What do you do?

    This case has a number of issues that need to be dealt with. You may consider whether the parents might object to this programming, as well as your own position on the use of dirty words. Some occupational therapists may be offended by the words, but may be comfortable programming them into the device as long as they don't have to hear them (although that's never a guarantee). Other occupational therapists may not want to even participate in the programming of such language. Remember, a cardinal rule is that an AAC user's vocabulary should be based on needs, interests, and vocabulary level and should be the primary consideration in programming. Certainly, motivation for use of a device for communication with others (interaction) will relate to how much it provides for the needs and interests of the AAC user. This may be a case of conflict between the AAC user's needs and your own moral code. One answer may be to have another person program the device and then request that the AAC user not use the language in your presence. Another option may be to program the words into the AAC user's device and then teach the use of language within proper social contexts as a part of his social development. For example, individuals must learn to be sensitive to others so they do not use language that may be perceived as offensive. With close friends, offensive language may be acceptable. Also, for some individuals, use of offensive language in private may serve as an emotional outlet.

5. A child's parents have been to a conference on facilitated communication and met some parents who are very enthusiastic about the use of it with their children. They ask you to implement such a program with their child who is enrolled in your special education program. They are very enthusiastic and willing to assist you in learning and using the techniques. What are your ethical options?

You have an ethical responsibility to use evaluation and treatment approaches that represent the best practices of the field. To do this, you must keep abreast of current practices through conferences, workshops, consultation with other professionals, and reading the available research. Although **facilitated communication (FC)** has enjoyed enthusiastic support from some special educators and speech-language pathologists, it has become very controversial. When Biklen introduced FC in the United States after observing its use by Crossley in Australia, there was a rapid growth of evangelistic-like activity. Many workshops were presented across the country and testimonials of success were bountiful. In some cases charges of child abuse were brought against parents or teachers because of the facilitated messages allegedly typed by the user (Seligman, 1992; Shapiro, 1992). When FC was subjected to scientific scrutiny, however, it did not hold up (Bligh & Kupperman, 1993; Cummins & Prior, 1992; Eberlin, McConnachie, Ibel, & Volpe, 1993; Shane, 1993, 1994; Thompson, 1993; Wheeler, Jacobson, Paglieri, & Schwartz, 1993). In carefully designed studies, the FC user and facilitator received different information; the message typed was that provided by the facilitator. For this reason, you must be cautious in using the technique without careful evaluation of its effectiveness. You also have a responsibility to share information regarding its effectiveness with the parents and to explain why you are or are not willing to use FC.

COMPETENCIES, CERTIFICATION, AND LICENSURE

AAC is a transdisciplinary field. Such a wide variety of professionals provide AAC services that there is no general agreement as to what qualifications are needed and who should lead the team. Although ASHA (1989) suggests that the speech-language pathologist is an appropriate professional to serve in this leadership capacity, in reality, the responsibility falls on the professional who has read enough and/or gained practical experience in AAC. In some cases this leadership has been provided by an occupational therapist, a special educator, a speech-language pathologist, or a rehabilitation engineer. Most professionals agree that each member of the team brings special skills or competencies that are critical to AAC assessment and intervention.

Many professionals believe that any individual who provides services to an AAC user should have a minimal set of competencies. Some have proposed that these competencies be articulated for certification/licensure. ASHA committees have been formed to consider specialty recognition. In 1994, RESNA received a grant to develop guidelines for certification/specialty testing in assistive technology. At first glance, RESNA certification seems appropriate for AAC professionals. However, the issue is complex. Professionals tend to examine the certification issue with a somewhat myopic view in terms of their individual training. The competencies to be specified, or the knowledge base to be tested, however, certainly must include basics of all relevant disciplines. For speech-language pathologists, this might mean a knowledge of anatomy of speech and hearing processes, language development, specialized language assessment procedures, and assistive communication devices. For the rehabilitation engineer, however, minimal competencies might include a knowledge of mechanics design, electronics, and computer programming. The challenge will be to agree on the fundamental concepts that should be common to all potential assistive technology participants, as well as specific additional competencies for the professional's area. This suggests a two-tiered certification process in which applicants demonstrate a basic knowledge across areas (e.g., occupational/physical therapy, technology), as well as specialized knowledge in their own professional domains (e.g., special education or speech-language pathology).

A general problem with certification/licensure is that it may do the opposite of what is intended. Most professionals maintain that licensure protects the client by ensuring that the provider of the service has minimal competencies. Many legislators, however, tend to view licensure as self-serving for the professional by protecting a domain of practice from outside intruders. The truth lies somewhere in between. However, if third-party payers limit payments to individuals who are certified/licensed, then licensure becomes important because it is linked to income. If a small number of individuals are licensed, the net effect may be restricted availability of services for the AAC user (which is likely because AAC is such a specialized area and a limited number of practitioners are considered to have expertise). If third parties recognize licensure, they will have to determine the rules under which payment will be made for services. Inasmuch as a team approach to assessment and intervention is gener-

ally recognized as the best practice, this approach should be recognized and reinforced. Therefore, an approach in which a program or delivery system is licensed in recognition that the AAC team comprises competent, licensed personnel may be more appropriate. In this case, reimbursement might well be to an AAC team-based program, not to an individual AAC provider.

SUMMARY

Many significant legal events have had an influence on the field of AAC. These new laws have introduced into the field the need for due process for testifying as an AAC witness. Organizations (e.g., ASHA, CEC, RESNA, USSAAC) whose professionals are involved in the delivery of AAC services have written codes of ethics to help professions with ethical dilemmas. New professionals are always encouraged to seek the counsel of experienced professionals as they pursue options for individuals needing AAC, and experienced professionals are encouraged to remain current. Certification and licensing continue to be an issue for AAC professionals.

CHAPTER 21

SERVICE DELIVERY AND FUNDING

CAROLE ZANGARI AND CHARLOTTE A. WASSON

Service delivery and funding are two areas of central importance to the field of **augmentative and alternative communication (AAC),** particularly as they relate to clinical and educational applications. In contrast to the early years of AAC service provision, which centered primarily on residential institutions and special schools, communication and other services are now provided in a wider variety of settings using one or more service delivery models. According to a recent survey, AAC services are now provided by approximately half of all facilities offering speech-language pathology services (Shewan & Blake, 1991). This chapter describes the characteristics, strengths, limitations, and challenges of the major models of AAC service delivery. Models are discussed in relationship to the settings in which AAC services are provided, and the major roles and responsibilities of team members are considered. Funding issues are discussed as they relate to (1) government sources building on the legal bases discussed in Chapter 20, (2) nongovernment sources, (3) the process, and (4) future directions.

SERVICE DELIVERY

Great diversity exists among the various approaches to delivering AAC services. One influential factor is that AAC involves many disciplines, with no one being fully equipped to provide the comprehensive services that are required by AAC users. AAC service delivery falls on a number of different turfs, including, but not limited to, occupational therapy, physical therapy, special education, speech-language pathology, and vocational rehabilitation.

A second factor influencing service delivery relates to the heterogeneity of individuals with AAC needs. For example, an individual with severe, multiple impairments may need comprehensive AAC services of long duration, which may include practice in accessing a device, learning its symbols, and using AAC in natural environments, whereas an individual with mild physical impairments may need only short-term AAC intervention that addresses only one aspect of communication, such as note taking or preparing messages. In addition, some AAC users have multiple needs (e.g., positioning, switch use, environmental control), whereas others need only communication services.

A third factor influencing AAC service delivery is that most AAC users require services across the life span, which usually brings with it varying teams, team philosophies, and team practices. Consider Lonnie, an individual born with multiple cognitive and physical impairments, who is identified as being at risk for severe communication disabilities. Both Lonnie and his family may begin working with early interventionists in the home setting before he attends an infant/toddler center-based program. He may then move on to a preschool program at age 3. In each of these early intervention settings, Lonnie is likely to receive services from a team of professionals working collaboratively with one another and with him and his family in an effort to meet his cognitive, communication, motor, self-help, and sensory needs. After preschool, he will probably continue to receive services in the public school system, where his multiple needs will be targeted by the local educational agencies (LEAs). After the school years, services may be provided either continuously or intermittently through a contractual arrangement with agencies that support Lonnie's living and vocational needs. At any time from birth until late life, AAC services may be a significant need for Lonnie. What models of service delivery are available to address these needs, and what are their characteristics? In what settings are they found, and what professionals will provide them?

Models of Service Delivery

Unidisciplinary Model. In some settings, AAC services are provided by one or more professionals operating independently of one another (McCormick, 1990a). In the **unidisciplinary model** or single-service provider model, each professional represents a specific discipline (e.g., occupational therapy or speech-language pathology) and provides services that are primarily specific to that discipline. However, occasional communication may occur between professionals on an as-needed basis. For example, James, a 58-year-old adult, has both severe aphasia and hemiplegia. He visits a university speech and hearing clinic for aphasia therapy, which includes AAC intervention. He receives occupational therapy in his home to help increase independent functioning in activities of daily living. Except for one instance when the occupational therapist called the speech-language pathologist to discuss James's speech and limb apraxia, the two professionals did not communicate. James and his family are quite comfortable with this model.

Multidisciplinary Team Model. The **multidisciplinary team model**, which grew out of a medical model, is composed of representatives from different professional domains who share information about a particular individual's status, intervention program, and progress on a regular basis (Locke & Mirenda, 1992; McCormick, 1990a; Yorkston & Karlan, 1986). Communication among team members exists with the expectation that shared information will lead to highly individualized and appropriate assessment and intervention programs. However, joint goal setting or

problem solving is not expected. Assessment and intervention activities are conducted separately by professionals in their respective areas of expertise. Results and recommendations are shared among group members through circulation of diagnostic reports, presentations at team meetings, or both. The multidisciplinary team model is used with Dee, a young woman with locked-in syndrome (LIS). She requires an alternative means of communication while she remains in the intensive care unit. Her service delivery team includes the occupational therapist, physician, respiratory therapist, and speech-language pathologist, and each evaluates her and develops recommendations, which are shared at her team conference. Each professional's recommendations then become a part of Dee's overall plan of care. The various professionals meet with her individually to address the goals and objectives detailed in their sections of the care plan. They also communicate their specific plans to appropriate individuals in Dee's present environment.

Interdisciplinary Team Model. The **interdisciplinary team model** also focuses on communication among team members, but differs from the multidisciplinary model in three primary ways (Locke & Mirenda, 1992; McCormick, 1990a; Yorkston & Karlan, 1986). First, the channels of communication among team members are formalized. Generally, a case manager is appointed to coordinate service delivery and manage the flow of information. Second, this model may include some form of consultation services, whereby some team members provide information and recommendations to others. Third, intervention programs may be planned jointly. Implementation of these programs are, however, still generally carried out by team members from specific disciplines who provide services in their particular areas. Clara, a 25-year-old woman who has had multiple strokes, for instance, receives services from an interdisciplinary team in the skilled nursing facility where she resides. In Clara's case, a rehabilitation manager coordinates the delivery of services. The occupational therapist, who is teaching Clara to use switches to activate a variety of assistive technology devices, consults with the speech-language pathologist for input regarding what communication devices can be used to best meet Clara's communication needs. The speech-language pathologist consults with the dietician regarding Clara's nutritional needs and incorporates this information into Clara's dysphagia treatment. Other collaborative meetings among service providers occur as needed.

Transdisciplinary Team Model.   The **transdisciplinary team model** focuses not only on communication among team members but also on collaborative team relationships and program planning (Locke & Mirenda, 1992; Lyon & Lyon, 1980; McCormick, 1990a; Yorkston & Karlan, 1986). Services developed under the transdisciplinary model represent the ultimate parity among members of the team. Team members work together to provide services, not just by sharing information, but also by jointly implementing assessment and intervention activities. A primary feature that distinguishes this team model from the multidisciplinary and interdisciplinary team models relates to the concept of **role release**, which provides for the crossing of traditional professional boundaries, leading to the transfer of knowledge and skills traditionally associated with a specific discipline to individuals outside of that discipline to improve the quality and functionality of service delivery (Lyon & Lyon, 1980). **Cotreatment** is a term that describes the joint delivery of services resulting from role release (Russell & Kaderavek, 1993).

Another feature of the transdisciplinary team model is continuous staff development. Team members teach one another about aspects of their own professional domains relevant to the assessment and intervention activities in which they are jointly engaged. A transdisciplinary team model is used by the AAC team working with Jason, a 15-year-old youth with autism who is preparing to participate in job training at a local hardware store. Initially, the team meets with Jason and his family to identify priority areas for intervention (e.g., job training and improvement in independent living skills). Team members then work together to assess Jason's strengths and specific needs within each of the priority areas. Because AAC skills are impor-

tant in each priority area, all team members help develop programs designed to improve communication skills within the broader context of service delivery. Once goals are identified and prioritized, a select few team members who spend the most time with Jason work to implement his communication programs. All have been provided with staff training by the speech-language pathologist. The job coach, for example, can help Jason learn to use a communication wallet to tell his boss when he has run out of supplies, his teacher can help him learn effective use of a picture menu to communicate food selections at the restaurant where he will eat lunch on workdays, and his parents can assist him in using a communication chart to choose his clothing the evening before each workday.

Related Forms of Service Provision.   In addition to the unidisciplinary, multidisciplinary, interdisciplinary, and transdisciplinary approaches, other service delivery approaches are noted in the literature. Several of these are actually a variation or a part of those already described. The transdisciplinary model, for example, is highly supportive of an integrated therapy approach. This collaborative approach centers around intervention that uses an individual's daily experiences as both a context and a focus (Albano, Cox, York, & York, 1981; Calculator & Jorgensen, 1991; Giangreco, York, & Rainforth, 1989). In this approach, just as in the transdisciplinary model, an individual's needs are identified and prioritized by the educational or treatment team. High-priority environments and activities are addressed first. Intervention goals and objectives are written to guide the development of skills required to participate or function in the prioritized environments, and activity plans are created. Intervention is programmatically integrated and infused into the individual's daily routines, and the effectiveness of the intervention program is evaluated in relation to the AAC user's performance in natural, daily environments (Calculator & Jorgensen, 1991). For example, a service delivery team may determine that independent transportation has the highest priority for an AAC user who needs increased opportunities to participate in integrated community activities. All prioritized goals and objectives for this AAC user would then relate directly to increasing independent transportation skills (e.g., telling the van driver the destination, scheduling times for pick-up, or communicating emergency messages).

Another variation of the transdisciplinary model, the **collaborative teamwork model**, was developed by professionals serving school-aged individuals with severe disabilities to stress team planning and decision making throughout assessment and intervention (Rainforth, York, & Macdonald, 1992; York & Vandercook, 1990). Students with severe disabilities provided with services via this model are integrated in typical educational settings. They are then provided with natural supports to assist them in learning social competence, improving levels of independence in daily routines, and developing special interests.

The collaborative teamwork model incorporates **collaborative consultation**, which has existed in general and special education for many years (Calculator & Jorgensen, 1991; Gibson, 1990a, 1990b; Idol, Paolucci-Whitcomb, & Nevin, 1986; Nelson, 1990; West & Idol, 1990). Broadly defined, collaborative consultation is "an interactive process that enables people with diverse expertise to generate creative solutions to mutually defined problems" (West & Cannon, 1988, p. 56).

The interdisciplinary model of service delivery, with its emphasis on shared information but not shared services, incorporates **expert consultation, systems consultation**, and **informational consultation** (Johnson, Pugach, & Himmitte, 1988). In expert consultation (or short-term consultation), a **consultant** who has been brought in as an AAC expert makes recommendations during the assessment, intervention, and evaluation phases of service delivery. The **consultee** then carries out these recommendations. In AAC service delivery, this consultee might, for example, be a classroom teacher, a parent, or a vocational training specialist. Expert consultation is usually of fixed duration and has no set procedures for follow-up.

In systems consultation the consultant is also viewed as an expert. As such, the consultant assesses, designs intervention, and then evaluates intervention effectiveness. Just as in expert consul-

tation, the consultee carries out the intervention. Unlike with expert consultation, however, systems consultation often includes specific mechanisms that support follow-up by the consultant. Systems consultation might occur when the AAC service provider who sees the AAC user only intermittently assists communication partners (e.g., parents and daily care staff) who frequently interact with the AAC user to understand their roles and responsibilities in carrying out interventions.

Informational consultation supports the consultant's attempts to share expert information that is narrow enough to meet the AAC needs of a particular individual, yet broad enough to be applied to the needs of other AAC users with similar challenges in similar situations. In this type of consultation unlike in expert and systems consultation, the consultee assumes responsibility for some of the assessment and most of the intervention and evaluation. The nature and extent of follow-up are at the discretion of the consultee, who will request additional consultant involvement as necessary. In AAC, informational consultation might, for example, involve a speech-language pathologist as the consultant and a vocational training agency's job coach as a consultee.

Strengths, Limitations, and Challenges of Service Delivery Models

Each of the four models of service delivery (unidisciplinary, multidisciplinary, interdisciplinary, and transdisciplinary) has strengths and limitations or challenges as applied to AAC (see Table 21.1). For example, a strength of the transdisciplinary model and its integrated therapy approach is that it uses the coordinated expertise of team members to facilitate the development of AAC skills within meaningful activities, thus minimizing problems of skill generalization. One limitation, however, is that this model requires administrative support and professionals from several disciplines who are willing and able to teach and learn from one another in a collaborative fashion. Another limitation is that, because services are generally provided within the context of the AAC user's daily activities, professionals must have

TABLE 21.1 Strengths and Limitations of Service Delivery Models

MODEL AND DESCRIPTION	STRENGTHS	LIMITATIONS
Unidisciplinary. One discipline is responsible for providing service.	Saves time because there is no time needed for coordination; reduces scheduling problems; links assessment and intervention.	Limits variety of professional knowledge, skills, and perspectives.
Multidisciplinary. Professionals from two or more disciplines working independently with each team member maintaining discipline boundaries; little, if any, service coordination.	May present minimal scheduling challenges because professionals do not need to be in close proximity; allows AAC user to seek services from preferred professionals.	Promotes dissection of services; may allow areas of great need to go unnoticed and untreated.
Interdisciplinary. Professionals from two or more disciplines working independently, but with formalized roles and coordinated information flow; coordinated by a team manager.	Provides for some coordination of assessment and intervention services; promotes coordinated management of information flow.	Challenges the linking of assessment and intervention because professionals from different professions may be responsible for each; charges professionals with implementing programming for which skills and supports may be lacking.
Transdisciplinary. Professionals from two or more disciplines engaging in joint functioning, continuous staff development and role release to promote arena assessments, integrated therapy, and consultation.	Eliminates isolation and/or redundancy of service delivery; promotes AAC user skill acquisition in natural environments; promotes parity among team members; provides necessary training to individuals charged with program implementation.	Requires team member and administrative support; presents scheduling challenges.

flexible schedules that fit the AAC user's typical routines.

The strengths and limitations of some models of service delivery are influenced heavily by the settings in which they are carried out. For example, a school-based program that employs a varied staff of professionals often has the personnel and administrative support to execute a transdisciplinary model of service delivery. On the other hand, a professional in private practice who may see AAC users in their home settings will probably find the logistics of transdisciplinary involvement problematic because of the isolated work environment.

Although some challenges are specific to the model of AAC service delivery being implemented, every model has similar challenges in varying degrees. Each team model challenges service providers to encourage and participate in open communication and collaboration among team members. Team functioning is enhanced by creative problem solving from different perspectives. Team skills, including negotiation and conflict resolution, are not often taught as a part of professional training, but such skills are essential to the success of each model. Frassinelli, Superior, and Meyers (1993) note that knowledge and skills in assessment and intervention in particular disciplines do not automatically lead to successful collaboration among members of service delivery teams. Training focused on developing communication skills that lead to effective collaboration and consultation must, therefore, become a key component of preprofessional and professional training programs.

AAC Service Delivery Settings

Although an individual can seek and find AAC services in numerous locations, all service delivery settings can be categorized as either off-site or on-site or, in some instances, both. Off-site services are provided in settings such as a university clinic, outpatient rehabilitation center, or private practice office, to which an AAC user must travel to get AAC services. On-site services are provided in a setting in which an AAC user regularly spends time, such as school, home, or the workplace. Generally, an AAC setting is selected based on the availability of services and the AAC user's needed level of care (i.e., frequency, intensity, and type of services).

Off-Site Services.

Center-Based Programs. In center-based programs, AAC users travel to agency settings where assessment and/or intervention services are provided. A hospital that provides individuals with both inpatient and outpatient services would be considered a center-based program. Here, outpatient AAC services and related services (e.g., occupational and/or physical therapy) may involve a few hours of treatment per day or week, or they may be as intensive as inpatient services, but with-

out the nursing and medical care component (Goldsmith, 1994). Examples of other common center-based program settings providing AAC services include clinics, rehabilitation centers, specialized schools, and universities (Locke & Miranda, 1992; Yorkston & Karlan, 1986).

Most center-based programs employ professionals from multiple disciplines who work together as an interdisciplinary or transdisciplinary team to provide AAC services. How often the AAC user attends center-based programs depends on the specific communication needs and logistics (especially distance to the site). Numerous center-based programs providing AAC services specialize in comprehensive evaluations of communication needs. These centers typically make recommendations for developing AAC programs, recommend assistive technology, and provide follow-up. The actual AAC intervention may be carried out by a separate agency, such as the LEA, which may look to the center-based program for training and/or technical support. In some instances, intervention will be offered at both the center-based program and the separate agency to provide more intensive services.

Center-based programs have a number of advantages, including the centralization of resources. Many center-based programs are well-equipped with AAC devices and other assistive technologies, such as page turners and environmental control units (ECUs). They also typically employ a professional staff from several disciplines with expertise in AAC who have experience working as a collaborative team. A drawback to center-based programs is the nonnaturalistic environment in which services are provided. Unless special arrangements are made to see the AAC user outside of the center, the staff may find it difficult to make accurate assessments of communication skills and needs in real-life situations and plan for generalization (Calculator & Jorgensen, 1991). In addition, some individuals who work closely with the AAC user may have difficulty coming to the center-based program, making the sharing of information among all team members problematic. This means that the individuals who work most closely with the AAC user in natural environments have little opportunity to provide center-based staff with critical information regarding the

AAC user's typical communication needs. Similarly, the center-based staff has little opportunity to teach strategies and techniques used in the center to individuals who work with the AAC user in natural environments.

Logistical arrangements related to center-based programs can also be problematic, particularly if the center is a great distance from the AAC user's home. Because many individuals with AAC needs fatigue easily, the time spent in travel may prevent them from arriving for an evaluation or therapy fresh and ready to put forth their best effort. If the AAC user has special transportation needs (e.g., an ambulance or travel attendant), additional time, discomfort, and expense may be involved. Teams need to develop creative solutions to all of these challenges. When distance prevents frequent communication partners from accompanying the AAC user, written and telephone communication can be useful. Videotaped examples of procedures being suggested by the center-based staff may clarify goals for those who cannot observe firsthand. Similarly, videotapes of the AAC user in natural settings can provide center-based staff with critical information not observable in the center. When AAC user fatigue is an issue, meetings should be arranged around optimal times.

Rehabilitation Centers.   Several levels of care, including levels of AAC assessment and intervention, may be provided by outpatient rehabilitation centers (Goldsmith, 1994). Some rehabilitation centers provide several levels of acute care to inpatients, along with a range of care levels to outpatients. At the most intensive level, rehabilitation centers or skilled nursing facilities may provide 24-hour rehabilitation programming to individuals residing at the center who need rehabilitative but not medical intervention. In these cases, the rehabilitation facilities would be considered on-site, rather than off-site, settings because the patients receiving such care are residing at the facility. In other cases, intense, whole-day rehabilitation services are provided to outpatients who need intensive interdisciplinary services, but not around-the-clock care. In these cases, the rehabilitation centers would be providing off-site services. Rehabilitation outpatients would typically arrive in the early morning,

receive aggressive therapies all day, and depart for their homes in the evening. In a less-intense form, outpatient rehabilitation programs may be provided by the full interdisciplinary or transdisciplinary team, but on a less frequent basis (e.g., a few hours 3 to 4 times per week). Still further, a select few members of the professional service delivery team may continue to see those outpatients who no longer require a full spectrum of services. For example, if occupational or physical therapy are no longer essential to achieve targeted AAC goals for a post-cerebrovascular accident (CVA) outpatient with severe aphasia, the speech-language pathologist alone may deliver AAC services, even though other professional services are still available at the facility.

On-Site Services.

School-Based Programs.   In many areas of the United States, a full range of AAC services are provided to preschool and school-aged children through individual school systems, consortiums, or cooperatives. In Broward County, Florida, for example, students with AAC needs may be referred to their region's Florida Diagnostic and Learning System (FDLS) office, which has on-staff professionals who are knowledgeable about AAC issues. Students may then be observed by the AAC specialist and other team members (e.g., assistive technology specialists, occupational therapists, or vision specialists), as necessary. These professionals work with each student's LEA team to develop an appropriate educational program (B. Sanders, personal communication, July 28, 1994). The AAC specialists may be involved in selecting and programming an electronic communication device, teaching the family and personnel from the LEA how to use it, and monitoring the student's AAC success. Other ways in which school-based programs provide AAC services include establishment of the following:

1. Specialized classrooms exclusively for students who have AAC needs, allowing intensive focus on developing AAC skills and competencies
2. Specialized teams of professionals who consult with and provide support to a student's primary educational team

3. Equipment loan programs
4. Educational networks that provide inservice training, resources, and/or technical support.

Like other service delivery settings, school-based programs have both strengths and limitations. This service delivery setting, in its optimal form, allows for integration of AAC services with other educational services, making AAC a means to an end (i.e., social and academic participation), rather than an end in itself (Calculator & Jorgensen, 1991). The school setting may also be more efficient because AAC and other educational services are provided by the same parent organization (i.e., schools). In many cases, the school-based services are more easily accessible to a student with AAC needs than services provided in other settings. An obvious limitation to this setting is the age restriction. A student who has benefited from high-quality AAC services as a student may graduate with a sophisticated, multicomponent AAC system, but must then find an alternative means and setting for service delivery. Another limitation relates to funding. Most school-based programs do not have an adequate financial base to acquire the full range of equipment needed for comprehensive AAC assessment and intervention services. Also, many school-based programs have been unsuccessful in billing Medicaid, a potential third-party payer, either for AAC services or devices.

Home-Based Programs.   Home-based programs use the AAC user's natural environment for service delivery. Although this service delivery setting is most frequently used with infants and toddlers or elderly individuals, home-based AAC services may also be appropriate for individuals discharged from inpatient programs who have acquired severe communication disabilities related to illnesses, injuries, or degenerative diseases. These individuals may require short-term, home-based AAC services prior to community and/or employment reintegration, or they may be candidates for long-term, home-based AAC services (Goldsmith, 1994). An obvious strength to home-based service delivery is that communication skills are targeted in an environment in which the AAC user is a daily participant. This practice not only promotes skill

generalization, but also helps interventionists identify communication goals and objectives that are most meaningful and functional (Calculator & Jorgensen, 1991; Goldsmith, 1994). Providing services within the home may also facilitate the use of a family-centered treatment approach, a consultative approach in which professionals outline treatments to be implemented by family members (Campbell, Draper, & Crutchley, 1991). Client fatigue is generally not an issue in home-based services, because the AAC user does not need to travel.

Disadvantages of service delivery in this setting include the time spent in travel by the AAC professionals and, in some cases, the need to transport equipment. Home-based service delivery may also present other time-related logistical problems. For instance, coordinating the schedules of all the professionals so that they can collaborate and/or cotreat in the AAC user's home can be difficult.

Private Practice and Contractual Services.   Individuals needing AAC services can also seek services from professionals in private practice. Private practitioners provide both direct and indirect services and can be contracted either by individuals or agencies (e.g., group homes, skilled nursing facilities, and school programs). Many facilities that serve individuals with little or no functional speech do not have the expertise within their own staff to provide their clients with the AAC services they require. Often, these facilities contract with AAC professionals to provide the required services under one of the several consultative models discussed earlier in this chapter. These consultative services range from direct contact with AAC users for evaluation, development, and implementation of AAC programs to indirect contact through inservice and staff development. Thus, contractual arrangements may not only provide for services to AAC users, but also serve to supplement the knowledge of general staff (as in informational consultation). This form of consultation has two distinct benefits. The first is directly to AAC users who gain needed communication skills because of the expertise of the consultant; the second is to staff members who gain skill in providing AAC intervention. Drawbacks of such consultation, however, also exist. First, program consultants may not be as familiar with the individual clients and/or the contexts for intervention as they would be if they were full-time employees. Second, some AAC users, families, or staff members may have a distinct bias against this type of service delivery, preferring a type in which an inherent long-term relationship exists between the service provider and AAC user.

Rural Service Delivery.   In rural areas, AAC users, families, and professionals may have difficulty getting together for AAC service delivery. Frequently, long distances, rugged terrain, or extreme weather conditions pose enormous challenges to the delivery of AAC services. Privratsky dealt with all three of these obstacles in addressing the AAC needs of rural Alaskans (Van Tatenhove, Kovach, Privratsky, & Costello, 1993). In this situation, professional members of the AAC service delivery team regularly traveled hundreds of miles to the communities in which AAC users lived, sometimes transporting their equipment and materials on sleds from the airstrips to the villages. Creative solutions unique to the circumstances can often be developed by dedicated service delivery teams to extend the resources of service providers and circumvent the obstacles that distances present. For example, in rural Texas, professionals with expertise in AAC can consult with AAC users and/or their local service providers via satellite conferencing (R. Linville, personal communication, March 14, 1995).

Combination Off-Site and On-Site Services.
Some approaches to service delivery that offer features of both off-site and on-site programs have previously been discussed. In some hospital and rehabilitation-based programs, for example, AAC users may be seen individually as outpatients, while also being served in a regular day program, such as a school. Sometimes this dual-site treatment approach may be delivered by the same service provider who is employed at both facilities. When the service provider works in both settings and is a full participant in developing the individual's service delivery plan, the individual with AAC needs can benefit from the advantages offered by both the center-based and school-based approaches. In some situations, this combination approach is favorable because drawbacks from one approach are offset by advantages of the other.

AAC Teams

Since the early 1950s, professionals have recognized that a team approach to service provision facilitates positive outcomes (Whitehouse, 1951). Currently, in most settings in which AAC services are provided, the AAC user, family members, and professionals from two or more domains work as a team to develop a course of action. In Chapter 11, teams were discussed with regard to the assessment process. Appendix D provides a listing of possible members on an AAC team. As in assessment, a subset of members often functions as a core team for intervention, with other members (e.g., audiologist, orientation and mobility [O & M] specialist, rehabilitation engineer, or vision specialist) being drawn in to meet specific needs of individual AAC users. In some settings, such as public schools, the function of the team is governed by specific policies and procedures. In other settings, such as the AAC user's home, teams may be more loosely structured.

Changes in health care and education have sparked a trend toward increased use of paraprofessionals or aides to provide AAC services previously provided by professionals. In some fields, such as occupational therapy, the use of assistants to provide services in a single domain is well established. More recently, therapy or rehabilitation assistants have been trained in a number of other domains to provide selected AAC services under the direction of qualified professionals. For example, a multiskilled assistant may position an AAC user based on the specifications of a physical therapist, use a communication board designed by a speech-language pathologist, reprogram a communication device with vocabulary selected by the special educator, or implement specific switch activities developed by the occupational therapist.

Rainforth, York, and Macdonald (1992) have suggested three types of service delivery roles that team members fill: (1) team members have generic roles and responsibilities, including active participation in making decisions, solving problems, sharing knowledge, supporting team efforts, and keeping current with their own professional literature; (2) members also have discipline-specific roles in which each professional is expected to contribute discipline-specific knowledge and skills for the benefit of AAC users being served; and (3) some members have related services roles, such as developing adaptations and/or equipment to encourage community participation, facilitating functional skills and abilities, and addressing other tasks as charged by other members of the service delivery team (Giangreco, 1990).

Misconceptions about "Experts"

A frequent misconception regarding AAC services is that the best ideas and solutions come from highly trained, professional experts. In reality, AAC has many experts, and the best solutions for effective and efficient service delivery are developed through collaboration among team members. Who are the "experts"? Certainly, professionals on the AAC service delivery team are expected to have expertise in their own areas. Not all practitioners in a specific discipline, however, have sufficient knowledge and skill to provide appropriate AAC assessment and intervention services. Some speech-language pathologists, for example, have commanding knowledge of communication development and disorders, but limited knowledge and experience with individuals with little or no functional speech. Similarly, educators may have extensive knowledge of content materials, curricular issues, and general principles of educational instruction, but lack experience in adapting the educational process to meet the needs of students with severe communication disabilities. Other professionals, on the other hand, may have in-depth knowledge and experience in AAC and should be sought to serve key roles in AAC service delivery, as long as that service delivery complies with the ethics of that specific professional discipline. Frequently, each profession's code of ethics will guide service providers in deciding whom and how to treat. See Chapter 20 for a discussion of professional ethics as they relate to AAC service delivery.

A second group of AAC "experts" whose contributions may be minimized because their areas of expertise are unrecognized or underacknowledged include AAC users' family members, peers, and paraprofessionals. Though not trained in professional disciplines, individuals close to the AAC user bring invaluable knowledge and experience to the AAC assessment and intervention processes. Their expertise is in their personal experiences and knowledge about individual AAC users, their communication needs, and the environments in which they live, work, and play. Without the information of these experts, accurately evaluating the AAC user's needs and abilities and determining the best plan of action are impossible.

"Expert" input most certainly comes from the AAC user. Often, the AAC user is capable of communicating prioritized goals and objectives and can provide insight into those environments most conducive and important for goal attainment.

Ideally, all the professional and nonprofessional members of the AAC service delivery team are recognized as experts. AAC users and their family members educate professionals on the AAC user's functional communication needs, and professionals educate AAC users and family members about communication options, strategies, and intervention techniques to meet those needs, thus forming a partnership that supports and promotes coinvolvement (Campbell, Draper, & Crutchley, 1991; Lloyd & Belfiore, 1994).

FUNDING

In addition to the challenges that AAC service providers experience in selecting and implementing appropriate services, teams face tremendous challenges in finding AAC **funding**. Because technology often plays a critical role in the lives of AAC users, service delivery teams traditionally think of AAC funding endeavors primarily as efforts directed toward acquisition of communication devices for particular AAC candidates. In this text, however, funding issues are addressed more broadly, recognizing that AAC service delivery requires provision of financial resources for a number of undertakings. Funding efforts typically include (1) gaining financial support for AAC user assessment and intervention, and (2) procuring monies that can be applied to AAC user-specific device acquisitions with both low technology and high technology, (3) in some cases, acquiring funds to seed or continue development of clinics and/or teams, and (4) procuring funding to support research and/or professional training (Church & Glennen, 1992; Cohen, 1986; Koul & Lloyd, 1994b; Lloyd & Belfiore, 1994). Developing comprehensive and effective funding plans for any and all of these activities, therefore, is one of the most critical elements of a comprehensive service delivery plan and requires significant time and energy from each AAC team. Efforts to secure funding are frequently exercises in patience, because no one systematic funding avenue currently exists. Skill, knowledge, and persistence are often required for a successful outcome (Hammond, 1992).

AAC Funding Team

Numerous members of the AAC team may hold significant roles throughout the funding process, regardless of which aspect of funding is being addressed. When funding searches are geared toward AAC assessment and/or intervention or communication device acquisition for a particular individual, the AAC user or candidate necessarily becomes the pivotal member of the team. Recent funding attention has, in fact, shifted away from focusing on recommendations of professional members of the team toward considering the needs and desires of AAC users (Franklin, 1993; Lahm & Elting, 1989; Morris, 1993b; Parette, Hofmann, & VanBiervliet, 1994). When the AAC user or candidate is unable to self-advocate during the funding process, then parent/guardian funding preferences should take priority (Parette, Hourcade, & VanBiervliet, 1993).

In addition to AAC users and individuals close to them, teams working toward AAC user-specific funding needs should consist of several professionals which may include the occupational therapist, physical therapist, physician, speech-language pathologist, teacher, and/or vocational rehabilitation counselor (see Appendix D for a more comprehensive listing of potential team members). The team's efforts will be most successful if one member is assigned to the leadership role of **funding coordinator** (Post & Crawford, 1992). This coordinator should be highly articulate, have knowledge of pertinent legislation regarding funding issues, and possess strong organizational and communication skills to guide the direction of the various funding activities. Often this team member is referred to as the "client advocate" (Ripley, 1989). Although the funding coordinator does advocate for the AAC user's funding needs, emphasis on consumer responsiveness is generally understood. The term *advocate* can be reserved for AAC users (consumers) and their caregivers, thus reflecting both a philosophical and procedural transfer of power in the service delivery structure (Morris, 1993b). Although occupational therapists, social workers, and speech-language pathologists have often served as funding coordinators, any skilled team member can potentially serve in this capacity. If a coordinator lacks funding experience, consultation with practiced funding coordinators from other teams is advisable.

If the goal of an AAC funding effort is to start up or continue developing an AAC assessment and/or intervention team, the team will consist primarily of only those professionals who serve as direct members of the assessment/intervention team. Typically, the AAC user will not be included. The team may still, however, be managed by a funding coordinator, but the coordinator's charge will be more global.

The AAC funding team working toward user-specific device acquisition often has the support of a second funding coordinator, employed by the manufacturer of the targeted communication device. The funding coordinator from the AAC team should work closely with the manufacturer's funding coordinator throughout the funding process to identify possible financial resources and coordinate time lines to avoid fragmentation in efforts that could lead to unnecessary funding delays (Post & Crawford, 1992; Prentke Romich Company, 1989; Ripley, 1989).

Securing resources to seed or continue the development of AAC training and research programs requires yet another team structure. Members of this team may be individuals who have AAC teaching and/or research duties (Lloyd & Belfiore,

1994). Again, a coordinator is needed to ensure that the goals and responsibilities of the training and research team are well served. Past experience and success in grant writing and program management are essential skills for this coordinator. Because only 30% of funding pools are awarded to new recipients, the coordinator may choose to find a mentor to assist in first-time funding endeavors. Mentors can be located by reviewing the public records of potential funding sources to identify individuals and/or institutions with recent grant success.

Disability Legislation

A review of potential AAC funding sources requires examining legal issues that either directly or indirectly affect funding. In the United States, for example, at least four recently enacted or amended pieces of federal disability legislation provide notable legal impetus for funding assistive technology devices and services in general, and AAC devices and services in particular. Most of these regulations affect user-specific AAC funding efforts. Although these pieces of legislation mandate services, they do not typically supply a funding base to support them. For a broader review of legal issues affecting AAC, see Chapter 20.

Technology-Related Assistance for Individuals with Disabilities Act.
The Technology-Related Assistance for Individuals with Disabilities Act (PL 100-407, 1988) or the Tech Act, as it is commonly called, was enacted to provide federal grant funds to various states to promote the provision of consumer-responsive services and assistive technology devices. A reauthorization of the Tech Act, the Technology-Related Assistance for Individuals with Disabilities Amendments (PL 103-218, 1994), includes broad-based mandates on each state's assistive technology projects to provide access to and funding reforms for assistive technology (Golinker, 1994). Presently all 50 states are voluntarily involved (Parette, Hofmann, & Van-Biervliet, 1994). Each state's Tech Act project has been charged to increase (1) awareness of need, (2) awareness of policy, and (3) opportunities to procure assistive technology devices and services

(Peter-Johnson, 1994; RESNA, 1993). Within each state, specific reform options have been developed across a wide variety of service delivery areas, including (1) public program focus, (2) interagency coordination, (3) protection and advocacy, (4) information awareness, (5) service capacity and consumer choice, (6) alternative financing options, and (7) alternative technology approaches (Moore, 1993).

Although the various state projects do not provide direct funding for AAC device acquisition, some states are making AAC devices and other assistive technologies accessible through regional assistive technology centers, so that individuals with disabilities can gain access to these devices without traveling long distances. Other states have suggested and are supporting innovative funding initiatives (Moore, 1993; RESNA, 1993). Additional systems changes for improving accessibility to technology and service are expected and will at least partially grow out of 16 specific policy recommendations that the National Council on Disability (NCD) provided to the United States President and Congress under Title II of the Tech Act (Morris, 1993b; Moore, 1993; RESNA, 1993).

A particularly important part of the Tech Act affecting AAC funding is the development and promotion of standard definitions of assistive technology devices and services (see Chapter 20 for definitions). These definitions have direct implications on the acquisition and use of AAC technologies because evaluation, device acquisition and training, therapy coordination, professional training, and technical assistance are specifically listed examples of services.

Because of the Tech Act's broad scope, legislation may have significant implications for each of the four types of AAC funding undertakings. Information regarding a particular state's Tech Act project may be obtained by contacting RESNA's Technical Assistance Project (see Appendix B-3). Most local and state educational agencies can also supply information about that state's Tech Act organization.

Americans with Disabilities Act.
The Americans with Disabilities Act (ADA) (PL 101-336,

1990), also referred to as the Civil Rights Bill for individuals with disabilities, is patterned after Sections 504 and 508 of the Rehabilitation Act (PL 93-112, 1973). The ADA offers broad protection to individuals with disabilities in public accommodations, employment, state and local government services, and transportation. Access to telecommunications, which most directly affects the communicative needs of AAC users, falls under Title IV, which specifies that telecommunication devices are to be accessible to individuals with hearing *and* speech disabilities. This accessibility is currently provided through Telecommunications Relay Systems (TRSs). The ADA also specifies that future technologies must also be accessible to individuals with disabilities, including those with little or no functional speech. Although direct funding for AAC devices and services is not provided by the ADA, "the ADA will make the link between equal opportunity access to assistive technology much stronger than ever before" (Williams, 1993, p. 7).

Individuals with Disabilities Education Act. The passage of the Individuals with Disabilities Education Act (IDEA) (PL 101-476, 1990) significantly expanded the well-known Education for All Handicapped Children Act (PL 94-142, 1975) and Education of the Handicapped Act (EHA) Amendments of 1986 (PL 99-457, 1986)[1] and adopted the definitions of assistive technology devices and services from the Tech Act. Further amended as PL 102-119 (1991), IDEA, along with the Letter to Anonymous (1991) from the Office of Special Education Programs (OSEP), clearly documented the right to assistive technology devices and services for children with disabilities (Brown, Perry, & Kruland, 1994; Morris, 1993a). Assistive technology devices and services may, in fact, be provided to children from birth through age 21 (Baldwin, Jeffries, Jones, Thorp, & Walsh, 1992; Parette et al., 1994). If a student's individualized education program (IEP) establishes that assistive technology devices and services are needed to pro-

vide free, appropriate public education (FAPE), the LEA may be required to fund such devices and services, or, at minimum, coordinate funding efforts. If use of the technology at out-of-school times is written into the IEP, the child should be allowed to take the device out of the school. If transportation of the device is impractical, then a second device for home use may have to be provided by the LEA (Beattie, 1993; Morris, 1993b). AAC devices and services have been funded on numerous occasions because of IDEA legislation.

Rehabilitation Act Amendments. The Rehabilitation Act Amendments of 1992 (PL 102-569, 1992) reflects several fundamental changes in the Rehabilitation Act of 1973 (PL 93-112, 1973), which directly affected AAC users who have vocational rehabilitation needs covered under state Vocational Rehabilitation Services (Button, 1993). For instance, the amendments provide for increased AAC user choice-making and control. These are based on the premise that individuals with disabilities are presumed capable of performing work tasks, unless a vocational rehabilitation agency can unequivocally prove otherwise. The amendments also grant increased access to technology devices and services by requiring that those devices and services necessary to the acquisition and/or retention of employment be included in the individualized written rehabilitation program (IWRP) (Project ACTT, 1993).

Although these four notable pieces of federal disability legislation address the need to provide assistive technology and services to individuals with disabilities, including those with little or no functional speech, they typically do not provide for a direct source of funding. Funding sources at the federal, state, and local levels, however, do exist. Although many of these public and private sources are tailored toward the funding of assistive technology devices and services for a specified individual, some have broader funding perspectives that meet the needs of AAC assessment and intervention teams and/or teams dedicated to AAC re-

---

[1]In this text, the term *disabilities* is used to be consistent with current terminology; however, *handicapped* is used when it is part of the title of laws.

search and professional training (Church & Glennen, 1992).

Funding Sources

Medicaid.   Although assistive technology is not specifically addressed under the federal and state-funded program of Medicaid, in at least 34 states, an individual who is currently receiving public assistance or Supplemental Security Income (SSI) or is in active treatment in an intermediate care facility (ICF) may qualify for technology devices and services (Golinker, 1994; Hammond, 1992; Markowicz & Reeb, 1988; RESNA, 1993; Rice, 1989). In several of these states, AAC devices and services may be funded through Medicaid if they are deemed to be medical necessities (i.e., durable medical equipment [DME]), and if payment is not covered by a third-party source (e.g., a private insurance carrier). In these states, a "speech prosthesis may be covered as a separate category to other benefits" (Brown et al., 1994, p. 6). Some states funding AAC devices under Medicaid do so under exclusionary policies. For instance, Illinois has funded AAC devices for residents of ICFs with cognitive impairments (mental retardation) and/or developmental disabilities (ICF/MR-DD), but for no one else. Although Medicaid's funding of AAC devices and services is not consistent, progress has been made and is expected to continue (Golinker, 1994).

Medicare.   In 1989, the funding of AAC devices and services under Medicare became more likely when the Six-Point Plan involving Medicare reimbursement took effect (Reimbursing Adaptive Technology, 1989; RESNA, 1993). Under this plan, which is a part of Medicare's Part B program, an individual may acquire assistive technology devices as DME if the equipment replaces a missing body part, is reusable, serves a primary medical need, and is usable in the home (Reeb, 1985). According to this plan, an AAC device for an individual who has been laryngectomized is likely to be covered, whereas a device for an individual who acquired a closed head injury (CHI) might not be. "Unfortunately, the evolution of Medicare policy has only reached the point where

funding will be approved on appeal" (Golinker, 1994, p. 23).

Veterans' Administration.   Based on a needs assessment conducted at a Veterans' Administration (VA) Medical Center, veterans with Type A service-related status qualify for assistive technology devices and services funding through the center's Prosthetics Activities Services and its Prosthetics Representative (Reeb & Stripling, 1989). Because not all veterans are eligible for all veterans' benefits, technology-related requests are handled on a case-by-case basis.

Workers' Compensation.   Workers' Compensation assistance, which can be awarded as either cash or medical benefits, can be used to procure AAC devices and/or services (Reimbursing Adaptive Technology, 1989; RESNA, 1993). In many instances, individuals who receive Workers' Compensation benefits because of a job-related disability qualify for all of the benefits related to vocational rehabilitation services, including those specific to assistive technology devices and services.

Social Security Administration.   Although the Social Security Administration (SSA) does not directly fund acquisition of assistive technology devices and services, as the largest single source of governmental payments, it does have provisions that allow an individual with assistive technology needs to become more self-sufficient without threat of losing Social Security Disability Income (SSDI) benefits. Specifically, SSDI permits an individual with disabilities to purchase assistive technology, such as an AAC device, and hold down employment, potentially earning more than the Substantial Gainful Activity (SGA) level (Reimbursing Adaptive Technology, 1989; RESNA, 1993).

Vocational Rehabilitation Services.   As noted above, enactment of the Rehabilitation Act Amendments of 1992 (PL 102-569, 1992) brought increased certainty for funding of AAC devices and other technologies for individuals covered under the Act. Devices and services necessary to the acquisition and/or retention of employment that are included in the IWRP are to be funded, because of an assumption that individuals with disabilities are capable of performing work tasks when given appropriate supports (Project ACTT, 1993).

Private and Group Insurance Carriers. Insurance companies vary dramatically in their coverage of many items, including AAC devices and other technologies and services. Some companies, for example, require that the condition creating the need for devices and services be medically related by being directly attributable to an illness, surgery, or accident. AAC devices would be covered under such headings as "speech prostheses." If AAC devices and other assistive technologies are not listed in the exclusionary clauses of a policy, individuals with technology needs are wise to apply (Church & Glennen, 1992; Hammond, 1992).

Corporate and Private Foundations. Both corporate and private foundations may meet the individual or group needs of persons with disabilities. Although corporate giving has decreased slightly in recent years (*RE:view*, 1994), substantial amounts of funds continue to be set aside as foundation resources. *The Foundation Directory*, which is updated every 2 years, is available through the sponsored program office at most universities and local libraries. It contains extensive information regarding foundation giving.

Subsidy Programs. Numerous subsidy programs, which offer low-cost or no-cost technology-related loans and financial awards, have been developed in an attempt to make technology products more broadly available to individuals with disabilities, as well as to groups serving the needs of individuals with disabilities (Lazzaro, 1993; Ward, 1989). Subsidies are offered, for example, by a number of private not-for-profit organizations (e.g., local service clubs such as the Lions or Kiwanis). Other subsidies are offered by wish granters, health organizations, manufacturers, charities, and partnerships between device manufacturers or retailers and volunteer organizations, as well as by private and public utility regulating agencies (Ward, 1989).

Personal and Budgetary Resources. Individuals in need of AAC devices and services may have personal resources that can fully or partially finance AAC devices and training. Although assets vary from person to person, AAC users should consider personal finances as a resource because of the sense of personal pride that comes from ownership (Lazzaro, 1993). AAC teams that provide AAC assessment and intervention, and AAC professional organizations that engage in AAC research and/or training may also set aside a portion of their budgets to support their own missions.

Funding Process

Although assistive technology financing provisions appear in several federal disability legislation, obtaining funding to support acquisition continues to be a challenge (Franklin, 1992; Golinker, 1994). As is noted throughout this text, AAC service delivery is built on the premise that all individuals with AAC needs should have access to quality learning and communication opportunities. Typically, these opportunities must include provision of potentially useful technologies and services. The service delivery team, therefore, is mandated to set bold agendas that will provide AAC users with appropriate AAC devices and services.

To date, however, the full application of available AAC technology has not been realized. Although clear policies govern the funding of AAC devices and other assistive technologies, practices and procedures to secure this funding are still failing (Parette et al., 1994). Lack of finances and lack of information are frequently cited as barriers to assistive technology acquisition (Uslan, 1992).

Several procedural factors must be considered in AAC user-specific funding endeavors, whether those endeavors are geared toward AAC device acquisition or services. Although in many instances, funding pursuits will be as individual as the person needing the funding, there is a common process. A procedural guide listing necessary funding activities can assist the funding coordinator and entire funding team (Table 21.2).

Release time from other duties for the funding coordinator and possibly other team members

TABLE 21.2 Procedural Guide for Seeking Funding for AAC User-Specific Technologies and Services

Gather information regarding the individual needing AAC device(s) and/or services.

Assign team membership and select funding coordinator.

Conduct a needs assessment and feature matching to determine appropriate device(s) and/or services.

Assign duties to team members for report-writing tasks.

Publish and/or announce time lines to all team members involved in funding requests.

File written justifications (e.g., reports and letters of support).

Follow up on status of requests.

If denied, appeal.

TABLE 21.3 Essential Information To Include in Funding Reports and Letters

Client description.

All necessary recommendations.

Reason for AAC device(s) and/or services funding request.

AAC user prognosis.

Listing of features of AAC device(s) and/or services.

Cost of AAC device(s) and/or services.

Listing of other potential funding streams being pursued.

Request for expected date of decision regarding funding.

could be essential to the acquisition of funding because of the amount of time that must be spent on the process. Gathering information; drafting reports, letters, and grants; and making phone and personal contacts with other team members and potential funding sources are typical time-consuming tasks.

Well-written reports and letters of request carry considerable weight in the positive outcome of funding requests (Lytton, 1994). Therefore, these requests must reflect terminology that specifically addresses the unique needs of the AAC user and, at the same time, reflect the activities and regulations of the agency being solicited (Lytton, 1994). Funding requests for Medicaid, Medicare, and private and group insurance companies, for example, need to focus on the medical necessities of the request. Requests to vocational rehabilitation service agencies, on the other hand, should demonstrate how a device or services will assist the individual with AAC needs in acquiring and/or keeping employment. Requests to public education agencies should detail how the device and services will facilitate the educational process. Table 21.3 details some of the areas that are typically included in AAC user-specific funding re-

ports and letters. Although details about requests differ from case to case, similar information should be incorporated into all requests.

Funding AAC Teams

When an AAC team has a more global focus to service delivery through provision of assessment and/or intervention to multiple AAC users or engagement in AAC professional training and/or research, numerous potential funding streams exist. Most of these, however, are directly accessed through successful grant writing. Several authors have addressed the general procedures involved in pursuing either private or public grant funds. Table 21.4 highlights the major activities of the grant-writing process (Catlett, 1989; Gelatt, 1989).

Certain AAC teams or team members may be eligible to seek funds through various disability legislation. For example, Part H, the Early Intervention Guidelines of IDEA, Section 303.12, specifically lists training or technical assistance for professionals and other persons working directly with children with disabilities as a mandatory technology service. Similar technical assistance and professional training is included in the Tech Act. Because the Tech Act is beginning to have far-reaching effects, the financial support for AAC team training may well show an increase (Morris, 1993a).

TABLE 21.4   Guide for AAC Grant Writing

Determine AAC grant funding team membership.

Select a funding coordinator.

Gather information about all potential sources of funding.

Educate the AAC funding team regarding potential grant funds.

Prioritize grant programs and select those most in line with AAC needs.

Aggressively pursue those grant programs most in line with AAC needs.

Review the AAC team's funding ideas with the funding agency before grant writing.

Write grant proposal, following grant criteria explicitly, including all information requested such as the abstract, need, methodology, evaluation, personnel, resources, and budget.

Write, read, rewrite, reread.

Seek feedback from successful grant writers.

Adhere to time lines.

If not funded, adhere to appeals/reapplication procedures, if such exist.

Adapted from Catlett (1989); Gelatt (1989).

Future Directions

Funding for appropriate AAC technology and services, AAC assessment and/or intervention teams, and AAC research and professional training will undoubtedly be a challenge to the AAC field for many years to come. Instances of successful funding of AAC devices and/or services may actually decrease before they increase. For example, although technologies to improve communication are booming, so is awareness. As individuals with AAC needs become more and more active as self-advocates and as teams become more responsive to AAC users, more demands will be placed on funding resources to purchase AAC devices and/or services. Yet, at the same time, both public and private institutions are facing budgetary cuts. Further, as more and more health agencies become involved in managed care, documenting the necessity of long-term AAC service may become increasingly more challenging for AAC teams. Concerted efforts will be required if the funding maze is to be conquered. Morris (1993a) notes the following:

> Who should bear the costs of assistive technology services and devices? There is no single response that will prove to be effective for all circumstances. There are instead a combination of strategies or approaches that build on the success of current public policy, public-private sector partnerships, selected state experience, and legal precedents to create a vision of an accessible American, with technology playing a critical role in changing the way individuals with disabilities interact with their social and physical environments. (p. 6)

SUMMARY

AAC service delivery is at the heart of every AAC activity. Team membership will include various professionals working collaboratively with individuals with AAC needs and their families and caregivers. Throughout the AAC service delivery process, which often spans a lifetime, many challenges arise. Open lines of communication and clear knowledge of the strengths and weaknesses of the service delivery model being employed will assist members of the service delivery team to provide effective and efficacious assessment and intervention.

Included in the challenges confronting AAC service delivery teams are those related to funding AAC assessment, intervention, device procurement and training, and/or research. Innovative means of support must be sought to provide the financial bases necessary to bring AAC devices and technology into the hands of individuals with little or no functional speech. Although funding requests can be challenging, AAC service delivery teams can meet this challenge.

CHAPTER 22

MULTICULTURAL ISSUES

GLORIA SOTO, MARY BLAKE HUER, AND ORLANDO TAYLOR

Augmentative and alternative communication (AAC) users come from many diverse cultural backgrounds, as do people in general. As AAC service providers work to facilitate and increase AAC users' opportunities for full academic, social, and/or vocational participation, they must become aware of cultural influences affecting their practices (Hetzroni & Harris, 1996).

Cultural and social factors underlie all AAC service delivery activities. They are present from the initial telephone inquiry for clinical/educational information or scheduling and continue during the assessment and intervention processes and parent/family counseling. Failure to recognize and take these cultural and social factors into account can diminish the effectiveness of clinical/educational services, even with state-of-the-art technology or the most up-to-date clinical/educational procedures (Taylor, 1989).

This chapter presents a cultural framework for viewing AAC and gives present and future service providers suggestions to work more effectively with culturally diverse AAC users and families.

CULTURE AND AAC

Most of what is known about **culture** has come from the knowledge base of cultural anthropologists in general, and ethnographers in particular. Although cultural anthropologists focus on various aspects of culture, they generally agree that culture can be defined as the total of beliefs, values, traditions, behaviors, and communication patterns that are shared by members of a community and are learned as a function of their social membership (Saville-Troike, 1989). Culture also encompasses all the human-made systems of "meaning," including language, laws, myths, religions, and special ways of understanding and organizing the social and natural environment.

Culture permeates most aspects of a developing individual, especially the development of an individual's identity. It functions as a framework that guides and shapes behavior. It is a lens through which individuals see themselves in relation to others and to the world.

An individual's culture, however, is not a diagnostic category that necessarily explains how an individual thinks or acts. Change and variability are intrinsic to culture. First, cultural groups are constantly evolving as a result of contact with other groups. Second, individuals vary in the degree to which they identify themselves with a particular group (Hanson, 1992). Factors such as age, education, gender, health, occupation, and socioeconomic status exert a powerful influence on how individuals view themselves and how families function. As a result of these factors, individuals in large cultural groups often form different social organizations, which result in natural groups or microcultures. Thus, individuals may actually belong to two (i.e., bicultural) or more (i.e., multicultural) cultural groupings.

In response to the growing awareness of cultural diversity, educators, health-care professionals, and politicians have begun to use the term *multiculturalism* in designing and discussing their programs and services. However, what is meant by this term is not always clear. For a program or a policy to be truly **multicultural**, there must first be an understanding of the diversity, not only between but also within cultural groups (Groce & Zola, 1993). For instance, African Americans are often discussed as members of a single group.

Although many African Americans may have confronted similar issues of racism and exclusion, the social service needs of a suburban, professional African American couple, for example, may be significantly different from those of a single, teenage mother living in an inner-city housing project. Likewise, such terms as *Hispanic* and *Asian* are often used both by researchers and individuals in the dominant culture to refer to individuals from any one of several dozen major countries and over a third of the world population. When researchers and politicians lump together non-European ethnic groups in such a manner, they clearly show a lack of understanding of these cultures and appreciation for the groups' internal diversity (Groce & Zola, 1993).

AAC users come from many different cultural groups. Their needs are as diverse and complex as the communities to which they belong. Their lives are affected by previously mentioned factors including age, education, gender, health, occupation, socioeconomic status, type of disability, and, of course, cultural membership. When working with culturally diverse individuals, AAC service providers should be aware that both their own and the AAC users' cultural practices, as well as personal and family characteristics, may influence the interaction between themselves and the individuals and families receiving services.

Every person involved in the clinical encounter comes with a set of cultural assumptions. These assumptions relate to attitudes, beliefs, perceptions, and values regarding at least the following areas (in alphabetical order) (Taylor, 1994): (1) attitude toward disability; (2) communication style and language use; (3) dress and personal appearance; (4) education; (5) explanation of natural and supernatural phenomena; (6) family structure and role of family members; (7) food preferences; (8) important events in life and rituals to honor them; (9) life expectations and aspirations; (10) perceptions of time and space; (11) perceptions of work and leisure; (12) religious beliefs; (13) rules for decorum and discipline; (14) rules for interpersonal interactions; and (15) standards for health and hygiene.

Culture pervades most aspects of human existence. Because cultural influences are such an integral part of everyone's personal life, they are often elusive and not easily recognized. Therefore, the first step for AAC service providers planning to provide quality services to culturally diverse AAC users is to examine and understand their own cultural assumptions and the cultural bases of their belief systems (Hanson, 1992; Lynch, 1992; Taylor, 1989). Conscious effort may be required to recognize and understand one's own cultural influences. Self-awareness of cultural influences starts by examining the beliefs, values, and patterns of behavior that are part of one's own cultural identity. Such introspection may not be easy because it requires the acknowledgment that one's own beliefs and behavior are not inherently right, but rather represent *only one* perspective.

Attitudes Toward AAC Intervention

Different cultures attach different meanings to the presence of disabilities and employ different ways to deal with them. These attitudes may range from emphasizing the role of fate and supernatural phenomena to placing responsibility on the person or the person's family (Groce & Zola, 1993; Hanson, 1992).

Understanding how a family perceives the cause of disability is critical to providing quality AAC services. Perceptions that permeate family and community attitudes toward persons with disabilities may influence the degree to which a family will initially seek help. How much and in what ways a family participates in the provision of services may also be influenced by these perceptions. Other cultural influences affecting family involvement in the provision of services include each family's perceptions of social participation and roles appropriate for children with disabilities, attitudes toward the use of technology, priorities with regard to services for their child, expectations for their child's survival, and so forth. AAC service providers should individualize and tailor services to address concerns and priorities to meet the needs of families from diverse cultures. Being sensitive, knowledgeable, and understanding of each family's cultural practices enhances this process (Hanson, 1992).

Changing Demographics

The cultural composition of the United States is increasingly becoming more diverse, and the number of children from families of non-European ancestry is expected to rise. These increases can be accounted for by the higher birth rate among women of color and increased immigration of non-Europeans (Adler, 1993; Battle, 1993; Langdon & Cheng, 1992). Based on projected demographic data and estimates of the total number of AAC users in the 1990s (Wasson, 1994a), Huer (1994) estimated numbers of AAC users across cultures for the years 2020 to 2050 (see Table 22.1).

The projected figures are based on scarce data and should, therefore, be interpreted with caution. Nevertheless, these numbers strongly suggest a need for multiculturalism in AAC service delivery. To meet the AAC needs of the growing number of individuals from diverse cultures, AAC personnel preparation programs should include coursework and practical experience with the languages, cultures, and communication styles and patterns of at least the major cultural groups in the United States (Huer, 1994).

Although the number of culturally diverse individuals with AAC needs is increasing, current professional organizations and existing training programs for AAC professionals still have relatively few members and students from cultures of non-European ancestry. Efforts to train minority students in AAC should be encouraged and supported (Huer, 1994). Culturally matching service providers and families, however, will not always be possible. A better plan may be to infuse multiculturalism and make it an integral part of *all* programs training professionals in AAC so that they can learn how to adapt their practices to address the needs, concerns, and priorities of the families with whom they work. Below are some suggestions for adapting AAC assessment and intervention procedures for working with culturally diverse individuals and their families.

CLINICAL ISSUES: ASSESSMENT AND INTERVENTION

The ultimate goals of AAC assessment and intervention processes is to increase the communicative competence and participation level of the AAC user. However, AAC service providers cannot contemplate communicative competence and participation without considering clients within their cultural contexts.

TABLE 22.1 AAC Users Across Cultures: Projected Demographic Data

	U.S. POPULATION, 1990	AAC USERS, 1990 (0.8%)	PROJECTED PERCENTAGE OF GROWTH (1990—2020)	PROJECTED U.S. POPULATION, 2020	PROJECTED AAC USERS, 2020 (1%)
European American	200,000,000	1,600,000	3.0%	206,000,000	2,060,000
African American	30,000,000	240,000	46.7	44,000,000	440,000
Hispanic/Latino	22,000,000	176,000	109.1	46,000,000	460,000
Asian/Pacific Islanders	7,300,000	58,400	122.2	16,206,000	162,060
American Indians	2,000,000	16,000	3.0*	2,060,000	20,600
Total	261,300,000	2,090,400	n/a	314,266,000	3,142,660

Adapted from Huer (1994).

*Projected growth estimates were not available for American Indians because of the large number of different tribes. This is a conservative estimate.

Assessment Issues

In general, AAC assessment is a dynamic process designed to gain information to aid in making decisions regarding the design of an appropriate and effective AAC intervention plan. The complexity of this process calls for a team of professionals using a variety of assessment tools and procedures to determine an individual's communication strengths and needs. As noted in Chapter 11, AAC assessment should be based on the AAC model that considers the multimodality of communication as well as the AAC user's partners and environments (see Chapter 3). This model considers the match or mismatch of the sender and receiver based not only on cognitive and physical characteristics, but also on linguistic, cultural, and experiential background.

Standardized Testing.   Assessing the abilities of individuals whose speech is severely limited can be an extremely difficult task (Nelson, 1992). Test performance is difficult to interpret because the examiner may not know how much performance is influenced by cognitive or physical impairments, limitations of communication ability, or limitations imposed by the responses required by the test. With AAC users who are culturally diverse, these limitations are further complicated by linguistic and cultural differences.

Standardized and formal tests have often been found to be invalid in assessing communicative competence for culturally diverse clients because test results may be biased by a discrepancy between the language and culture assumed by the test and the language and culture of the test taker, as well as by the lack of normative data from culturally diverse populations (Hernandez, 1994; Taylor, 1986; Taylor & Payne, 1983). Some of the potential biases include (1) communication style bias—confusion or misunderstanding created by the communication style expected by the test and the cultural communication style of the test taker; (2) directions/format bias—confusion or misunderstanding created by the use of unfamiliar or ambiguous directions or test formats, including the use of procedures that may conflict with an individual's cultural rules for social interaction with

adults; (3) linguistic bias—mismatch between language/dialect required in the test in phonology, grammar, and/or vocabulary and language/dialect of the test taker; (4) response bias—mismatch between the response mode required by the test and the abilities and/or culturally preferred style for communication interaction and responses of the test taker; and, (5) values bias—mismatch between the values assumed in test items and the values of the test taker.

To determine whether assessment instruments and/or test procedures are biased against a particular client, AAC service providers should analyze the tests/tasks for specific cultural content, communication style, and responses expected from the test taker (Erickson & Iglesias, 1986; Hernandez, 1994). Before using any test, the service provider should examine each item to evaluate whether the AAC user has had access to the information being tested, can comprehend what is being asked, and has a reliable means to respond. If the test is biased in any of these areas, testing procedures should be modified. Modifications will vary depending on the source of bias, but they may include providing more time to complete the task, rewording or translating items, and/or providing for alternative means of responding (Erickson & Iglesias, 1986; Hernandez, 1994). All modifications must be documented and described on the test protocols and assessment report. Adapting tests nullifies standardization.

Clinicians and educators continue to rely heavily on standardized and formal tests to identify disabilities, make educational placement decisions, and design AAC systems and intervention programs. To obtain more accurate and culturally valid results, however, even adapted standardized tests must be combined with information obtained through the use of such qualitative approaches as observation, inventories, and interviewing.

Observation.   Consistent with the assessment approach discussed in Chapter 11, observation should be conducted in environments where individuals typically participate, such as home, school, after-school programs, community, and vocational settings. Parameters of observation should include (1) quality and quantity of partner-AAC user and partner-peer communicative interactions (also parent-sibling if observing at home); (2) partner expectations and demands on the AAC user's communicative performance; (3) partner use of communication training techniques and communication breakdown repair strategies; and (4) variation across situations in which different communicative functions are emphasized (Soto, 1995).

Before making an observation, the AAC service provider must understand not only **verbal**, but also **nonverbal**[1] forms of communication that are meaningful to a particular cultural group, because (1) nonverbal forms of communication are a critical component of the communicative repertoires of AAC users, and not being aware of culturally meaningful forms of nonverbal communication would lead to misinformation about an individual's current communication skills; (2) AAC intervention builds on existing communication skills, both verbal and nonverbal; and (3) AAC intervention should not only respect, but also enhance culturally appropriate ways to communicate (Soto, 1995).

Inventories. Inventories can be used to collect information to analyze an individual's level of functioning and participation in typical activities and environments. Beukelman and Mirenda (1992) describe an activity/standards inventory designed to identify discrepancies between the individual's and peers' levels of participation and to determine opportunity and access barriers that may account for these discrepancies. When making observations and creating inventories, service providers must be sure that they have a clear understanding of the activities being observed and analyzed if they are unfamiliar with them because of cultural diversity.

Interviewing. Interviewing individuals who know AAC users best is another critical component of AAC assessment. When interviewing parents and family members who are culturally diverse, the AAC service provider must be respectful of culturally appropriate ways to communicate (Erickson & Iglesias, 1986; Rosado, 1994). Thus, before interviewing, service providers should attempt to gather some information on family preferences for ways of greeting (e.g., formal versus informal), type of dress (e.g., formal versus more casual), degree of eye contact to be made with the person with whom they are talking, and appropriate ways to gather and transmit information (e.g., spoken versus written). The first interaction with a family may determine whether an effective working relationship will be established. Understanding and respecting the communication styles practiced by various families will facilitate this process (Hanson, 1992; Harry, 1992; Lynch, 1992; Rosado, 1994). If information cannot be gathered before interviewing, service providers should use the "safest" communication style, in which they use a tone of absolute and genuine respect for the client and the family, and avoid the use of technical jargon, which often alienates the family from participating in the assessment process.

AAC service providers should be aware of differing communication styles resulting from high- and low-context cultures. Members of high-context cultures (e.g., most African American, Arab, Asian, Latino, Mediterranean, and Native American) tend to rely heavily on common understanding through implicit information shared by nonverbal cues and messages (Lynch, 1992). Members of low-context cultures, (e.g., Anglo-American, Flemish, German, Northern-European American and Scandinavian), on the other hand, tend to rely more on verbal or linguistic communication and less on gestures, environmental clues, and nonverbal messages that are critical to effective communication in high-context cultures.

Communication between members of high- and low-context cultures can lead to misunderstanding and dissatisfaction by both parties (Lynch, 1992). Members of high-context cultures tend to

[1]Although this book in general has avoided the use of the terms *verbal* and *nonverbal*, it seems appropriate to use them in this chapter as they relate to cultural issues. As discussed in Chapter 4, *verbal* indicates linguistic communication, and *nonverbal* indicates nonlinguistic communication. In this chapter, the use of *verbal* typically refers to spoken languages, but it may also refer to the sign languages of different cultures/nations.

be more formal and more reliant on hierarchies, whereas members of low-context cultures are more informal and allow more equality in interaction. Experts in multicultural intervention (Harry, 1992; Lynch, 1992; Taylor, 1986, 1994; Taylor & Clarke, 1994) recommend that service providers become aware of the level of context that families use in their communication with outsiders and adapt to the style that is comfortable for the family.

The task of communicating with a parent or family member about their child's disability is by nature a *high-context* activity, in which complex, subtle personal and cultural information is open to interpretation (Harry, 1992; Rosado, 1994; Westby, 1990). To approach such a task with precise, direct, low-context communication may set the stage for communication breakdown if used with families from high-context cultures.

Use of Interpreters.   Ideally, culturally diverse families would be paired with service providers who speak their language and understand their culture (Lynch, 1992). However, service delivery frequently falls short of reaching such an ideal, and interpreters are called in to assist. Communicating through an interpreter is a complicated task. Using an interpreter necessarily slows down and changes the dynamics of communication, making the interaction more cumbersome and open to misinterpretation. It also deprives family members of the privacy they may need to discuss their child's needs. Service providers must recognize and be sensitive to these difficulties. To help ensure that interpreters will be effective, they should be (a) **bilingual** (i.e., proficient in both the language of the family and the service provider) and (b) **bicultural** (i.e., able to understand and appreciate the culture of both parties and able to convey the subtle nuances of each). In addition, the interpreter should understand the function of and professional jargon used in clinical/educational programs (Erickson & Iglesias, 1986; Hanson, 1992).

Given the lack of fully qualified bilingual, bicultural interpreters, service providers may be tempted to seek the assistance of bilingual family members to act as interpreters. Using family members and relatives as interpreters can, however, be problematic. Difficulties may arise from role conflicts and personal relationships within the family, a lack of training as an interpreter, and a lack of knowledge of the content of the issues to be addressed. In addition, parents may feel embarrassed to discuss intimate matters with family members. In turn, family members may wish to censor or reinterpret what is disclosed to minimize family shame (see Lynch, 1992, for extensive information on working with interpreters).

Intervention Issues

When working with AAC users who are culturally diverse, the AAC service provider should have two kinds of simultaneous intervention goals (Soto, 1995): (1) to increase the client's communicative competence and participation levels while respecting culturally appropriate rules for social interaction and social participation, and (2) to facilitate family participation by providing families with opportunities to learn about educational/clinical programs so that they can exercise their rights.

Increasing Communicative Competence and Participation Levels.   As noted in Chapter 15, some of the critical aspects of AAC intervention include (1) providing a means to communicate; (2) providing opportunities to communicate; and (3) having partners with whom to communicate. For AAC intervention to be culturally valid, however, AAC service providers must also have an understanding of the cultural backgrounds of AAC users and act on this knowledge through the following strategies:

1. **Providing a culturally appropriate means to communicate.** If the AAC user is a member of a bilingual (e.g., Spanish and English) or bidialectal (e.g., African American English and Standard English) family, the service provider should accommodate the linguistic preferences of the family by developing a bilingual/bicultural AAC system for school/work and for home (Harris, 1995; Soto, 1995). A bilingual/bicultural AAC system should include culturally appropriate vocabulary (accommodating the primary language or dialect of the AAC user's immediate cultural group), culturally appropriate and meaningful means of representation (i.e., symbols), and culturally appropriate

strategies for functional AAC use (Harris, 1995; Soto, 1995).

Culturally appropriate vocabulary could be gathered by sampling the language and/or dialect of siblings and peers (Harris, 1995). (See Chapter 12 for a more thorough discussion of vocabulary selection.) The vocabulary should allow AAC users to communicate about things considered important in their culture (Soto, 1995). Vocabulary and symbol selection (Chapter 13) should always be reviewed by a person highly familiar with the client's native language and culture (Harris, 1995; Soto, 1995). Language is one of the most critical elements by which individuals are socialized into their culture. Thus, not having access to a bilingual/bicultural AAC system may cause further cultural/social isolation, identity conflicts, and increase the sense of being different (Harris, 1995).

2. **Providing opportunities to communicate.** Culturally valid intervention should take into account the rules of social and communicative interaction as defined by the AAC user's cultural group (Taylor & Clarke, 1994). Even with AAC, communication is a social event with an identifiable set of rules, values, expectations, and roles, depending on topic, situation, and participants (Taylor, 1994). Therefore, AAC strategies for intervention at home should be built on and include (1) culturally meaningful nonverbal forms of communication, (2) communicative functions most frequently used at home, (3) primary language used at home, and (4) discourse strategies most commonly used by family members (Soto, 1995). Intervention strategies to increase the AAC user's opportunities for participation at home should respect cultural norms of participation and customary ways of interacting. For example, with families having a long tradition of family interdependence (e.g., Latino and Asian American), child independence and assertiveness may not be valued. Intervention strategies that promote these behaviors may be considered inappropriate (Harry, 1992). To increase the use of the AAC system, AAC intervention for children at home should respect and enhance cultural communication styles and communicative functions most often used with children (e.g., book reading, story telling). Service providers should avoid basing AAC intervention on communicative functions that are not culturally appropriate.

3. **Having partners with whom to communicate.** The ultimate purpose of AAC intervention is to en-

able AAC users to establish cultural/social membership in their communities (Beukelman & Mirenda, 1992; Ferguson, 1994). Achieving membership for AAC users, however, can be challenging. In general, culture affects what academic, social, and vocational roles a person with a disability can hold in a society. Traditionally, persons with severe impairments have been excluded from access to economic, social, and vocational participation in society (Braithwaite, 1991). Yet, by using an AAC system, users can overcome some of the barriers associated with their disabilities.

When working with culturally diverse parents, service providers may encounter families whose expectations for their child's social participation are different from their own. A family may be reluctant to support AAC intervention because social participation for their child is understood differently. Again, in this case, the service provider can opt for designing a bicultural AAC intervention plan that allows the AAC user to function and participate in two cultures. The bicultural intervention plan would include objectives and approaches that respect the values, attitudes, and wishes of the AAC user's culture for intervention at home (Soto, 1995). However, at school and in other mainstream settings such as leisure and vocational settings, AAC intervention would revolve around the communication needs and demands for academic and social participation in those environments (Soto, 1995).

Facilitating Parent and Family Participation. Parent and family participation and involvement in the AAC intervention process increases the chances of intervention effectiveness, generalization, and maintenance (Beukelman & Mirenda, 1992). Yet, research shows that parents of children with disabilities tend to have limited knowledge about the services their children need and how they can procure these services (Harry, 1992; Harry, Allen, & McLaughlin, 1995; Rosado, 1994). They also encounter barriers that tend to limit their power and authority in the decision-making process. This limited authority is often exacerbated in culturally diverse families by the perceived "disadvantaged" status of being a minority and results in a lower level of involvement of culturally diverse parents in the special education process (Harry, 1992; Harry et al., 1995; Rosado, 1994).

Research on parent participation suggests that culturally diverse parents often (1) hold different perceptions of their child's disability than those held by service providers, (2) view themselves as inadequate to the task of collaborating with professionals, (3) perceive parent participation as intimidating or inappropriate, (4) may have overwhelming life circumstances, and/or, (5) are disillusioned with clinical/educational programs (Harry, 1992; Harry et al., 1995; Rosado, 1994). Harry and her colleagues (1995) found that parent disillusionment was paralleled by decreasing levels of participation and noncompliance. Perceptions of being provided inadequate and unsatisfactory services and of being looked down on or not being acknowledged as legitimate participants in the intervention process often elicited noncompliant behaviors that, in turn, engendered nonsupportive responses by service providers (Harry et al., 1995).

As AAC service providers plan for family collaboration, they must honor and respect the values, beliefs, child-rearing practices, parent–child interaction styles, interpersonal styles, attitudes, and behaviors of the families that they serve (Anderson & Battle, 1993; Lynch & Hanson, 1992). To increase parent participation, service providers should recognize that culturally diverse AAC users are members of cultures (e.g., home and school) that may hold different and sometimes competing sets of assumptions regarding perceptions of disability, disease and health, and need for services (Cummins, 1986). The quality of the interaction dynamics among these cultures in relation to AAC users may yield results that either empower clients and their families or disable them even further (Cummins, 1986). The degree to which an intervention will be effective is a function of the nature and quality of these interaction dynamics.

Soto (1994) described strategies that AAC service providers can use to facilitate culturally diverse parent participation in the AAC process. Several of these strategies are listed below.

1. *Listen* to parents' priorities, their expectations and preferences regarding AAC systems, and *act* on this knowledge by designing a system that accommodates these preferences.
2. *Ask* parents about their family structure and roles, and *act* on this knowledge by inviting and including input from other influential family members as appropriate. This is particularly important when working with clients from cultural groups in which the extended family is the family unit. In these groups, young parents may be considered too inexperienced to make major decisions on behalf of their children. Key decisions are typically made in consultation with older relatives within the larger family unit. Care, assistance, and financial support frequently come from the extended family network.
3. *Recognize* and *respect* that issues of family survival may take priority over educational concerns.
4. *Respond* to family needs in terms of meeting times and other logistics.
5. *Avoid* the use of technical jargon that may be a barrier to understanding.
6. *Present* results and recommendations clearly so parents understand and can become actively involved in the provision of services.

SUMMARY

Several issues pertaining to multiculturalism and AAC must be considered when designing culturally valid AAC assessment and intervention. Recognizing diversity between cultures is critical to the provision of appropriate AAC services; however, service providers must also recognize the inherent variability within members of the same cultural group.

Working with culturally diverse families requires an understanding of one's own culture and how it influences clinical interaction. The changing demographics in the United States bring professionals new demands and challenges. Cultural understanding and respect are crucial to the provision of effective AAC services for culturally diverse individuals.

CHAPTER 23

LITERACY

MARTINE M. SMITH AND DOREEN M. BLISCHAK

Few reading this text will be conscious of the skills they are using as they read its pages, or of the process by which they acquired these skills. For most readers, the primary focus will be on evaluating the content or style of the information presented, with some perhaps taking notes on a writing pad or in the margins of the text. For such readers, these dual processes of reading (decoding) and writing (encoding) have long become subservient to the goal of acquiring or exchanging information, maintaining social contact, evaluating perspectives, or simply passing time. In Western cultures, literacy is an important key to opportunities in all aspects of life. Without this key an individual faces many barriers, from difficulties selecting television programs to difficulties seeking employment.

Literacy is especially critical for **augmentative and alternative communication (AAC)** users. Many AAC users have severe physical impairments that limit vocational options to jobs that require literacy skills over manual skills. For individuals with developmental disabilities whose life experiences from birth have been severely restricted, literacy opens many doors to new, otherwise inaccessible experiences. AAC users with acquired disabilities may find that literacy is the only realm of expertise in which their former levels of competence are retained. Literacy may provide an important psychological link with their former functioning in society.

Although literacy skills clearly are important in AAC interventions, attention in the literature to the role of literacy and AAC is relatively recent, dating substantially from the mid-1980s. In many ways, interest has remained relatively isolated within the confines of the field of AAC, although

nonetheless shadowing developments in mainstream literacy research. One of the challenges to researchers on both sides of this divide is to effect greater crossover of information exchange.

MAINSTREAM LITERACY RESEARCH

Largely because of economic and cultural pressures, interest in reading and writing development in Western societies has a long history. However, despite considerable government efforts, 20% of the American adult population has severe problems with even the most common reading activities (Blachman, 1991). Controversy and debate surrounds the reasons for such failure to develop functional reading and writing skills. Although reading appears to be a rather simple process of extracting meaning from print, it is actually highly complex, requiring synthesis of visual and auditory information. Both modalities are critical in developing reading and in explaining difficulties in reading, but the proportion of responsibility of each modality is a source of much controversy. Considerable early interest centered around the visual demands of reading and writing as explanatory factors. More recent research indicates that, although visual acuity and visual perceptual problems clearly interfere with the mechanics of interpreting orthography, disordered eye movements are typically a byproduct of reading difficulty, rather than an underlying cause (Pumfrey & Reason, 1991; Willows, 1991).

Research focus has now shifted primarily to the language demands of reading and writing. Deficiencies in semantic processing (Denckla & Rundel, 1976; Ellis, 1981; Silva, Williams, & McGee, 1987), syntactic processing (Catts &

Kamhi, 1986; Shankweiler & Crain, 1986), and more recently, **metalinguistic abilities** such as phonologic processing (Shankweiler & Crain, 1986) have all been found to correlate with difficulties in reading and writing. Of particular interest recently is **phonologic awareness** (sometimes referred to as "phonemic awareness"), which "involves the more or less explicit understanding that words are made of discrete units" (Ball, 1993, p. 130). The size of the subword unit may vary, referring to syllables, **onset–rime** boundaries (e.g., c-at; tr-uck), or phonemes (Hjelmquist, Sandberg, & Hedelin, 1994). Evidence is growing that sophistication of knowledge about phonologic structure is a critical factor in successfully learning to read and write alphabetic languages (e.g., Bradley & Bryant 1983, 1985; Lundberg, Olofsson, & Wall, 1980). Lack of an awareness of the phonologic structure of language makes it particularly difficult to learn the correspondence between alphabet letters and the speech sounds they represent (Catts, 1989; Jorm & Share, 1983). In fact, measures of phonologic awareness administered in kindergarten have predicted first-grade reading ability as well as, or better than, measures of intelligence or traditional reading readiness tests (Tunmer, Herriman, & Nesdale, 1988; Wagner & Torgeson, 1987). One factor that perhaps clouds the issue is that the relationship between phonologic awareness and reading ability is considered to be reciprocal, with phonologic awareness facilitating the development of reading, but benefiting also from reading experience (Goswami & Bryant, 1990).

Concurrent with the focus on the metalinguistic skills involved in the reading process, interest in the contexts in which reading and writing develop has also come to the fore, in an area often referred to as *emergent literacy*. Teale and Sulzby (1989) outlined four areas of change in literacy research, including (1) a broadening of the age range of interest down to 14 months or younger; (2) the conception of literacy as a social-linguistic-psychological activity, occurring in many different contexts and environments; (3) consideration of both home and school environments as centers of learning; and (4) a new focus on literacy learning from the perspective of the child actively engaging in the learning process. This shift in focus has implications that Galda, Cullinan, and Strickland (1993) suggested have become widely accepted.

1. Literacy learning begins early in life and is ongoing. "As children search for patterns and make connections, they bring what they know to each new situation and apply their own childlike logic to make sense of it" (Galda et al., 1993, p. 75).
2. Literacy develops concurrently with oral language. Harste, Woodward, and Burke (1984) referred to the "linguistic data pool" from which children draw to support their literacy development and to which they add, based on their literacy experiences.
3. Learning to read and write are both social and cognitive endeavors, and children are active participants in the process.
4. Literacy learning is a developmental process.
5. Storybook reading, particularly within the family, has a special role in young children's literacy development.
6. Literacy learning is deeply rooted in the cultural milieu and in the family communication patterns.

Models of Literacy Learning

In reviewing models of literacy learning, Pumfrey and Reason (1991) distinguished between top-down and bottom-up approaches. Top-down approaches emphasize the reader's use of background information and world knowledge to derive meaning from text, only rarely deciphering individual words. A bottom-up approach, on the other hand, emphasizes the complex component skills involved in reading, which are presumed to operate in a building-block system, each step in the process contingent on successful completion of the previous step (Ellis, 1993). In many respects the contrast between the two approaches reflects a distinction between reading for meaning at the text level and single-word recognition. The picture is further complicated by the fact that reading and writing change developmentally. Reason (1990) has suggested an interactive framework (see also Dechant, 1991) that incorporates a combination of both approaches and takes the form of an inverted triangle, as illustrated in Figure 23.1.

The first (and largest) section of the triangle refers to previous and present life experiences and

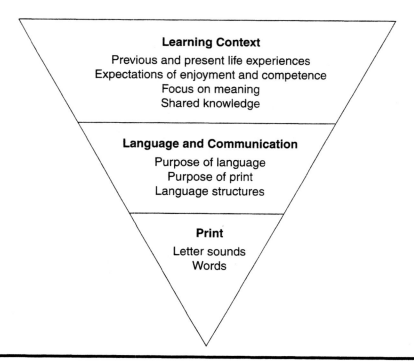

FIGURE 23.1   Ingredients of Literacy.

expectations, which determine whether the reader will be able to make sense of the thoughts of the writer. The second section links with top-down approaches, emphasizing the function of print over its form, promoting active involvement with print from the start, and viewing literacy development as proceeding alongside language development. Print form comprises the small, but essential third segment of the triangle, dependent on the larger sections above, but providing the key to successful independent literacy experiences. At this level bottom-up components, such as the ability to handle **graphophonic elements** of print, become critical. Pumfrey and Reason (1991) suggested that, for some readers, particularly those struggling with decoding orthography, this triangle may become inverted, so that graphophonic elements occupy the largest segment.

Such a model emphasizes that a combination of factors influences the development of literacy over an extended period, starting with a child's first encounters with language. Some of these factors are intrinsic to the individual, such as perceptual, linguistic, and metalinguistic abilities. Others may be considered extrinsic, relating more to the environment in which the individual functions and the importance attached to literacy in those primary environments. Clearly, whatever model is adopted, it must accommodate these intrinsic and extrinsic factors and must address the key points discussed under the next five headings.

Reading and Writing as Developmental Skills.
In outlining "how far the beginner travels in learning to read," Ehri (1991, p. 64), citing the work of Chall, suggested four stages in reading development. With minor modifications, the sequence outlined is as follows. At stage 1, the *prereading* or *emergent reading stage*, background literacy skills are developed. Here, children learn key ideas about reading: print carries the message; books and print have a certain orientation and must be

read in a particular order—front to back, word by word, left to right, top to bottom; readers use print and pictures differently; particular vocabulary is used to talk about reading and print (e.g., *page*, *word*); and, the language of books sometimes differs from spoken language (Galda et al., 1993). At this stage, reading is logographic, based on salient visual cues, such as the golden arches behind McDonalds (Ehri, 1991). At stage 2, the *decoding stage*, the link between specific grapheme and phoneme elements is established. Sight word reading begins to take account of letters rather than other visual cues, signaling the beginning of the alphabetic or phonetic cue stage of word identification. Initially, only a few letter cues are used in word identification, and gradually apprentice readers become able to read words "by storing in memory complete associations between specific spellings and their pronunciations" (Ehri, 1991, p. 73). During stage 3, the *fluency stage*, these skills are consolidated and expanded. Words are processed as single units, and patterns within words are the basis for word identification, in what is referred to as the orthographic phase. Successful progress into this stage allows for reading by analogy to develop, where shared spelling patterns within words can form the basis for identification of unfamiliar words. The final stage, stage 4, is termed the *reading to learn stage*, where the process of reading is subservient to the goals of reading.

A similar developmental sequence occurs in writing or encoding skills. In the first stage, background principles similar to those of stage 1 in reading are established, with the additional complication of learning the motor and perceptual skills necessary for pen control. Gillam and Johnston (1992) suggested that children initially investigate the equivalencies of speaking and writing as they interweave playing, talking, drawing, and writing. Gradually, spelling skills develop, through a series of stages from **semiphonetic spelling** to conventional spelling (Gentry, 1982). The modality differences between spoken and written language become more important, and the unique conceptual, linguistic, and mechanical constraints posed by written language are accommodated with increasing sophistication.

Not all authors agree with the delineation of stages in reading and writing. Ellis (1993), for instance, argued that the stages reflected teaching approaches in vogue at the time of study, rather than universally based developmental stages. Nonetheless, certain key concepts about print and a degree of awareness of the structural aspects of language facilitate progress in developing competency in written language.

Changing Needs at Different Stages. One of the advantages of a developmental perspective is that it allows the consideration of changing needs and skill bases. Ehri (1991) suggested that although there is clearly an overlap and interaction between stages, different factors become critical to further progress at each stage. At stage 1, background experience and environmental influences are key. At stage 2, where the alphabetic principles of the language are being mastered, actual teaching time is deemed critical. Ehri (1991) proposed that the crossover from logographic word reading to phonetic cue reading is contingent on developing the ability to be analytical about print, paying attention to letter units and their correspondences to sounds. "The way that movement from stage 1 to stage 2 occurs is by acquiring letter knowledge and rudimentary phonemic segmentation skill" (Ehri, 1991, p. 74). At this stage, the overlap between the decoding and encoding processes of reading and writing is most evident, with spelling practice facilitating important phonologic awareness and analytical skills. Although clearly essential at all stages, at stage 3, opportunities to practice are critical, using easy texts so that reading can become more automatic. Transition to stage 4 is contingent on simultaneous increases in sophistication in cognitive and language development.

Reading and Writing as Learned Skills. Although reading is clearly a language-based activity, reading and speech are not equivalent forms of development and all children do not learn both "in the same natural unconscious way" (Liberman & Liberman, 1990, p. 56). Written language has historically been viewed as heavily dependent on spoken language, yet there are compelling reasons to consider spoken and written language as complex symbol systems with their own distinctive characteristics (Gillam & Johnston, 1992). Furthermore, as Ellis (1993) pointed out, it is only within the last 100 years or so that universal literacy has been a declared aim of many societies. Learning to read and write requires exposure to models of competent readers/writers, direct instruction, and specific skill development relating to orthographic processing, along with opportunities to learn and to practice.

Literacy as a Complex Integration. Stanovich (1986) emphasized that many factors are linked with success or failure in learning to read and write, but whether these links reflect causative, correlational, or "bootstrapping" relationships is unclear. Success in interpreting and producing written language requires a complex integration of cultural, social, cognitive, perceptual, linguistic, and metalinguistic information. Gillam and Johnston (1992) outlined the complexities of such integration in relation to reading and writing:

> Conceptually, writers create communicative context, project the information needs of an imagined audience, reflect and rereflect on intended meaning, elaborate their messages, and shape their texts in accordance with genre-specific organizational schemata. Linguistically, they make lexical choices that convey intended meanings and mood, and formulate sentences that best convey the interconnections between propositions. Mechanically, they deal with the perceptual and motor requirements of handwriting while they adhere to spelling, capitalization and punctuation convention. (p. 1304)

Purpose of Literacy Activities. Reading and writing are means to an end, not ends in and of themselves. Meaningful literacy activities are goal directed, although goals may change as literacy skills develop. Becoming functionally literate may be linked with long-term goals that relate to cultural, social, communication, vocational, and recreational issues, but within that framework, each literacy activity has a more immediate goal, whether it relates to ensuring no essential purchases are forgotten, operating a new kitchen appliance, or filling a page with colorful patterns. More abstract goals include the following:

- Expanding communication options (both face-to-face and distance)
- Broadening experiences and world knowledge
- Enhancing educational participation
- Providing vocational opportunities
- Developing recreational options
- Facilitating participation in society
- Increasing independence

The wealth of information on literacy development in the general population can serve as a useful point of departure for investigation of literacy development in AAC users.

LITERACY DEVELOPMENT IN AAC USERS

Although some have achieved mastery levels (e.g., Fourcin, 1975; Nolan, 1987), research to date suggests that the majority of AAC users face significant difficulties in achieving functional literacy. Many studies have been carried out with individuals with congenital impairments, particularly cerebral palsy. Estimates of prevalence of reading difficulties range from 33% (Asher & Schonell, 1950) to as high as 90% (Barsch & Rudell, 1962) even where traditional measures of intelligence would lead one to expect higher levels of functioning (Berninger & Gans, 1986a; Dorman, 1985; Kelford-Smith, Thurston, Light, Parnes, & O'Keefe, 1989; Seidel, Chadwick, & Rutter, 1975; Smith, 1990). For a more comprehensive review of findings in this area, see Koppenhaver and Yoder (1992a).

Intrinsic Factors

Early attempts to explain such limited literacy attainment have focused on factors known from mainstream literacy research to be related to literacy achievement. This equates broadly with the emphasis on intrinsic factors, which can be broadly divided into four areas of impairment: physical, sensory/perceptual, language, and cognitive. Many AAC users have multiple impairments, each of which alone, or in combination with other impairments, may hamper literacy development.

Physical Impairment. Schonell (1956) reported a clear and negative correlation between extent of physical impairment and reading achievement.

From an early age, children with physical impairments encounter reduced opportunities to interact with the environment, severely restricting their sensorimotor experiences (Carlson, 1987). Thus, the physical impairment itself might be more appropriately thought of as the first link in a chain of second-order effects, including reduced opportunities for stimulation and interaction, restricted experiences, and changed expectations for educational placement and achievement. These, along with the increased time demand for activities of daily living, often result in decreased emphasis on literacy experiences and development for children with physical impairments (Light & Kelford-Smith, 1993).

Sensory/Perceptual Impairment.   In addition to the obvious effects of visual acuity difficulties on accessing print, evidence suggests that children with severe visual impairments may also experience restricted opportunities for sensorimotor interactions. They may encounter differences in linguistic experiences important in the development of literacy, such as reduced language input and difficulties matching language input to an object, person, or event (Blischak, 1995).

From the few studies to date, no firm connection has been established between visual-perceptual and/or visuomotor difficulties and reading difficulties. For example, Jones et al. (1966) reported that disordered eye movements were likely to impair reading rate, but not text comprehension. Katayama and Tamas (1987) suggested that abnormal eye movements, coupled with difficulty maintaining postural control of the head and neck in children with cerebral palsy may increase visual-perceptual difficulties as well. However, eye movement patterns may be more a symptom of reading difficulty than a cause.

As with visual impairment, the effects of hearing impairment on literacy development are well documented. By age 18, deaf students typically achieve a fourth or fifth grade reading level and demonstrate dramatic differences in producing written language compared with hearing peers. Experience with auditory language lies at the very heart of reading development and, as such, is dramatically reduced or unavailable for deaf children.

Hearing children internalize spoken language, providing them with a real-world knowledge base for top-down reading. Deaf children "lack this auditory language and its associated experiential, cognitive, and linguistic skills. Thus, for them, learning to read becomes also a process of experience building, cognitive development, and language learning" (King & Quigley, 1985, p. xi).

Deaf individuals are also expected to have difficulty with bottom-up reading processes that depend on knowledge of the sound structure of the spoken language. Recent evidence has shown, however, that some individuals with prelingual, profound deafness have demonstrated skill in phonologic awareness (Hanson, 1991; Hanson & Fowler, 1987). These findings provide additional evidence to support the tenet that internalizing phonologic information does not necessarily depend on intelligible speech production.

Language Impairment.   Some children with intact hearing may experience difficulties in language comprehension and production that, in turn, affect literacy development. Mainstream research indicates that a high proportion of children with reading disabilities have difficulty processing and producing spoken language, exhibiting difficulties at all levels—semantic, syntactic, phonologic, and metalinguistic. Severe speech impairment may also be a causative factor in failure to achieve appropriate literacy levels, with particular interest in a link between severe speech impairment and phonologic awareness skills (Bishop, 1985, 1988; Bishop, Byers-Brown, & Robson, 1990; Bishop & Robson, 1989; Foley, 1989). Although some individuals with severe speech impairments demonstrate skill in phonologic awareness, results from these studies remain inconclusive.

Cognitive Impairment.   Cognitive impairment may create developmental delays, affecting physical, sensory/perceptual, and/or language abilities and may also coexist with other impairments. Studies have reported that approximately 60 to 70% of children with cerebral palsy, for example, demonstrate some degree of cognitive impairment (Koppenhaver & Yoder, 1992a). Impairment of specific cognitive abilities, such as attention and memory, have also been reported (Parker, 1987). AAC users are at risk for many intrinsic factors that may interact in complex ways to impede literacy development. However, such influences may further interact with factors extrinsic to the individual, creating a complex web of first- and second-order effects.

Extrinsic Factors

Home Environment.   Emergent literacy research shows that children learn to read and write by active participation in meaningful, functional literacy activities, such as storytelling and nursery rhyme games. Under such circumstances, adults and children engage in prolonged discussions about what has been read, an activity that, although involving the repetition necessary for language learning, is not merely a repetitious exercise. Children internalize these dialogues and engage in **protoreading**, a constructive process in which the child orally recreates the story, facilitating progression ultimately to conventional literacy. Typically, AAC users have less time available for participation in these types of activities (Light & Kelford-Smith, 1993), and when they do, experiences may be dramatically different from those of children without disabilities. Positioning a child with physical disabilities and reading materials simultaneously while maintaining dialogue is extremely difficult. Similar practical difficulties are encountered when trying to engage in writing activities, which require a much greater degree of motor skill.

Further, parental priorities for children with speech impairments may emphasize other aspects of development over literacy. In the Light and Kelford-Smith study (1993), parents of preschool children without disabilities considered learning to read and write to be second in importance only to making friends and learning to communicate effectively. Parents of preschool AAC users from similar family groups considered learning to communicate effectively to be the most important priority, with independent mobility, feeding, and toilet-training coming next on the list. Lowest priority was given to reading and writing. Similar patterns were reported by Light and McNaughton

(1993), citing a survey of older AAC users carried out by Light, Koppenhaver, Lee, and Riffle. Only 9 of 59 students over the age of 9 (15%) were reported to be able to read the newspaper or more complex texts and almost a quarter (24%) of the parents indicated that they did not expect any improvement in their children's current level of literacy by age 25. This extension of different priorities beyond the preschool years suggests a life-span effect of differing expectations and priorities. Coleman (1992) referred to the cumulative effects of reduced opportunities for active participation, lower expectations, and different priorities as an equation summing to "literacy lost."

School Environment.   For most students, school is the primary context for formal literacy instruction. Although much can be done in preparation at home, much can also be compensated for in a school environment that provides a knowledgeable and enthusiastic teacher to guide; an environment that encourages social interaction around books; a structure that allows students to make choices about what they will do with books; and the time and the materials to allow students to read and respond to what they read (Galda et al., 1993). Paradoxically, practice in reading is one of the best predictors of reading ability (Anderson, Wilson, & Fielding, 1988; Galda et al., 1993). Stanovich (1986) coined the phrase "Matthew effects" to describe this cumulative advantage effect, after the Gospel according to Matthew: "Unto every one that hath shall be given, and he shall have abundance; but from him that hath not shall be taken away even that which he hath" (XXV; 29). Good readers read, and thereby improve their reading. Poor readers read less, practice less, and therefore fall further behind. As mentioned previously, such practice is particularly critical in transitioning to the fluency stage of reading.

AAC users may require extra practice, simply to survive educationally. Furthermore, given the many challenges they face, explicit instruction on the specific skills involved in reading and writing is essential. In reality, they may receive even less instructional time than peers who do not have disabilities. Koppenhaver and Yoder (1992a, 1992b) reviewed a number of studies of classroom literacy instruction time available to students with speech impairments and concluded that substantial proportions of instructional time may be lost to noninstructional activities, such as transportation within and between rooms, feeding, toileting, and therapies. Koppenhaver (1991) found that students spent more time in nonliteracy activities (up to 38%) than any single literacy activity during their literacy instruction time. Much of the time lost in such situations resulted from the typically high number of extra pieces of equipment necessary for functioning in the classroom, all of which are susceptible to breakdown. Additional time may be spent in trying to resolve communication problems or breakdowns.

Koppenhaver (1991) also reported that the instructional focus during the period of observation was primarily geared toward words and sentences in isolation, fill-in-the-blank exercises, and spelling practice, seldom including reading more than paragraphs or writing more than sentence-length passages. As Koppenhaver and Yoder (1992a) pointed out, research with speaking children has shown these to be the least effective strategies for improving literacy. Effective strategies include building background knowledge, setting purposes for reading (generic, specific, and student-generated), and using easy materials and tasks. Furthermore, a substantial body of research indicates the value of including explicit instruction in phonologic awareness as part of literacy programs (for review, see Adams, 1990).

So What Works?

Given the recency of interest in literacy and AAC, little documented evidence exists as to which assessment and instructional approaches might best accommodate the needs of AAC users. What is particularly needed at this stage is longitudinal research documenting the effects of varying approaches. Until such information is available, however, clinicians/educators must continue to borrow from research with individuals without disabilities within the framework of a theoretical model of reading and writing that accommodates the similarities and differences of individuals using AAC. The relative influence of both intrinsic and extrinsic factors, while taking into account that literacy is a developmental, learned skill must guide both assessment and intervention.

ASSESSMENT

Certain general principles guide assessment of literacy at all stages of development. Across the span of development, all three ingredients shown in Figure 23.1 are relevant: (1) learning context, (2) language and communication, and (3) print. Literacy assessment which must be viewed in the context of overall language and communication development and assessment must be ongoing. It must reflect the unusual reciprocal relationship between AAC users and print: AAC use provides access to otherwise unobtainable literacy experiences, and written language provides a powerful means of expression for individuals with little or no functional speech. Thus, the assessment process must view both AAC and literacy as goals and as tools. In addition to the 10 AAC assessment principles discussed in Chapter 11, clinicians/educators must also consider the five literacy assessment principles discussed below.

Assessment Principles

Principle 1. Assessment must recognize that literacy involves an integration of many intrinsic and extrinsic factors. Literacy achievement reflects the complex interaction among the reader/writer, the text, and the context. Above all, competence in literacy must not be viewed as static. Every reader adapts and accommodates to different situations and demands. For example, skilled readers may simply slow their rate of reading in response to difficult texts or distracting environments. Less-skilled readers may abandon the task altogether. Thus, assessment must be conducted across a variety of situations and settings.

Principle 2. Assessment must provide a guide to intervention, rather than establish a list of deficits. Pumfrey and Reason (1991) referred to this as the "symbiotic relationship" between assessment and intervention. Within this framework, the strengths, abilities, and strategies being used by the individual are the focus of attention. This approach relies heavily on criterion- rather than norm-referenced assessment tools, and much of the information gathering is based on observation, rather than direct formal evaluation.

Principle 3. Assessment must be goal driven and reflect the varied functions of literacy in relation to current and future needs. On the one hand, AAC can be used to access literacy, such as using a voice output communication aid (VOCA) to allow a child to participate in group book reading. On the other hand, literacy skills may form the basis for use of an AAC method, such as logical letter coding to produce spoken and written language. Thus, assessment must reflect current and future AAC and literacy functions.

Principle 4. Assessment should, where appropriate, reflect the developmental nature of literacy attainment. Both the forms and the functions of literacy change as individuals become more competent. Skills that are relevant at the emergent literacy stage, such as scribbling, turning pages, exploring pictures, and playing with sounds, have far less relevance at later stages. Assessing knowledge of grapheme-phoneme correspondence makes little sense when a child still does not understand that the print, rather than the picture in a book, is the focus of attention. Task difficulty, whether in decoding or encoding, interacts in complex ways with the reader's/writer's abilities. Thus, an individual may have certain skills, but not be able to use them effectively in all contexts. Several developmental stages may be observed as text demands change. A rigid application of developmental stages, therefore, is often not the most appropriate framework for assessment or intervention.

Principle 5. Assessment should consider the adaptations required by AAC users and the extent to which those adaptations may change task demands. Many tasks involved in reading assessment require a spoken response. Thus, for many AAC users, obtaining a measure of letter or word identification is difficult. Although some AAC users may be able to produce a recognizable word approximation, others may not. Providing choices ultimately changes an identification task to a closed-set recognition task. The change in task demands, plus the potential cognitive load imposed by use of AAC makes generalization from typically developing readers difficult. Assessment procedures that require the fewest adaptations are suggested (Blischak, 1994).

General Procedures

In undertaking literacy assessment, both the tools available and the contexts in which those tools are used must be considered. As discussed in Chapter 11, many different types of assessment tools exist, including formal norm- and criterion-referenced assessments, observation checklists, questionnaires, protocols developed by individual practitioners, interview formats, and unstructured observations. The choice of tools will vary depending on the information sought, the context of the assessment, the abilities/disabilities of the individual being assessed, and the personal preferences of the assessor.

The context and focus of the assessment warrant careful consideration. Many authors stress the need to consider not only the individual, but also the environments in which individuals function (Koppenhaver & Yoder, 1992b; Light & McNaughton, 1993). Often, the environment is a starting point for assessment, as immediate suggestions for intervention may become obvious. This may provide motivation for others to continue participating in the assessment process. Regardless of the specific nature and context of assessment, however, extrinsic factors must be considered if assessment is to be functional.

Environmental Assessment: Extrinsic Factors. Beukelman and Mirenda (1992) outlined a participation model for communication assessment that is easily adaptable within the context of literacy. They suggested that at least three critical factors be considered: opportunities, needs, and barriers.

Assessment of *opportunities* can be considered under all three sections of Figure 23.1, both broad headings and specific literacy-related factors. The largest segment of Figure 23.1 indicates the importance of a broad range of life experiences if the reader is to be able to relate to the thoughts and purposes of the author. Therefore, the different environments and experiences available to the person being assessed must be considered.

At the second segment, experience with language forms and uses, allied with opportunities to participate in various communication situations, is considered. More specifically, opportunities to observe literate adults engaging in reading and writing, to participate actively in meaningful literacy activities, and to independently explore literacy materials are important considerations. The availability of reading and writing materials within the home should be explored, given the finding of Koppenhaver, Evans, and Yoder (1991) that a print-rich environment was part of the early experiences of adults who were successful in achieving literacy. Opportunities to visit libraries, to purchase books, and to develop specific interests in reading and writing should also be considered (Smith, 1992).

Finally, the bottom segment of the triangle must be addressed through assessment of opportunities to explore the sound system of the language. Opportunities to engage in sound play, and in directed activities involving rhyming, segmentation and analysis, and production of vocalizations or synthetic speech output should also be assessed.

Most people read or write to fulfill definite *needs* or purposes, which dictate the nature and form of the literacy activity selected. Assessment of an individual's needs to engage in literacy activities should consider a variety of overlapping purposes of literacy, such as self-regulation (e.g., writing a reminder to oneself), social interaction (e.g., writing a letter to a friend), education (e.g., obtaining or transmitting information), employment (e.g., developing a mailing list), and recreation (e.g., enjoying poetry).

AAC service providers must identify needs that are currently being met, as well as those that are currently unmet and those that are expected to be unmet in the future. A restricted range of identified needs suggests a lack of awareness of the many functions of print. Given that literacy learning ideally occurs in the context of functional, meaningful experiences, the service provider may want to explore broadening the range of needs before addressing the issue of literacy learning itself.

Subtle philosophical *barriers* may relate to beliefs, policies, and practices, whereas more obvious practical barriers refer to the physical characteristics of the environment. In relation to beliefs, the study by Koppenhaver et al. (1991) of literate adults clearly indicated the importance of parental and teacher expectations in shaping the perceptions of individuals of themselves as readers/writers. Light and McNaughton (1993) reported that other outcomes, such as independence, may supersede literacy in the hierarchy of parental and professional priorities. Questionnaire or interview approaches with parents and professionals may yield important insights into their beliefs regarding literacy development and the priority attached to literacy achievement.

Beliefs themselves often guide policies. For example, if the expectation is that all children will learn to read and write, then inclusion of children with disabilities in mainstream education is required. If expectations are low, or if physical independence is considered to be of primary importance, then withdrawal from reading class for physical or occupational therapy is acceptable. Clearly, for individuals with such diverse needs as those typically presented by individuals with severe speech impairments, expectations and priorities must be determined on an individual basis. Thus, the formulation of policy and methods of intervention based on beliefs about such a heterogeneous group is risky, at best. Practices may closely mirror policy, or may operate almost in direct opposition to stated policy, even though this opposition may not be conscious or deliberate. For example, a child with a speech impairment may be placed in a mainstream class, and withdrawal for therapies may not be allowed, but there may still be little real participatory inclusion.

Careful observation of school and/or work environments should indicate whether philosophical barriers exist relating to beliefs about needs, ways of learning, and expectations for learning. Practical barriers, such as physical positioning in a classroom, may be more easily identified. For example, Eileen, described by Smith (1991) attended a small rural school, with narrow aisles between desks. To accommodate her wheelchair within the class, it was placed in the front of the class, facing her peers. This not only made peer interaction difficult, but also physically placed Eileen closer to the teacher, thereby emphasizing her exclusion from her classmates. Assessment of extrinsic barriers is best accomplished in collaboration with the individuals who can actually effect change.

Frequently, simply being asked to consider and write down specific information regarding accessibility is sufficient to spark change. However, both interview and direct observation are important in determining the interactions between beliefs and expectations, policy, and actual practice.

Individual Assessment: Intrinsic Factors. Assessment of barriers must also include consideration of factors intrinsic to the individual. As discussed previously, potential intrinsic barriers to literacy include physical, sensory/perceptual, language, and/or cognitive impairments. When an individual experiences one or more intrinsic barriers to literacy, extrinsic factors should be modified or adapted to help overcome the effects of the impairments. Literacy assessment should be conducted in conjunction with assessment of the whole person, with appropriate team members contributing expertise in evaluating skills related to these identified areas of impairment and recommending appropriate extrinsic adaptations.

Physical impairments may range from minor difficulties with fine motor tasks to severe restrictions on all types of voluntary movement. For all AAC users with physical impairments, seating and positioning are of primary importance in maximizing opportunities and abilities to interact with print. Careful consultation with occupational and physical therapists and rehabilitation engineers is essential to assess both intrinsic limitations and use of appropriate extrinsic modifications, such as adapted seating, page turners, and switches.

Sensory/perceptual impairments, which may significantly interfere with an AAC user's access and ability to interpret print, are easy to overlook. As a minimum requirement, consideration must be given to assessment of visual acuity, visual field, and the ability to bifocally coordinate eye movement, alignment, fixation, and focus. Likewise, assessment of both hearing sensitivity and functional use of hearing are imperative. This requires involvement of both hearing (e.g., audiologist, educator for deaf individuals and individuals with hearing impairments) and vision (e.g., ophthalmologist, optometrist, educator for blind individuals and individuals with visual impairments) support personnel for assessment of sensory/per-

ceptual abilities and recommendations for adaptations such as amplification, corrective lenses, and/or enlarged print.

Given that many different aspects of *language* comprehension and production may affect literacy learning, careful gathering of information regarding functioning across the language areas of semantics, **syntax-morphology**, phonology, and pragmatics is often recommended. Such information should be sought only if it is perceived to fulfill a specific purpose, for example, to determine the appropriate language level of reading materials to be provided. Otherwise, information may be gathered simply for its own sake, thereby sacrificing valuable intervention time for questionable gain.

Of more immediate relevance is the individual's experience with a range of language forms and functions. Galda et al. (1993) asserted that "when teachers observe children's oral language, they need to focus on what children *do* with language rather than merely what they know about it" (p. 335). In observing language use, service providers must consider AAC users' abilities to use language to direct their own behavior and that of others, to report on past and present experiences, to imagine, to predict, to elicit information, and to solve problems. For many AAC users, the range of communication functions they can fulfill is influenced by the modes of communication available to them and by the characteristics of the type(s) of AAC they use. Vocabulary and communication functions may be extremely restricted.

Specific information regarding speech production abilities is important as well. The myth that reading and writing difficulties can be explained simply and exclusively in terms of motor speech difficulty has been laid to rest. However, the exact nature of the relationship between speech production and factors implicated in reading and writing (such as phonologic awareness, memory, verbal rehearsal) is as yet unresolved. Furthermore, research suggests that access to speech output, whether through natural or synthetic means, may facilitate literacy (Koke & Neilson, 1987).

A speech-language pathologist may not only assist in gathering information regarding language functioning across all levels and interactions between language functioning and the individual's communication system, but may also make recommendations for expanding the current system to increase literacy opportunities. The extent to which the use of fingerspelling may facilitate phonologic awareness (Koehler, Lloyd, & Swanson, 1994), the contribution of graphic symbols (McNaughton, 1993; Rankin, Harwood, & Mirenda, 1994), the opportunities to produce synthetic speech (Foley, 1993), or the introduction of a method to produce print (Berninger & Gans, 1986b) may be assessed as means of reducing restrictions to language/literacy experiences.

Few individuals are too cognitively impaired to benefit from some type of literacy experiences. Thus, assessment of *cognitive* abilities should extend beyond traditional measures of intelligence, mental age, and adaptive behavior, and aim to yield information about the literacy experiences likely to be of most benefit. Although providing experiences that are both age and cognitively appropriate is often difficult, observation of the experiences and materials enjoyed by same-aged peers is an important step in the assessment process, in conjunction with gathering information regarding the AAC user's current literacy opportunities and participation (Rainforth, York, & Macdonald, 1992). Input from team members such as parents and other caregivers, early childhood educators, psychologists, reading specialists, and special educators can help determine how best to provide literacy experiences that meet the criteria of both age and cognitive appropriateness.

Performance Assessment. Direct observation and evaluation is necessary to determine the stage of literacy that has been achieved. The AAC team must identify the individual's awareness of the functions, conventions, and units of written language; the alphabetic/symbolic principles involved; and the structural principles that differentiate spoken and written language (Galda et al., 1993). Performance in each of these areas must be considered in the light of potential physical, sensory/perceptual, language, and cognitive impairments that may serve as barriers to the development of literacy.

Specific Procedures

Assessment procedures are described according to general literacy requirements across age span for four groups: young preschool, preschool–early elementary school, later elementary school, and adolescence-adulthood. Suggestions for assessment include specific procedures and questions that relate to consideration of opportunities, needs, and barriers (both intrinsic and extrinsic); assessment of materials; consideration of present AAC use; and development of an individual performance profile. Clearly, this list provides only a starting point for developing a profile of abilities and potential intervention points for any one individual.

Young Preschool. Independent access to print materials is critical in developing an early enjoyment of literacy. Many literacy activities at this age revolve around storybooks, early drawing and scribbling, and independent handling of books and other print materials. Repetition of familiar stories is an important factor in determining the level of sophistication with which a young child engages in storybook activities, including the level of dialogue surrounding the activity (Clay, 1991). Table 23.1 provides a list of specific questions for use with young preschool children that may be answered via questionnaires, interviews, and observation of children across caregivers (e.g., parents, extended family, daycare providers, teachers) and environments.

Preschool–Early Elementary School. During this time, as some children are beginning to read, others are catching up on missed emergent literacy activities. As such, literacy experiences in formal preschool settings and early elementary school involve activities just described for young preschoolers as well as explicit instruction in the specific skills involved in literacy. Needs become more evident as literacy is increasingly required for school and social participation. Assessment of skills such as naming alphabet letters and knowing their associated sounds, often enters the assessment picture at this time. Table 23.2 provides questions for use with preschool–early elementary

TABLE 23.1   Literacy Assessment of Young Preschool Children

OPPORTUNITIES	NEEDS	BARRIER REDUCTIONS
Are storybooks read frequently to the child at home? In other settings? By whom?	What are the different literacy needs throughout the day?	Is importance attached to literacy in the home? In other environments?
Does the child have a favorite storybook? Are stories reread?	How is the child encouraged to or assisted in participating in literacy activities (e.g., reading recipes, writing lists, looking up telephone numbers, sending greeting cards, reading maps)?	Do caregivers believe that the child can attain literacy? How important is literacy within the total framework of the child's needs?
Does the child actively participate in the reading activity? Does the child assist in turning pages? Ask questions? Comment?	Does the child know the front from the back of books? Top from bottom? Can the child turn the pages? Point to print vs. picture?	Are there barriers in the child's positioning during reading and writing activities? Can the child see the text? The reader's face?
Does the child handle books and other print materials?	Does the child differentiate writing from drawing? Know that writing can be read?	Is an assistive communicative device used? How does the child typically communicate during literacy activities?
Does the child have a variety of writing opportunities? Scribbling? Painting?	Does the child understand that during reading, some elements are repeated? Does the child recognize adults' mistakes in reading?	Are adaptations such as amplification or magnification provided?
Does the child have opportunities to observe adults engaging in literacy activities?	Does the child engage in fingerplays, rhymes, and sound play?	Are activities interesting? Relevant to the child's experiences? At a suitable language level? Are writing materials adapted?

school children, bearing in mind that questions from Table 23.1 may apply as well.

Later Elementary School.   It is during this period that students begin "reading to learn." Those who are not fluent readers have a special need for concentrated, direct instruction and practice in reading and writing, although as emphasized throughout, instruction and practice are important at all stages of the journey toward literacy mastery. Assessment of this age group thus requires not only observation of opportunities to engage in literacy experiences, but also documentation of both *quantity* and *quality* of literacy instructional time. Unfortunately, Koppenhaver and Yoder (1993) concluded that "school-aged children with severe disabilities appear to receive less literacy instruction than do their nondisabled peers, participate in

that instruction in fairly passive ways, seldom interact with peers during instruction, and experience frequent and regular interruptions despite receiving that instruction most often one-to-one or in small groups" (p. 5). Given this finding, comparisons need to be made between scheduled literacy activities and actual time spent in literacy instruction. As part of the assessment process, teachers may themselves be encouraged to monitor the number of interruptions to their schedules, taking note of each interruption as it occurs during the school day. Alternatively, Koppenhaver and Yoder (1993) suggested setting an alarm watch for regular intervals throughout the day. As the alarm goes off, the teacher notes exactly what is occurring in the class, paying particular attention to the AAC user. Over a period of time, a profile of time organization should emerge. Allowing the teacher

TABLE 23.2   Literacy Assessment of Preschool–Early Elementary School Children

OPPORTUNITIES	NEEDS	BARRIER REDUCTIONS
Is the school environment print-rich? Does the school have a literacy center with available reading and writing materials? Is the child encouraged to view educational television programs that feature explicit exposure to literacy? Independently? With adult interaction and discussion? Are children encouraged to engage in literacy experiences in pairs, groups, or individually? Is group discussion encouraged? Are visits to the library included as part of the home or school curriculum? How often? Are books purchased or borrowed? Does the child have a personal book collection? A favorite book?	Are reading activities built around a language theme or do they occur independently of other school activities? Does the child attend to or identify print in the environment on possessions (e.g., bookbags, lunchboxes), in personal areas (e.g., lockers), and other areas of the school and classroom (e.g., boys' and girls' restrooms)? Does the child identify the alphabet? Associate letters with sounds? Recognize words by sight? Demonstrate beginning word-attack skills? Does the child print letters to represent sounds, syllables, or words? Write from left to right? Write words? Sentences? Use invented spellings? Can the child retell familiar stories? Remember and/or predict outcomes?	What is the prevailing philosophical approach to literacy development in the school? Is there a lessening in emphasis on readiness for determining when to introduce literacy materials? Are reading/writing materials physically accessible? Does the application of technology provide physical access? Can the child participate in literacy experiences to the extent that typical peers do? Are appropriate communication messages available via an AAC device? How are changes in message needs managed?

to monitor such time use is less intrusive than introducing an outsider or teaching assistant as the observer, and results of the observation may be more easily accepted. Questions for use with later elementary school children are provided in Table 23.3.

Adolescence-Adulthood. Typically, adolescents and young adults decide what independent literacy opportunities they wish to explore. At this major stage of personal development and conscious exploration of self-image, reading and writing may play an important role, either through correspondence with peers or through journal writing and reading. Of crucial importance are opportunities for privacy in reading and writing. Therefore, although many of the opportunity questions raised in relation to younger age groups may be asked,

AAC service providers must also explore the opportunities for and barriers to producing and reading private texts.

During adolescence and young adulthood, literacy for vocational and daily living needs becomes important, as well as for higher education, where appropriate. Barriers that may arise at this time include an overreliance on a developmental framework of literacy development, with an insistence on orderly progression through each of the stages, ignoring the fact that typical development is characterized by overlapping abilities across stages. Persistence with such a rigid application of a developmental model may result in little functional gain for some students, leading to frustration and an eventual rejection of all literacy-related activities. Furthermore, the student's self-perception as a potentially functional reader/writer may be

TABLE 23.3   Literacy Assessment of Later Elementary School Children

OPPORTUNITIES	NEEDS	BARRIER REDUCTIONS
Does the child have opportunities to engage in different types of reading/writing activities?	What are the literacy needs/tasks of same-aged peers as they relate to academic, social, and extracurricular participation (e.g., while working in content areas such as social studies, mathematics, music, art; corresponding with an electronic pen pal; playing board or card games; participating in school performances such as plays or concerts; viewing, participating in, or discussing sports)?	Is the use of AAC linked with the literacy demands of the classroom?
Does the child spend the most time on skill building with word- or sentence-level tasks?		Is technology easily integrated and readily expanded? Are backups provided in case of equipment breakdown?
How frequently does the child produce text that is longer than a paragraph?		Are appropriate adaptations provided for test taking, completing homework, independent study, and text production?
Does the child have opportunities to independently read text of personal interest within his ability range? Is adult guidance provided? Is the teacher aware of the child's interests?	Does the child comprehend extended written text? Answer questions? Discuss what has been read?	
Does the child have opportunities for discussing literature and suggesting future reading?	Can the child compose coherent text with few spelling errors? Edit independently? Revise both mechanical errors and writing content/style?	
	Can the child access dictionaries, encyclopedias, and other reference materials?	

seriously undermined. Here, again, individualized assessment is called for, with careful evaluation of the student's current and future literacy needs and how they relate to total functioning in relevant situations and environments.

Another group of potential adolescent-adult AAC users includes individuals with acquired disabilities, such as those occurring as a result of a cerebrovascular accident (CVA), traumatic brain injury (TBI), or such neurological conditions as multiple sclerosis (MS) and Parkinson's disease. Much of the assessment information to be gathered will mirror that described previously, including consideration of opportunities, needs, and barriers to reading and writing. However, additional intrinsic factors must be considered; first and foremost, the individual's premorbid literacy skills. This information must be obtained to establish a

point of reference from which to conduct the present assessment and determine appropriate AAC intervention. An individual for whom literacy was critical for employment and recreational participation presents quite a different picture from an individual who experienced past difficulty in achieving even a basic level of literacy.

Some individuals with acquired disabilities, particularly those with stroke or TBI, may have visual (e.g., Padula & Shapiro, 1993) or physical impairments such that application of technology is required for access to reading and writing. For further discussion of issues surrounding assessment of individuals with acquired disabilities, see Chapter 19.

In summary, of critical importance in literacy assessment is the recognition that the previously described general principles serve as a guide throughout the process. AAC service providers must recognize the complexity and nature of literacy development, the interaction between intrinsic and extrinsic factors that influence that development, the contributions of various types of AAC, and the reciprocal relationship between assessment and intervention.

INTERVENTION

Few areas of educational intervention are as fraught with controversy as approaches to literacy instruction (Ellis, 1993). Many different approaches have been in vogue in this century (see Adams, 1990, for a more complete description of their rationales and effectiveness). A brief summary of some of the more common approaches is presented here.

Whole word approaches, sometimes referred to as *look-and-say*, dominated in the United States in the 1930s (Ellis, 1993) and still prevail (Adams, 1990). Such methods encourage the learner to focus on the visual unit as a direct route to word identification. The aim is to develop a comprehensive sight vocabulary through the use of, for example, flashcards and environmental labels, with an expectation that sight vocabulary will provide the basis for generalization to unfamiliar words. No explicit reference is made to **grapheme-phoneme correspondence**.

Phonics approaches are frequently viewed as the antithesis of look-and-say methods in that the primary focus is on teaching letter-sound correspondences, with gradual increases in difficulty of materials to incorporate irregular patterns. Such approaches emphasize the bottom-up aspects of decoding and encoding referred to earlier in this chapter. As learners master the decoding steps, they gradually bypass this indirect route of word identification and develop a sight word vocabulary that can be accessed directly, while retaining their decoding skills as a backup for analysis and identification of unfamiliar words.

Language experience approaches emphasize the integration of listening, speaking, reading, and writing. Learners are encouraged to select their own topics and use their own vocabulary. Although the relationship between spoken and writ-

ten words is made explicit, the correspondences between individual letters and sounds are not (Ellis, 1993).

Whole language approaches emphasize top-down reading processes in which reading and writing are viewed as natural outgrowths of spoken language development. Learners are surrounded with print and given opportunities to use it functionally and purposefully. Little if any exposure to basal readers, spelling programs, or handwriting practice is provided. Learners are encouraged to discover literacy through experiences with spoken language, predictable books, creative writing, and invented spellings (Goodman, 1986).

Ellis (1993) suggested that battles over the most effective approach have raged primarily among overzealous "experts," whereas educators have freely incorporated elements from different approaches. Furthermore, the developmental nature of emergent literacy makes it likely that different strategies may be effective at different stages in the reading process. One fact remains: many children have become and continue to become competent readers regardless of the teaching approach(es) employed. Others, despite adequate intelligence, opportunities, and instruction demonstrate a persistent failure to master basic literacy skills. When an individual has such difficulties, questions must be asked as to the effectiveness of the teaching approach(es) being used and their applicability to the specific individual. Although research results have provided some bases for selecting some approaches over others, results are as yet sufficiently tentative to warrant incorporating elements from different approaches, rather than strictly adhering to one particular approach. In addition to the 14 general AAC intervention principles discussed in Chapter 15, the four literacy intervention principles discussed below were developed to guide clinicians/educators in their use.

Intervention Principles

Principle 1. Intervention programs should recognize that good literacy intervention practices apply across all types of literacy instruction with clients with all types of disabilities. Certain characteristics are desirable across all instructional programs and may be of particular importance to individuals using AAC. These include

a. a view of reading and writing as interactive, constructive processes, where the reader/writer is actively engaged in the process (Clay, 1975; Galda et al., 1993; Koppenhaver, 1992; Watson, Layton, Pierce, & Abraham, 1994).

b. a primary focus on meaning, as suggested in the first segment of the triangle of Figure 23.1 (Forester, 1988; Musselwhite, 1992; Pumfrey & Reason, 1991).

c. an emphasis on the integration of language skills, both spoken and written, while building on life experiences and knowledge (Blackstone, 1989; Foley, 1993; Koppenhaver, Pierce, Steelman, & Yoder, 1994; Pumfrey & Reason, 1991). This incorporates the first two segments of Figure 23.1. Crucially, consideration must also be given to the final segment, encompassing analytic skills relating to grapheme-phoneme correspondence. Thus, an instructional program built around this model requires the integration of both holistic and analytic components.

d. dual recognition of the importance of the *functions* and *forms* of print (Galda et al., 1993; Koppenhaver, Coleman, Kalman, & Yoder, 1991; Teale & Sulzby, 1987).

e. a focus on providing strategies, rather than teaching splinter skills (Crain, 1988). Galda et al. (1993) suggested that "as children acquire strategies, they automatically acquire skills" (p. 106).

f. consideration of the linguistic/communication context of literacy learning, as well as the social and physical contexts. Thus, active participation in communication surrounding literacy activities is encouraged (Galda et al., 1993); perceptions and expectations for reading and writing are addressed (Koppenhaver & Yoder, 1992a; Musselwhite, 1992); and, the availability and accessibility of literacy materials and literate models are considered (Steelman, 1992).

g. a focus on the individual learning style of the apprentice reader/writer (Koppenhaver et al., 1994), rather than adopting a prescriptive approach to reading/writing instruction.

h. recognition of both the similarities and the differences between spoken and written language (Gillam & Johnston, 1992).

i. fostering of "safe" learning—building on success and current levels of functioning (Forester, 1988), with the goal of allowing learners control of their own learning.

j. provision of materials that are of personal interest (Forester, 1988) and appropriate difficulty (Koppenhaver & Yoder, 1992b; Steelman, 1992).

Principle 2. Intervention programs should recognize that although reading and writing emerge in a developmental sequence, in some cases application of a developmental framework is less appropriate than a functional approach. Reading instruction that uses developmental information, emphasizing the building of skills in a sequence, is most often the method of choice. However, at some point a more functional approach to reading may be implemented, particularly for individuals with cognitive impairments or older individuals with a long history of reading failure. Such approaches emphasize, for example, the development of an individualized sight word vocabulary, deemphasizing analysis and segmentation. In the past, some sight word instruction has used behavioral techniques such as **stimulus shaping**, **time delay**, and **errorless learning** (Conners, 1992; Lalli & Browder, 1993). Recently, learning to read "survival" words (e.g., informational signs, cooking, and shopping words) to promote independence in the community has been emphasized for many individuals with cognitive impairments.

A functional approach relies on careful task analysis of specific literacy requirements for the individual and the development of appropriate materials directly related to the demands placed on the individual (Cornell, 1988). The emphasis is on action-oriented rather than passive educational tasks. A functional approach incorporates teaching specific occupation-related literacy strategies, such as locating information for immediate use, "rather than the traditional classroom goal of internalizing content for future reference" (Phillippi, 1988, p. 660). As pointed out by Browder and Lalli (1991), instruction should extend beyond nonfunctional "word calling" into comprehension and use of written words in meaningful contexts. Sight word approaches to literacy instruction have been criticized in the past on the basis that such approaches provide the reader with few strategies for dealing with unfamiliar words, limiting independence (Ellis, 1993). On the other hand, approaches that emphasize bottom-up skills have been accused of focusing on form over function, with poor readers frequently overrelying on word analysis, while ignoring other sources of information (Smith, 1982; Stanovich 1986).

The decision to employ a strictly functional approach to reading instruction for AAC users should not in any case be determined merely on the bases of cognitive level and/or educational placement. Conners (1992) reported that some individuals with a moderate degree of cognitive impairment have learned to read using a word analysis approach. With maximum opportunities for participation in literacy experiences, many AAC users may also become productive, competent readers. However, at times casting off a developmental approach becomes the appropriate choice, one that should involve, first and foremost, assessment of past opportunities to develop literacy. Untreated sensory impairments, exposure to sporadic instruction, lack of exposure to explicit skill instruction (with particular reference to phonologic segmentation and analysis skills), poor implementation of instruction, and/or passive learning experiences should always be considered as contributing factors in reading difficulties and be managed accordingly. As is the case with developing intelligible speech, a developmental approach may be frustrating and futile for a person who is approaching adulthood and has had adequate opportunity for developing word analysis skills. Conners' (1992) statement referring to individuals with moderate cognitive impairments may also apply broadly to others experiencing reading difficulty:

> Given that many children with moderate mental retardation can learn word analysis, a question still remains as to whether it is wise to teach them this skill. On the one hand, the major goal in educating such children is to increase their ability to function independently in society. Word analysis represents a more independent form of reading than does sight-word recognition. If a child can sound out, then he or she has a chance of reading new words. To have the skill allows much more flexibility than to know a finite set of words by sight. On the other hand, children with moderate mental retardation will take much longer than children without mental retardation to learn the skill of word analysis. . . . before they have the skill, they will need to find the restroom and the exit. (p. 593)

Conners (1992) recommended concurrent instruction in word analysis and sight word instruction, a recommendation not unlike that proposed for AAC users (Blau, 1986; Foley, 1993). Use of such an approach may also set the stage for moving into greater emphasis on functional reading if and when it is determined to be appropriate for a particular individual.

Because writing and spelling depend on the development of reading and physical, language, and cognitive abilities, even competent readers demonstrate broad variability in writing abilities. Quite likely, the same is true of AAC users, although less information is available regarding their writing skills and appropriate instructional methods. Some individuals with severe physical impairments may not be able to use handwriting at all and may rely on other means to produce functional writing in activities of daily living, such as signing one's name or making shopping lists. Various alternative methods to actual handwriting can be employed, which accordingly depend on reading skills and some degree of physical ability. For example, a rubber stamp can be used for producing a signature, a checklist for constructing a grocery list, a typewriter for addressing envelopes, and a computer for writing personal letters. Many individuals use a multimodal approach to written communication. As with reading, an instructional approach that emphasizes both skill development and functional outcomes may be most beneficial to AAC users with writing difficulties.

Principle 3. Intervention programs should be based on appropriate assessment. This is not to suggest that exhaustive assessment should precede any attempt at encouraging literacy development. This text has emphasized the symbiotic relationship between assessment and intervention; ongoing intervention-focused assessment, generally carried out informally through observation of literacy behaviors, is needed.

Principle 4. Intervention programs should consider factors intrinsic and extrinsic to the individual. The ultimate goal should be to maximize opportunities to participate in literacy activities, while minimizing barriers to active participation, in a format that is tailored to the needs of each individual AAC user. Intrinsic needs related to physical, sensory/perceptual, language, and cognitive impairments as well as extrinsic needs related to environments must be continuously evaluated so that adjustments can be made throughout the intervention process.

Procedures

The intervention procedures outlined here are based on the model of reading presented in Figure 23.1, addressing the three segments of the triangle: the learning context, language and communication, and print. Some useful intervention procedures are suggested, based on a wide range of resources and clinical experience.

Learning Context.   As suggested by emergent literacy research, consideration of environmental experiences is important in developing an effective intervention program. This includes the previous and present experiences of life, which form the basis of shared knowledge in contexts such as the home, school, or workplace. The current state of knowledge of the experiences of young AAC users suggests that many do not have access to experiences that facilitate literacy development (e.g., Light & Kelford-Smith, 1993). Thus, a priority in intervention must be to increase not only the *opportunities* available to AAC users, but their *access* to active participation in literacy activities. Recognition of both intrinsic and extrinsic barriers is often a crucial first step, and potential immediate solutions should be explored. For young children, this may simply mean changing the physical context of storytelling, so that they are positioned closer to the reader. Developing specific book-related communication boards, adapting VOCA vocabulary, adapting reading style to accommodate the communication demands faced by young AAC users, and encouraging multiple book readings can all serve to alleviate barriers to active participation. Introducing activities focusing specifically on increasing phonologic awareness in a fun context can help develop skills known to be predictive of reading progress, skills that may be particularly

difficult for children with severe speech impairments to access. For older children, scheduled reading and writing instruction time should be sacrosanct. As with all ages, interruptions should be kept to a minimum, and when a teacher has observed that frequent interruptions have become the norm, consideration should be given to changing the schedule.

Every effort should be made to ensure that reading materials reflect the real-life experiences of AAC users, because meaning may be more readily accessed if the content of a text is related in some way to the reader's life experiences. Texts specifically related to AAC users or other individuals with disabilities are few and far between, although some excellent ones, such as *Nick Joins In* (Lasker, 1980) (Figure 23.2) and *On Being Sarah* (Helfman, 1992), are available.

Differences in life experiences, which may inhibit easy access to the content of other texts may be minimized by adequate discussion and introduction. Unfamiliar texts offer access to vicarious experiences, which may otherwise remain inaccessible to AAC users. As Galda et al. (1993) suggested, "books provide 'virtual experience,' thereby adding to knowledge of the world, leading to an increase in possibilities for responding to the world, thereby increasing a child's storehouse of information, leading to better comprehension in reading new texts, in a cycle of mutual reciprocation" (p. 107).

Research results indicating that expectations of enjoyment and competence may be low for AAC users must be disseminated, along with a changing perspective of literacy that emphasizes a continuum of development rather than "reading readiness." Parents, caregivers, and professionals may come to value literacy behaviors that they previously disregarded and may be more aware of the need to provide opportunities for participation in literacy activities. Similarly, AAC users need help to recognize how much they already know about print, so that they come to view themselves as readers and writers. Forester (1988) has suggested that this is a key factor in working with adults with literacy difficulties. Specific intervention suggestions regarding learning context are described in Table 23.4.

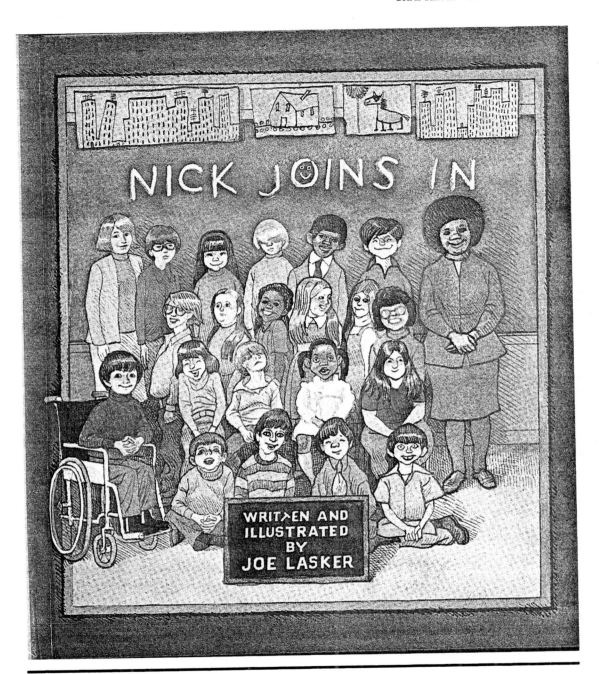

FIGURE 23.2   *Nick Joins In.*

Cover illustration from *Nick Joins In* by Joe Lasker. Copyright © 1980 by Joe Lasker. Published in hardcover by Albert Whitman & Company. All rights reserved.

TABLE 23.4   Learning Context: Some Specific Suggestions for Intervention

PREVIOUS AND PRESENT LIFE EXPERIENCES

PRESCHOOL AGE	SCHOOL AGE	ADOLESCENT/ADULT
Create a print-rich environment by displaying literacy materials at an appropriate level; providing a range of books and drawing/writing equipment; making available alphabets, printed names, and labels; and encouraging parents to watch programs such as Sesame Street with their child.	*Consider how time is being used* and, where necessary, adapt the daily schedule. *Fill in gaps in life experiences* by providing experiences or through preparatory discussion before reading or writing about a topic.	*Evaluate current life experiences*; analyze typical weekly schedule, preferred activities, and interests, and select reading materials accordingly; encourage students to draw on their own experiences in writing through use of a private journal.
Encourage storybook reading, using adaptations such as page fluffers or tabs, so that the child can assist in turning pages; develop individualized photo books for personal interest; use materials that reflect the child's experiences or consider how new experiences might be provided—by a shopping trip, visit to the park, going to a birthday party—and refer back to the experience when reading.		*Provide vicarious experience* through "wide reading," supplemented with discussion, audiovisual materials, etc.
Encourage multiple readings of books, allowing time for discussion, retelling the story at other times during the day, predicting what will happen next, and misreading key parts in a playful manner.		
Provide a means of control, including messages such as "My turn," "Stop," and "I want to turn the page" on communication displays.		
Encourage active participation by providing thematic communication displays.		
Provide models of reading/writing, such as reading notes, writing lists, signing one's name.		
Encourage drawing and scribbling, using fingerpaints, sponges, or other adaptive tools.		

EXPECTATIONS OF ENJOYMENT AND COMPETENCE

PRESCHOOL AGE	SCHOOL AGE/ADOLESCENT/ADULT
Share information about the value of early literacy experiences and caregiver involvement.	*Help students realize how familiar they are with print.*
Provide "intergenerational" literacy instruction as necessary.	*Encourage co-reading* and small group reading/writing, balancing abilities within the group.
Foster positive and appropriate expectations.	*Select materials carefully*, ensuring plenty of success; if necessary, devise materials on an individual basis.
Provide experiences of success; use stories with repeated lines, such as "I'll huff and I'll puff . . ." from the Three Little Pigs with the repeated line programmed into a VOCA, so that the AAC user can participate actively, and help "read" the story.	

TABLE 23.4   (*Continued*)

FOCUS ON MEANING

PRESCHOOL AGE	SCHOOL AGE/ADOLESCENT/ADULT
Encourage paraphrasing of stories where possible; mix up story endings and discuss; use multiple readings so stories are familiar; before reading notes, introduce a question such as "I wonder what this is about," or "What does Daddy need today?" *Encourage acting out the stories* that are read. *Plan and discuss messages* that are to be written, such as shopping lists, checking cupboards for items needed, repeating item names as they are written down, and referring frequently to the list when shopping.	*Frame content* of a text, outlining the organizational structure; make students aware of how much they already know about the topic before they engage in reading/writing, discussion, taking quizzes, etc.; check how much they can predict about a story, accepting all predictions, and rechecking after reading for accuracy of predictions. *Scan texts* before starting to read, encouraging students to pick out any unfamiliar vocabulary that may cause problems in comprehending the text. *Role-play* major parts from a story, presenting an alternative viewpoint, such as courtroom dramatization of such fairy tales as Hansel and Gretel. *Value content over form in written output*; encourage risk taking and extended text output, emphasizing content and ignoring grammatical or spelling errors, allowing time for editing and correction of specific errors *after* content has been completed and evaluated; minimize form demands by focusing on one type of error only in editing. *Rewrite familiar stories from a different perspective*, for example, Jack and the Beanstalk from the point of view of the giant.

SHARED KNOWLEDGE

PRESCHOOL AGE	SCHOOL AGE/ADOLESCENT/ADULT
Build around life experiences, selecting materials accordingly.	*Brainstorm* a particular topic before coming to the written task, encouraging students to build semantic maps of concepts related to the topic; use probe questioning to determine any areas of difficulty, where background knowledge needs to be developed; identify possible questions students may have about the topic.

Compiled from Forester (1988); Funk (1988); Galda, Cullinan, & Strickland (1993); Light & McNaughton (1993); Nickse, Speicher, & Buchek (1988).

Language and Communication. Literacy skills draw heavily on the spoken language resources of the learner, within the context of communication (Galda et al., 1993). Therefore, the related *purposes* of spoken and written language must be made explicit. AAC users may be advantaged in development of this concept, given their exposure to the use of graphic symbols for communication; however, caution is urged by Bishop, Rankin, and Mirenda (1994) in accepting "the overall assertion that graphic symbol use facilitates reading acquisition" (p. 123). The role of the graphic symbol system is discussed in greater detail below.

The transition into literacy from use of non-orthographic AAC must be given careful consideration, although research addressing this issue is only in the initial stages. Koehler et al. (1994) have suggested that the use of fingerspelling may be particularly beneficial in facilitating phonologic awareness, grapheme-phoneme correspondence, and spelling. Because assistive communication devices (both manual and electronic) often contain written words and the alphabet, their use requires careful advance planning to integrate communication and literacy intervention.

The term *language structures* is used here to refer to experience with, and knowledge of, the structural aspects of language: syntax, morphology, and phonology. For typically developing children, spoken language development provides a rich resource supporting top-down text processing. In later development, experience with written language has important benefits in increasing vocabulary (Nagy & Anderson, 1984) and encouraging complexity in sentence level language development (Gillam & Johnston, 1992).

Although research into language development in AAC users is still in its infancy, certain trends have been suggested, including a tendency to rely on short utterances and restrictions in sentence structure, with a predominance of simple syntactic structures (e.g., Kelford-Smith et al., 1989; Smith, 1994; Spiegel, Benjamin, & Spiegel, 1993; Udwin & Yule, 1990). Distinguishing between such performance restrictions and potential underlying competence is extremely difficult. Use of reduced sentence length and simple structures

may be a response to pragmatic constraints, reminiscent of pidgin language strategies (von Tetzchner, 1985). On the other hand, access to complete sentences through single keystrokes (e.g., via an electronic assistive communication device) may have implications for language development that have remained as yet relatively unexplored. Given the uncertainty surrounding these issues, expanding experience in communicative use with a range of syntactic structures and inflections may be an important focus in literacy intervention. Furthermore, the questions previously recommended in relation to intrinsic and extrinsic factors should help focus distinctions between underlying competence and performance limitations (see Intervention Principle 4).

In relation to the role of **phonology** in literacy development, attention is given here only to the metalinguistic skill of phonologic awareness. For a review of the literature in this area, with specific reference to AAC, see Blischak (1994) and Hjelmquist et al. (1994). Although a severe speech impairment does not necessarily inhibit the development of phonologic awareness, AAC users face greater challenges in developing this critical skill. For *all* beginning readers, Adams (1990) has concluded, "The evidence is compelling: toward the goal of efficient and effective reading instruction, explicit training of phonemic awareness is invaluable" (p. 331). For young AAC users, instruction may focus on encouraging parents and caregivers to engage children in reading nursery rhymes, an activity that may be otherwise overlooked for children with severe speech impairments. For older learners, sound play activities specifically targeting manipulation of the phonologic structure of words should be an integral part of instruction. Such practice is more effective if the connections between phonologic segments and letters are made explicit (Blachman, 1991), therefore linking with print, the final segment of Figure 23.1. Goswami (1994) stated, "successful training programs teach children about both phonology and orthography, and stress the link between rhyming sounds and spelling patterns for rimes" (p. 23). Specific suggestions for intervention at all levels of language are outlined in Table 23.5.

TABLE 23.5 Language and Communication: Some Specific Suggestions for Intervention

PURPOSE OF LANGUAGE

PRESCHOOL AGE/SCHOOL AGE/ADOLESCENT/ADULT

Maximize opportunities to engage in communicative interaction with a range of communication partners, ensuring that a range of communicative functions can be met.

PURPOSE OF PRINT

PRESCHOOL AGE	SCHOOL AGE/ADOLESCENT/ADULT
Describe and demonstrate purposes; encourage caregivers to express a reason for using print, such as "Let's read a book, just for fun," "I need to find out Anna's phone number," "I have to remember what to buy."	*Brainstorm*, encourage students to list where around them they see print—in a particular room, within their home, in their neighborhood; discuss what that print means; list possible reasons for reading and writing in their own daily lives; discuss who they see reading and writing, when they themselves read or write, and why; discuss when they would like to read or write; if appropriate, list the reading/writing requirements of employment.
Recap purpose after a task has been completed: "So that's what happened to the bad fox," "Now I can phone Anna," "Gerard's birthday card is ready now."	
Label and indicate printed message on AAC displays, whether the word is written with a graphic symbol or is presented on a VOCA screen.	*Provide the alphabet on communication displays*, ensuring format (upper or lower case) is the same as that of instruction, adapting VOCA overlays/screens as necessary.
	Highlight orthography on a communication display, through color emphasis, and draw attention to the printed message output, whether presented in a visual display or printed as hard copy.
	Encourage use of orthographic strategies in communication to communicate messages otherwise unavailable through first-letter cueing; if necessary, elicit vocabulary through semantic strategies, then model first-letter cueing strategies.

LANGUAGE STRUCTURES: SYNTAX-MORPHOLOGY

PRESCHOOL AGE/SCHOOL AGE/ADOLESCENT/ADULT

Be aware of the expressive language level of the AAC user.

Model a range of syntactic structures, using the learner's own communication display; rephrase and/or expand on learner's own output to encourage greater syntactic and morphologic complexity.

Foster experience with as broad a range of sentence types as possible.

TABLE 23.5 *(Continued)*

LANGUAGE STRUCTURES: PHONOLOGY/PHONOLOGIC AWARENESS		
PRESCHOOL AGE	**SCHOOL AGE**	**ADOLESCENT/ADULT**
Encourage caregivers to engage in nursery rhyme activities as they would with a child who was developing speech, pausing at predictable points, even if the child is unable to produce an intelligible vocalization; mix up rhymes, for example, "Jack and Jill went up the . . . mountain!" and monitor responses; program rhymes into VOCAs, if possible, ideally where one activation yields the full rhyme. *Segment words* into onset and rime, in "silly talk," prolonging the initial phoneme, starting with continuants, such as /s/, /m/, etc., so that "sun" is produced as "ssssun".	*Hide objects or pictures of rhyming objects* around the room to foster rhyme recognition, present a sample of the target rhyme (e.g., cat); have students gesture, eye gaze, etc., to objects that rhyme (hat, mat, bat, etc.); present two spoken words; have students indicate by gesture, manual sign, switch activation, yes/no signal whether words rhyme; sort objects according to rhyme (e.g., only things that rhyme with "mat" get put on a mat, those that rhyme with "sack" go in the sack); have students indicate by eye gaze or gesture where each object should go. *Produce target rhyme*, then list other words; have students indicate by gesture, manual sign, buzzer when adult gets one wrong. *Provide spoken word; students find rhyming word* on communication board or VOCA, with semantic clues given as necessary. *Have students sort objects into groups* on the basis of the number of syllables each word contains, indicating through pointing, eye gaze, etc., to foster segmentation—syllables. *Have a bag for "sound of the day"* to foster segmentation—onset-rime identification with only words beginning with that sound going into the bag; have students indicate through yes/no response. *Choose one student's name*, identify initial phoneme(s); have students then identify other items in room that share the same onset to foster segmentation—onset-rime alliteration. *Use activities similar to those outlined above* to practice segmentation—phoneme level, moving from onset phoneme as singleton to initial consonant clusters, final phoneme, and medial phoneme in (C)CVC words; student response based on identification through gesture, eye gaze, yes/no response.	*Remember that focusing on developing phonologic awareness may not be appropriate,* as a developmental model of intervention may not be the model of choice. However, where indicated, similar activities to those suggested already may be adapted with age-appropriate materials, such as rap songs or limericks.

Print. However facilitative background information and spoken language proficiency may be, the reader is still faced with the task of decoding orthography and the writer with encoding messages into orthography. As Stanovich (1986) stated, "a beginning reader must at some point discover the alphabetic principle: that units of print map onto units of sound" (p. 363). Thus, any effective instructional program must incorporate analytical elements that focus on the specific skills needed for both decoding and encoding. As mentioned above, explicit instruction in phonologic awareness is particularly relevant for AAC users, who typically are restricted in their ability to engage in sound play in early development, or in "sounding out" at a later stage (i.e., exploring the relationship between sounds, motor movements, and grapheme representations).

The value of writing is frequently overlooked, partly due to difficulties that may arise in providing access to independent writing. The reciprocal relationship between reading and writing is particularly critical in the early stages of development. Ellis (1991) suggested that knowledge gleaned from spelling contributes to reading in the early stages, but the reverse is not necessarily true. He attributes this to the fact that spelling acts as a mediator for the influence of explicit phonologic awareness on reading. Within this context, invented spelling plays a particularly important role (Ellis, 1991).

Therefore, access to written output must be provided as early as possible, whether this is achieved via a VOCA, word processing, or low technology options such as adapted writing materials. Few studies have been carried out on the differential effectiveness of instructional techniques and spelling for AAC users. McNaughton and Tawney (1993) compared a copy-write-compare (CWC) method and a student-direct cueing (SDC) method for two adult AAC users, and found only minor differences in rates of acquisition, although a retention advantage for the SDC method was observed. This finding supports the position that effective instructional practice drawn from mainstream research is effective for AAC users; the primary challenge is to creatively provide practice for individual learners.

Concurrent with a focus on the analytical skills necessary for decoding and encoding orthography, AAC users must be encouraged to develop additional alternative strategies for word identification, such as a sight word vocabulary. Opportunities may be present in many school environments, where names are placed on chairs and hooks for coats, or labels are placed on play materials.

Just as no recipe consists of a single ingredient, no instructional approach is effective if it reduces the complexities of reading and writing to a specific set of skills. Of far greater importance is a focus on developing flexible strategies that accommodate both analytical and holistic components. Galda et al. (1993) suggested that "as children acquire strategies, they automatically acquire skills" (p. 106). However, assuming skill development in AAC users may be dangerous unless such skills are specifically targeted. Specific skill instruction such as letter identification and sound-letter correspondence is recommended in the context of meaningful literacy events. Frequently, criticisms of instructional approaches that incorporate analytical components, such as explicit instruction in grapheme-phoneme correspondence, have arisen out of overzealous emphasis on the final segment in Figure 23.1, combined with inappropriate methods of instruction. However, as Blachman (1991) pointed out, in relation to phonologic awareness activities

> . . . no one has suggested that these activities provide a complete diet or encompass the child's entire day. Ideally, one would want phonologic awareness activities to be incorporated into a classroom where storybook reading was common-place, spoken language experiences were valued, basic concepts about print (e.g., how to hold a book) and the functions of reading and writing were developed, and children had opportunities both to talk and to write about their experiences. (p. 63)

A balanced diet of intervention requires consideration of all the components of Figure 23.1. For AAC users, certain aspects of the diet may be missing due to both intrinsic and extrinsic factors, and therefore, dietary supplements must be provided, targeting particular risk areas such as experience with print, expressive language development, and explicit instruction in phonologic awareness. Suggestions for intervention surrounding print are described in Table 23.6.

Role of Technology. Technology can provide AAC users with opportunities for independent, active participation in all types of literacy experiences, overcoming many of the previously discussed barriers to literacy. Various types of technology to support literacy are readily available, with new ones being developed almost daily. Indeed, keeping abreast of the latest developments in microcomputer hardware, software, and adaptations that are appropriate for AAC users can be difficult. Organizations (e.g., Closing the Gap, Communication Aid Manufacturers Association [CAMA], RESNA), publications (e.g., *Communication Outlook*), and educational software catalogs and exhibits are available to assist members of the AAC team in product selection. As always, determining appropriate use of technology requires careful assessment of individual short-term and

long-term needs, including opportunities afforded to typical peers and barriers experienced by AAC users.

Technology to support literacy—computer hardware and software, as well as dedicated communication devices—can be divided into three broad categories, with considerable overlap among them. These include technology that provides opportunities for (1) early literacy experiences; (2) skill development; and (3) text composition, editing, and printing. Technology that uses personal microcomputers and software for these purposes can be broadly referred to as computer-assisted instruction (CAI).

Technology for Young Children. The use of technology by young children should promote emerging literacy and provide reading and writing experiences through interactive learning with typical peers (Steelman, Pierce, & Koppenhaver, 1993). Preschool children, who typically engage in emergent literacy experiences such as independent book handling, rhyming and alliterative songs and

TABLE 23.6 Print: Some Specific Suggestions for Intervention Using Letter Sounds

PRESCHOOL AGE	SCHOOL AGE
Name letters in titles of favorite books; draw attention to letter at beginning of own name, family members' names. *Specify section of communication display for letters*, adding letters as they are encountered in activities as above, such as first letter of own name, Mommy, Daddy.	*Incorporate letters onto communication displays*; demonstrate access to letters in high-technology devices; ensure format (upper or lower case) is compatible with that known to student. *Encourage sound play* by using VOCAs; activate spell mode; encourage students to explore letter sounds, selecting sequence of letters, then activating speak function. *Encourage invented spelling*, particularly with voice output; encourage students to explore spelling options. *Provide word ending/rime* (e.g., -an); have students try different onset letters with VOCA and decide whether output is a word or nonword. *Engage in "change a word" activity*; provide a CVC word (e.g., *cat*), then give semantic clue to related word that requires one letter change only (e.g., "you use it in baseball > *bat*"; "the opposite of good > *bad*").

poems, alphabet learning, and drawing/writing activities, may use both low and high technology such as switches, tape loops, computers, synthetic speech output, enlarged keyboards, touch screens, and specialized software.

Experience with books may be enhanced for young AAC users by various types of technology. A child must be provided with a means to independently choose a desired book and the desired activity with the book via an appropriate AAC mode, such as a graphic symbol communication board or VOCA. Preprogrammed messages such as "Read to me," "I want to look at a book," and names of available books should be readily accessible to the child. Some children with physical impairments may independently interact with books using modifications such as page tabs, page separators, and/or thickened pages. Others with more severe physical disabilities may use switches to operate page turners, books on color slides (King-DeBaun, 1990) or videos, or computer software with graphics and synthetic speech output. Books on cassette tapes that are commercially available for independent listening come with printed and illustrated text. For persons with visual and/or physical impairments, free books on tape are also available (Cassette Books, 1992).

Active participation during storybook reading can be facilitated by use of a VOCA or a computer with an adapted keyboard. A cassette tape loop can be created to contain repeated or predictable text (e.g., "Then I'll huff, and I'll puff . . ."). VOCAs with digitized speech are particularly useful in that they may be programmed quickly with any voice (e.g., another child's). Graphic symbols used to access the voice output may be placed on pages of the book to assist the child in selecting the appropriate utterance. During storybook reading, typically developing children frequently comment and ask questions, later reenacting the story alone or with another child. Unfortunately, these spontaneous uses of language are particularly difficult to provide for AAC users. Children who are afforded opportunities for extended interaction with typical peers are at a distinct advantage, as they can benefit from models of others' questions, comments, and protoreadings. Further, utterances produced

by peers can be preprogrammed into VOCAs for activation during both interactive and independent storybook reading. Preprogrammed VOCA messages with accompanying graphic symbols should also be provided so that young AAC users can participate in a broad variety of imaginative play experiences that promote functional literacy, such as ordering food in a restaurant or writing tea party invitations (Koppenhaver et al., 1991; Pierce & McWilliam, 1993).

Technology may also be invaluable in providing opportunities for early drawing and writing experiences for AAC users—a challenging, yet critical aspect of literacy development. Low-technology adaptations such as splints that allow a child to hold a crayon or paintbrush independently may be used, along with fingerpaints, rubber stamps, felt or magnetic boards, or with unconventional drawing/writing materials (e.g., shaving cream). Children who have severe physical impairments may be limited to experiencing writing in a more indirect manner by using switch activated or touch-screen software to draw, select graphic symbols (e.g., cartoon figures, orthography), and compose lists of simple word/picture stories, using talking word processing software. Like early reading activities, drawing and writing activities may occur as part of an interactive group project (e.g., writing a language experience story after a cooking activity) or for independent exploration (King-DeBaun, 1990).

Skill Development.   Classroom computers, with appropriate software designed for vocabulary, word recognition, and spelling instruction, can be of benefit for many students in that they provide motivational opportunities for independent work with consistent, objective feedback (Beukelman & Mirenda, 1992) (see Appendix C-9 for examples of literacy software). As previously emphasized, skill development should be used only in conjunction with interactive learning in meaningful contexts. Steelman et al. (1993, p. 79) provide a list of desirable characteristics to guide software selection.

1. Easy to use
2. Clear documentation
3. Flexible, allowing for individual modification

4. Interactive, altering the format in response to student input
5. Supports classroom curriculum
6. Interesting to students
7. Appropriate to student age and abilities
8. Includes record keeping
9. Uses multimedia (e.g., graphics, synthetic speech)

Text Preparation. Beukelman and Mirenda's (1992) suggestions for text preparation for students with learning disabilities may certainly apply to many AAC users:

> Individuals whose progress with handwriting instruction has not matched their writing needs or who write very slowly may benefit tremendously from word processing programs operated through standard keyboards or alternative input devices. It simply does not make sense to deprive children or adults of the enjoyment of writing simply because of their poor handwriting. Unfortunately, however, many professionals are reluctant to allow access to a keyboard for young children in particular, possibly because they fear that the computer will become a permanent crutch and that handwriting will not develop as a result. As with all such decisions, this one need not be made on an either/or basis. (p. 240)

In the past, many literate AAC users with physical impairments tediously composed text letter-by-letter using one- or two-finger typing or a headstick. In this age of technology one can admire, if not marvel at, their perseverance in that time-consuming and no doubt fatiguing and frustrating process. Communication acceleration techniques such as **semantic compaction** (Baker, 1982), and **word prediction** (e.g., Newell et al., 1992) were designed to eliminate or save keystrokes in generating novel messages in conversation and in text composition.

Semantic compaction is a specific semantic association approach. Chapter 8 discussed semantic association as a part of semantic and conceptual encoding in which individuals associate multiple meanings to graphic symbols (icons). These associations can result in keystroke savings.

Word prediction, sometimes referred to as **lexical prediction**, is one of the most common

methods for increasing speed of message preparation (see Chapter 8). Here, the software in the assistive communication device is set up to provide the user with a group of likely choices after selecting (using an input method such as typing or scanning) the first letter(s) of the word. Some software programs also speak the predicted words via synthetic speech. The user then selects the whole word. For example, the user may select the letter D, whereby the words "Darlene, David, Dear, Denny's, Denver" appear, usually in a window that is separate from the message. Most lexical prediction programs contain a stored dictionary of words, updated according to a particular user's most frequently used words. Entire messages, such as a name and address, may also be stored and accessed with a few keystrokes.

Keystroke savings, however, is only one measure of efficiency of text generation. Extra time requirements (e.g., to scan a visual array; produce switch hits) and increased cognitive demands (e.g., memory) may work against acceleration for some individuals (e.g., Levine, Gauger, Bowers, & Khan, 1986; Venkatagiri, 1993).

Most reported uses of communication acceleration techniques for text preparation have been by AAC users who had prior literacy abilities. As such, little is known about their effects on individuals who are developing literacy. For extensive descriptions of other methods of communication acceleration, see Church and Glennen (1992), Higginbotham (1992), and Chapter 10.

Role of Synthetic Speech. Although little has been reported regarding the benefits of synthetic speech in literacy development, opportunities to produce synthetic speech may foster the development of top-down and bottom-up reading processes and assist in text preparation. For example, Foley (1993) has suggested that AAC users with poor decoding skills may make use of a talking word processing program to increase comprehension by independently listening to and reading previously entered text. Synthetic speech produced via a VOCA or during CAI may also contribute to the development of word recognition (Romksi & Sevcik, 1993b) and phonologic awareness skills

(Barron et al., 1992; Foley, 1993), particularly when combined with print.

In producing text, synthetic speech feedback (with or without word prediction) may provide assistance in selecting words for AAC users with poor reading and/or spelling skills. Teaching approaches to text preparation that emphasize *process* over *product*, often used with students with learning disabilities, make use of this technology so that the writer can devote greater cognitive energy to the actual process of composition. Here, software that allows pertinent vocabulary (e.g., science words) to be entered prior to student use may be employed (Beukelman & Mirenda, 1992; McGinnis & Beukelman, 1989). Synthetic speech feedback allows writers to hear their written work to assist in text editing.

Role of Graphic Symbols.   One area specific to AAC that has just begun to be the focus of research and clinical interest, is the role of graphic symbols employed by an AAC user (Bishop et al., 1994; McNaughton, 1993; McNaughton & Lindsay, 1995; Rankin et al., 1994). Given the previous discussion on the importance of early language and communication experiences to literacy development, arguing against use of graphic symbols by prereading children to promote independent communication would be difficult. However, the specific processes involved when children produce language using nonorthographic means is currently unknown. McNaughton (1993) described the holistic processing required when a young child is communicating with pictographic symbols and the visual analysis opportunities afforded by symbols containing sequenced components. She suggested that use of graphic symbols may differentially contribute to literacy development according to the type of symbol introduced at different developmental stages. McNaughton regarded AAC users as having "a radically different developmental experience to that of the nondisabled child" (p. 60). The extent to which graphic symbol use may affect development of linguistic and metalinguistic underpinnings of literacy, however, remains open to question. Bishop et al. (1994) speculated that the use of graphic symbols may support development of print awareness in young children, but that benefits may not extend to other processes involved in beginning reading.

Arguments against the contribution of graphic symbols to the development of print awareness, in particular for children with developmental disabilities, emerge from early work in reading instruction in which pairing pictures with written words actually impairs sight word acquisition (e.g., Samuels, 1967; Saunders & Solman, 1984; Singh & Solman, 1990, as reviewed by Blischak & McDaniel, 1995). In opposition to this, Romski and Sevcik (1993b) reported results of a 2-year study involving graphic symbol and synthetic speech use by adolescents with severe developmental disabilities. Here, without direct instruction in reading, participants recognized at least 60% of the words printed on their communication displays. Exposure to print in the context of meaningful communication interactions, along with the benefits of voice output, may have contributed to word recognition, in contrast to previously cited studies in which sight words were taught in drill-type activities. However, until further research has been conducted, young AAC users should be provided with experiences that are known to promote the development of language and literacy.

SUMMARY

Throughout this text, the interrelationship between spoken and written language has been emphasized. For AAC users, this relationship is particularly critical because, to a great extent, aided AAC users are dependent on literacy for access to an open-ended communication system. Maintaining the delicate balance between a focus on encouraging communication and an emphasis on the development of literacy can be difficult. Using assistive communication devices to promote literacy development may lead to viewing the device as an academic, rather than a communication tool. Thus, one aspect of communication may be overemphasized, resulting in reduced opportunities to communicate across a broad range of settings and functions. Literacy development should not take precedence over more traditional communication intervention, but rather the long-term impact of literacy on communicative competence should be recognized from the start. As with so many intervention issues with AAC users, a simple either/or position is ultimately disadvantageous to the AAC user. What is required is a holistic communication-centered perspective that recognizes the interdependence of communication and literacy without neglecting the unique demands specific to both. This requires consideration of the communication and learning environments of AAC users, as well as the resources they bring to the dual tasks of communication and literacy development.

CHAPTER 24

COMMUNICATION-BASED APPROACHES TO PROBLEM BEHAVIOR

RALF W. SCHLOSSER

In the last two decades, the emphasis in the assessment and treatment of **problem behavior** has shifted from a focus on the form of the behavior toward a focus on the functions that the problem behavior may serve for individuals. Interventions are then based on the identified functions of the problem behavior and teaching alternative and more socially acceptable behavior. This chapter is specifically concerned with replacing problem behavior with communicative alternatives in individuals who require **augmentative and alternative communication (AAC)** intervention. It provides an overview of AAC selection considerations so that professionals with an AAC background can assume a more active role in intervention development for individuals with little or no functional speech who also engage in problem behavior. These considerations are derived from existing research on **communication-based approaches to problem behavior** and from recent AAC intervention research. This chapter is not intended to provide an overview of the entire assessment and intervention processes for communication-based approaches to problem behavior (for such information, see Carr et al., 1994; Durand, 1990; Reichle & Wacker, 1993). Rather, it provides information that can aid in understanding the relationship between communication and problem behavior and how to effect change in problem behavior through communication-based approaches.

PROBLEM BEHAVIOR

Aggression, autistic leading, disruptive behavior, self-injurious behavior (SIB), stereotypic behavior, tantrums, and **unconventional verbal behavior** are considered problem behaviors. Aggression includes behaviors directed toward other persons (e.g., kicking, punching, scratching, biting) or things (e.g., property destruction). Autistic leading is a nonlinguistic form of requesting in which individuals take communication partners by the wrist, lead them to a desired object, and then place the partners' hands on the object (Carr & Kemp, 1989; Rutter, 1978). Disruptive behavior may include falling on the floor or manipulating lights in the classroom (Durand, 1990; Hunt, Alwell, & Goetz, 1988). SIB includes headbanging, self-biting, self-slapping, pica, vomiting, rumination, and other forms (see Fee & Matson, 1991; Schlosser & Goetze, 1992). Stereotypic or self-stimulatory behavior includes behaviors such as incessantly rocking back and forth, repetitiously moving fingers in front of the eyes or flapping hands in the air (Koegel & Koegel, 1989). Tantrums involve prolonged screaming and crying and may be accompanied by one or more of the other behaviors (Carr et al., 1994). Unconventional verbal behavior includes immediate echolalia, delayed echolalia, perseverative speech, and incessant (repetitive) questioning. Whether unconventional verbal behavior represents a problem to communication partners hinges on the degree of the conventionality, intelligibility, and interactiveness of the speech (Prizant & Rydell, 1993).

COMMUNICATIVE NATURE OF PROBLEM BEHAVIOR

As documented by Durand (1990), the communicative nature of problem behavior in some individuals has a long-standing history, as evidenced by anecdotal observations (Plato, 348 B.C./1960), theoretical accounts (e.g., Ferster, 1965; Minuchin, 1974), and empirical reports (Bates, Camaioni, & Volterra, 1975; Schlosser & Goetze, 1991; Talkington, Hall, & Altman, 1971). Before addressing the communicative nature of problem behavior in individuals with disabilities, this issue will be reviewed as it relates to typical child development.

Evidence from Typically Developing Children

The philosophers Plato (348 B.C./1960) and Rousseau (1762/1979) observed that typically developing infants may cry to get their caregivers to fulfill their needs (see Durand, 1990). However, there has long been discussion regarding the intentionality of such behaviors. Intentionality, a mentalistic concept, may be inferred, but not observed (Bates et al., 1975; Day, Johnson, & Schussler, 1986). Evidence suggests that although problem behavior may not be initially intentional, it may turn intentional as a result of attributing meaning to these behaviors (Bates et al., 1975; Carr et al., 1994; Day et al., 1986; Hart, 1980). For instance, a caregiver may respond to an infant's cry by saying "She is hungry; she wants a bottle" and providing a bottle. The pragmatic concept of perlocutionary behaviors (Bates et al., 1975) has been found useful in conceptualizing this stage toward intentionality: problem behaviors are ". . . perlocutionary in that their communicative value was more the result of the perceptions of the audience, than actual intent on behalf of the infant" (Day et al., 1986, p. 122). Over time, the child may learn that behavior A, exhibited in the presence of a communication partner, leads to response B by that partner. Eventually, the child will learn that behavior can be used to cause others to respond accordingly. In reviewing the typical child development literature, Carr et al. (1994) conclude that problem behavior serves a purpose for the individual exhibiting it; moreover, as children acquire socially more appropriate ways (e.g., speech) to achieve their goals, they tend to give up their old means (e.g., crying) of reaching those goals.

Evidence from Individuals with Disabilities

Among individuals with language disorders, developmental disabilities, and other psychiatric disorders, several findings suggest that the severity or frequency of problem behavior is related to the severity of communication disability (Aram, Ekelman, & Nation, 1984; Baker & Cantwell, 1982; Cantwell, Baker, & Mattison, 1980; Caulfield, Fischel, DeBaryshe, & Whithurst, 1989; Schlosser & Goetze, 1992; Shodell & Reiter, 1968; Stevenson & Richman, 1978; Talkington et al., 1971). For example, Talkington et al. (1971) observed an increased incidence of aggression among persons with cognitive impairments and severe communication disabilities. Shodell and Reiter (1968) noted more SIB in schizophrenic individuals with little or no functional speech as opposed to individuals with speech. Recently, Schlosser and Goetze (1992) found that 50% of the participants in intervention studies involving SIB had little or no functional speech, and 81% of the participants reportedly were not provided with AAC, as reported in original intervention studies.

In summary, evidence from typical child development and from the relationship of communication disability to problem behavior in individuals with disabilities demonstrates that problem behavior may be communicative in nature. Children without disabilities seem to engage in problem behavior for similar reasons as individuals with disabilities but gradually replace problem behaviors as they acquire more acceptable forms of communication (i.e., speech). Individuals with disabilities and more severe communication disabilities seem to exhibit more problem behaviors with increased severity than those with intact communication skills. Because many individuals with little or no functional speech may never develop functional speech to replace problem behavior, AAC can play a role in replacing problem behaviors with functionally equivalent, socially acceptable response alternatives.

COMMUNICATION-BASED APPROACHES

Despite the strong correlation between the degree of communication disability and the degree of problem behavior exhibited, only recently has the development of communication-based assessment and intervention procedures increased. In their meta-analysis of intervention studies addressing SIB published between 1976 and 1990, Schlosser and Goetze (1991, 1992) found that only .9% of the studies employed communication-based approaches despite the large number of subjects who reportedly had little or no functional speech. This has changed dramatically in recent years (Table 24.1). Prior to the widespread use of communication-based approaches, problem behaviors were largely addressed through other interventions, including differential reinforcement of other behavior, overcorrection, time-out, exercise, extinction, medication, restraint, and contingent electric shock (Durand, 1990; Schlosser & Goetze, 1992). These traditional approaches focused on reducing problem behavior without considering what types of skills needed to be taught to bring about the *permanent* replacement of problem behavior (Carr et al., 1994). Results from the meta-analysis of intervention studies addressing SIB support this notion in that only a small percentage of studies based their intervention on a functional assessment and reported maintenance data (Schlosser & Goetze, 1992).

This chapter uses the term *communication-based* approaches rather than *communication* approaches to problem behavior. Communication-based approaches consider communication issues in the assessment and intervention processes (Carr et al., 1994), but may also include other behavioral, or operant, strategies to address the problem behavior (e.g., extinction, tolerance for delay). Because this chapter focuses on communication-based approaches to problem behavior that involve AAC (see Lloyd & Blischak, 1992), the term **AAC-based approaches to problem behavior** is used. Communication-based approaches involve assessing the functions of the behaviors and subsequently replacing the problem behavior by teaching an alternative behavior that serves the same communicative function.

Functional Equivalence and Response Efficiency

The relationship of the alternative behavior to the problem behavior is known as **functional equiva-**lence (Carr, 1988). The interventionist attempts to ensure that obtaining reinforcers or other desirable consequences by the individual proves more successful through the use of appropriate communicative behaviors than through problem behavior (Carr et al., 1994; Donnellan, Mirenda, Mesaros, & Fassbender, 1984; Doss & Reichle, 1989; Durand, 1990; Durand & Berotti, 1991; Durand, Berotti, & Weiner, 1993; Johnston & Reichle, 1993). Whether the replacement behavior can address the function of problem behavior depends on the efficiency of the alternative response (Horner & Day, 1991). In other words, from the learner's perspective the replacement behavior must be as good a deal as the problem behavior. Three variables affect **response efficiency**: (1) the **physical effort** required to perform the response (the calories of energy expended), (2) the **schedule of reinforcement**, and (3) the **time delay** between presentation of the discriminative stimulus for a target response and delivery of the reinforcer for that response (Horner & Day, 1991; Horner, Sprague, O'Brien, & Heathfield, 1990):

> Head hitting and signing BREAK may both serve as responses that result in the removal of a difficult task. Signing BREAK may be more efficient if it requires less effort than head hitting, is followed by a break each time the response is emitted, and the learner gets the break immediately after requesting. On the other hand, head hitting may be more efficient if signing BREAK must be done several times to get the teacher's attention (or if signing is followed by significant delays) whereas head hitting gets immediate results. (Horner & Day, 1991, p. 720)

Communicative Functions

Four major areas of communicative function have been identified and addressed in communication-based approaches, including getting or maintaining social attention, getting or maintaining tangible consequences, escaping from demands, and obtaining sensory consequences or automatic reinforcement (Durand, 1990). Both social attention and tangible consequences contingent on problem behavior may positively reinforce problem behavior (Mace & Roberts, 1993).

TABLE 24.1 Studies of AAC-Based Interventions to Problem Behavior

AUTHOR(S) AND NUMBER OF SUBJECTS	NAME(S) AND BEHAVIOR(S)	FUNCTION(S)[1] ASSESSMENT	COMMUNICATION-BASED INTERVENTION	EXISTING COMMUNICATIVE REPERTOIRE (INCLUDING FUNCTIONS)	COMMUNICATION INTERFACE SELECTED[2] AND RATIONALE; MEANS TO REPRESENT, SELECT, TRANSMIT
Bird, Dores, Moniz, & Robinson (1989); N = 2	*Name:* Greg *Behavior:* SIB	*Function:* Escape from task deands *Assessment:* MAS[3]; direct observation	AAC, positive reinforcement, & demand fading or AAC & positive reinforcement (preferred reinforcers)	*Receptive:* Understands simple one-step directions *Expressive:* Says 15 one-word utterances (often not intelligible); initiates rarely	*Represent:* Aided. Not reported; the means to transmit may have served as a representation in and of itself ("break"); rationale not reported *Select:* Unaided. Direct select (handing over the token); rationale not reported *Transmit:* Aided. Plastic token; rationale not reported
	Name: Jim *Behaviors:* SIB; aggression	*Functions:* 1. Escape from task demands 2. Tangible consequences *Assessment:* MAS; direct observation	1. AAC & demand fading 2. AAC	*Receptive:* Understands simple two-step directions *Expressive:* Performs two signs (BATHROOM, FOOD), is seldom spontaneous; grabs; requests	*Represent:* Unaided. 1. sign (BREAK) 2. signs (MUSIC, FOOD, WORK, BATHROOM) Rationale not reported *Select:* Unaided *Transmit:* Unaided
Carr & Kemp (1989); N = 4	*Name:* Cal *Behavior:* Autistic leading	*Function:* tangible consequences *Assessment:* Not reported	AAC	*Receptive:* 14 mos. (Communication Evaluation Checklist) *Expressive:* Has little or no functional speech; 14 mos. (Communication Evaluation Checklist)	*Represent:* Unaided. Speech, gestures (pointing); rationale not reported *Select:* Unaided *Transmit:* Unaided
	Name: Mike *Behavior:* Autistic leading	*Function:* Tangible consequences *Assessment:* Not reported	AAC	*Receptive:* 13 mos. (Communication Evaluation Checklist) *Expressive:* Has little or no functional speech; 13 mos. (Communication Evaluation Checklist)	*Represent:* Unaided. Speech, gestures (pointing); rationale not reported *Select:* Unaided *Transmit:* Unaided
	Name: Jim *Behavior:* Autistic leading	*Function:* Tangible consequences *Assessment:* Not reported	AAC	*Receptive:* Not reported *Expressive:* Makes nonsensical vocalizations; imitates vocally; has little or no functional speech; functions not reported	*Represent:* Unaided. Speech, gestures (pointing); rationale not reported *Select:* Unaided *Transmit:* Unaided

Study	Name/Behavior	Function/Assessment	Intervention	Communication	Represent/Select/Transmit
Day, Rea, Schussler, Larsen, & Johnson (1988); N = 1	*Name:* Sue *Behavior:* Autistic leading	*Function:* Tangible consequences *Assessment:* Not reported	AAC	*Receptive:* Not reported *Expressive:* Makes spontaneous echoic approximations; has little or no functional speech; functions not reported	*Represent:* Unaided. Speech, gestures (pointing); rationale not reported *Select:* Unaided *Transmit:* Unaided
	Name: Mary *Behavior:* SIB	*Functions:* 1. Escape from task demands 2. Tangible consequences *Assessment:* Functional analyses	1. AAC (protest training) 2. AAC (request training)	*Receptive:* Not reported *Expressive:* Performs a few signs; makes one-word verbalizations; labels objects	*Represent:* Unaided. 1. Spoken "no" (protest) 2. Hand-clap, manual sign, spoken label for objects (request) Rationale not reported *Select:* Unaided *Transmit:* Unaided
Doss (1988); N = 3	*Name:* D.D. *Behavior:* Food stealing	*Function:* Tangible consequences *Assessment:* Not reported	AAC (request training), response interruption (extinction), differential reinforcement, & stimulus fading	*Receptive:* 2 yrs., 6 mos. (PPVT)[4]; functions not reported *Expressive:* 39 (TARC[5]-Subscore); has little or no functional speech; uses a communication wallet; requests assistance and objects with wallet; requests successfully, asks for permission only with difficulty	*Represent:* Aided. Graphic symbol (generalized "want"); rationale: Response recognizability (practicality of one generalized request for several tangibles) *Select:* Unaided. Direct select (pointing); rationale not reported *Transmit:* Aided. Communication wallet; rationale not reported
	Name: P.P. *Behavior:* Food stealing	*Function:* Tangible consequences *Assessment:* Not reported	AAC (request training), response interruption (extinction), differential reinforcement, & stimulus fading	*Receptive:* 2 yrs., 8 mos. (PPVT); functions not reported *Expressive:* 42 (TARC-Subscore); has little or no functional speech; performs a large number of idiosyncratic signs; requests objects and/or assistance via idiosyncratic signs; requests infrequently, does not distinguish situations requiring permission	*Represent:* Aided. Graphic symbol (generalized "want"); rationale: Response recognizability (practicality of one generalized request for several tangibles) *Select:* Unaided. Direct select (pointing); rationale not reported *Transmit:* Aided. Flashcard (initially); wallet (later); rationale not reported
	Name: L.K. *Behavior:* Food stealing	*Function:* Tangible consequences *Assessment:* Not reported	AAC (request training), response interruption (extinction), differential reinforcement, & stimulus fading	*Receptive:* 2 yrs., 3 mos. (PPVT); functions not reported *Expressive:* 30 (TARC-Subscore); vocalizes "no"; ASL sign TOILET; points to watch and tugs staff; protests via "no"; requests access (toilet), lunch break (pointing to watch), excursions (tugs staff); requests infrequently, distinguishes situations requiring permission	*Represent:* Unaided. ASL sign approximation (WANT); rationale: Response recognizability (practicality of one generalized request for several tangibles) *Select:* Unaided *Transmit:* Unaided

TABLE 24.1 (*Continued*)

AUTHOR(S) AND NUMBER OF SUBJECTS	NAME(S) AND BEHAVIOR(S)	FUNCTION(S) ASSESSMENT	COMMUNICATION-BASED INTERVENTION	EXISTING COMMUNICATIVE REPERTOIRE (INCLUDING FUNCTIONS)	COMMUNICATION INTERFACE SELECTED AND RATIONALE; MEANS TO REPRESENT, SELECT, TRANSMIT
Durand (1993); N = 3	*Name:* Michelle *Behavior:* Problem behavior (SIB, crying)	*Functions:* Escape from demands; social attention *Assessment:* MAS	AAC (both)	*Receptive:* Levels not reported; function: opposition to requests *Expressive:* Has no functional speech; uses head nods and pointing inconsistently; uses device unsuccessfully; functions not reported	*Represent:* Aided. Not reported *Select:* Aided. Direct select (head pointer); rationale: Difficulty using her hands to point *Transmit:* Aided. VOCA (Wolf™—synthetic speech); rationale: Response recognizability (not available with manual signs), cost, durability, intelligibility of speech output to others
	Name: Peter *Behavior:* SIB	*Function:* Escape from demands *Assessment:* MAS	AAC	*Receptive:* Not reported *Expressive:* Has no formal system; unsuccessful speech and sign training; has not used any device previously; functions not reported	*Represent:* Aided. Not reported ("I want to take a break"); rationale not reported *Select:* Unaided. Direct select (hand); rationale: Ability to select with hand *Transmit:* Aided. VOCA (Introtalker™—digitized speech); rationale: Response recognizability (not available with manual signs), cost, durability, intelligibility of speech output to others
	Name: Joshua *Behavior:* Problem behavior (aggression, crying)	*Function:* Tangible consequences *Assessment:* MAS	AAC	*Receptive:* Not reported *Expressive:* Has no formal system; has not used device previously; functions not reported	*Represent:* Aided. Not reported ("I want more"); rationale not reported *Select:* Unaided. Direct select (hand); rationale: Ability to select with hand *Transmit:* Aided. VOCA (Wolf—synthetic speech); rationale: Response recognizability (not available with manual signs), cost, durability, physical demands to operate, intelligibility of speech output to others

Study	Name/Behavior	Function/Assessment	Curriculum recommendations		
Durand & Kishi (1987); *N* = 5	*Name:* Tina *Behavior:* Aggression	*Function:* Escape from demands *Assessment:* MAS; CRMC[6]	Curriculum recommendations	*Receptive:* Vocabulary not reported; has no verbal or nonverbal imitation skills; functions not reported *Expressive:* Not reported	*Represent:* Aided. TO ("I want a break"); rationale: Unsuccessful in speech and signing, intelligibility (written message) *Select:* Unaided. Direct select (handing over a card); rationale not reported *Transmit:* Aided. Nonelectronic (flashcard); rationale: Teachability, facilitated intelligibility by allowing a written message
	Name: John *Behavior:* Aggression	*Function:* Escape from demands *Assessment:* MAS; CRMC	Curriculum recommendations	*Receptive:* Vocabulary not reported; has no verbal or nonverbal imitation skills; functions not reported *Expressive:* Not reported	*Represent:* Aided. TO ("I want a break"); rationale: Unsuccessful in speech and signing, intelligibility (written message) *Select:* Unaided. Direct select (handing over a card); rationale not reported *Transmit:* Aided. Nonelectronic (flashcard); rationale: Teachability, facilitated intelligibility via a written message
	Name: Lew *Behavior:* SIB	*Function:* Tangible consequences *Assessment:* MAS; CRMC	Curriculum recommendations	*Receptive:* Vocabulary not reported; has no verbal or nonverbal imitation skills; functions not reported *Expressive:* Not reported	*Represent:* Aided. Not reported; rationale: Unsuccessful in spoken language and manual signing, teachability, intelligibility (written message) *Select:* Unaided. Direct select (handing over a card); rationale not reported *Transmit:* Aided. Nonelectronic (flashcard); rationale: Teachability, facilitated intelligibility via a written message
	Name: Jim *Behavior:* SIB	*Function:* Tangible consequences *Assessment:* MAS; CRMC	Curriculum recommendations	*Receptive:* Vocabulary not reported; has no verbal or nonverbal imitation skills; functions not reported *Expressive:* Not reported	*Represent:* Unaided. Manual signs (message not reported); rationale: Unsuccessful in speech, teachability, intelligibility *Select:* Unaided *Transmit:* Unaided
	Name: Kim *Behavior:* Aggression	*Function:* Social attention *Assessment:* MAS; CRMC	Curriculum recommendations	*Receptive:* Vocabulary not reported; has no verbal or nonverbal imitation skills; functions not reported *Expressive:* Not reported	*Represent:* Unaided. Manual signs (message not reported); rationale: Unsuccessful in speech, teachability, intelligibility *Select:* Unaided *Transmit:* Unaided

TABLE 24.1 *(Continued)*

AUTHOR(S) AND NUMBER OF SUBJECTS	NAME(S) AND BEHAVIOR(S)	FUNCTION(S) ASSESSMENT	COMMUNICATION-BASED INTERVENTION	EXISTING COMMUNICATIVE REPERTOIRE (INCLUDING FUNCTIONS)	COMMUNICATION INTERFACE SELECTED AND RATIONALE; MEANS TO REPRESENT, SELECT, TRANSMIT
Dyer, Dunlap, & Winterling (1990); *N* = 2	*Name:* Mary *Behaviors:* Problem behavior; aggression	*Function:* Not identified *Assessment:* Informal preference of tasks and reinforcers	AAC, contingent exercise, & positive practice over-correction	*Receptive:* Not reported *Expressive:* Says 10 words; requests	*Represent:* Aided. Objects; rationale not reported *Select:* Unaided. Pointing; rationale not reported *Transmit:* Aided
	Name: Lori *Behavior:* Problem behavior	*Function:* Not identified *Assessment:* Informal preference of tasks and reinforcers	AAC & interruption	*Receptive:* Not reported *Expressive:* Has little or no functional speech; uses gestures, manual signs; functions not reported	*Represent:* Aided. Objects: rationale not reported *Select:* Unaided. Pointing; rationale not reported *Transmit:* Aided
Fisher et al. (1993); *N* = 4	*Name:* Bob *Behavior:* SIB	*Function:* Escape from task demands *Assessment:* Functional analysis	AAC and/or AAC & punishment	*Receptive:* Not reported *Expressive:* Reaches; requests preferred objects	*Represent:* Unaided. Not reported; rationale not reported *Select:* Unaided *Transmit:* Unaided
	Name: Jan *Behavior:* Destructive behavior	*Functions:* 1. Escape from task demands 2. Social attention 3. Tangible consequences *Assessment:* Functional analysis	For all three, AAC, AAC & extinction, and/or AAC & punishment	*Receptive:* Not reported *Expressive:* Reaches; request preferred objects	*Represent:* Unaided. Sign (MORE); sign (FINISHED); clapping (to get attention) and signing (GO) (to change environments); rationale not reported *Select:* Unaided *Transmit:* Unaided
	Name: Art *Behaviors:* SIB; aggression; disruption	*Function:* Escape from task demands *Assessment:* Functional analysis	AAC & extinction, AAC & punishment, and/or demand fading	*Receptive:* Not reported *Expressive:* Has no functional speech; has no gestures, signs, or words; functions not reported	*Represent:* Unaided. Sign (GO); rationale not reported *Select:* Unaided *Transmit:* Unaided
	Name: Abe *Behavior:* SIB	*Function:* Tangible consequences *Assessment:* Functional analysis	AAC, AAC & extinction, AAC & punishment, and/or helmet fading	*Receptive:* Not reported *Expressive:* Has no functional speech; has no gestures, signs, or words; functions not reported	*Represent:* Unaided. Sign (MORE); rationale not reported *Select:* Unaided *Transmit:* Unaided

Study	Name/Behavior	Function/Assessment	Intervention	Receptive/Expressive	Represent/Select/Transmit
Horner & Budd (1985); N = 1	*Name:* Not given. *Behavior:* Grabbing or yelling	*Function:* Not reported. *Assessment:* Observation of antecedents & consequences	AAC (request training)	*Receptive:* Has good receptive skills; functions not reported. *Expressive:* Does not use conventional signs; has not been exposed to manual sign training; functions not reported	*Represent:* Unaided. ASL signs (JUICE, TIMER, CHOOSE, BOTTLE, FOLDER); rationale: Functional means to communicate, teachability. *Select:* Unaided. *Transmit:* Unaided
Horner & Day (1991); N = 3	*Name:* Paul. *Behavior:* Aggression	*Function:* Escape from demands (difficult tasks). *Assessment:* Structured interviews; functional analyses	AAC	*Receptive:* Understands simple language; understands requests. *Expressive:* Uses 20 manual signs; requests objects	*Represent:* Unaided. ASL sign (I WANT TO GO PLEASE); ASL sign (BREAK); rationale not provided. *Select:* Unaided. Sentence signing (I WANT TO GO PLEASE); key word signing (BREAK); rationale: Response efficiency (i.e., physical effort) examination. *Transmit:* Unaided
	Name: Peter. *Behavior:* SIB	*Function:* Tangible consequences (access to assistance). *Assessment:* Structured interviews; functional analyses	AAC & interruption/blocking	*Receptive:* Understands simple language; understands requests. *Expressive:* Uses gestures; functions not reported	*Represent:* Unaided. ASL sign (HELP); rationale not provided. *Select:* Unaided. *Transmit:* Unaided
	Name: Mary. *Behaviors:* SIB; aggression	*Function:* Escape from demands (difficult tasks). *Assessment:* Functional analyses	AAC & interruption	*Receptive:* Understands simple language; understands requests. *Expressive:* Says single words; functions not reported	*Represent:* Aided. TO ("break"). *Select:* Unaided. Direct select (handing over a card). *Transmit:* Aided. Nonelectronic (flashcard)
Horner, Sprague, O'Brien, & Heathfield (1990); N = 1	*Name:* David. *Behavior:* Aggression	*Function:* Escape from tasks. *Assessment:* Structured interview; functional analyses	AAC	*Receptive:* Not reported. *Expressive:* Has little or no functional speech; not reported whether the VOCA has been used; functions not reported	*Represent:* Aided. TO ("Help please"); color (red) ("Help please"); rationale: Difficult to sign due to motor limitations, response efficiency examination. *Select:* Unaided. Direct select; spelling complete message; prestored message retrieval; rationale: Response efficiency (i.e., physical effort) examination. *Transmit:* Aided. VOCA (Canon Communicator™—synthetic speech & print output); rationale: Spelling capacity, single key retrieval of prestored messages

TABLE 24.1 *(Continued)*

AUTHOR(S) AND NUMBER OF SUBJECTS	NAME(S) AND BEHAVIOR(S)	FUNCTION(S) ASSESSMENT	COMMUNICATION-BASED INTERVENTION	EXISTING COMMUNICATIVE REPERTOIRE (INCLUDING FUNCTIONS)	COMMUNICATION INTERFACE SELECTED AND RATIONALE; MEANS TO REPRESENT, SELECT, TRANSMIT
Hunt, Atwell, & Goetz (1988); N = 3	*Name:* Paula *Behaviors:* Disruptive behavior; unconventional verbal behavior	*Function:* Social attention *Assessment:* Observation of antecedents & consequences	AAC & extinction	*Receptive:* Understands up to two or more word combinations; uses gestures and context clues in response to complex speech; 2 yrs. to 2 yrs., 6 mos. (TACL[7]); functions not reported *Expressive:* Deletes pronouns and morphological detail; displays stereotypical speech; lacks verbal fluency; functions not reported	*Represent:* Aided. Graphic symbols; rationale: Recognizability *Select:* Unaided. Direct select; rationale not reported *Transmit:* Aided. Communication book; rationale: Recognition memory (cues and comments for appropriate answer)
	Name: Peter *Behaviors:* Aggression; disruptive behavior; unconventional verbal behavior	*Function:* Social attention *Assessment:* Observation of antecedents & consequences	AAC & extinction	*Receptive:* Exceeds production greatly; 3 yrs. (TACL); functions not reported *Expressive:* Displays echolalic speech; has poor intelligibility; uses spontaneous speech rarely; functions not reported	*Represent:* Aided. Graphic symbols; rationale: Recognizability *Select:* Unaided. Direct select; rationale not reported *Transmit:* Aided. Communication book; rationale: Recognition memory (cues and comments for appropriate answer)
	Name: Mary *Behavior:* Disruptive behavior	*Function:* Social attention *Assessment:* Observation of antecedents & consequences	AAC & extinction	*Receptive:* 3 yrs. (TACL); understands only stereotyped phrases and labels for concrete referents *Expressive:* Not reported	*Represent:* Aided. Graphic symbols; rationale: Recognizability *Select:* Unaided. Direct select; rationale not reported *Transmit:* Aided. Communication book; rationale: Recognition memory (cues and comments for appropriate answer)
Northup et al. (1991); N = 2	*Name:* Curtis *Behavior:* Aggression	*Function:* Escape from task demands *Assessment:* (Brief) functional analysis	AAC & guided compliance (extinction)	*Receptive:* Not reported *Expressive:* Has no formal communication system; functions not reported	*Represent:* Unaided. Sign (PLEASE as generalized request to escape); rationale: Practicality of generic sign in initial training *Select:* Unaided *Transmit:* Unaided

Study	Name/Behavior	Functions/Assessment	Intervention	Communication	Representation model
	Name: Heidi *Behavior:* Aggression	*Functions:* 1. Escape from task demands 2. Tangible consequences *Assessment:* (Brief) functional analysis	For both, AAC & guided compliance (extinction)	*Receptive:* Not reported *Expressive:* Has no formal communication; functions not reported	*Represent:* Unaided. Sign (PLEASE as generalized request for tangibles); rationale: Practicality of generic sign in initial training *Select:* Unaided *Transmit:* Unaided
Schlosser & Karlan (1994); *N* = 1	*Name:* Sam *Behaviors:* SIB; aggression; maladaptive behavior	*Functions:* 1. Tangible consequences 2. Social attention *Assessment:* Qualitative interview; document analysis	1. AAC 2. AAC & choice-making	*Receptive:* Understands multiword instructions; functions not reported *Expressive:* Has few word approximations; uses 15 manual signs, gestures (pointing), leading; functions not reported	*Represent:* Unaided. Sign (WANT as generalized request) plus pointing, signing, vocalizing, or leading; rationale: Multimodality, recognizability, existing repertoire *Select:* Unaided (specific request: want plus item) *Transmit:* Unaided
Steege et al. (1990); *N* = 1	*Name:* Ron *Behavior:* SIB	*Function:* Escape from task demands *Assessment:* Functional analysis	AAC & guided compliance (extinction)	*Receptive:* Not reported *Expressive:* Has no independent communication skills; ability to activate switch not reported; functions not reported	*Represent:* Aided. Not reported *Select:* Aided. Direct select (activation of a switch); rationale not reported *Transmit:* Aided. Battery-operated tape recorder ("Stop"); rationale: Potential for assertiveness
Wacker et al. (1990); *N* = 3	*Name:* Jim *Behavior:* Aggression	*Function:* Escape from demands *Assessment:* Functional analysis	AAC & guided compliance, AAC, or guided compliance	*Receptive:* Not reported *Expressive:* Signs PLEASE and EAT; requests objects	*Represent:* Unaided. Manual sign (PLEASE as generalized request to escape; EAT to escape); rationale: Existing training repertoire *Select:* Unaided. Rationale: Existing training repertoire *Transmit:* Unaided. Rationale: Existing training repertoire
	Name: Bobby *Behavior:* SIB	*Function:* Tangible consequences *Assessment:* Functional analysis	AAC & guided compliance, AAC, or guided compliance	*Receptive:* Not reported *Expressive:* Has 1 sign approximation; requests	*Represent:* Unaided. Sign approximation (generalized WANT); rationale: Existing repertoire, teachability (resisted hand-over-hand guidance to teach other signs) *Select:* Unaided. Rationale: Motoric ability *Transmit:* Unaided. Rationale: Motoric ability

TABLE 24.1 *(Continued)*

AUTHOR(S) AND NUMBER OF SUBJECTS	NAME(S) AND BEHAVIOR(S)	FUNCTION(S) ASSESSMENT	COMMUNICATION-BASED INTERVENTION	EXISTING COMMUNICATIVE REPERTOIRE (INCLUDING FUNCTIONS)	COMMUNICATION INTERFACE SELECTED AND RATIONALE; MEANS TO REPRESENT, SELECT, TRANSMIT
Wacker et al. (cont.)	*Name:* Barb *Behavior:* Stereotopy	*Function:* Sensory reinforcement *Assessment:* Functional analysis	AAC & guided compliance, AAC, or guided compliance	*Receptive:* Not reported *Expressive:* Has no signs or gestures; accesses toys via switch (cause-effect); functions not reported	*Represent:* Aided. Not reported ("I am tired of rocking, somebody give me something to do?"); rationale: No success with sign training *Select:* Aided. Direct selection via switch; rationale: Existing motoric repertoire *Transmit:* Aided. Tape loop; rationale: Potential for assertiveness

[1]The functions were cross-referenced to the communication-based interventions. For example, subject Jim's (Bird et al., 1989) problem behavior was motivated by (1) escape from task demands, and (2) tangible consequences. AAC and demand fading addressed the first function (1), whereas AAC intervention addressed the second function (2).

[2]Only the communicator interface selected to be taught was included; communicative responses that were only monitored were not included.

[3]Motivation Assessment Scale

[4]Peabody Picture Vocabulary Test

[5]Topeka Association for Retarded Citizens

[6]Communicative Response Modality Checklist

[7]Test of Auditory Comprehension of Language

Social Attention.   Some problem behavior may be positively reinforced by social attention, suggesting that the problem behavior may be used to elicit, or to request, attention (Carr & Durand, 1985a). For example, a student may engage in **social-attention-motivated problem behavior** whenever the teacher directs attention away from the student to engage in another activity (e.g., writing on the blackboard) or whenever the teacher divides attention between a student and another individual (e.g., peer) (Lalli & Goh, 1993). If the teacher redirects attention back to the student, the problem behavior is reinforced and is likely to occur more frequently.

Tangible Consequences.   Tangible consequences (e.g., food, toys, activities) may also serve as positive reinforcement for problem behavior (e.g., Doss & Reichle, 1989). Individuals may engage in **tangible-consequences-motivated problem behavior** when (1) they are denied access to a preferred or requested item or activity, (2) an item that they had inappropriately manipulated or obtained is removed, or (3) delays occur between the requested and the actual presentation of the requested item (Lalli & Goh, 1993). For example, a resident in a group home liked to put on layers of clothing that belonged to other residents. When this was discovered by staff and he was asked to return the clothing items, he would engage in an episode of SIB. Frequently, staff did not follow through, and the resident was allowed to keep the clothing.

Escape.   Some problem behavior may also be maintained by **negative reinforcement** in that individuals have learned to terminate or postpone demands and caregiver expectations for performance by engaging in problem behaviors (Carr & Durand, 1985b; Mace & Roberts, 1993). Thus, **escape-motivated problem behavior** serves as a request to terminate, postpone, or withdraw from ongoing activity or interaction. For example, to terminate a personal-care activity prematurely, a child may engage in aggressive behavior (Lalli & Goh, 1993). When the caregiver reduces expectations for the child to perform the personal-care activity, the child may have learned that by engaging

in problem behavior the caregiver would stop making demands. In other words, the child was negatively reinforced for engaging in problem behavior by the caregiver's withdrawal of aversive demands.

Sensory Consequences/Automatic Reinforcement. In addition to these socially mediated functions, **sensory-consequences-motivated problem behavior/automatic-reinforcement-motivated problem behavior** may be maintained by sensory consequences (e.g., auditory, visual, tactile) provided automatically by engaging in problem behavior (e.g., Rincover & Devany, 1982). For example, a student may obtain such external stimulation as auditory feedback from banging objects against a hard surface or visual feedback from a spinning object (Rincover & Devany, 1982). A student engaging in stereotypic body rocking may be reinforced by such internal stimulation as kinesthetic feedback from the trunk and/or vestibular feedback from the inner ear (Lovaas, Newsom, & Hickman, 1987).

When Communicative Functions Cannot Be Honored.   In communication-based approaches, appropriate communicative responses that serve the same function as the problem behavior are taught. For example, an individual may be taught to request objects by pointing rather than engaging in problem behavior (i.e., tangible consequences). An individual whose problem behavior is escape motivated may be taught to request a break or to request assistance by using manual signs. However, in some situations the functions that problem behaviors serve cannot always be honored (Fisher et al., 1993). For instance, caregivers may not always be able to provide attention or access to preferred objects every time the individual communicates appropriately. Staff in a group home cannot always provide a van ride whenever one of the residents requests one. Also, in community settings, it may be inappropriate for an individual to escape nonpreferred activities (e.g., brushing teeth, taking medicine) through communication because of missed learning opportunities (e.g., learning to brush teeth) or harmful consequences (e.g., more seizures) (Fisher et al., 1993).

In these situations intervention strategies can be used in conjunction with teaching communicative alternatives. Teaching tolerance for delay is one such strategy that may be accomplished through demand fading and reinforcement fading (Bird, Dores, Moniz, & Robinson, 1989; Fisher et al., 1993). In demand fading, the individual is required to complete one or few task steps before the communication will function to allow escape. For instance, an individual in a vocational program may be required to sort a predetermined number of items before signing FINISHED results in an escape from the task. Then the number of requested things to sort before escaping through signing FINISHED would be gradually increased. A recent application of demand fading was presented in a study of three children with developmental disabilities (Lalli, Casey, & Kates, 1995). Procedures included requests to the subjects to perform task steps, a stated criterion for earning a break, and pointing to the instructional materials related to the specified criterion. Contingent on the performance of the appropriate communicative behavior (i.e., saying "no" to escape), the therapist said "Good saying 'no,' but you have to do (task step). Then you can ask for a break." With reinforcement fading, the individual may be required to wait a few seconds after emitting the appropriate communicative response (e.g., signing FINISHED) associated with the positive reinforcer (escape). The length of delay would then be gradually increased.

FUNCTIONAL ASSESSMENT

To design and implement communication-based interventions, **functional assessment** techniques are required; these are the full range of strategies used to develop and test hypotheses regarding antecedents and consequences that control problem behavior. Functional assessment is considered an ongoing process in designing initial intervention and in keeping pace with continuing changes in behavior during intervention (see Horner, 1994). Available techniques are reviewed only briefly here along with examples of their applications. For more comprehensive reviews of these techniques, see Iwata, Vollmer, and Zarcone, 1990; Lennox

and Miltenberger, 1989; Mace, Lalli, and Shea, 1992; O'Neill, Horner, Albin, Storey, and Sprague, 1990; Schlosser, 1993b.

Hypotheses Development

Hypotheses development focuses on identifying the possible functional relations between a problem behavior and naturally occurring environmental events. Hypotheses may be developed through indirect methods or through direct, descriptive methods.

Indirect Methods. **Indirect methods** include rating scales (Durand & Crimmins, 1992), structured interviews (Bailey & Pyles, 1989; O'Neill et al., 1990; Schuler, Peck, Willard, & Theimer, 1989), and qualitative interviews (Schlosser, 1993; Schlosser & Karlan, 1994). These indirect methods are typically completed by or with partners who are familiar with the individual.

Motivation Assessment Scale. The Motivation Assessment Scale (MAS) is a rating scale widely used to develop initial hypotheses regarding the functions of problem behavior (Durand & Crimmins, 1992). Three of the AAC-based intervention studies of problem behavior summarized in Table 24.1 employed the MAS. The MAS is a 16-item survey with four questions within each of four groups of motivational factors (stimulus events): sensory feedback, escape, social attention, and tangibles. One MAS per target behavior per setting is administered to a number of individuals who are familiar with the individual being assessed. Each question in the MAS is scored on a scale from 0 (never) to 6 (always) and totals are derived for each of the four motivational factors. Higher scores for a particular factor establish the hypothesis that the problem behavior may be maintained by this motivational factor. The MAS has undergone psychometric validation; for critical reviews, however, see Bihm, Kienlen, Ness, and Poindexter, 1991; Crawford, Brockel, Schauss, and Miltenberger, 1992; Durand and Crimmins, 1988; Kearney, 1994; Newton and Sturmey, 1991; Singh et al., 1993; and Zarcone, Rodgers, Iwata, Rourke, and Dorsey, 1991. Overall, researchers agree that although the MAS is useful in generating initial hypotheses, it should be used only in conjunction with other assessment methods (Durand & Crimmins, 1992; Kearney, 1994).

Communicative Response Modality Checklist. Although the MAS is not designed to provide information regarding AAC variables that may be important for designing communication-based interventions, Durand (1990) suggests that using the Communicative Response Modality Checklist (CRMC) to guide the decision-making process might help to establish potential modalities for AAC-based intervention. The conclusions from the CRMC, which are based on staff responses, are used for designing interventions, which are based on the following assumptions: First, in order for intervention to be successful, it should build upon the existing communicative repertoire. For instance, if a student uses unaided means to represent in order to communicate on a regular or occasional basis, then, unaided means should be considered as a response modality. Second, intervention should build on existing successes and emphases from the individual's speech-language therapy; that is, if unaided means to represent have been used successfully, such means should be considered as a response modality. However, if the individual has been found, in therapy, to be unsuccessful with unaided means to represent, then aided means to represent should be used.

Functional Analysis Interview. The Functional Analysis Interview (FAI) (O'Neill et al., 1990) is one of the available structured interviews. The FAI was used in two of the studies summarized in Table 24.1. The FAI includes sections describing the problem behavior, the potential ecological events affecting it, the events and situations that predict its occurrences, its functions, its efficiency, the primary ways of communicating, the events (actions and objects) perceived as positive, the functional alternative behaviors known by the person, and a history of the behavior and previous intervention attempts. Noteworthy from a communication perspective are the sections on the primary ways of communicating and the functional alternative behaviors known by the person. Included are questions regarding existing expressive communication strategies and their consis-

tency, receptive communication (following verbal directions and gestural/signed instructions, making yes/no responses, and imitating models), and the behaviors used to express various communicative functions.

Communication Interview. The Communication Interview (CI) (Schuler et al., 1989) is another structured interview. None of the studies summarized in Table 24.1 has employed the CI, which requires the person interviewed to indicate, for each communicative function item, the communicative behavior(s) most frequently used to express it. Communicative function items include requests for affection/interaction, requests for adult action, requests for tangibles (food, objects, or things), protests, and declarations/comments. For each of these functions, the form provides several contexts that may apply to that function. For example, the section "request for affection" includes an item asking how the individual requests an adult to sit nearby. The communicative behaviors include both problem and appropriate behaviors.

Qualitative Interviews. Qualitative interviews were used in only one of the summarized studies (Schlosser & Karlan, 1994). Like structured interviews, qualitative interviews are employed with partners who are familiar with the individual. Unlike structured interviews, qualitative interviews use open-ended, guiding questions. Data from various sources are used to strengthen the credibility of the findings. Schlosser and Karlan (1994) used interview transcripts and group home documents. Both were analyzed using constant comparative analysis (Glaser & Strauss, 1967) to derive common themes or categories. The categories derived related to stimulus events (e.g., escape, tangible consequences), the existing communicative repertoire, the signing competence among direct care staff, and interaction patterns with the individual. Although qualitative interviews are believed to have several advantages over structured interviews, they are very time consuming (Schlosser, 1993b).

Direct Methods. Hypotheses developed from indirect methods may be further refined through **direct methods**. Direct methods have seldom been employed in communication-based research (see

Table 24.1). Direct methods include techniques such as scatterplot analyses (Touchette, MacDonald, & Langer, 1985), antecedent-behavior-consequence (ABC) charts, and other direct observations (Bijou, Peterson, & Ault, 1968). The purpose of direct observation is to identify the natural covariation between the problem behavior and environmental events occurring prior and subsequent to it. For a recent review of direct methods, see Lalli and Goh (1993).

Hypotheses Testing

The hypotheses developed from indirect and/or direct methods need to be tested through a functional analysis (Iwata, Dorsey, Slifer, Bauman, & Richman, 1982). **Functional analysis** involves the experimental manipulation of environmental aspects that represent the hypothesized functions of the problem behavior. For example, if direct observation suggests that an individual engages in problem behavior to escape difficult tasks, situations will be created that manipulate the difficulty of the tasks presented to the individual while assessing its effect on problem behavior. Functional analysis might be required to clarify the relationship between two differing events when indirect methods cannot. For example, if interviews indicate that the problem behavior might be functionally related to both keeping adult attention (social attention) and task demand (escape), then one might, in one manipulation, provide constant attention while changing between high-demand and low-demand activities. Then, in another manipulation, one might change from high adult attention to low adult attention during a low-demand activity.

DEVELOPING INTERVENTIONS: REPRESENTING, SELECTING, AND TRANSMITTING FUNCTIONALLY EQUIVALENT RESPONSES

The development of AAC-based interventions involves several sets of considerations beginning with the outcomes of the functional assessment (e.g., Doss & Reichle, 1991a; Durand, 1990; Mace & Roberts, 1993; Repp, Felce, & Barton, 1988). The central consideration is selecting a response

that is functionally equivalent but more efficient than the problem behavior. For individuals with little or no functional speech, AAC is the key to functional equivalence and response efficiency. In selecting equivalent and efficient responses, interventionists must make important decisions regarding the **means to represent, means to select,** and **means to transmit** (Lloyd, Quist, & Windsor, 1990). Any response conveyed through AAC consists of these three components of the AAC transmission processes and interface.

Several authors have addressed considerations in selecting communicative responses as alternatives to problem behaviors (e.g., Carr et al., 1994; Durand, 1990; Durand et al., 1993; Horner & Day, 1991; Horner et al., 1990). For instance, response recognizability (Durand et al., 1993, p. 329) and interpretability (Carr et al., 1994, p. 133) have been suggested as important considerations in selecting communicative responses. Durand et al. (1993) state that "if the trained response is not easily recognizable by significant others in the environment, then these other people will not respond and challenging behavior will not be reduced" (p. 329). Although response recognizability relates to the intelligibility of the response in its entirety and includes the means to represent, select, and transmit, these and other authors have not necessarily approached this issue from an AAC perspective per se. Their recommendations, therefore, do not always address the three components of the AAC transmission processes and interface. Thus, the considerations from the literature on communication-based intervention to problem behaviors must be supplemented with those reported in the AAC literature and integrated conceptually with the means to represent, the means to select, and the means to transmit.

Means to Represent

An initial consideration in designing an AAC-based intervention involves deciding between aided (e.g., graphic symbols) and unaided (e.g., manual signs) means to represent. Subsequent considerations involve selecting among (1) unaided means, (2) aided means, and (3) multimodal means to represent.

Natural Speech. Generally, the intervention team has the option of choosing between aided (e.g., graphic symbols) and unaided (e.g., gestures, manual signs, natural speech) means to represent the message inherent in the functionally equivalent response. Certainly, natural speech is the preferable and most acceptable means to represent ideas. However, poor intelligibility often does not permit the reliance on residual speech in individuals with severe communication disabilities. Intelligibility refers to the recognizability of all means to represent, but most often refers to the *speech* symbol, that is, either the natural speech symbol or the synthesized or digitized speech symbol (Beukelman & Mirenda, 1992). Thus, the selection of an intelligible means to represent may be crucial if problem behavior is to be replaced (Carr et al., 1994).

With individuals who have little or no functional speech, natural speech may be a poor choice as the *only* means to represent, because the lack of intelligibility may hinder partners from recognizing the response, and hence, hinder the success of the intervention. For instance, Durand and Carr (1991) observed that after the initial success of intervention involving vocalizations, a boy had resumed SIB. Their analysis determined that the teacher failed to respond to his requests for assistance because she could not understand what he was saying. The boy resumed hitting himself because the teacher did not provide assistance when he asked for it. Carr et al. (1994) described a similar situation involving Juan, who was taught to request breaks from exercise routines via natural speech ("Take a break"). Functional assessments had determined that he used aggressive behavior to end the exercise. Although he was unable to say the request in its entirety, he managed to say "Takee." This request resulted in decreased aggressive behavior, but there was only one staff member who regularly understood and accepted this approximation and consistently delivered the requested break. Whenever other staff were on duty, Juan's requests were either ignored or misunderstood. Although articulation training may lead to intelligible vocalizations and replacement of problem behavior with some individuals (for an example, see Durand & Carr, 1991), frequently the problem behavior is dangerous and warrants faster solu-

tions than extensive articulation training can provide. Thus, other means to represent, such as graphic symbols (aided) or manual signs (unaided), need to be given careful consideration as replacements for or supplements to the individual's residual natural speech.

Unaided vs. Aided Symbols.

Intelligibility. As with natural speech, the intelligibility (iconicity) of symbols is important to the effectiveness of communication. The majority of AAC-based intervention studies of problem behavior selected unaided rather than aided symbols (see Table 24.1). Unaided means such as manual signs, however, may not be sufficiently intelligible to allow many communication partners to understand and make appropriate responses (Durand, 1993; Durand et al., 1993). Unlike graphic symbols, whereby communication partners can rely on a gloss to determine what the AAC user is communicating, manual signs are usually not accompanied by a gloss; thus, manual signs must be highly guessable. Durand (1993) opted against the use of manual signs for three individuals because of this lack of recognizability of manual signs. The guessability of manual signs in general may be further diminished when they become idiosyncratic (Durand, 1993; Fay & Schuler, 1980). Fay and Schuler (1980) noted that the prevalence of inappropriate hand movements among students with autism may further impair comprehension of their manually signed responses. One adult with moderate cognitive impairment engaged in aggressive behavior and had a large expressive repertoire of signs and sign phrases from Signing Exact English (SEE-II) (Gustason, 1990). However, according to staff reports, none of the direct care staff could recognize his signs because he had developed such idiosyncratic signs that only his father, who had taught him these signs initially, was able to recognize their meanings. Manual signs that may have been initially guessable by partners may become less so over time or in other instances if the AAC user produces the signs inconsistently (e.g., due to changes in motoric abilities). Graphic symbols, on the other hand, are consistent because they are selected rather than formed (Lloyd & Kangas,

1994). Finally, the guessability of manual signs may be further diminished due to the lack of sign training among communication partners. Research indicates that the receptive signing competence among immediate teaching and care personnel is often insufficient (Bryen & McGinley, 1991).

Communicative Effectiveness. During interactions, the lack of guessability of manual signs impedes communicative effectiveness. If the trained means to represent are not easily recognizable by communication partners, then these partners will not respond and the problem behaviors will not be replaced (Durand et al., 1993). Although there is a lack of research comparing the effects of manual signs versus graphic symbols in communication-based approaches to problem behavior, one can extrapolate communicative effectiveness in terms of request behavior. Rotholz, Berkowitz, and Burberry (1989) assessed the effect of using manual signs versus graphic symbols transmitted via a communication book on the percentage of successful requests when ordering meals at fast-food restaurants with two individuals with severe disabilities. Successful requests were defined as the receipt of a requested food item. Both individuals used manual signs as their primary means of communication prior to the onset of intervention; John's signing and Sam's signing were 75% and 54% intelligible to their teachers due to interfering hand movements and poor production. The use of a communication book with graphic symbols for food-related vocabulary was trained prior to the onset of community-based probes in fast-food restaurants. Results indicate that the communication book did yield more successful requests than manual signing. Although manual communication was not effective prior to the intervention due to the lack of intelligibility to even familiar partners, the counter persons probably would not have recognized more signs if the sign production had been better, because they were not trained to understand manual signs at all. These findings indicate that selecting graphic symbols transmitted via a communication book would be more effective than manual signing in community settings that involve partners who are generally not trained in manual communication.

Learnability. Learnability of the means to represent is another important consideration. Whether manual signs are easier to learn than graphic symbols depends on the background of the person exhibiting problem behavior. With individuals who exhibit severe problem behaviors, intervention teams should spend as little time as possible teaching new communicative forms as replacements for the problem behavior. Whether the existing communicative repertoire consists of manual signs or graphic symbols, for individuals with escape-motivated behavior, selecting a means to represent that already exists in the communicative repertoire and/or is easy to learn is particularly important. Introducing means to represent that may be difficult to learn may place an additional demand on a person who resorts to problem behaviors to escape demands in the first place. Thus, the means chosen to represent should, if possible, build on the existing communicative repertoire of an individual.

Existing Communicative Repertoire. The **existing communicative repertoire** involves those receptive skills (understanding of vocabulary and functions) and those expressive skills (production of symbols and functions) that the individual has already learned. Certainly, if the individual already has a repertoire of graphic symbols, the intervention team should build on it. However, many individuals with developmental disabilities who have spent time in residential facilities, including group homes, already have a manual sign repertoire prior to the onset of communication-based intervention. Although, as argued above, graphic (aided) symbols might be preferable to manual signs, if the intervention is to build as much as possible on an existing repertoire, then aided symbols might be considered as a duplicate mode or as part of a multiple mode. Several communication-based studies have built on existing gesture or sign repertoires (e.g., Schlosser & Karlan, 1994; Wacker et al., 1990). Sometimes the intervention team might wish to build on an existing sign repertoire but also teach graphic symbols because of the shortcomings of using manual signs in the individual's particular environment. In such a situation, the intervention team might use the graphic representations of the manual signs as found in the instructional book

Signing Exact English (Gustason, 1990). These representations permit an individual to build on an existing sign repertoire because the representations show both the movement and handshapes of the signs while providing the gloss to help direct care staff understand messages. Dictionaries of various manual sign systems or graphic symbols that represent the individual's existing sign repertoire are other sources to consider (Bornstein, Saulnier, & Hamilton, 1983; Cregan & Lloyd, 1990).

With individuals who have an existing manual sign repertoire but who also have motoric difficulties, new manual signs may be difficult, if not impossible, to learn and, therefore, would be less preferable than graphic symbols. Individuals with autism, for example, frequently lack the dexterity to produce signs (Fay & Schuler, 1980). Because of such motor limitations, Horner et al. (1990) opted against manual signs for their subject and chose to use traditional orthography (TO) and color as means to represent. Even with individuals who have motor skills intact and for whom graphic symbols and manual signs are viable options, graphic symbols are believed to be easier to remember than manual signs (see Lloyd & Kangas, 1994; Reichle, 1991).

Projectability.   **Projectability** of the means to represent is one of the more critical variables. Gestures and manual signs project better than graphic symbols if the latter are transmitted through a non-electronic communication device (e.g., communication board). For example, if an individual engages in problem behaviors to escape demands, gestures and manual signs (e.g., STOP) project better because they can be seen from across the room (Doss & Reichle, 1991a). However, if graphic symbols are converted to acoustic symbols through voice output communication aids (VOCAs), their projectability relative to manual signs is altered, and perhaps equalized.

Required Specificity.   A selection consideration that applies to both aided and unaided symbols is the **required specificity of the means to represent** (e.g., a symbol representing "pants" versus one representing "jeans"). As a guiding principle, regardless of means to represent, symbols should be sufficiently generic to allow the user to communicate in a large range of contexts while being sufficiently specific to minimize the communicative burden on the partner (O'Neill & Reichle, 1993). For example, a symbol for "coffee" may be sufficiently specific regardless of the context, but using the symbol "soda" (versus "Coke") in a fast-food restaurant would not be sufficiently specific and would place considerable burden on the counter person. In the fast-food restaurant, appropriate communication (e.g., a request) may not be successful (e.g., no receipt of requested item). Also, different means to represent may have different potentials to represent specificity. Unaided symbols may not be able to represent a particular type of pants (e.g., jeans, the subordinate category item) because the subordinate sign does not exist. Such specificity may also be problematic with graphic symbol sets. For instance, most iconic symbol sets (e.g., Picture Communication Symbols [PCS]) do not provide representations at the subordinate level of specificity (jeans), and if they are at all available, they are difficult to distinguish from the next higher level (e.g., pants, the basic level concept) (Schlosser, 1993a, 1997a, 1997b). Therefore, most communication-based studies have used generic means to represent (see Table 24.1). If specificity is required, O'Neill and Reichle (1993) suggest using a product logo (e.g., Coke™). Alternatively, symbols may be selected from a system that permits sufficient specificity, such as Blissymbols (Schlosser, 1993a, 1997a, 1997b; Schlosser & Lloyd, in press). Selecting the means to represent with the required degree of specificity may be guided by its implications for opportunities to teach an initial communicative repertoire. O'Neill and Reichle (1993) provide an excellent table describing the advantages and disadvantages of general versus specific vocabulary. Specific symbols may serve the learner best in community settings and may lessen the burden placed on the partner. In some conditions, however, they recommend the use of a more general symbol for individuals who require a large number of teaching opportunities to establish discrimination because of the potential for satiation and reinforcer shifts.

For example, consider an individual who likes a particular diet soda but after several sips desires no more. For this individual, there may be a small window of opportunity for the interventionist to implement meaningful instructional opportunities. In other instances, a shift in reinforcer preferences may render a previously explicit symbol relatively useless. A learner who found a particular brand of soda to be a preferred beverage may sample a new soft drink. Having done so, the learner establishes a preference for the new beverage over the formerly preferred brand. (p. 211)

For these reasons general symbols such as generic "want" or "please" undoubtedly seem essential during initial intervention for many individuals. However, the long-term outcomes are unknown and warrant careful consideration of the implications for an overall communication program (Northup et al., 1991; Sigafoos, Doss, & Reichle, 1989). Studies are needed to document how participants in communication-based studies move from the initial intervention toward a more complete communication program. For example, how will participants of communication-based studies expand their communicative repertoire from using a generic "want" to making specific requests that minimize the communicative burden placed on unfamiliar partners? How will these participants expand their communicative repertoire to other communicative functions not served by the problem behavior? In absence of such reports, long-term considerations may not be as important as immediate considerations with individuals who exhibit problem behavior.

Long-Term Considerations. Nonetheless, long-term considerations should not be entirely ignored in communication-based interventions. Long-term considerations for selecting among means to represent involve both their expansion capability and their effectiveness with potential partners. Graphic symbol systems, unlike symbol sets, have rules for expansion and allow the expression of virtually any thought. Manual signs also provide rules for expansion if they are taken from a system such as American Sign Language (ASL) (see Fuller et al., 1994; Chapters 5, 6, 7, and 13). Gestures do not have such rules for expansion. In terms of effectiveness with communication partners, manual signs are generally less recognizable by potential partners, especially in community-based settings

(Bryen, et al. 1988; Bryen & McGinley, 1991). One solution to this difficult and multidimensional decision may be the selection of multiple means to represent as a long-term consideration in meeting future communication needs while successfully managing problem behavior.

Unaided Means to Represent. If the intervention team has opted for gestures or manual signs, a number of issues need to be considered in selecting the specific means to represent. A review indicates that, although manual signs were selected in several studies (see Table 24.1), the specific type of manual signs selected were often not reported (Bird et al., 1989; Northup et al., 1991; Wacker et al., 1990). Specifically, the question arises: What sign or signs should be selected if several alternatives are available to represent the same referent, message, or function?

Existing Communicative Repertoire. The learnability of the gestures or manual signs, especially within the context of developing a functionally equivalent response, seems to be a crucial consideration for selecting initial manual signs. The intervention team must avoid, to the maximum extent possible, the introduction of new manual signs or gestures where there is an existing sign repertoire. Wacker et al. (1990) taught Jim to use the manual signs PLEASE as a generic request and EAT as a request for food to escape demands. Even though Jim had not been observed to produce these signs, he had received training at school to sign PLEASE and EAT prior to the development of the communication-based intervention. For another participant, Wacker et al. selected an existing sign approximation to represent requests for a desired item. Schlosser and Karlan (1994) taught one individual to use the manual sign WANT as part of a multimodal representation to express generalized requests even though he did not use manual signs functionally in any of his daily environments (group home, community, community-based workshop). However, Sam was able to produce the sign WANT when asked "Show me the sign for want" prior to intervention. Selecting the sign WANT permitted the intervention team to build on an existing, albeit not functional, communicative repertoire. As mentioned previously, for individuals with escape-motivated behavior, the training of new signs may constitute a new demand in addition to the demands that induced the problem behavior in the first place, further increasing the probability that the problem behavior will occur (Fisher et al., 1993). Thus, for demand-escape situations, the intervention team should select manual signs that (1) already exist in the person's repertoire, (2) are approximations of actual signs, and (3) are easy to produce.

Physical Features.   In addition to the existing communicative repertoire, several parameters have been empirically determined to influence the relative physical ease of production of manual signs (Doherty, 1985). However, these parameters (e.g., contact, handedness, symmetry, and handshape) generally have not been reported as rationales for selecting manual signs (see Table 24.1) and have yet to be systematically manipulated in communication-based intervention research to problem behavior. Thus, although they are not recommended for wholesale adoption until empirical support becomes available, they are discussed here as considerations when choosing an initial sign vocabulary. (For complete definitions for each parameter, see Chapter 7.)

Based on her review, Doherty (1985) recommends that contact signs be selected over noncontact signs. Further, symmetric signs should be selected over asymmetric signs. In addition, she suggests that translucent signs be selected over opaque signs for signs produced with one hand. Finally, she encourages that one-handed signs be selected over two-handed signs because they are easier to produce. With respect to the handshapes that are used to produce manual signs, Doherty (1985) made a number of recommendations. First, she suggested selecting signs with handshape features that are less difficult to produce. Signs at Boyes-Braem's (1973) stage 1 (i.e., A, S, L, baby O, 5, C, G) and stage 2 (B, F, O) of handshape difficulty are believed to be acquired more readily than those at stage 3 (I, D, Y, P, 3, V, H, W) and stage 4 (8, 7, X, R, T, M, N, E). Second, she recommended that motoric capabilities to form handshapes and conduct movements be tested to determine which signs

should be avoided initially and which signs would be acceptable to approximate.

Teachability.   The teachability of manual signs is a consideration intrinsically related to their learnability. Teachability can refer to the potential to use commonly accepted practices to introduce manual signs (e.g., hand-over-hand guidance). The study by Wacker et al. (1990) illustrates how teachability may be considered in selecting manual signs. Because one of their participants resisted hand-over-hand guidance when new sign teaching was attempted, they opted to accept an existing sign approximation (e.g., lightly touching or brushing the chin with one finger) to represent a generalized request (WANT). Teachability can also refer to the previous effectiveness of manual sign teaching. Horner and Budd (1985) initially selected manual signs because they were taught successfully on earlier occasions.

Iconicity.   The iconicity of the individual manual signs *as perceived by partners* may be crucial if the functionally equivalent communicative behavior is to be recognized by partners. The literature (see Doherty, 1985; Chapters 7 and 13) overwhelmingly supports the facilitative effect of iconicity on sign comprehension by individuals with cognitive impairments (e.g., potential peers) and individuals without disabilities (e.g., potential caregivers). In addition, because they are usually not accompanied by the referent, manual signs must remain highly guessable. Thus, although the specific effects of varying degrees of iconicity of manual signs on appropriate communicative behavior and problem behavior have not been studied, response recognizability has been purported as a precondition to response success, which refers to whether partners respond to the trained communicative responses (Durand et al., 1993). Thus, the selection of highly guessable signs as the means to represent is suggested to increase the probability that partners will recognize and respond to the communication.

Aided Means to Represent.   If the intervention team has decided to employ aided means, a number of issues may need to be considered in choosing the specific means to be used. A review of the literature indicates that aided means to represent have been used in only a few studies (see Table 24.1). These studies have used graphic symbols (Doss, 1988), TO (Horner & Day, 1991; Horner et al., 1990), color (Horner et al., 1990), and objects (Dyer, Dunlap, & Winterling, 1990). Durand (1993) also employed aided means to represent with three participants, although it is not reported whether graphic symbols or TO were used. Robinson and Owens (1995) used photographs with an adult with cognitive impairment; however, their study was of a pre-experimental nature.

Existing Communicative Repertoire.   As with unaided means, decisions must be made by the intervention team concerning both which aided sets/systems to choose and which particular symbols within the aided set/system to select to represent the various referents, messages, or functions to be used by an individual. As with unaided means, the considerations relating to these decisions include the issues of teachability and learnability.

Certainly, as discussed above for unaided means, in designing the AAC-based intervention, the team should determine whether the individual has previously learned to use any aided means and, if so, how they were used. Sometimes, interventionists may not be aware of an existing repertoire. For example, Reichle (1991) reported an anecdote of an individual who, surprisingly, discriminated equally well among line drawings as he did among color photographs. The individual's mother then explained that she had used line drawings of specific toys over 3 years to indicate the contents of various plastic containers.

Interestingly, none of the studies summarized in Table 24.1 reported that the individuals had a pre-existing aided symbol repertoire. However, the individuals may have manipulated objects in the environment as attempts to communicate that were unrecognized, leading to the problem behavior. For example, if a student grabs a magazine to indicate a desire to escape from a demand and flips through the magazine during the time spent away from a demand task, the partner may not recognize this as a request to escape and takes the magazine away, resulting in an episode of SIB (which in turn temporarily ends the demand task).

Thus, objects may not only be unrecognized in specific instances of communication, but they can also be overlooked in studies of communication-based intervention as constituting an existing repertoire of potentially functionally equivalent responses.

Iconicity.   The intervention team may choose a specific aided means to represent from an array that varies in the degree of iconicity present to promote both recognizability and learnability. Iconicity is a powerful variable in graphic symbol learning in that more iconic symbols (across and within symbol sets and systems) are more readily learned than opaque symbols (see Chapters 6 and 13). As a general guiding principle, therefore, intervention teams should select iconic symbols over opaque symbols for the initial repertoire of communicative alternatives to problem behavior.

Other Considerations.   The relative importance of iconicity among other selection considerations is yet unknown. The reinforcing value of the referent (motivation) might have a greater effect on the rate at which a symbol is acquired than its iconicity (Reichle, 1991). Schlosser and Karlan (1994), for instance, worked with one individual who engaged in problem behavior that was reinforced by obtaining and keeping tangibles, (e.g., the clothing of other residents). This individual may more readily acquire a highly opaque symbol for a pullover (e.g., a lexigram) than a highly iconic symbol for a newspaper (e.g., PCS) because the pullover was more motivating.

In addition, other individual difference variables may be more important than iconicity when the team makes a selection decision. For instance, individuals who do not have receptive knowledge of the referent, that is, they cannot point to a picture of the referent when asked (e.g., "point to shoe") may not be able to benefit from iconicity in associating a symbol with a referent (Sevcik, Romski, & Wilkinson, 1991). For these individuals, opaque symbols such as lexigrams may be more successful in communication intervention (for a review, see Romski & Sevcik, 1992). Graphic symbols in general, and opaque symbols in particular, have rarely been selected in communication-based intervention studies and, thus, communication-based intervention research has yet to provide sufficient documentation of receptive vocabulary skills of their participants to enable more informed selection decisions (see Table 24.1).

Multimodal Means to Represent.   A few of the studies summarized in Table 24.1 have used multimodal means to represent as an alternative communicative response (Day, Rea, Schussler, Larsen, & Johnson, 1988; Schlosser & Karlan, 1994). Multimodal means to represent may incorporate any combination of (1) aided means (e.g., graphic symbols and objects), (2) unaided means (e.g., pointing, reaching, leading, and manual signs), or (3) aided and unaided means to represent (e.g., graphic symbols and manual signs). **Multimodal approaches** provide the team with ways of combining several of the considerations discussed above within the same intervention. Day et al. (1988) taught Mary to request tangibles using a combination of unaided means, including a hand-clap to gain the trainer's attention, and manual signs and/or spoken labels for the items requested. Although no rationale was reported (see Table 24.1), this particular multimodal approach is noteworthy in that it successfully addresses the problem that manual signs are limited in the initial attaining of attention. Teaching Mary to use a hand-clap before signing ensured that she had the trainer's attention. Also, instructing Mary to use either manual signs or spoken labels permitted her to build on her existing sign (a few signs) and speech repertoire (one-word verbalizations).

In another study, Schlosser and Karlan (1994) taught Sam to request tangibles by using a combination of unaided modalities. He could request objects using the sign WANT in addition to any communicative form that would specify the object for the partner, including a sign of the object's name, vocalizing, using gestures (e.g., pointing), or leading the partner to the object. This approach was selected because it allowed Sam to build on his existing multimodal repertoire. It also reduced the

communicative burden placed on direct-care personnel by increasing the recognizability of the entire response. First, the use of only one known manual sign as a "generalized want" addressed the lack of signing competence among direct-care staff. Second, supplementing this one sign with transparent communicative behaviors (e.g., pointing) further increased the recognizability of the means to represent.

Fisher et al. (1993) employed a similar approach with Jan in one of the study phases. Jan was taught to use a hand-clap to gain the trainer's attention and to sign GO to change the environment. This approach differs from the one employed by Day et al. (1988) and Schlosser and Karlan (1993) in one respect. In the latter two studies, all modalities served as an alternative to one function, that is, to request tangibles. The hand-clapping merely served to prepare the partner for the request of a tangible. In the Fisher et al. (1993) study, the hand-clap served a social attention function whereas the sign GO served a tangible function (to request a different environment).

These studies employed only combinations of unaided means; none of these studies combined several aided means or aided and unaided means to represent. As a means to represent, sign-linked Sigsymbols (Cregan & Lloyd, 1990) may lend themselves to being combined with unaided means to represent (manual signs) because they were specifically designed for use in combination with manual signs.

In light of the widely proposed benefits of a multimodal approach to AAC intervention (e.g., Grove & Walker, 1990; Hamre-Nietupski, Nietupski, & Rathe, 1985; Hooper, Connell, & Flett, 1987; Kiernan & Jones, 1985), the use of multimodal means to represent may warrant further exploration in communication-based approaches to problem behavior. A multimodal approach is based on the notion that individuals who are using AAC effectively do not rely solely on one mode[1] of communication but rather on a combination of modes, as demanded by their needs with different

---

[1]"Mode" is used in a generic sense; it may incorporate the means to represent, select, and transmit (see the Means to Transmit section for a further discussion of multimodal means to transmit).

communication partners in a variety of environments. Differential means to represent may be required when partners or settings change from familiar to unfamiliar ones. For instance, familiar partners may understand a user's idiosyncratic manual signs, whereas unfamiliar partners may not. Differential means to represent may also be necessitated by the changing availability of the means to transmit (e.g., devices). Horner et al. (1990) provided initial data of such multimodal use (i.e., TO with a VOCA, gestures, and manual signs) within the realm of communication-based approaches to problem behavior. They reported a collateral increase in an untrained means to represent (i.e., gesturing and signing) in situations when the trained means to represent (i.e., TO) could not be used because the VOCA was unavailable. Thus, the selection of multiple means to represent and training their differential use are important considerations if communication-based approaches to problem behavior are to generalize to community settings with unfamiliar partners.

Means to Select

Having selected a means to represent the referents, messages, or functions for which the intervention team wishes to develop functionally equivalent responses, consideration must next be given to the means by which the individual will select the represented message before transmitting it to the partner. According to Lloyd et al. (1990), the means to select refers to the strategies used to indicate particular symbols (e.g., direct selection, scanning) and may also include encoding techniques and prediction techniques as discussed in Chapter 8. Messages that are represented in unaided forms require no external aids or techniques, whereas those represented through aided means require that external elements be considered during the design of the communication-based intervention.

Manual Signs.   The means by which manual signs needed for a message are selected involves no external aids, but rather recall memory. With graphic symbols, on the other hand, recognition memory is sufficient. Selection is facilitated by the

display of symbols on the aid which require only recognition, not recall. Because individuals must rely primarily on more difficult recall memory in using signs expressively, an important consideration is whether to use manual signs (1) for an entire English sentence (sentence signing) or (2) for only one or a few representative signs via **key word signing** (BREAK standing for "I want to go, please") or generalized requests (e.g., MORE, PLEASE).

Key Word Signing vs. Sentence Signing: Physical and Mental Effort.   Horner and Day (1991) examined the effects of sentence signing (I WANT TO GO, PLEASE) versus key word signing (BREAK) on problem behavior, on attempts to complete tasks, and on requesting with Paul, one of their participants. Results indicate that key word signing, in contrast to sentence signing, resulted in increased requesting, increased attempts to complete tasks, and decreased aggression. In addition, during the key word signing, Paul never resorted to sentence signing. Horner and Day (1991) concluded that only key word signing could compete with aggressive behavior in terms of the physical effort required to perform the response. Although this conclusion is accurate from the perspective of applied behavior analysis, a cognitive perspective may add to the understanding of this phenomenon. From such a perspective, sentence signing may also have placed a greater mental effort on Paul because he needed to select several signs in correct order from memory. In key word signing, however, he had to select only one sign (BREAK). Aggressive behavior, in Paul's case, was already established as an effective means of escaping, thus it already had **response efficiency**. Therefore, due to the lower mental effort, only key word signing, as a new response, could compete with the response efficiency of the aggressive behavior.

Key word signing has been used in the reported studies summarized in Table 24.1 to represent specific consequences or referents. For example, Horner and Day (1991) used "BREAK" as a key word for requesting leave from a task; Day et al. (1988) used manual signs for specific objects to request particular tangibles.

Generalized Request Signing: Physical and Mental Effort.   As another approach to making the means to select the message more efficient than the existing problem behavior, a number of studies have employed generalized requests (1) to escape (e.g., FINISHED, GO [Fisher et al., 1993], PLEASE [Northup et al., 1991], WANT [Wacker et al., 1990]), (2) for assistance (e.g., HELP [Horner & Day, 1991]), and (3) for tangibles (e.g., MORE [Fisher et al., 1993], PLEASE [Northup et al., 1991]). Wacker et al. (1990) is particularly noteworthy in that they employed two signs (PLEASE, EAT), which both served as a request to escape a task by receiving a break.

Although generalized requests have been shown to be effective when establishing functionally equivalent responses, no consideration has apparently been given to what happens if the desired object or consequence of the generalized request is unclear to the communication partner. What, for example, would happen in community environments when more than one object is present and the partner is unaware of the individual's known preferences? Also, what would happen if an unfamiliar partner were to respond to the use of PLEASE as though it were a request for an object and not a request for a break? In these instances, the individual might revert to the problem behavior, largely as a result of the lesser specificity of the generalized request. Thus, researchers need to empirically scrutinize the relative physical and mental effort associated with using briefer, more generalized means of selecting (key signs or generalized requests) versus lengthier, more specific responses (e.g., sentence signing or combining a generalized want and the sign for the object) relative to the problem behavior.

Aided Symbols.   The major techniques involved in selecting aided symbols are direct selection and scanning (Reichle, 1991). To compete with problem behavior, the symbols representing the desired consequences must be selected as quickly as possible with minimum physical and mental effort, yielding a functional equivalent and more efficient response. The means to select should also place as little burden on the partner as possible.

Direct selection for a nonelectronic communication board requires adequate visual acuity and only the physical capabilities required to point to a symbol (Reichle, 1991). Direct selection via a VOCA requires the physical abilities to perform a key-activation response. Direct selection was found to result in better recall of graphic symbols than row-column scanning from an array of 40 symbols, suggesting that direct selection is cognitively less difficult than scanning with typically developing preschoolers (Mizuko, Reichle, Ratcliff, & Esser, 1994; Ratcliff, 1987). Direct selection techniques are also quicker and place less of a burden on the partner than scanning (Reichle, 1991).

All studies summarized in Table 24.1 involving aided communication used direct selection to select symbols or objects. Various techniques were used including pointing with a head pointer (Durand, 1993), pointing with hands or fingers (Durand, 1993), and activating a switch for a recorded message (Steege et al., 1990; Wacker et al., 1990). Physical considerations were used to support direct selection as the means to select in several studies. With Michelle, Durand (1993) chose a head pointer for selecting because of her difficulties in using her hands. With Peter and Joshua, Durand (1993) chose to have the participants use their hands to select because they were able to point. In another study, the participant had been taught to activate a microswitch prior to the onset of intervention, so this means to select was chosen (Wacker et al., 1990).

Encoding: Physical and Mental Effort.   Encoding techniques (see Chapter 8) may provide a viable option to further increase the efficiency of direct selection. Horner et al. (1990) compared the effects of a no-encoding condition with a color-encoding condition on escape-motivated problem behavior exhibited by one individual with moderate cognitive impairment. Using a VOCA, the first condition involved spelling out the complete message by pressing one key for each letter ("Help, please"), whereas the second condition involved activating one colored key representing the prestored message ("Help, please"). An underlying assumption was that spelling the message was less efficient than the problem behavior, and that problem behavior was less efficient than pressing one key that resulted in assistance. Results demonstrated that the low-efficiency response (spelling a message) did not replace aggression in the long term, whereas the high-efficiency response (activating one key) seemed to decrease aggression and increase use of appropriate communication. As mentioned earlier for manual sign selection, the differences may also be due to the varying levels of mental effort required, as the no-encoding condition required greater recall memory (recall of the phrase and recall of how to spell the words in the phrase) than did the color encoding (recall of the phrase and recognition of one color associated with the phrase).

Two directions for further research seem critical. First, the relative efficiency of scanning techniques in competing with problem behavior needs to be examined. Some individuals have upper extremity motor impairments that do not permit direct selection. Second, the relative efficiency of other encoding and prediction techniques (as discussed in Chapter 8) in competing with problem behavior need to be studied.

Means to Transmit

The means to transmit a message may involve interfaces such as electronic and nonelectronic communication devices or no interfaces at all as, for example, when manual signs are used. Unaided transmission (e.g., with manual signs) is always direct, and hence does not involve any aid external to the user's body (Lloyd et al., 1990). Thus, discussion will focus on the means to transmit for aided communication, including electronic devices (e.g., VOCAs, tape players, loops tape) and nonelectronic devices (e.g., communication boards, communication books, and flashcards). VOCAs (Durand, 1993; Horner et al., 1990), tape players (Steege et al., 1990), and tape loops (Wacker et al., 1990) have been used successfully in communication-based approaches to problem behavior. In the absence of comparative research on the effects of electronic versus nonelectronic devices in communication-based approaches to problem behavior, extrapolations are being made from general research on the effectiveness of various means to

transmit (Schlosser, Belfiore, Nigam, Blischak, & Hetzroni, 1995; Soto, Belfiore, Schlosser, & Haynes, 1993), previous reviews (Doss & Reichle, 1991a), and reported rationales for selecting means to transmit in communication-based research (e.g., Durand, 1993; Horner et al., 1990; Steege et al., 1990; Wacker et al., 1990).

Pairing Graphic and Acoustic Symbols. The selected means to transmit may have an effect on the learnability of the means to represent and the potential for communication-based intervention to problem behavior. Graphic symbols (e.g., lexigrams) were learned more efficiently by two out of three individuals with severe to profound cognitive impairments when they received augmented input and feedback through speech output from a VOCA compared to when the speech synthesizer was turned off (Schlosser et al., 1995). The efficacy of the VOCA-transmission was attributed to the provision of auditory stimuli in the form of augmented input and feedback during training. Thus, one might expect that individuals who exhibit problem behavior and whose characteristics are similar to those of the participants in this study may learn the means to represent more readily with a VOCA.

Projectability and Assertiveness. The selected means to transmit may also alter the projectability (see Chapter 13) of the means to represent and therefore alter the user's potential assertiveness. **Assertiveness** may be defined as the degree to which the means allows the user to influence interactions through initiations or interruptions, to ward off interruptions from others, or to protest something.

Doss and Reichle (1991a) suggested that graphic symbols require that the partner be fairly close to the user to be understood and may therefore be less suitable for individuals whose problem behavior is escape-motivated and who might be aggressive toward others; under such circumstances they recommend using gestures (e.g., STOP) that can be discerned from a distance. To increase the projectability when graphic symbols are transmitted via nonelectronic systems, O'Neill and Reichle (1993) recommend using a separate response to obtain the partner's attention (e.g., activating a buzzer) before emitting a more complete response. Another option may be to transmit the selected message via a VOCA or electronic signaling device. For example, a worker who runs out of materials may request assistance even if the supervisor is across the room. Steege et al. (1990) selected a battery-operated tape recorder to teach an individual with escape-motivated problem behavior to activate "Stop." They argued that the activation of pretaped messages may be made as assertive as needed by adjusting the volume, whereas signs could go unnoticed or be ignored. Reporting a similar rationale, Wacker et al. (1990) selected a tape loop with a recorded message ("I am tired of rocking; somebody give me something to do") to allow one of their participants to appropriately leave an activity. With individuals who are taught appropriate means to request attention, graphic symbols transmitted through a VOCA may indeed project better than either nonelectronic communication devices or manual signs because the communication partner does not need to face the individual to receive and respond to the request. This may be crucial in classroom situations where teachers cannot face a particular student all the time because their attention needs to be distributed among many students.

Assertiveness and Time Delay.

Horner and Day (1991) demonstrated indirectly the importance of assertiveness to appropriate communicative behavior and its control over problem behavior. In one study, they instructed a partner to systematically vary the delay (1 second or 20 seconds) between the participant handing over a card (with the word *break*) or engaging in aggression and the delivery of the break. The 20-second–delay condition may be viewed as a simulation of low assertiveness; that is, the communicative behavior is not assertive enough to yield a more immediate response from the partner. Results indicate that the 20-second delay resulted not only in increased aggression but also in markedly decreased use of the card. The 1-second delay, on the other hand, resulted in increased use of the card and a marked decrease in aggression. Horner and Day (1991) concluded that the longer delay could not compete with the problem behavior; the problem behavior

resulted in quicker receipt of the break than the use of the card. In other words, the learner did not perceive it as a good deal to have to wait 20 seconds for the break after communicating appropriately.

Assertiveness and Schedule of Reinforcement.

Schedule of reinforcement refers to the number of appropriate communicative responses required to obtain the requested consequence. In a second study, Horner and Day (1991) demonstrated what might happen relative to signing, task completion, and problem behavior if an individual is required to sign several times to receive teacher assistance. They provided teacher assistance on a picture-matching task any time the participant engaged in SIB or if he signed HELP once (FR1) or three times (FR3) during the trial. Repeating the same sign simulates a situation in which the partner responds to request only after appropriate communicative behavior is repeated. Using a reversal design, results for FR1 demonstrated that the participant signed for help on nearly every trial, attempted the tasks in every trial, and engaged in no SIB. Despite initial improvements in the first FR3 phase, a later phase indicated a drop in the attempts to complete the task, a substantial increase in problem behavior, and a dramatic reduction in the use of the sign. Horner and Day (1991) concluded that FR3 was less efficient than problem behavior in that the participant needed to sign several times to obtain teacher attention whereas SIB resulted in immediate attention. This study demonstrates that the intervention team needs to select a means to transmit that permits partners to respond quickly and frequently to the appropriate communicative behavior for appropriate communication to compete with problem behavior.

Assertiveness Potential of Different Means to Transmit.

The assertiveness potential of different means to transmit in relation to problem behavior remains to be examined. In the absence of such research, extrapolations are again being made from AAC intervention research. A comparison of a VOCA (Wolf™ with Echo synthesized speech) with a communication board involving one participant with profound cognitive impairment indicated that there were no differences in terms of the percentage of successful requests for objects and activities (Soto et al., 1993). In both conditions, the individual was taught to make specific requests by pointing to or pressing graphic symbols ("want" + item) on each of the two devices that were familiar to the communication partner.

Doss et al. (1991) implemented an initial study comparing the effectiveness and efficiency of various means to transmit while ordering fast food from unfamiliar partners (i.e., counter clerks). Effectiveness was defined by the number of requests for clarification from the clerks. Efficiency was defined by the length of time it took to order a meal. A comparison of a communication wallet with a VOCA (LightTalker™ with Echo synthesized speech) in experiment 1 indicated that with both devices, all items requested were obtained. Results also showed that the communication wallet was more effective and more efficient than the VOCA. Doss et al. (1991) attributed these differences to the low intelligibility of the Echo synthesized speech. These findings seem to suggest that, when unfamiliar partners are involved, a nonelectronic system may be more effective and efficient than a VOCA with low-intelligibility synthesized speech (Doss et al., 1991). When familiar partners are involved, no differences existed between a nonelectronic device and a VOCA with low-intelligibility synthesized speech (Soto et al., 1993).

Experiment 2 (Doss et al., 1991) examined differences among a communication wallet, an Alltalk™ with digitized speech, a RealVoice™ with good synthesized speech and a printer, and a RealVoice with good synthesized speech without a printer. These chosen means to transmit unfortunately used neither the same means to represent (e.g., PCS for the wallet and TO for the electronic devices) nor the same means to select, so no firm conclusions can be drawn from this study. No significant differences were found in effectiveness in terms of the number of clarifications required. Doss et al. (1991) attributed this lack of differences in experiment 2 compared with differences in experiment 1 to the increased intelligibility of the speech output. Although the efficiency results yielded several significant comparisons (both the communication wallet and the Alltalk were more efficient than the RealVoice with printer), Doss et al. (1991) believe that these differences are not clinically meaningful. Although preliminary, this study suggests that electronic and nonelectronic means to transmit can be equally effective in requesting food from unfamiliar partners if the electronic devices (1) employ either digitized speech or good synthesized speech; and (2) the speech output is optimized through inserting pauses between items ordered, ensuring correct pronunciation of each word, and conducting tests on its validity. Future researchers need to examine how these different means to transmit may affect appropriate communicative behavior and compete with problem behavior.

User Preference. User preference for a certain means to transmit is a selection consideration frequently ignored. A review of the literature indicates that no communication-based study has selected the means to transmit based on user preference or has systematically explored the effects of preferred versus nonpreferred transmission means on problem behavior (see Table 24.1). However, communication effectiveness research indicates that preference may be an important consideration, especially when there are no effectiveness advantages for a particular means to transmit as occurred in the Soto et al. (1993) study previously discussed.

Durability and Replaceability. Durability and replaceability may be another set of variables to consider when selecting devices for communication-based intervention for problem behavior. In developing a program for an adult who engaged in aggressive behavior and property destruction (e.g., his radio), durability and replaceability became primary considerations for selecting an appropriate means to transmit. After a decision was made to opt for an aided means to transmit, consideration was given to a VOCA versus a nonelectronic device. After consultation with the individual's direct-care staff, however, a communication wallet was recommended because it would be more durable and easier to replace than a more sensitive and costly electronic device. The AAC user was involved in developing the wallet. He helped select vocabulary and photographs of his favorite celebrities to be put in the wallet and helped select a cover that would be durable. It was hypothesized that the AAC user's input would enhance his sense of ownership and reduce the chance that the wallet would be destroyed. When VOCAs are being selected, a nonelectronic communication board must be available as a backup in case the VOCA needs repair. Unlike an AAC user who does not engage in problem behavior, the individual who has learned to communicate with a VOCA instead of engaging in problem behavior may regress substantially if a backup system is not immediately available.

Key Activation and Physical Effort.   Physical effort may be another important consideration when selecting aided means to transmit. Communication boards and books accessed via direct selection require merely pointing to the appropriate square containing the graphic symbol, whereas VOCAs require a key-activation response. Different VOCAs vary in the degree of effort required to activate keys, with some VOCAs allowing for adjustment. Durand (1993), for example, selected an IntroTalker™ rather than a SuperWolf™ for one of his participants because it required less physical effort to activate. To date, the effects of varying degrees of physical effort required for activation of prestored messages by different or the same transmission means have not been examined in communication-based studies of problem behavior. Basic research examined the effects of response effort on choice behavior by varying the pressure required to depress a response key (Bauman, Shull, & Brownstein, 1975). Findings suggest that subjects preferred the lower response effort. The chosen means to transmit may affect how well graphic symbols are learned and used. In addition, the preference for a means to transmit may also affect the individual's use of that means. Sometimes selecting the means to transmit might also call for a reevaluation of those selection considerations that favored unaided over aided means to represent.

SUMMARY

A review of studies of communication-based approaches to problem behavior with individuals who have little or no functional speech (see Table 24.1) indicated that researchers frequently provide insufficient information regarding the participant's existing communicative repertoire, which is the basis of one of the more important AAC selection considerations in designing interventions. Further, rationales for selecting AAC means to represent, means to select, and means to transmit are provided only in a few studies and do not nearly reflect the range of the considerations proposed here. Both of these findings may be in part explained by the apparent underutilization of the range of available assessment methods, especially those that are more useful in AAC-based intervention development (e.g., CI, CRMC, FAI). Teams designing communication-based interventions for individuals with little or no functional speech may therefore benefit from including professionals who are well-versed with AAC selection and development considerations. The considerations proposed in this chapter are not complete and warrant conceptual integration in terms of relative importance as further research becomes available. Nonetheless, this overview of the range of AAC considerations may allow professionals with an AAC background to assume a more active role in intervention development for individuals with little or no functional speech who exhibit problem behavior.

CHAPTER 25

EPILOGUE

LYLE L. LLOYD, RAYMOND W. QUIST, AND HELEN H. ARVIDSON

The field of **augmentative and alternative communication (AAC)** evolved out of a growing need to meet the clinical and educational needs of individuals with little or no functional speech. The early AAC knowledge base was derived from clinical experience, observation, and the perceptions of outcomes for AAC users. Although a considerable amount of research related specifically to AAC has emerged during the last two decades, more solid empirical knowledge about the basic elements of communication technology and assessment and intervention strategies and techniques is needed to build a firm foundation on which the field can continue to grow. This chapter looks at some of the research needs and current issues that relate to the many aspects of AAC that have been discussed in this text.

FOUNDATIONS AND FRAMEWORK

Over the years, the need for AAC services has increased as advances in medicine have improved survival rates of medically fragile infants and infants with severe disabilities. Improved medical care and drugs that allow individuals to live longer have increased the need for AAC services for older individuals. Documentation about the effects of drugs and the changing needs of individuals whose abilities decline as a result of progressive diseases such as multiple sclerosis (MS) and Parkinson's disease, and individuals whose abilities improve as a result of recovery from medical events such as traumatic brain injury (TBI) or a cerebrovascular accident (CVA) has aided clinicians/educators in developing and implementing AAC services.

Research

The basic research that guided the early development of AAC was borrowed from a variety of other disciplines (Lloyd, 1993; Zangari, Lloyd, & Vicker, 1994). Current clinical/educational practice evolved from the building blocks of learning theory and behaviorism (Baer, Wolf, & Risely, 1968; Carr & Durand, 1985a, 1985b; Carr & Kologinsky, 1983; Carrier, 1974, 1976; Guess, Sailor, & Baer, 1976; Premack, 1970; Remington, 1991a, 1991b, 1994; Schlinger, 1992; Sidman, 1971, 1986; Sidman & Cresson, 1973; Sidman & Tailby, 1982; Sigurdardottir, Green, & Saunders, 1990; Skinner, 1938, 1957, 1969, 1974, 1989; Stromer & Mackay, 1993). Skinner's research provided a basis for developing operant/behavior modification programs, single-subject designs, and specialized programs such as Sidman's stimulus equivalence paradigm, which has been used with individuals with severe cognitive impairments (Remington, 1994; Sidman, 1971, 1986; Sidman & Cresson, 1973; Sigurdardottir, Green, & Saunders, 1990). Research in visual perception (E. Gibson, 1969; J. Gibson, 1966) played a role in the development of teaching strategies. Research in linguistics (Stokoe, 1969) influenced the use of symbols in AAC. Both basic and applied research on speech and speech intelligibility conducted by Bell Laboratories and other programs during the first half of the twentieth century (Cooper, DeLattre, Liberman, Borst, & Gerstman, 1952; DeLattre, Liberman & Cooper, 1955; Dudley, Reisz, & Walkins, 1939; Egan, 1948; Fant, 1960, 1969; Fletcher, 1929; French & Steinberg, 1947; Hirsh, 1952; Licklider & Miller, 1951; Miller, 1951; Miller, Heise, &

Lichten, 1951; Peterson & Barney, 1952; Potter, Kopp, & Green, 1947; Potter & Peterson, 1948; Stevens & House, 1956, 1961) laid the groundwork for the development of voice output communication aids (VOCAs). More recent research in a wide variety of areas such as electronics, biomedical prostheses, and miniaturization and computerization have continued to contribute to the development of the wide variety of VOCAs that are in use today.

Research Needs

A considerable amount of knowledge about the communication process, symbol characteristics, vocabulary selection, literacy, features and functions of VOCAs, educational approaches, and communicative competence has emerged since the 1980s as a result of both borrowed and AAC-specific research. As the field expands, however, more research is needed in these and other areas if the needs of individuals with little or no functional speech are to be fully met. In an editorial in *Augmentative and Alternative Communication*, Lloyd (1989) stated the following:

> Although much progress has been made in AAC, as a new field we are still operating from a limited empirical base and a number of critical issues remain to be addressed. In other words, the educational and clinical application of AAC approaches have far out-distanced our knowledge about AAC symbols and systems. Some of the most critical research issues and needs that must be addressed in AAC during the next decade are related to (a) selection of symbols/systems (and symbol/system characteristics); (b) modification of symbols/systems; (c) symbol/system acquisition and generalization; (d) use of multiple symbols/systems; (e) development of successful social facilitation of communication (e.g., communicative competence and interaction); (f) selection of initial lexical items; (g) involvement of staff, parents, and significant others; (h) application of microcomputer and other technology (considering factors such as intelligibility, preference, and speed/rate); (i) artificial intelligence; (j) literacy; and (k) vocational and quality of life considerations. Other statements of AAC research issues and needs have typically in-

cluded one or more of the above. For example, the August 1987 AAC Think Tank reaffirmed several of these as continuing AAC issues in need of further research. . . . (p. 83)

Almost a decade later, many of these issues remain. Research needs have been discussed in a number of articles and at a variety of seminars, conferences, and presentations (Beukelman & Ansel, 1995; Beukelman, et al., 1989; Lloyd, 1989, 1993; Lloyd, Romski, Beukelman, & Higginbotham, 1993; Mineo, 1990). In 1994, the National Institute of Deafness and Other Communication Disorders (NIDCD) organized a one-day working meeting on AAC research, which was summarized by Beukelman and Ansel (1995). They highlighted six needs:

1. To study the impact of AAC technologies on the development of communication, language, natural speech, and discourse skills of persons with severe communication disorders.
2. To study the influence of user variables (for example, knowledge, skill, and learning style) on AAC system use.
3. To investigate the impact of AAC system features on communicative competence and interaction skills of users.
4. To develop tools and strategies to validly and reliably measure communicative, operational, linguistic, strategic, and social competence of children and adults who use AAC systems.
5. To investigate the effectiveness of AAC interventions by studying users of a variety of ages, etiologies, and social contexts and to determine those factors that are related to success and failure of AAC use.
6. To encourage the academic development of researchers with a focus in AAC by establishing predoctoral and postdoctoral research and training opportunities.

AAC Model

These NIDCD priorities provide a broad, comprehensive research agenda consistent with the institute's mission and focus on language and communication and can serve as a general guide for researchers seeking to expand the empirical knowledge base of AAC. The need for research, however, can be organized more specifically. One organizational scheme, for example, already exists within the major elements of the AAC communication model proposed by Lloyd, Quist, and Windsor (1990) and summarized in Chapter 3. According to the model, communication must have a purpose; that is, the sender must have a reason to communicate. In the communication model, the sender formulates a message and then uses AAC to represent, select, and transmit it through signal channels or transmission environments to a receiver who decodes it. Research related to the means to represent, select, and transmit, as well as research into the use of multiple modes of communication, can be organized under the heading of the sender (message encoder). Typical speakers use a variety of modes such as affect, gestures, and speech to communicate. Research into determining and teaching the most effective modes of communication for individual AAC users is critical as clinicians/educators strive to provide services that have successful outcomes. Research into the physical conditions through which acoustic and visual signals are transmitted can be categorized under a heading such as signal channels or transmission environments. The receiver (message decoder) provides the heading for research into aspects of receiving messages. All these elements interact with the others across communication partners and environments to create research questions related to humanistic aspects of communication. Feedback from communication partners aids the sender in determining which communication modes are most effective. Although a VOCA may be more effective in gaining attention in relatively quiet environments, signing or using a symbol board may be more effective and may elicit more positive feedback from a communication partner in a noisy environment. Questions related to external feedback from the receiver and internal feedback from the sender can be organized under feedback.

The model provides one systematic way to organize specific research questions for AAC professionals who have typically had trouble focusing on developing a prioritized list. The critical components of the communication process need to be identified so that the research base can grow and the field can continue to move forward.

SYMBOLS

The selection and use of symbols are basic components of the communication process. Understanding the characteristics of a wide variety of symbol sets and systems and why they may or may not be the most appropriate for any given AAC user is critical to the successful design and use of an AAC system. Investigation into effective ways to select, teach, and promote the generalization of both iconic and opaque symbols across communication partners and environments continues to be needed.

To date, most of the research paradigms and knowledge base for AAC symbol characteristics are still borrowed and/or extrapolated from the fields of audiology, human communication, electrical engineering, linguistics, and cognitive and perceptual psychology. Most of the knowledge about graphic symbols comes from perceptual psychology. Much of the knowledge about unaided symbols comes from the fields of linguistics, human communication, and psychology. Basic knowledge of speech synthesis comes from the fields of audiology, electrical engineering, and psychology.

Schlosser and Lloyd (1993a) distinguished a number of variables that play a role in the symbol learning process of AAC. They include (1) symbol variables (e.g., investigator-defined complexity, configuration, symbol organization, or taxonomy); (2) referent variables (e.g., frequency of occurrence); (3) learner variables (e.g., experiential background, cognitive functioning); (4) instruction variables (e.g., teaching strategy, context); (5) communication interaction variables (e.g., social regulation functions, communicative functions); and (6) outcome variables (e.g., receptive and expressive acquisition and generalization, language acquisition and development, cognitive development, and literacy). At present, however, there is little empirical knowledge about how these variables may interact.

The only interaction that has been studied to

date is that of symbol, referent, and learner variables evident in the iconicity phenomenon. Investigation into the interaction of iconicity (translucency and transparency) and the outcome variables of symbol learning and retention, for example, has provided considerable evidence that high translucency AAC symbols (both manual signs and Blissymbols) are easier to learn and retain than low translucency symbols. This finding holds true for both children and adults with and without cognitive impairments (Lloyd & Fuller, 1990). Interaction effects of iconicity, however, warrant further attention because of a lack of data on the effects of the experiential and cultural backgrounds of learners. Gestures and other communicative behaviors have been found not to have universal iconicity but rather are strongly influenced by culture (Morris, Collett, Marsh, & O'Shaughnessy, 1979). Brown (1977, 1978) hypothesized that iconicity was bound by culture, experience, age, and time; however, none of the studies to date dealing with age, cognitive level, or implied experiential differences related to disability have demonstrated qualitative differences in the influence of iconicity in learning Blissymbols or manual signs, for example. Culture, per se, has not yet been investigated.

Another area that needs research is the use of manual signs. Except for the evidence supporting the role of iconicity, not much has been learned about manual sign characteristics since Doherty published her review in 1985. There is still a lack of knowledge about manual signs and their use as AAC. Individuals are sometimes reluctant to use manual signs because they believe that this means giving up on their ability to acquire natural speech. This misconception persists even though research indicates this is not the case (for a summary see Silverman, 1980, 1989, 1995).

Other areas in need of research involve the effects of symbol variables on indicators of cognitive ability and successful language acquisition (Schlosser, 1993a, 1997a, 1997b; Sevcik, Romski, & Wilkinson, 1991) and how symbol sets (e.g., Picture Communication Symbols [PCS]) differ from symbol systems (e.g., Blissymbols, Sigsymbols) in facilitating categorical perception and cat-

egory learning (Schlosser, 1993a, 1997a, 1997b). No major research regarding the role of graphic symbols in the development of literacy has been conducted to guide clinicians/educators in making decisions about when to use symbol sets and when to use symbol systems. However, it seems that literacy could be facilitated more by the use of graphic symbol systems (e.g., Blissymbols) than by the use of graphic symbol sets (e.g., pictographs) (McNaughton, 1993). Another aspect of literacy concerns the relationship between graphic symbols and printed words. Pairing pictures with printed words, for example, has been a common practice among clinicians/educators for many years, even though it has been found to be a relatively ineffective method of teaching reading (Blischak & McDaniel, 1995). The less widely used practice of embedding pictures in print to increase the association (e.g., iconicity phenomenon) between words and referents, on the other hand, has been found to facilitate some types of literacy tasks (Blischak & McDaniel, 1995; McDaniel, Blischak, & Einstein, 1995). More research leading to published findings can help educators/clinicians make better decisions on methods for teaching literacy skills.

TECHNOLOGY

Despite the fact that technology is just one of the components of AAC, in recent years it has assumed a dominant role. The refinement of synthesized speech and the emergence of VOCAs during the 1980s represent a significant milestone in the development of AAC. In the last 15 years, improvements in synthetic speech received considerable attention. Many studies have focused on evaluating intelligibility of synthetic speech (Kangas & Allen, 1990; Koul & Allen, 1993; Logan, Greene, & Pisoni, 1989; Mirenda & Beukelman, 1990). Although early speech synthesizers had poor intelligibility, contemporary synthesizers such as DECtalk™ have been found to be 90 to 95% intelligible under laboratory conditions (Logan et al., 1989).

Although high intelligibility is desirable for any communication device, a number of factors interact and affect both the intelligibility and the effectiveness of a VOCA for individual AAC users. Environmental sounds and different signal-to-noise ratios, for example, affect intelligibility. Understanding the effects of varying pitch, rate, intensity, and prosody on intelligibility and meaning (emotion and emphasis) has practical implications for AAC users and their communication partners. Research on the effects of varying these parameters is needed. More sophisticated suprasegmental rules may need to be developed to improve the intelligibility of VOCAs as they are used in real-world environments.

More studies that simulate real-world environments for individuals with disabilities who use synthetic speech need to be conducted (Koul & Allen, 1993). Future studies should include systematic evaluation of synthetic speech in real-world environments under conditions in which cognitive loads of receivers are varied. Studies should include diverse populations of children and adults with disabilities (e.g., individuals with cognitive impairments and cerebral palsy) and individuals with progressive neurological disorders such as amyotrophic lateral sclerosis (ALS) and MS. Research into the ways in which speech recognition systems can interpret and translate distorted utterances for individuals with neurologically impaired speech is needed. The effects of hearing impairment in both VOCA users and their communication partners also needs further investigation if high technology is to be used to its full advantage.

The role of technology, especially VOCAs, relative to graphic symbol learning and literacy has received some attention to date. For example, VOCAs may enhance the learning of opaque graphic symbols (Romski & Sevcik, 1992; Schlosser, Belfiore, Blischak, Nigam, & Hetzroni, 1993; Schlosser et al., in press) and improve interaction (Healy, 1994; McGregor et al., 1992; Schepis & Reid, 1995). The use of graphic symbols to represent signs (and other gestures) has also been reported in the literature (e.g., Cregan, 1980a, 1980b, 1982, 1993; Cregan & Lloyd, 1984, 1990). However, more empirical research is needed to aid in understanding how this multimodal approach can be best used. Most approaches to graphic symbol learning currently practiced by professionals in the field today are still based on assumptions rather than research.

High technology may be an appropriate component of an AAC system for many, but not for all. More information is needed on the use and effectiveness of low technology to aid in system development and intervention programming for individuals for whom low technology is more appropriate, for individuals who use low technology for backup, and for individuals who prefer low technology as their primary mode of communication.

AAC ASSESSMENT

Assessing the communication needs of individuals with little or no functional speech is a complex process that requires knowledge and skill from many disciplines. Part of the complexity of assessment is due to the fact that individuals come to the assessment process with a wide range of strengths and needs. An individual with severe visual impairment, for example, requires that special consideration be given to selecting the most appropriate means to represent. The selected symbols must have features appropriately matched with the strengths and needs of the AAC user. A blind individual with AAC needs, for example, may require symbols that can be identified by touch. An individual with severe motor impairment would need special consideration given to the means to select. Recommendations might include the use of eye gaze, a head pointer, or any one of a number of switches. The interaction of physical strengths and needs with cognitive abilities makes an assessment all the more complex.

Changes in physical condition and cognition that affect the strengths and needs of AAC users are additional challenges of the assessment process. Knowledge of recovery of function from medical events and decline of function from progressive diseases that influence long- and short-term recommendations is imperative.

Matching the strengths and needs of individuals with the means to represent, the means to select, and the means to transmit requires knowledge about symbols, vocabulary, access, and both aided (using low and/or high technology) and unaided approaches to AAC, but there is another critical component. As the model described in Chapter 3 illustrates, the sender must have a reason to communicate (Lloyd et al., 1990). The reason(s) for communication will influence the assessment process. Recommendations related to the means to represent, select, and transmit for an individual who wants to communicate only for social closeness will be different from those for an individual who wants to continue working as a supervisor directing the activities of others.

Assessing strengths and needs, matching features, collecting and evaluating data from trial use of devices, and making final recommendations is a complex process. Research can broaden the knowledge base and improve the process and outcomes of designing a system that enhances the ability of AAC users to communicate and more fully participate in activities of choice.

AAC INTERVENTION

Assessment and intervention have been presented in two units in this text. They should not, however, be viewed as two separate and distinct processes. Assessment is an ongoing process that does not stop when intervention begins. It must be ongoing not only because of change in the status of individual strengths and needs, but also because of change in the status of knowledge and technology. Assessment must be ongoing to determine how well the intervention process is helping AAC users reach their goals. Data and information regarding the efficacy of intervention must be collected and evaluated so that adjustments can be made. One often thinks about assessment preceding intervention. In certain circumstances, however, a specific intervention may be introduced before assessment. Goossens' (1989), for example, described the introduction of intervention designed to teach a young girl with cerebral palsy how to use a switch in order to conduct a better switch assessment. Assessment and intervention often become entwined. One can facilitate the other.

Both assessment and intervention occur over time. In some instances, when individuals are diagnosed with severe communication disabilities due to congenital disorders, their AAC needs are assessed when they are young and may be reassessed as they mature into adulthood and even old age. In this event, typical aging that may contribute to changes in memory and linguistic skills must be considered. The occurrence of an acquired disorder in addition to a congenital disorder affects assessment and intervention even more.

As discussed earlier in this chapter, many of the strategies used in AAC intervention have come from the research of learning theory and behaviorism. Individuals with severe communication disabilities, however, typically bring additional factors to the learning situation. More research is needed to determine the best strategies for teaching so that AAC users can develop their maximum potential alongside their typically developing peers.

However, learning and developing effective communication can be exceedingly slow. Sometimes expectations that technology can remove all barriers result in setting unrealistic goals for AAC users who are educated with typically developing peers. In some cases, pressure builds and counterproductive frustration filters down to the AAC user.

CURRENT ISSUES AND TRENDS

Because AAC is a relatively new field that requires a high level of expertise, concerns exist about the varying levels of knowledge and skills among clinicians/educators. Many practitioners have not had formal preparation in AAC. Many have been prepared to work in other areas and have become involved in AAC as a result of their changing work environments. For example, speech-language pathologists who have worked in the public schools for many years may not have been trained in AAC, because at the time they entered the school setting, children who needed AAC were not on their caseloads. Now, however, with more and more children with severe disabilities being educated in their home schools, speech-language pathologists have more need to provide AAC services. The need for preprofessional preparation is essential. Clinicians/educators entering practice must have a sufficient knowledge base and skills to provide quality services.

Preservice Education

In the United States, AAC still does not constitute a significant part of the preservice programs in either speech-language pathology or special education. A survey of universities found that less than 50% of programs in speech-language pathology and less than 30% of programs in special education provide even one course in AAC (Koul & Lloyd, 1994b). Related AAC professionals (e.g., occupational therapists, physical therapists, rehabilitation specialists) receive even less coursework specifically in AAC. Other professionals, such as nurses, physicians, and psychologists receive virtually none. Although opportunities for classroom instruction are often limited, opportunities for practicum experiences with individuals with AAC needs are even more scarce. Because the field is relatively young, new professionals often find themselves the "designated AAC professional" even though their coursework and clinical experiences are limited. They often enter the field without a role model or appropriate supervision from experienced professionals.

Even in programs in which training in AAC is considered to be a necessary part of preservice education, there is often no clearly defined agreement as to how it should be included in the curriculum. Many faculty do not consider AAC a specialty, field, or discipline. They feel it should be subsumed within disorders courses and considered as one of many approaches for a given disorder (e.g., aphasia, dysarthria). Other faculty, however, recognize AAC as a complex field that cuts across areas and requires intensive training in many of its aspects in order to be effective. There is no evidence as to which approach provides the best training to make the AAC clinician/educator competent to provide quality services. As long as preservice preparation remains limited, however, professionals will continue to enter the workforce ill prepared and in need of continuing or inservice education.

Continuing Education

Continuing or inservice education (e.g., conferences, seminars, workshops) is often available to provide practicing professionals with opportunities to acquire updated information on relevant topics,

develop new skills, and meet ongoing continuing education requirements for certification or licensure. Continuing education serves to maintain and upgrade the skills of professionals who have had training in AAC and develop new skills in professionals who have not. It can be especially important in maintaining and developing the skills of staff at a facility with a high rate of turnover. Continuing education (in whatever form it is provided), however, is usually expensive when one considers cost in tuition or grant supports to pay for accommodations, instructors, and substitute personnel. Sometimes working professionals are discouraged from taking advantage of such continuing education or inservice opportunities. The whole area of cost effectiveness and quality of programming of continuing education must be examined; however, the fact that many preservice preparation programs turn out professionals with neither the knowledge nor the skills to provide quality services in AAC demands solution.

Continuing education should not, however, be considered a long-term solution to the problem of inadequately trained professionals. Little is actually known about the effectiveness of continuing education programs. Most data collected on continuing education (generally via evaluation forms) are general assessments of participants' perceptions of the continuing education process (e.g., content, delivery) and of how much they feel they have learned. No data exist on how the information obtained in this instruction is subsequently used by the participants with their clients or how the well-being of their clients improves as a result of the newly learned information.

Many continuing education programs involve a single presentation by an "expert" with little or no follow-up. Practitioners typically do not have the opportunities to confirm understanding of the material when they receive it or to validate the effectiveness of the training after they have had an opportunity to apply it in their particular settings. The planners and implementers of continuing education should consider what has been learned in the field of education regarding individual learning styles and instructional methodologies. Certainly individual professionals should not be expected to learn equally well from any one approach any more than individual AAC users should be expected to learn equally well from any one approach. Continuing education should include a variety of approaches.

Because so many practicing clinicians/educators received their original preservice preparation prior to the inclusion of academic coursework and practica in AAC in university training programs, a real need exists for educational opportunities. However, the major role of continuing education should not be to make up for the inadequacies of preservice training. The major goals in continuing education should be to provide information about the latest research findings, evaluation of the newest techniques and procedures, and insight into the major components of communication (the means to represent, the means to select, and the means to transmit). This will certainly include information about new and emerging technologies and how they can be used to improve the communication skills of AAC users, but this should be only part of it. Learning about *how* to use new technology in AAC can be exciting, but this is not enough. Clinicians/educators must acquire a solid understanding as to *why* AAC technologies should or should not be used. At the most basic level, practitioners need to understand not only the *how* of therapy, but also the *why*. Researchers (especially university faculty and staff in laboratory settings) need to have a solid understanding of the most critical application issues and needs to ensure a good degree of external validity. Researchers are frequently quite thorough in their consideration of internal validity, but sometimes at the expense of external validity. Practitioners in the field working with AAC users should have a solid understanding of both internal and external validity.

Continuing education should include information on the scientific bases for the clinical/educational practice of AAC research methodologies. Methodologies should be practiced because research has shown them to be effective. If methodologies are being practiced on the basis of assumptions, it should be with the full knowledge that the research base is lacking and the understanding that empirical data is needed. Unfortunately, many clinicians/educators use certain approaches with neither a research base to support

them nor a clear understanding of the assumptions from which they were derived. Clinicians/educators should be sufficiently well-versed in data collection and analysis to investigate the comparative effectiveness of the specific therapy approaches they employ. Too often, clinicians/educators rush to use various techniques or approaches without systematic evaluation of their efficacy.

Facilitated communication (FC) is a classic example of an approach that clinicians/educators began using without a research base (Shane, 1994). Although some professionals regarded FC as a method of choice for some individuals with little or no functional speech, it turned out to be harmful for others. The allegations of physical and sexual abuse that came out of the use of FC caused irreparable damage to many individuals. Implementing approaches/techniques that are not supported by research can be a dangerous practice.

Credentialing

Credentialing of professionals is typically accomplished through certification by professional organizations and licensing by state agencies. This is generally considered necessary to safeguard consumers from incompetent service delivery. Certification/licensure assures the public that professionals have met certain minimum standards (academic coursework and practica) needed to deliver appropriate services. The setting of minimum standards for professional practice is generally done by practicing professionals using their best judgment based on their experience. Although there is a general assumption that this ensures consumers quality services, there are no objective data yet to demonstrate that practitioners in states that require licensure provide better quality services than those in states that do not.

Although most professionals are certified and/or licensed in their broad areas of professional practice (e.g., special education or speech-language pathology), there is currently no form of credentialing for AAC. Organizations such as the American Speech-Language-Hearing Association (ASHA), Rehabilitation Engineering and Assistive Technology Society of North America (RESNA), and the United States Society for Augmentative and Alternative Communication (USSAAC), however, have formed committees to consider the possibility of some type of AAC credentialing.

Collaboration and Support Services

The movement away from providing services to individuals on a one-to-one basis or in small segregated groups toward providing services to individuals within classroom settings, illustrates an increasing appreciation for developing functional communication skills within a natural environment. Increasingly, this model depends on the collaborative efforts of the classroom teacher, special educator, speech-language pathologist, and a host of other communication partners who interact with AAC users during day-to-day routines. The special educator and speech-language pathologist serve increasingly as consultants and less often as direct service providers. There are many subjective reports on the increased effectiveness of this approach. No objective, controlled data on the comparative effects of services delivered directly and services delivered through collaborative/consultant approaches, however, have been made available. Similarly, relatively little information exists on the relationship between the support of administrators, teachers, parents, and community on the availability and effective use of AAC. Data on these relationships are needed to understand the parameters that will increase the acceptance and effective use of AAC.

Funding

Although laws are in place that outline the rights of individuals with disabilities to services, the laws are interpreted, implemented, and enforced in a variety of ways. Various associations such as the American Association on Mental Retardation (AAMR), ASHA, Council for Exceptional Children (CEC), and RESNA, as part of their legislative and government agendas, must make AAC research one of their most critical priorities in order to build a more solid, uniform foundation on which to make judgments that will improve services for individuals with severe disabilities.

Federal vs. State Control of Funding. Political changes surrounding issues of integration throughout the 1960s had an impact on individuals with disabilities in the 1970s. These political forces led to legislation for educating individuals with disabilities, eliminating discrimination in the workplace, increasing accessibility of buildings, and facilitating the use of technology. In the 1990s, changes in the political makeup of Congress and the philosophies of newly elected representatives are having significant effects on the funding of a number of programs, including health care and special education. Much of the legislation that parents and professionals vigorously fought for is in danger of being severely reduced, altered in form, or even eliminated. Proposed actions threaten the well-being of individuals with disabilities. Although the federal government has played a significant role in developing these programs to benefit individuals with disabilities in the past, the trend is toward more state control of monies. Some judgments on the potential effects of these changes can be surmised by examining the status of services prior to the 1960s, but it is too soon to predict the consequences. The legislation and practices of the past 30 years may influence state officials to maintain quality services in the future, but this is not ensured. Comparing the extent and quality of services funded and controlled by the federal government with those funded and controlled by the state government may provide interesting insights as to which is really better. The underlying issue in such a comparison is whether the AAC user's needs can be met in a cost-effective manner.

School vs. Medical Funding. Funding of communication devices has generally come from a variety of sources. An advantage of funding devices through third-party providers such as Medicaid, Medicare, or private insurance has been that they are considered the property of AAC users and can be used in every setting. The underlying justification for procuring communication devices in most cases, however, has been medical need. When schools have funded devices, they are often available to children only at school. A major result of the Tech Act (PL 100-407, 1988) and a series of interpretations by the Office of Special Education Programs (OSEP), however, resulted in an increase in the number of schools that make communication devices available to children for use both in and out of school. The determination of funding in these cases is made on the basis of educational need as determined by the individualized education program (IEP).

Financial need has typically not been a consideration in securing funding to purchase a communication device. As funds become more difficult to obtain, however, this may change. Data will be needed to determine how funding affects the availability of communication devices. As cost factors are considered, effective use of funded devices becomes an increasingly important consideration. Expensive communication devices bought for AAC users end up on storage shelves for a variety of reasons (e.g., clinicians/educators may find them too difficult to operate or too inconvenient for use in daily routines). Trial use of devices through loan programs or lease options from manufacturers can increase the probability of an appropriate match of client needs and device features, and better understanding of the use of the device by the clinician/educator or caregiver. Data on the effectiveness of loan programs and long-term device usage by AAC users, caregivers, and members of the educational/rehabilitation team are needed.

Effectiveness, Efficacy, and Outcome Measurement

With changes in health-care policies and the expressed needs of third-party providers for cost-effectiveness, therapy outcome evaluation is in increasing demand. One form of outcome evaluation is functional assessment, which is based on observational judgment ratings of an individual's effectiveness of communication in natural, daily activities. Functional assessment is based on neither individual disabilities nor potential. In response to these pressures, ASHA has developed the Functional Assessment of Communicative Skills (FACS), which has four assessment domains: (1)

social communication, (2) communication of basic needs, (3) reading, writing, and number concepts, and (4) daily planning (Frattali et al., 1995).

The FACS was developed by examining functional assessments already in use for specific disorders and developing a similar tool that addressed their limitations. The resulting instrument was refined according to the comments of peer reviewers. Among advantages of the FACS are its administration time (20 minutes), ease of administration and scoring, and more general assessment of functional communication based on observations of performance in common situations. The fact that rated levels of performance are described increases the reliability of administration and scoring. Overall, there is a potential for comprehensive data collection on therapy approaches used with a number of individuals with a wide variety of communication disabilities. On the down side, however, because the FACS is relatively short and nonspecific to disorders, it has limited sensitivity to gradations of behavior change and is not useful for analyzing differences resulting from treatment interaction with the characteristics and functions of individuals with specific disorders. Therefore, the FACS may be of value as a general measure of pre- and post-therapy skills but not as an ongoing measure of progress throughout therapy. Research comparing the results of this instrument with others will be needed to understand the relationships and the meanings of change across instruments.

Another form of outcome measurement involves goal attainment scaling (Granlund, 1993), which involves rating the attainment of goals not according to norms or criterion, but rather according to expectancy. The goals that have been established are periodically rated as having been attained below, at, or above the expected level.

SUMMARY

AAC is not an end in itself, but rather the means to an end. It goes far beyond enabling individuals to gain attention, make choices, and express wants and needs. The purpose of AAC is to enable individuals who cannot communicate through natural speech and/or writing to communicate through augmentative and/or alternative means as effectively as possible with whomever they choose in whatever environments they choose. AAC provides the means to initiate and maintain interactions that provide opportunities to influence others and assume status in society. AAC is the means to an end of acquiring fuller participation in endeavors of choice and enjoying a richer quality of life.

APPENDIX A

CHARACTERISTICS AND FEATURE GUIDES

This appendix includes characteristic and/or feature guides for the analysis of both specific components and multicomponent aspects of augmentative and alternative communication (AAC) systems. Appendices A-1, A-2, and A-3* provide guides to assist clinicians/educators in identifying and describing features of AAC devices, switches, and symbols. Appendices A-4[†] and A-5[‡] provide guides for viewing the broader aspects of AAC components and systems. Appendix A-6 provides a feature checklist for matching AAC technology to the strengths and needs of the AAC user.

*Developed by Karen Kate Kellum and Amy Waller as part of the AAC Personnel Preparation Program at Purdue University, which is partially funded by the U. S. Department of Education OSERS/OSEP Grant No. HO29B20148-95 (L. L. Lloyd & H. H. Arvidson, project co-directors). However, the contents of this material do not necessarily represent the policy of that agency nor endorsement by the federal government. The developers acknowledge the contributions of several of the chapter authors of this text and members of the Purdue AAC Group, especially Lyle L. Lloyd, Lisa Pufpaff, and Raymond W. Quist.

†Previously published by Vanderheiden & Lloyd (1986) in the introductory AAC text published by the American Speech-Language-Hearing Association.

‡From AAC feature-matching software (McNairn & Smith, 1996) produced by Doug Dodgen & Associates.

Appendix A-1 AAC Symbol Set and System Guide

Symbol Set/System _____   Publisher/Vendor _____

DIRECTIONS: CHECK ALL THAT APPLY

_____ aided

    _____ objects

    _____ photographs

    _____ colored pictures

    _____ detailed line drawings

    _____ line drawings

    _____ pictographs

    _____ graphic representations of manual signs or gestures

    _____ logographs

    _____ modified symbols

    _____ modified orthography

    _____ traditional orthography

    _____ graphic representations of fingerspelling

    _____ tactile, static codes (e.g., Braille)

    _____ electronic tactile codes

    _____ synthetic speech

    _____ other _____

_____ set

_____ system

_____ dynamic

_____ static

_____ primarily iconic

    _____ primarily transparent

    _____ primarily translucent

_____ primarily opaque

_____ symbols are modifiable

_____ symbols are easy to produce/draw in real time

_____ unaided

    _____ gestures

    _____ manually coded languages (e.g., Signed English)

    _____ fingerspelling or manual alphabet

    _____ eye-blink, gestural, and/or vocal alphabet codes

    _____ vibrotactile codes (e.g., Tadoma)

    _____ hand-cued speech

    _____ vocalizations

    _____ natural speech

    _____ other _____

    _____ symbols can represent concrete ideas

    _____ symbols can represent abstract ideas

_____ gloss present

    _____ above symbol

    _____ below symbol

    _____ English

    _____ other language(s)

    _____ modifiable

_____ two-colored (e.g., black and white)

_____ multicolored

_____ commercially available

_____ fabricated

_____ idiosyncratic

DIRECTIONS: COMPLETE ADDITIONAL INFORMATION

Estimated dimensions: _____   Modifiable? _____

Describe the iconicity (if any) of this symbol set/system:

Describe the complexity of this symbol set/system:

Describe the perceptual distinctiveness of this symbol set/system (e.g., presence of minimal pairs):

Describe other visual characteristics of this symbol set/system (e.g., contrast, boldness):

Describe a distinctive feature of this symbol set/system:

Describe a possible reason you might choose this symbol set/system:

Describe a possible reason you might not choose this symbol set/system:

Selected Reference

Lloyd, L. L., & Kangas, K. K. (1994). Augmentative and alternative communication. In G. H. Shames, E. Wiig, & W. Secord (Eds.), *Human communication disorders* (4th ed., pp. 606–657). Boston: Allyn & Bacon. (Originally published by Merrill/Macmillan Publishing Co.)

Appendix A-2   AAC Switch Guide

Name of Switch _____   Manufacturer/Vendor _____

DIRECTIONS: CHECK ALL THAT APPLY

Input Type

_____ contact (zero pressure)

_____ eye movement/eye gaze

_____ motion (e.g., changes in switch orientation)

_____ photosensitive

_____ physioelectric (muscle contraction)

_____ pneumatic

_____ pressure sensitive

_____ sound (e.g., vocalization, noise)

Output Type

_____ dual switch (e.g., rocking)

_____ joystick

_____ multiple switches (e.g., armslot)

_____ single switch

Type of Feedback

_____ auditory

_____ tactile

_____ vibrotactile

_____ visual

DIRECTIONS: COMPLETE ADDITIONAL INFORMATION

Estimated amount of force necessary to activate switch: _____

Estimated travel (distance from resting position to actual switch closure): _____

Estimated weight: _____   Estimated dimensions: _____

Estimated size of activation surface: _____   Moisture resistant? _____

Possible body sites:

Describe how this switch can be mounted:

Describe other features of this switch:

Describe a distinctive feature of this switch:

Describe a possible reason you might choose this switch:

Describe a possible reason you might not choose this switch:

Selected References

Brandenburg, S. A., & Vanderheiden, G. C. (Eds.). (1987). *Communication, control, and computer access for disabled and elderly individuals: Switches and environmental controls.* Boston: College-Hill Press.

Goossens', C., & Crain, S. S. (1992). *Utilizing switch interfaces with children who are severely physically challenged.* Austin, TX: Pro-Ed.

Appendix A-3   AAC Device Guide

Name of Device _____   Manufacturer/Vendor _____

DIRECTIONS: CHECK ALL THAT APPLY

Input Methods

_____ contact (e.g., membrane)

_____ eye movement/eye gaze

_____ joystick

_____ mouse

_____ photosensitive

_____ pressure (e.g., keyboard)

     _____ modifiable pressure

_____ speech recognition

_____ switch

     _____ single

     _____ multiple

_____ trackball

_____ trackpad

Selection Techniques

_____ direct selection

_____ scanning

     _____ auditory

     _____ visual

        _____ automatic linear

        _____ directed

        _____ frequency of use

        _____ inverse

        _____ step linear

Interface Capabilities

_____ computer/command language

     _____ Apple

     _____ Macintosh

     _____ DOS

     _____ Windows

_____ directly to external printer

Encoding/Retrieval Methods

_____ memory-based encoding (e.g., alpha and/or numeric encoding, abbreviations, logical letter coding)

_____ conceptual/semantic encoding (e.g., icons or pictures)

_____ visual/motor coding (e.g., HANDS, VoisShapes)

_____ chart/display-based

_____ levels

_____ message prediction

_____ Morse code

_____ other _____

Output Capabilities

_____ auditory

     _____ digitized

     _____ synthesized

        _____ stored (e.g., VoCaid)

        _____ phonetic (e.g., Echo II)

        _____ phonetic systems using linear predictive coding (e.g., DECtalk)

_____ visual display

     _____ cathode-ray tube

     _____ light-emiting diode

     _____ liquid crystal display

     _____ plasma

     _____ monochrome

     _____ color

     _____ backlit

     _____ sidelit

_____ printed

     _____ internal

     _____ external

DIRECTIONS: COMPLETE ADDITIONAL INFORMATION

Vocabulary size: _____   Amount of time: _____   Number of messages: _____

Estimated weight: _____   Estimated dimensions: _____

List available overlay configurations for this device (e.g., 2 locations, 32 locations, customized):

List any preprogrammed vocabulary/symbols that may be available for this device:

Describe how a switch can be interfaced/mounted:

Describe the portability of this device:

Describe a distinctive feature of this device:

Describe a possible reason you might choose this device:

Describe a possible reason you might not choose this device:

Selected References

Beukelman, D. R., & Mirenda, P. (1992). *Augmentative and alternative communication: Management of severe communication disorders in children and adults.* Baltimore: Paul H. Brookes.

Brandenburg, S. A., & Vanderheiden, G. C. (Eds.). (1987). *Communication, control, and computer access for disabled and elderly individuals: Switches and environmental controls.* Boston: College-Hill Press.

Church, G., & Glennen, S. (1992). *The handbook of assistive technology.* San Diego: Singular.

Goossens', C., & Crain, S. S. (1992). *Utilizing switch interfaces with children who are severely physically challenged.* Austin, TX: Pro-Ed.

PennTech (1991). *Self-guided device feature worksheet.* Harrisburg, PA: Author.

Appendix A-4   AAC Multicomponent Communication System Requirements

A multicomponent system has different symbols, techniques (with aids as required), and strategies that are used together to meet an individual's overall needs and constraints. The following checklist is useful in evaluating the systems of individual clients. Remember that the questions apply to the overall system of symbols, techniques, and strategies, not just to a single symbol/technique.

Checklist for Client's System

Yes	No	
		A. PROVIDES FULL RANGE OF COMMUNICATIVE FUNCTIONS - Communication of basic needs - Conversation - Writing and messaging - Drawing - Computer access (electronic communication, learning, and information systems) **B. COMPATIBLE WITH OTHER ASPECTS OF INDIVIDUAL'S LIFE** - Seating system and *all* other positions - Mobility - Environmental controls - Other devices, teaching approaches, etc., in the environment **C. DOES NOT RESTRICT COMMUNICATION PARTNERS** - Totally obvious yes/no for strangers (from 3–5 feet away) - Usable/understandable with strangers and those not familiar with special techniques or symbols - Promotes face-to-face communication - Usable with peers/community - Usable with groups **D. USABLE IN ALL ENVIRONMENTS AND PHYSICAL POSITIONS** - Always with the person (always working) - Functions in noisy environments - Withstands physically hostile environments (sandbox, beach, travel, classroom) **E. DOES NOT RESTRICT TOPIC OR SCOPE OF COMMUNICATION** - Any topic, word, idea can be expressed - Open vocabulary - User definable vocabulary **F. EFFECTIVE** - Maximum possible rate (for both Quicktalk and Exacttalk) - Very quick method for key messages (phatic, emergency, control) - Yes/no communicable from a distance - Basic needs communicable from a distance - Ability to interrupt - Ability to secure and maintain speaking turn (e.g., override interruptions) - Ability to control message content (e.g., not be interpreted) - Ability to overlay emphasis or emotion on top of message - Low fatigue - Special superefficient techniques for those close to individual **G. ALLOWS AND FOSTERS GROWTH** - Appropriate to individual's current skills - Allows growth in vocabulary, topic, grammar, uses - New vocabulary, aspects easily learned **H. ACCEPTABLE AND MOTIVATING TO USER AND OTHERS** - Individual - Family - Peers/friends - Education or employment environment **I. AFFORDABLE** - Purchase - Maintenance

Appendix A-5   Functional Dimensions of Individual System Components

DIMENSION	DEFINITION	IMPORTANCE/IMPACT
Functionality/Ability to Meet Needs		
Openness	Ability to express any thought	Reduces topic limitations Allows individual to advance on own
Speed	Rate of communication	Provides more effective system Easier for younger and retarded
Assertability	Ability to interrupt; resist interruptions; and control conversation	Provides more effective system Prevents frustration, shutdown
Display permanence	Permanence of the presentation or display (temporary dynamic, temporary static, displayed, printed)	Meets writing needs Provides time to decipher Provides access to other words through cues Improves rate of communication; not necessary to wait for message receiver Provides feedback for growth, learning
Projection	Ability to communicate from a distance	Allows communication to/with groups Allows communication at a distance
Correctability	Ability to unambiguously repair or correct utterances	Improves clarity Allows accurate representation Facilitates learning Increases motivation
Expandability	Ability of users to expand the vocabulary	Allows user to expand topics Allows vocabulary growth
Availability/Usability		
Portability	Ability to conveniently stay with the person at all times	Can be with user in all environments
Position independence	Ability to be used in any and all positions (wheelchair, couch, standing, lying down)	Increases availability Allows use with people available only in certain environments
Independence	Ability to be used without an assistant or interpreter	Increases effectiveness Increases motivation Lowers cost to use
Intelligibility/obviousness	Ability to be understood by strangers	Increases potential communication partners, strangers Facilitates learning
Appropriateness	Appropriate to individual's current and future abilities (physical, cognitive, language, etc.)	Increased effectiveness Facilitates growth
Durability	Ruggedness, reliability	Is more often available for use (not broken) Can go with user to more places
Total cost	Cost of purchase, maintenance, training, and assistants or aides required for use	Decreases cost
Acceptability/Compatibility with Environment		
Cosmesis	Appearance, attractiveness	Improves acceptability to user, others Increases communication partners (e.g., isn't removed in public)
Materials/practice compatibility	Compatibility of technique with materials and practices of educational or employment settings	Facilitates use at school or job Increases acceptability to teachers, employers
Similarity	Similarity to communication system of peers and community	Allows more communication partners Increases number of models for the user Is more acceptable
Training	Amount of training required of user, clinicians, others	Improves ability to learn how to use the system when resources are limited Reduces cost overall
Adaptability	Ability to be customized to individual's needs, abilities, and constraints	Facilitates adaptation to user's other aids Facilitates vocabulary customization Allows fine tuning for speed, function
Interdevice compatibility	Ability to use with other standard devices in the environment	Allows access to electronic communication, learning, or information systems in environment Allows control of devices in environment
Computer compatibility	Ability to implement the technique (or symbols) on standard computers	Provides low-cost writing system Allows computer-aided teaching

Appendix A-6   Feature Checklist

Device Evaluation Sheet

Device Type: _____

Vendor: _____

Phone: _____   Fax: _____

Language Organization/Encoding Methods

☐ Abbreviation expansion   ☐ Levels/themes/pages   ☐ Symbols

☐ Branching   ☐ Numeric codes   ☐ Symbol sequencing

☐ Letters/words   ☐ Photographs   ☐ Word prediction

Additional Language Features

☐ Foreign language capabilities   ☐ Language application program

Speech Output

☐ Digitized   Digitized memory: _____

☐ Synthesized   Synthesized memory: _____

☐ Adjustable volume   ☐ Multiple voice option   ☐ Expandable digitized memory

Direct Select Input

☐ Alternate keyboard   ☐ Uses direct select input   ☐ Remote infrared system

☐ Auditory prompts   ☐ Infrared system   ☐ Standard keyboard

☐ Eye gaze   ☐ Optical pointer   ☐ Touch screen

Scanning/Switch Input

☐ Auditory scanning   ☐ Uses scanning/switch input   ☐ Predictive

☐ Auto   ☐ Column/row   ☐ Quarter/row/column

☐ Block/row/column   ☐ Inverse/hold   ☐ Row/column

☐ Centering   ☐ Linear   ☐ Step

☐ Circular   ☐ Morse code

Keyboard

☐ Standard   ☐ Membrane   ☐ Variable key size

☐ Keyguard

Keys

Size/selection area: _____   Sensitivity: _____

Feedback

☐ Auditory feedback   ☐ Tactile feedback   ☐ Visual feedback

Device Evaluation Sheet (*continued*)

Switch Types

Switch count:

☐ Cheek

☐ Cup

☐ Joystick

☐ Light touch

☐ Leaf

☐ Mercury

☐ Mouse

☐ Photo cell

☐ Pillow

☐ Plate

☐ Pneumatic/sip-and-puff

☐ Pressure

☐ Rocking lever

☐ Sensor

☐ Toggle

☐ Tongue

☐ Trackball

☐ Wobble

Display Type

☐ Active matrix color

☐ Passive matrix color

☐ LCD

☐ Display available

☐ Monochrome

☐ Static display

☐ Display backlighting

☐ Dynamic display

Display Size: _____

Printer

☐ Built-in

☐ External interface

Mounting Options Available

☐ Belt

☐ Carrying case

☐ Desktop mounting

☐ Strap

☐ Walker mounting

☐ Rigid wheelchair mounting

☐ Swing-away wheelchair mounting

Power Sources

☐ AC power supply

Battery Type

☐ Alkaline

☐ Nicad

☐ Lead

☐ Other

☐ Lithium ion

Battery Replacement

☐ Field replacement

☐ Factory replacement

Battery life: _____

Additional Features

Price: _____

Weight: _____

Programming difficulty: _____

Dimensions: _____

☐ Calculator

☐ Computer interface

☐ Environmental control interface

☐ Icon prediction

☐ Notebook function

☐ Scratch pad

☐ Warranty

Support Options

☐ Manuals

☐ Training

☐ Video

AAC RESOURCES AND ORGANIZATIONS*

This sample of resources includes the names, addresses, and phone numbers of companies and organizations related to augmentative and alternative communication (AAC). It is not intended to be comprehensive. The resources are organized into four groups.

Appendix B-1   Developers, Manufacturers, and Vendors

This appendix lists a variety of companies and organizations that develop, manufacture, and/or market products for individuals with a variety of communication disabilities including individuals who use AAC. It includes information about companies referred to in Chapter 10 and Appendix C. Some of the entries include notations in italics referring to the general types of products available (e.g., adaptive equipment, VOCA, aided symbols) or list specific equipment (e.g., Switch 'n See, AudioScan, Readman). This terminology is consistent with the text, with two major exceptions: (1) *VOCA* is used to refer only to high technology devices that have voice output, and (2) *communication aid* refers to low technology items such as rotary scanners and communication boards. A few other terms merit descriptions: (1) *manual communication* refers to all types of unaided communication including sign languages, fingerspelling, and gestures, (2) *vision technology* refers to items intended for persons with visual impairments except for those items specifically noted as Braille products, and (3) *resource material* refers to print items. Some notations include only specific items associated with a particular company or organization. Companies that are members of the Communication Aid Manufacturers Association (CAMA) are indicated in bold.

Ability Research, Inc., PO Box 1721, Minnetonka, MN 55345; Tel. 612-939-0121; *Action Voice*

AbleNet, Inc., 1081 Tenth Ave. SE, Minneapolis, MN 55414-1312; Tel. 800-322-0956, 612-379-0956, Fax 612-379-9143; *mounting systems, switches, toys, aided symbols, input adaptations, resource materials, environmental control*; CAMA Member

Access Unlimited, 3535 Briarpark Dr., Suite 102, Houston, TX 77042-5235; Tel. 800-848-0311, 713-781-7441; *Proword Talking Word Processor*

Acrontech International, Inc., The Williamsville Executive Center, 5500 Main St., Williamsville, NY 14221; Tel. 716-854-3814, Fax 716-854-4014; *vision technology*

Activating Children Through Technology, Project ACTT, 27 Horrabin Hall, Western Illinois University, Macomb, IL 61455; Tel. 309-298-1014; *Switch 'n See*

ADAMLAB, Wayne County RESA, 33500 Van Born Rd., Wayne, MI 48184; Tel. 313-467-1610, Fax 313-326-2610; *VOCAs, communication aids*

AdaptAbility, PO Box 515, Colchester, CT 06415-0515; Tel. 800-243-9232, 203-537-3451; *communication aids, adaptive equipment*

*Compiled by Lisa Pufpaff and Lyle L. Lloyd. The compilers acknowledge the contributions of several of the chapter authors in this text and members of the Purdue AAC Group, especially Colleen Haney, Raymond W. Quist, and Amy Waller. The development of these resource lists was partially supported by the U.S. Department of Education's Office of Special Education Programs (OSEP) funded project for master's students titled An Augmentative and Alternative Communication Preparation Program for Special Educators and Speech-Language Pathologists (Lyle L. Lloyd and Helen H. Arvidson, project co-directors), and the Indiana Department of Education's Division of Special Education through a subcontract from the Technology/Communication Project (T/CP) of the Porter County Education Interlocal (Nancy Martin, project director). Funding of these agencies does not necessarily imply endorsement of the views of the presenters or the content of the material presented.

Adaptive Aids, Inc., 1716 E Glen, Tucson, AZ 85713; Tel. 602-745-8112, 800-223-5369 Ext. 357, Fax 602-745-9749; *switch interface, switches*

Adaptivation, PO Box 1401, Sioux Falls, SD 57101-1401; Tel: 800-723-2783, 605-335-4445, Fax: 605-335-4446; (e-mail: adaptaac@aol.com; Web site: http://users.aol.com/adaptaac); **CAMA Member**

Adaptive Communication Systems (ACS) Technologies, Inc., 1400 Lee Dr., Suite 3, Corapolis, PA 15108; Tel. 412-269-6656, Fax 412-269-6675; *VOCAs, speech synthesizers, environmental control*

AdaptTech, Inc., ISU Research Park, 2501 North Loop Dr., Ames, IA 50010; Tel. 800-723-2783, 515-296-7171, Fax 515-296-9910; *communication aids, switches*; **CAMA Member**

AICOM Corporation, 1590 Oakland Rd., Suite B112, San Jose, CA 95131; Tel. 408-453-8251; *speech synthesizers*

American Guidance Service (AGS), Inc., 4201 Woodland Rd., PO Box 99, Circle Pines, MN 55014-1796; Tel. 800-328-2560; *resource materials and tests*

American Printing House for the Blind, 1839 Frankfort Ave., PO Box 6085, Louisville, KY 40206-0085; Tel. 502-895-2405; *Speaqualizer*

Apple Computer Disability Solutions Store, The, PO Box 898, Lakewood, NJ 08701-9930; Tel. 800-600-7808; 800-755-0601(TDD)

Apple Computer, Inc., Worldwide Disability Solutions Group, One Infinite Loop, MS 38DS, Cupertino, CA 95014; Tel. 800-600-7808, 408-974-7910(V); 408-974-7911(TDD); *Closeview*

Arkenstone, 1390 Borregas Ave., Sunnyvale, CA 94089; Tel. 800-444-4443, 408-752-2200, Fax 408-745-6739; *vision technology*

Arroyo & Associates, Inc., 2549 Rockville Centre Pkwy., Oceanside, NY 11572; Tel. 516-763-1407, Fax 516-766-4119; *aided symbols, input adaptations*

Artic Technologies International, Inc., 55 Park St., Suite 2, Troy, MI 48083; Tel. 313-588-7370, Fax 313-588-2650; *speech synthesizers, vision technology*

Artificial Language Laboratory, Michigan State University, 405 Computer Center, East Lansing, MI 48824-1042; Tel. 517-353-5399; *photoelectric switch*

Arts Computer Products, Inc., 33 Richdale Ave., PO Box 604, Cambridge, MA 02140; Tel. 800-343-0095; *Perfect Scribe*

Assistive Technology, Inc., 850 Boylston Street, Chestnut Hill, MA 02167-2402; Tel: 800-793-9227, 617-731-4900, Fax: 617-731-5201; (Web site: http://www.assistivetech.com/); **CAMA Member**

Attainment Company, Inc., PO Box 930160, Verona, WI 53593-0160; Tel. 800-327-4269, 608-854-7880; *Picture Cue Dictionary, Picture Prompt System*

Automated Functions, Inc., 6424 N 28th St., Arlington, VA 22207; Tel. 703-536-7741; *SmarTalk*

Automated Voice Systems, Inc., See TBS Marketing; *environmental control*

Baggeboda Press, Route 1, Box 2315, Unity, ME 04988; Tel. 207-437-2746, Fax 207-437-2404; *PICSYMS Dictionary, DynaSyms*

Berkeley Systems, Inc., 2095 Rose St., Berkeley, CA 94709; Tel. 510-540-5535, Fax 510-540-5115; *vision technology*

Blissymbolics Communication International (BCI), 1630 Lawrence Ave. West, Suite 104, Toronto, Ontario, M2J 4S9, Canada; Tel. 416-242-2222; *Blissymbols*

BrainTrain (tash), 727 Twin Ridge Lane, Richmond, VA 23235; Tel. 800-446-5456, 804-320-0105; *software, resource material*

Bright Star Technology, 1450 114th Ave. SE, Suite 200, Bellevue, WA 98004; Tel. 206-562-6050

Burkhart, Linda J., 8503 Rhode Island Ave., College Park, MD 20740; Tel. 301-345-9152; *resource materials, switches, adaptive equipment*

Canon USA, Inc., One Canon Plaza, Lake Success, NY 11042; Tel. 516-488-6700; *VOCAs, adaptive equipment*

C.J.T. Enterprises, 3625 W MacArthur Blvd., Suite 301, Santa Ana, CA 92704; Tel. 714-751-6295, Fax 714-751-5775; *mobility products*

Cleo, Inc., 3957 Mayfield Rd., Cleveland, OH 44121; Tel. 800-321-0595, 216-382-9700, Fax 216-382-1934; *rehabilitation equipment*

Communication Aids, 324 Acre Ave., Brownsburg, IN 46112; *aided symbols*

Communication Devices, Inc., 421 Coeur d' Alene Avenue, Ste. 5, Coeur d' Alene, ID 83814-2862; Tel: 800-60-HOLLY, 208-765-1259, Fax 208-765-1529; (e-mail: hollycom@nidlink.com); **CAMA Member**

Communication Skill Builders. See Psychological Corp.; Tel. 800-866-4446(V/TDD) (e-mail: dawn_dunleavy.@hbtc.com); *resource materials*

Compeer, Inc., 1409 Graywood Dr., San Jose, CA 95129; Tel. 408-255-3950; *PC-Voice, Porta-Voice*

COMPIC Development Association, PO Box 351, N. Baldwyn, Victoria 3104, Australia; *COMPICS*

ComputAbility Corp., 40000 Grand River, Suite 109, Novi, MI 48375; Tel. 800-433-8872, 313-477-6720, Fax 313-477-6324; *aided symbols, input adaptations, hardware, software, speech synthesizers, environmental control, mounting systems, switches*

Computer Conversations, 6297 Worthington Rd. SW, Alexandria, OH 43001; Tel. 614-924-2885, 614-924-3325; *Verbette Mark I and II*

Computers to Help People, Inc., 1221 West Johnson St., Madison, WI 53715; Tel. 608-257-5917; *hardware, speech synthesizers, software*

Consultants for Communication Technology, 508 Bellevue Terrace, Pittsburgh, PA 15202; Tel. 412-761-6062, Fax 412-761-7336; *Handy Speech Communication Aide, environmental control*; **CAMA Member**

Covox, Inc., 675 Conger St., Eugene, OR 97402; Tel. 503-342-1271; *Speech Thing*

Creative Communicating, PO Box 3358, Park City, UT 84060; Tel. 801-645-7737; (e-mail: Playware@aol.com); *software, adaptive equipment*

Creative Switch Industries, PO Box 5256, Des Moines, IA 50306; Tel. 800-257-4385, 515-287-5748; *environmental control, mounting systems, switches*

Crestwood Company, 6625 N Sidney Place, Milwaukee, WI 53209-3259; Tel. 414-352-5678, Fax 414-352-5679; *communication aids, input adaptations, switches, Talking Pictures, VOCAs, toys*; **CAMA Member**

DawnSignPress, 9080 Activity Road, Suite A, San Diego, CA 92126-4421; Tel. 619-549-5330(V/TDD), Fax 619-549-2200; *manual communication products, resource materials*

Designing Aids for Disabled Adults, 249 Concord Ave, #2, Toronto, Ontario M6H 2P4, Canada; Tel. 416-530-0038; *keyboard interface, alternate keyboard*

Detroit Institute for Children, 5447 Woodward Ave., Detroit, MI 48202; Tel. 313-832-1100; *AudioScan*

Dickey Engineering, 3 Angel Rd., North Reading, MA 01864; Tel. 508-664-2010, Fax 508-664-4467; *input adaptations, switches*

Digital Equipment Corporation, 146 Main St., Maynard, MA 01754; *DECtalk*

Don Johnston Incorporated, PO Box 639, 1000 N Rand Rd, Bldg 115, Wauconda, IL 60084-0639; Tel. 800-999-4660, 708-526-2682, Fax 708-526-4177; (e-mail: DIDE@aol.com; Web site: http://www.donjohnston.com); *aided symbols, assessment tools, adaptive input, mounting systems, switches, environmental control, hardware, software, resource materials, speech synthesizers*; **CAMA Member**

Dragon Systems, Inc., 320 Nevada St., Newton, MA 02160; Tel. 617-965-5200, Fax 617-527-0372; (e-mail: info@dragonsys.com; Web site: www.dragonsys.com); *voice recognition*

DU-IT Control Systems Group, 8765 Twp. Rd. 513, Shreve, OH 44676-9421; Tel. 216-567-2906; *hardware, input adaptations*

Dunamis, Inc., 3580 Hwy. 317, Suwanee, GA 30174; Tel. 800-828-2443, 404-932-0485, Fax 404-932-0486; (e-mail: dunamis@aol.com); *adaptive input, alternative keyboard*

Duxbury Systems, Inc., 435 King St., PO Box 1504, Littleton, MA 01460; Tel. 508-486-9766, Fax 508-486-9712; *Braille products*

Ednick Communications, Inc., PO Box 3612, Portland, OR 97208; *aided symbols, manual communication products*

EduQuest Courseware Center (IBM), 101 Union St., PO Box 1000, Plymouth, MI 48170-9989; Tel. 800-426-4338; *Primary Editor Plus*

EKEG Electronics Co. Ltd., PO Box 46199, Station G, Vancouver, B.C., Canada V6R 4G5; Tel. 604-273-4358, Fax 604-273-1148; (e-mail: richmush@Direct.ca); *alternate keyboards, input adaptations, hardware*

Electronic Speech Enhancement, Inc., 143 McDonnell Boulevard, Bldg. B, St. Louis, MO 63042-2309; Tel: 888-463-7353, 314-731-1000, Fax 314-731-1130; (Web site: http://www.SpeechEnhancer.com); **CAMA Member**

ENABLE, Schneier Communication Unit, 1603 Court St., Syracuse, NY 13208; Tel. 315-455-7591; *software (environmental control, scanning, direct selection)*

Enabling You, 4024 Black Hawk Rd., Rock Island, IL 61201-7164; Tel. 309-788-9775, Fax 309-788-8680; *adaptive equipment*

First Byte, Inc., 19840 Pioneer Ave., Torrence, CA 90503-1660; *Kid Talk, SmoothTalker, Speller Bee*

Franklin Learning Resources, 122 Burrs Rd., Mt. Holly, NJ 08060; Tel. 800-525-9673, 609-261-4800, Fax 609-261-8368; *Language Master*

Gallaudet University Press, Kendall Green, PO Box 300, Washington, DC 20002; *manual communication products*

Ginny Brady-Dobson, 89623 Demming Rd., Elmira, OR 97437; *Brady-Dobson Alternative Communication (B-DAC) Symbols*

Great Talking Box Co., The, 2211B Fortune Dr., San Jose, CA 94043; Tel. 800-361-8255, 408-456-0133, Fax 408-456-0134; *input adaptations, VOCA (EasyTalk)*

Gus Communications, Inc., 3838 W. King Edward Ave., Vancouver, B.C. V65 1N1 Canada; Tel. 604-224-6699, Fax 604-224-5516; (e-mail: gus@gusinc.com; Web site: http://www.gusinc.com); **CAMA Member**

GW Micro, Inc., 310 Racquet Dr., Fort Wayne, IN 46825; Tel. 219-483-3625, Fax 219-484-2510; (e-mail: support@gwmicro.com; Web site: www.gwmicro.com); *vision technology*

Handicapped Childrens Technical Services, Box 7, Foster, RI 02825; *switches, toys, hardware, software, environmental control*

Health Concepts, Inc., 19 E Central Ave., Paoli, PA 19301; Tel. 800-721-4848, Fax 610-640-4488; *UltraVoice*

HEARIT Co., 8346 North Mammoth Drive, Tucson, AZ 85743-1046; Tel: 800-298-7184, 520-579-2026, Fax: 520-579-3363; **CAMA Member**

Helen Keller National Center, 112 Middle Neck Rd., Sands Point, NY 11050-1299; Tel. 800-255-0411 Ext. 311; *deaf/blind materials*

H.K. EyeCan Ltd., 36 Burland St., Ottawa, Ontario K2B 6J8 Canada; Tel. 800-356-3362, 613-828-0056, Fax 613-356-3362; *VisionKey*

Hooleon Corporation, 260 Justin Dr., Cottonwood, AZ 86326; Tel. 800-937-1337, 602-634-7515, Fax 602-634-4620; *keyboard enhancement products*

HumanWare, Inc., 6245 King Rd., Loomis, CA 95650; Tel. 800-722-3393, Fax 916-652-7296; (Web site: http://humanware.com); *aided symbols*

IBM Educational Systems, PO Box 950, Internal Zip 5432, Boca Raton, FL 33432; Tel. 800-284-9482(TDD), 800-426-2133, 407-982-9099; *IBM AccessDOS, IBM Personal dictation system*

Imaginart Communication Products, 307 Arizona St., Bisbee, AZ 85603; Tel. 800-828-1376, 602-432-5741, Fax 602-432-5134; (e-mail: imaginart@aol.com); *instructional materials, software, resource materials, assessment tools, aided symbols*; **CAMA Member**

INCAP, GmbH; Wohlichstr 6-8, 75179 Pfrozheim, Germany; Tel. 49-7231-0, Fax 49-7231-9463-0; (e-mail: INCAP@T-online.de; Web site: http://www.incap.de); *Micro Keyboard, software for communication boards*

Independent Living Aids, Inc., 27 East Mall, Plainview, NY 11803; Tel. 800-537-2118, Fax 516-752-3135; *vision technology*

Infogrip, Inc., 5800 One Perkins Pl., Suite 5F, Baton Rouge, LA 70808; Tel. 504-766-8082; (e-mail: infogrip@infogrip.com; Web site: http://www.infogrip.com.infogrip); *The BAT (one-handed keyboard)*

INMAC, 2465 Augustine Dr., PO Box 58031, Santa Clara, CA 95052-9941; *keyboard skins*

Innocomp, 26210 Emery Rd., Suite 302, Warrensville Heights, OH 44128, Tel. 800-382-8622, 216-464-3636, Fax 216-464-3638; (e-mail: Innocomp@aol.com; Web site: http://www.sayitall.com); *software, aided symbols, mounting systems, switches, environmental control*; **CAMA Member**

Innovative Products, Inc., 830 South 48th St., Grand Forks, ND 58201; Tel. 800-950-5185, Fax 701-772-5284; *toys, switches*

Institute of Applied Technology, Children's Hospital, Boston, MA 02115; *Multi Voice, Write Away*

IntelliTools, Inc., 55 Leveroni Court, Suite 9, Novato, CA 94949; Tel. 800-899-6687, 415-382-5959, Fax 415-382-2250; (e-mail: info@alphasmart.com; Web site: http://www.alphasmart.com); *Intellikeys, Intellitools software*; **CAMA Member**

Interactive Products, Inc., 1600 Valley River Dr., Suite 170, Eugene, OR 97401; Tel. 503-341-4964, Fax 503-341-4965; *VoiceMouse*

International Communication Learning Institute, 7108 Bristol Blvd., Edna, MN; *Visual Phonics*

Intex Micro Systems Corporation, PO Box 12310, Birmingham, MI 48012; Tel. 810-540-7601; *Talker II*

In Touch Systems, 11 Westview Rd., Spring Valley, NY 10977; Tel. 914-354-7431, 800-332-MAGIC; *Magic Wand Keyboard*

InvoTek Corporation, 700 W 20th St., Engineering Research Center, Fayetteville, AR 72701; Tel. 501-575-7446; *Talking Eye Point Board*

Jesana Ltd., PO Box 17, Irvington, NY 10533; Tel. 800-443-4728, Fax 914-376-0021; *communication aids, software, environmental control, switches, toys*

Kapable Kids/Able Child, PO Box 250, Bohemia, NY 11716; Tel. 800-356-1564; *resource materials, communication aids, switches, toys*

Kinesis Corporation, 22232 17th Ave. SE, Bothell, WA 98021; Tel. 800-454-6374, 206-402-8100, Fax 206-402-8181; *ergonomic keyboard*

Language Research Center, Project FACTT, Georgia State University, Atlanta, GA 30303; *Yerkish/Lana Lexigrams*

LC Technologies, Inc., 9455 Silver King Court, Fairfax, VA 22031; Tel. 800-733-5284, 703-385-7133, Fax 703-385-7137; *eyegaze systems, environmental control*

Lighthouse Low Vision Products, 36-02 Northern Blvd., Long Island City, NY 11101; Tel. 800-453-4923, Fax 718-786-0437; *vision*

LS&S Group, PO Box 673, Northbrook, IL 60065; Tel. 800-468-4789; *communication aids, speech synthesizers*

Luminaud, Inc., 8688 Tyler Blvd., Mentor, OH 44060-4348; Tel. 216-255-9082, Fax 216-255-2250; *communication aids, switches, aided symbols, input adaptations*; **CAMA Member**

Maddak, Inc., 6 Industrial Rd., Pequannock, NJ 07440; Tel. 800-443-4926, 201-628-7600, Fax 201-305-0841; *adaptive equipment*

Madenta Communications, Inc., 9411A - 20 Ave., Edmonton, Alberta T6N 1E5, Canada; Tel. 800-661-8406, Fax 403-988-6182; (e-mail: madenta@madenta.com); **CAMA Member**

Magic Laboratories, Inc., 1733 Woodside Rd., Suite 315, Redwood City, CA 94061; Tel. 415-368-9498, Fax 415-368-4535; (e-mail: gordonhc@aol.com); *Voice Bachs*

Makaton Vocabulary Development Project, 31 Firwood Dr., Camberley, Surrey GU15 3QD, England; *Makaton materials*

MarbleSoft, 12301 Central Ave. N.E., # 205, Blaine, MN 55434; Tel. 612-755-1402; (e-mail: mail@marblesoft.com; Web site: http://www.learningco.com); *software and overlays*

Maxi-Aids, PO Box 3209, Farmingdale, NY 11735; Tel. 800-522-6294, 516-752-0521; *vision technology*

Mayer-Johnson Co., PO Box 1579, Solana Beach, CA 92075-1579; Tel. 619-550-0084, Fax 619-550-0449; (e-mail: mayerj@aol.com); *software, Picture Communication Symbols (PCS), resource materials*; **CAMA Member**

McIntyre Computer Systems, 22809 Shagbark, Birmingham, MI 48025; Tel. 810-645-5090, Fax 810-645-6042

Med Labs, Inc., 28 Vereda Cordillera, Goleta, GA 93117; Tel. 805-968-2486, Fax 805-968-2486; *Scan Com-PS*

Meeting The Challenge, Inc., 3630 Sinton Rd., Suite 103, Colorado Springs, CO 80907; Tel. 800-864-4264, 719-444-0269; *Key Ability*

Merrill Publishing Company, 1300 Alum Creek Dr., PO Box 508, Columbus, OH 43216; *input adaptations, hardware*

Microflip, Inc., 112111 Pentworth Ln., Glen Dale, MD 20769-2017; Tel. 301-262-6020, Fax 301-262-4978; (e-mail: microflip@microflip.com); *telecommunications products*

Microsystems Software, Inc., 600 Worcester Rd., Framingham, MA 01701-5342; Tel. 800-828-2600, 508-879-9000, Fax 508-626-8515; (e-mail: hware@microsys.com; Web site: http://www.handiware.com); *software (Handikey, Handiword, MAGic), hardware, environmental control*; **CAMA Member**

Modu-Tray, The, 9 Orlando Dr., Chattanooga, TN 37415; Tel. 615-870-3245, Fax 615-265-2127; *wheelchair tray system*

NanoPac, Inc., 4833 South Sheridan Rd., Suite 402, Tulsa, OK 74145-5718; Tel. 918-665-0329; *Cintex, software, environmental control*

Oakland Schools Communication Enhancement Center, 2100 Pontiac Lake Rd., Waterford, MI 48328; Tel. 313-858-1901; *Oakland Picture Dictionary, resource materials*

OMS Development, 1921 Highland Ave., Wilmette, IL 60091; Tel. 708-251-5787, Fax 918-665-0361; (e-mail: info@nanopac.com; Web site: http://www.nanopac.com); *KeyCache*

Optelec USA, Inc., 4 Lyberty Way, Westford, MA 01886; Tel. 800-828-1056, 508-392-0707, Fax 508-692-6073; (e-mail: optelec@optelec.com); *large print DOS*

Personal Data Systems, Inc., PO Box 1008, Campbell, CA 95009; Tel. 408-866-1126, Fax 408-866-1128; *Audapter Speech System, telecommunications software*

Philips Electronics N.V., Groenewoudseweg 1, 5621 BA Eindhoven, Netherlands; Tel. 800-422-2066, Fax 212-825-5398; (Web site: http://www.philips.com); *Clarity*

Phonic Ear, Inc., 3880 Cypress Dr., Petaluma, CA 94954-7600; Tel. 800-227-0735, 707-769-1110, Fax 707-769-9624; *communication aids, aided symbols, resource materials, software, mounting systems;* **CAMA Member**

Pictogram Centre, Saskatchewan Association of Rehabilitation Centres, Saskatoon, Saskatchewan, Canada; *Pictogram Ideogram Communication (PIC)*

Plum Enterprises, Inc., 9 Clyston Circle, PO Box 283, Worcester, PA 19490; Tel. 215-584-5003; *headgear for children*

Pointer Systems, Inc., 1 Mill St., Burlington, VT 05401; Tel. 800-537-1562, 802-658-3260; *input adaptations, hardware, software, switches*

Prentke Romich Co. (PRC), 1022 Heyl Rd., Wooster, OH 44691; Tel. 800-262-1984, 216-262-1984, Fax 216-263-4829; (e-mail: kgerrior@aol.com); VOCAs, *input adaptations, environmental control, aided symbols, hardware, software, speech synthesizers, communication aids, mounting systems, switches;* **CAMA Member**

Preston, 60 Page Rd., Clifton, NJ 07012; *adaptive equipment*

Products for People with Vision Problems, American Foundation for the Blind, 100 Enterprise Place, PO Box 7044, Dover, DE 19903-7044; *vision technology*

Pro-Ed, 8700 Shoal Creek Blvd., Austin, TX 78757-6897; Tel. 512-451-3246; (Web site: http://www.proedinc.com); *aided symbols, manual communication products, assessment tools, tests*

Psychological Corporation (Harcourt Brace), Tel. 800-866-4446(V/TDD); *Tangible Symbols, tests and resource material*

RC Systems, Inc., 121 W Winesap Rd., Bothell, WA 98012; Tel. 206-672-6909; (e-mail: rcsys@sprynet.com); *software, hardware*

R. D. Clark, Inc., 1902 East Cove Court, Findlay, OH 45840-6607; *NU-VUE-CUE*

REACH, Inc., 890 Hearthstone Dr., Stone Mountain, GA 30083; Tel. 404-292-8933; *resource materials, communication aids, hardware, software, environmental control, switches*

Repro-Tronics, Inc., 75 Carver Ave., Westwood, NJ 07675; Tel. 800-948-8453; (Web site: http://www.repro-tronics.com/); *Braille products, vision technology, tactile graphics, The Bumpy Gazette*

Rhamdec, Inc., 476 Ellis St., Mountain View, CA 94043-2240; Tel. 800-428-0620, 415-965-3251, Fax 415-965-0705; *accessible desks, mounting systems*

RJ Cooper and Associates, 24843 Del Prado #283, Dana Point, CA 92629; (e-mail: rj@rjcooper.com; Web site: http://www.rjcooper.com); *adaptive equipment, software*

ROHO, Inc., PO Box 658, Belleville, IL 62222; Tel. 800-851-3449, 618-277-9150, Fax 618-277-6518; *wheelchair cushioning and seating products*

Safko International, Inc., 1438 W. Broadway, #B240, Tempe, AZ 85282; Tel. 602-731-9805, Fax 602-731-9835; *Sen-Sei System*

Schamex Research, 19443 Superior St., Northridge, CA 91324; Tel. 818-772-6644; *Readman*

Semantic Compaction Systems, 801 McNeilly Rd., Pittsburgh, PA 15226; Tel. 412-885-8541, Fax 412-885-8548; *Minspeak*

Sentient Systems Technology, Inc., 2100 Wharton St., Suite 630, Pittsburgh, PA 15203; Tel. 800-344-1778, 412-381-4883, Fax 412-381-5241; (e-mail: sstsales@sentientsys.com); *VOCAs, input adaptations, mounting systems;* **CAMA Member**

Shea Products, 1721 W Hamilton Rd., Rochester Hills, MI 48309; Tel. 313-852-4940; *VOCAs, communication aids*

Sighted Electronics, Inc., 464 Tappan Road, Northvale, NJ 07647; Tel. 800-666-4883; (Web site: www.sighted.com/); *Braille products, vision technology*

Signit Project, Arnold Derrymount School, Nottingham, England; *HANDS*

Ski Soft Publishing Corporation, 1644 Massachusetts Ave., Suite 79, Lexington, MA 02173; Tel. 800-662-3622, 617-863-1876; *Eye Relief*

Slater Software, 351 Badger Land, Guffey, CO 80820-9106; Tel. 719-479-2255, Fax 719-479-2254; (e-mail: jimslater@earthlink.net; Web site: http://home.earthlink.net/jimslater); **CAMA Member**

Society for Visual Education, Inc., Dept. BV, 6677 N Northwest Hwy., Chicago, IL 60631; Tel. 800-829-1900; *vision technology*

Spastic Centre of New South Wales, New South Wales, Australia; *Mosman Sounds and Symbols*

Special Designs, Inc., PO Box 130, Gillette, NJ 07933; Tel. 908-464-8825, Fax 908-464-8251; *positioning equipment*

Speech Plus, Inc., PO Box 3703, 1293 Andiwood Dr., Sunnyvale, CA 94088-3703; Tel. 408-428-3701; *speech synthesizers*

Stanton Magnetics, 101 Sunnyside Blvd., Plainview, NY 11803; Tel. 516-349-0235; *speech amplifier*

Street Electronics Corporation, 6420 Via Real, Carpinteria, CA 93013; Tel. 805-684-4593, Fax 805-684-6628; *ECHO products for Apple II, speech synthesizers*

SWITCHWORKS, PO Box 64764, Baton Rouge, LA 70896; Tel. 504-925-8926; *switches, toys*

Synergy, 66 Hale Rd., East Walpole, MA 02032; Tel. 508-668-7424, Fax 508-668-4134; *Synergy PC*

Syntha-Voice Computers, Inc., 125 Gailmont Dr., Hamilton, ON L8K 4B8, Canada; Tel. 800-263-4540, Fax 905-662-0568; (e-mail: help@synthavoice.on.ca; Web site: http://www.synthavoice.on.ca); *Panorama*

Tapeswitch Corp. of America, 100 Schmitt Blvd., Farmingdale, NY 11735; Tel. 516-694-6312, Fax 516-694-6304; *switches*

TASH International, Inc., Unit 1 - 91 Station St., Ajax, Ontario, L1S 3H2 Canada; Tel. 800-463-5685, 905-686-4129, Fax 905-686-6895; (e-mail: tashcan@aol.com); *input adaptations, aided symbols, speech synthesizers, mounting systems, switches, hardware, software, environmental control*; **CAMA Member**

TBS Marketing, 17059 El Cajon Ave., Yorba Linda, CA 92686; Tel. 714-524-4488; *environmental control*

Telesensory Systems, Inc., PO Box 7455, Mountain View, CA 94043; Tel. 800-227-8418; (e-mail: sclark@telesensory.com; Web site: www.telesensory.com); *speech synthesizers, vision technology*

Therapeutic Toys, Inc., PO Box 418, Moodus, CT 06469-0418; Tel. 800-638-0676, 203-873-9509, Fax 203-873-2388; *environmental control, switches, toys, VOCAs, communication aids*

Therapy Skill Builders, 3830 E Bellevue, Dept. C, Tucson, AZ 85716; *aided symbols, resource materials, manual communication products*

Tiger Communication System, Inc., 155 E. Broad St. #325, Rochester, NY 14604; Tel. 800-724-7301, Fax 716-454-3631; *software, VOCAs*

T.J. Publishers' Catalog of Publications, 817 Silver Spring Ave., Suite 206, Silver Spring, MD 20910-4617; Tel. 800-999-1168, 301-585-4440; *manual communication products*

Toby Churchill Ltd., 102 Christchurch Rd., Winchester, Hanis So23 9TG, England; Tel. 011-44-962-862340, Fax 011-44-962-8549; **CAMA Member**

Tolfa Corporation, 1001 N Rengstorff Ave., Mountain View, CA 94043; Tel. 415-390-9566; *Lingraphica*

Tomor Zavalani, 14664 Rosco Blvd., #33, Panorama City, CA 91402; *CyberGlyphs (aka Jet Era Glyphs)*

Toys for Special Children-Enabling Devices Inc., 385 Warburton Ave., Hastings-on-Hudson, NY 10706; Tel. 800-832-8697, 914-478-0960, Fax 914-478-7030; *aided symbols, input adaptations, hardware, environmental control, mounting systems, switches, toys*

Trace Research and Development Center, University of Wisconsin—Madison, S-151 Waisman Center, 1500 Highland Ave., Madison, WI 53705; Tel. 608-262-6966, 608-263-5408(TDD); (e-mail: info@trace.wisc.edu; Web site: http://trace.wisc.edu); *input adaptations, resource materials, hardware, Hyper-ABLEDATA*

UCLA Intervention Program for Handicapped Children, 1000 Veteran Ave., Rm. 23-10, Los Angeles, CA 90024; Tel. 310-825-4821; *Sight Words*

Ultratec, Inc., 450 Science Dr., Madison, WI 53711; Tel. 608-238-5400(TDD), Fax 608-238-3008

Visually Impaired Student's Initiative ON Science (VISIONS) Laboratory, Purdue University, 1393 BRWN Box 88, West Lafayette, IN 47907-1393; Tel. 765-496-2865; (Web site: chem.purdue.edu/facilities/sightlab/index.html); *vision technology including braille products and tactile graphics*

VME Technologies, Inc., 5202 Westland Blvd., Baltimore, MD 21227; Tel. 410-455-6397; *ViewKey*

Voice Connection, 17835 Skypark Cir., Ste C, Irvine, CA 92714; Tel. 714-261-2366; *HAL Entry System, IntroVoice, environmental control*

Votrax, Inc., 30777 Schoolcrest Rd., Lavonia, MI 48150; Tel. 800-521-1350; *speech synthesizers*

Vysion, Inc., 30777 Schoolcraft Rd., Livonia, MI 48150; Tel. 313-522-3300; *Personal Speech System*

WesTest Engineering Corporation, 1470 N Main, Bountiful, UT 84010; Tel. 801-298-7100; *DARCI*

Wisconsin Assistive Technology Initiative, CESA #8, Attention: Jane Bubolz, PO Box 320, Gillett, WI 54124; *Voice-in-a-Box*

Words+, Inc., 40015 Sierra Hwy., Bldg. B-145, Palmdale, CA 93550; Tel. 800-869-8521, 805-266-8500, 805-266-8896 (BBS), Fax 805-266-8969; (e-mail: phil@words-plus.com; Web site: http://www.words-plus.com); *input adaptations, aided symbols, software, hardware, VOCAs, speech synthesizers, mounting systems, switches, environmental control*; **CAMA Member**

World Communications, 245 Tonopah Dr., Fremont, CA 94539; Tel. 510-656-0911; *Help U Type and Speak, MouseKeys for Windows, Freedom Writer*

Worldsign Communication Society, Perry Siding, Winlaw, British Columbia V0G 2J0, Canada; *Worldsign*

X-10 USA, Inc., PO Box 420, Closter, NJ 07624-0420; Tel. 800-526-0027, 201-784-9700; *Home Automation*

Xerox/Kurzweil Computer Products, Personal Reader Department, 185 Albany St., Cambridge, MA 02139; *vision technology*

Zygo Industries, Inc., PO Box 1008, Portland, OR 97207-1008; Tel. 800-234-6006, 503-684-6006, Fax 503-684-6011; *input adaptations, aided symbols, hardware, communication aids, VOCAs, mounting systems, switches*; **CAMA Member**

Appendix B-2   Software Developers and Vendors

This appendix lists a variety of companies and organizations that develop, manufacture, and/or market software that may be appropriate for AAC including all of the companies referred to in Chapter 10 and Appendix C. Some of the entries include notations in italics referring to the following: (1) public domain (free), (2) shareware (nominal fee), (3) general software (e.g., language development), (4) specific software titles (e.g., KidsWord), (5) operating systems (Macintosh, DOS), and (6) catalog only.

Ability Systems Corporation, 1422 Arnold Ave., Roslyn, PA 19001; Tel. 215-657-4338; *KeyUp*

AccessDOS, Trace & Developmental Center, University of Wisconsin, Madison, WI 53705-2280; Tel. 800-426-7282; *free software for IBM keyboard*

Access Unlimited, 3535 Briarpark Dr., Suite 102, Houston, TX 77042-5235; Tel. 800-848-0311, 713-781-7441; *Adaptive Firmware Card setups*

ACL, 1601 Fulton Ave., Suite 10, Sacramento, CA 95825; Tel. 916-973-1851; *shareware*

Adaptive Computers, 11 Fullerton St., Suite 110, Albany, NY 12209; Tel. 518-434-8860; *One-Switch Paintbrush*

Advantage Computing, 6172 Bollinger Rd., Suite 106, San Jose, CA 95129; Tel. 800-356-4666; *public domain (Apple II, Commodore, IBM)*

Affordable Software, 1421 N 1725 West, Layton, UT 84041; *public domain (IBM and compatible)*

Ai Squared, PO Box 669, Manchester Center, VT 05255-0669; Tel. 802-362-3612; *Zoom Text*

Allegiant Systems, Inc., 9740 Scranton Rd., Suite 300, San Diego, CA 92121; Tel. 800-225-8258, 619-587-0500, Fax 619-587-1314; *SuperCard*

Assistive Device Center, School of Engineering and Computer Science, California State University, Sacramento, CA 95819; Tel. 916-278-6422; *switch training software*

A. V. Concepts, 1917 West 1st Street, Tempe, AZ 85281; Tel. 800-473-6828, 602-894-6642, Fax 602-894-8376; (Web site: webmaster@avconcepts.com); *literacy and language development software*

Berkeley Macintosh Users Group (BMUG), 1442 A Walnut St., #62, Berkeley, CA 94709-1496; Tel. 510-549-2684; *public domain (Macintosh)*

Borland International, Inc., 100 Borland Way, Scotts Valley, CA 95066; Tel. 408-431-1000; *dbase for Windows, Paradox for Windows*

Boston Computer Society, 385 Elliot St., Newton, MA 02164; *IBM PC users group software exchange*

Bradley Murray, S. J., 5704 Roland Ave., Baltimore, MD 21210; Tel. 410-435-1833; *CTRL, ALT, and SHIFT key adaptations*

Broderbund Software, Direct Dept. 93EC, PO Box 6125, Novato, CA 94948-6125; Tel. 800-521-6263; *software (Bankstreet Writer)*

Cambridge Development Laboratory, Inc., 86 West St., Waltham, MA 02154; Tel. 800-637-0047, 617-890-4640, Fax 617-890-2894; *special education software*

Center for Computer Assistance to the Disabled, 1950 Stemmons Frwy., Suite 4041, Dallas, TX 75207-3109; Tel. 214-746-4217, 214-746-4203(TDD), 817-429-5327(BBS); *Stickey*

CE Software, Inc., PO Box 65580, West Des Moines, IA 50265; Tel. 800-523-7638, 515-221-1801, Fax 515-221-2258; *DOS and Macintosh*

Chariot Software Group, 123 Comino De La Reina, West Bldg., San Diego, CA 92108-3002; Tel. 800-242-7468; *Macintosh*

Claris Corporation, PO Box 526, Santa Clara, CA 95052-9870; Tel. 800-628-2100 Ext. 92; *Claris Works, Filemaker Pro*

Colorado Easter Seals Society, Center for Adaptive Technology, 5755 West Alameda, Lakewood, CO 80226; *public domain (Apple)*

Compu-Teach, 16541 Redmond Way, Suite 137C, Redmond, WA, 98052; Tel. 800-44T-EACH, 206-885-0517, Fax 206-883-9169

Connecticut Rehabilitation Engineering Center, 78 Easter Blvd., Glastonberry, CT 06033; Tel. 203-659-1166

Continental Press, Inc., 520 E Bainbridge St., Elizabethtown, PA 17022; Tel. 800-233-0759; *literacy and language development software*

Corel Corporation, Corporate Headquarters, 1600 Carling Ave., Ottawa, Ontario, KIZ 8R7, Canada; Tel. 613-728-8200, Fax 613-728-9790; (Web site: www.corel.com); *Lotus Approach, Wordperfect*

Creative Learning, Inc., PO Box 829, North San Juan, CA 95960; Tel. 800-576-0538, 916-292-3001, Fax 916-292-4262; *software (multisensory)*

Discount Software House, PO Box 93, Winnebago, WI 54985; Tel. 414-231-1696; *discount software catalog*

Doug Dodgen & Associates, PO Box 180503, Arlington, TX 76096; Tel. 817-467-0627; *AAC feature match software*

Edmark, PO Box 97021, Redmond, WA 98073-9721; Tel. 800-362-2890, 206-556-8400, Fax 206-556-8430; *software (Assessment, TouchWindow)*

Educational Resources, 1550 Executive Dr., Elgin, IL 60123; Tel. 800-624-2926, 708-888-8300, Fax 708-888-8499; *discount software catalog*

Egghead Software, 29777 Telegraph Rd., Suite 3651, Southfield, MI 48034; Tel. 313-352-6790; *discount software catalog*

Exceptional Children's Software, PO Box 487, Hays, KS 67601; Tel. 913-625-9281; *Rabbit Scanner*

Humanities Software, PO Box 950, Hood River, OR 97031; Tel. 800-245-6737; *Write On!*

IBM Educational Systems, PO Box 1328, Internal Zip 5432, Boca Raton, FL 33432; Tel. 800-284-9482, 407-982-9099, 800-426-2133(TDD); *IBM Linkway*

Judy Lynn Software, 278 Dunhams Corner Rd., East Brunswick, NJ 08816; Tel. 908-390-8845; *switch activated software*

Kentucky Special Education, Technology Training Center, c/o Margaret Shuping or Marie Keel, Department of Special Education—University of Kentucky, Lexington, KY 40506-0001; *public domain*

Kidsview Software, PO Box 98, Warner, NH 03278; Tel. 800-542-7501, 603-927-4428; *KidsWord*

KidTECH/Soft Touch, 21274 Oak Knoll, Tehachapi, CA 93561; Tel. 805-822-1663; *literacy and language development software*

Laureate Learning Systems, Inc., 110 East Spring St., Winooski, VT 05404-1837; Tel. 800-655-4755; *developmental software*

LCSI, PO Box 162, Highgate Springs, VT 05460

Learning Company, 6493 Kaiser Dr., Fremont, CA 94555; Tel. 800-852-2255, 510-792-2101; *literacy and language development software*

Learning Lab Software, 21000 Nordhoff St., Chatworth, CA 91311; Tel. 800-899-3475

Lekotek of GA Public Doman Library, 3035 N. Druid Hills Rd., Atlanta, GA 30329; *public domain (Apple)*

Life Science Associates, 1 Fenimore Rd., Bayport, NY 11705; Tel. 516-472-2111; *cognitive rehabilitation software*

Logo Foundation, 250 W 57th St., Suite 2603, New York, NY 10107; Tel. 800-321-LOGO, 212-765-4918

MACWAREHOUSE, 1690 Oak St., Lakewood, NJ 08701; Tel. 800-255-6227, Fax 908-905-9279; *discount software catalog*

Marblesoft, 12301 Central Ave. NE #205, Blaine, MN 55434; Tel. 612-755-1402; *developmental software*

MECC, 6160 Summit Dr., N, St. Paul, MN 55430; Tel. 612-569-1640; *literacy and language development software*

Microsoft Corporation, One Microsoft Way, Redmond, WA 98052; Tel. 800-876-4726, 206-454-2030; (Web site: http://www.microsoft.com); *ballpoint mouse, application software (Word, Works, Excel)*

Micro Star, 2245 Camino Vida Roble, Suite 100, Carlsbad, CA 92009, Tel. 800-444-1343; *IBM, Macintosh*

MicroWarehouse, PO Box 3014, 1690 Oak St., Lakewood, NJ 08701-3014; Tel. 800-367-7080, Fax 908-905-5245; *discount software catalog*

Mindscape Educational Software, 6677 N Northwest Hwy., Chicago, IL 60631; Tel. 800-829-1900

Optimum Resource, Inc., 10 Station Pl., Norfolk, CT 06058; Tel. 800-327-1473; *literacy and language development software*

Orange Cherry Talking Schoolhouse Software, PO Box 390, 69 Westchester Ave., Pound Ridge, NY 10576; Tel. 800-672-6002, 914-764-0104

Parrot Software, PO Box 1139, State College, PA 16804-1139; Tel. 800-727-7681, 814-237-7282

PC-SIG, 1030D East Duane Ave., Sunnyvale, CA 94086; Tel. 800-245-6717

PEAL Software, PO Box 8188, Calabasas, CA 91372; Tel. 800-541-1318, 818-883-7849, Fax 818-992-4368; *early language software*

Productivity Software International, 211 E 43rd St. #2202, New York, NY 10017-4707; Tel. 800-533-7587, 212-967-8666; *Keylock, abbreviation expansion software*

Public Band Software/Shareware, PO Box 51315, Indianapolis, IN 46251

Realtime Learning Systems, 2700 Connecticut Ave. NW, Washington, DC 20008-5330; Tel. 800-832-2472, 202-483-1510, Fax 202-328-6681

Research Design Associates, Inc., 10 Boulevard Ave., Greenlawn, NY 11740; Tel. 800-654-8715, 516-754-5280; *literacy and language development software, telecommunications software*

Roger Wagner Publishing, Inc., 1050 Pioneer Way, Suite P, El Cajon, CA 92020; Tel. 800-421-6526; *HyperStudio*

Scholastic Software, PO Box 7502, 2931 E McCarty St., Jefferson City, MO 65102; Tel. 800-541-5513; *software (voice output, large print, literacy and language development)*

Softkey International, Inc., 201 Broadway, Cambridge, MA 02139; Tel. 800-323-8088, 800-227-5609; *Product Information*

Software To Go, Gallaudet University, 800 Florida Ave, NE, Washington, DC 20002

Sunburst Communications, 101 Castelton St., Pleasantville, NY 10570-3498; Tel. 800-628-8897, 914-747-3310

Sunset Software, 9277 E. Corrine Dr., Scottsdale, AZ 85260; Tel. 602-451-0753; *cognitive rehabilitation software*

Teacher Support Software, 1035 NW 57th St., Gainesville, FL 32605-4486; Tel. 800-228-2871, 904-332-6404, Fax 904-332-6779; *software (Apple, Mac, DOS)*

Technology for Language and Learning, Special Education Public Domain Project, PO Box 327, East Rockaway, NY 11518; Tel. 516-625-4550

Techware Corporation, PO Box 151085, Altamonte Springs, FL 32715-1085; Tel. 800-34-REACH; *Hypermedia*

Tell'em Ware, 1714 Olson Way, Marshalltown, IA 50158; Tel. 515-752-9667

Tom Snyder Productions, 80 Coolidge Hill Rd., Watertown, MA 02172; Tel. 800-342-0236

Wings for Learning/Sunburst, PO Box 660002, Scotts Valley, CA 95067; Tel. 800-321-7511, 408-438-5502

Appendix B-3   Organizations, Centers, and Electronic Resources

This appendix lists professional and nonprofessional organizations, national advocacy groups, centers, and electronic resources related to AAC and AT. These sources provide assistance, printed information, and/or products.

AAMR Communication Disorders Division; *offers several AAC sessions at the annual AAMR convention*

Alliance for Technology Access, 1307 Solano Ave., Albany, CA 94706; Tel. 415-528-0747, Fax 415-528-0746; (e-mail: atafta@aol.com; Web site: http://www.atacess.org)

ALS Association, 21021 Ventura Blvd., Ste. 321, Woodland Hills, CA 91364; Tel. 818-340-7500, Fax 818-340-2060; (e-mail: eajc27b@prodigy.com; Web site: http://www.alsa.org)

American Association on Mental Retardation (AAMR), 444 North Capital St. NW, Suite 846, Washington, DC 20001-1512; Tel. 800-424-3688, Fax 202-387-2193

American Foundation for the Blind, Technology Center, 11 Penn Plaza, Ste. 300, New York, NY 10001; Tel. 212-502-7642, Fax 212-502-7773; (e-mail: techctr@afb.org; Web site: http://www.asb.org/afb)

American Occupational Therapy Association (AOTA), PO Box 31220, 4720 Montgomery Ln., Bethesda, MD 20824-2682; Tel. 301-652-2682, Fax 301-652-7711

American Physical Therapy Association (APTA), 1111 N Fairfax St., Alexandria, VA 22314; Tel. 703-684-2782, Fax 703-684-7343; (Web site: http://www.apta.org)

American Speech-Language-Hearing Association (ASHA), 10801 Rockville Pike, Rockville, MD 20852; Tel. 301-897-5700(V/TDD), Fax 301-571-0457; (Web site: http://www.asha.org)

ASHA Special Interest Division 12, Augmentative and Alternative Communication; *publishes quarterly newsletter*

Augmented Communicators On-Line Users' Group (ACOLUG): listserv@vm.temple.edu (type "subscribe firstname lastname" in the body of the message)

Blissymbolics Communication International (BCI) (previously known as Blissymbolics Communication Institute), 1630 Lawrence Ave. West, Suite 104, Toronto, Ontario M2J 459, Canada; Tel. 416-242-2222; (e-mail: ortckse@oise.on.ca; Web site: http://home.istar./~bci)

Closing the Gap, 526 Main Street, PO Box 68, Henderson, MN 56044; Tel. 612-248-3294; (e-mail: info@closingthegap.com; Web site: www.closingthegap.com)

Communication Aid Manufacturers Association (CAMA), 518-26 Davis St., Evanston, IL 60201; Tel. 800-441-2262, Fax 708-869-5689; (e-mail: cama@northshore.net)

Council for Exceptional Children (CEC), 1920 Association Dr., Reston, VA 22091-1589; Tel. 703-620-3660, Fax 703-264-1637; (e-mail: cecpubs@cec.sped.org; Web site: http://www.cec.sped.org)

CSUN Center on Disabilities, 18111 Nordhoff, Northridge, CA 91330; Tel. 818-885-2869, Fax 818-885-4929; (e-mail: ltm@csun.edu; Web site: http://www.csun.edu/cod/)

Cued Speech Center, PO Box 31345, Raleigh, NC 27622

EARO, The Resource Centre, Black Hill, Ely, Combridgeshire, England

Electronic Industries Association, Consumer Electronics Group, 2500 Wilson Blvd., Arlington, VA 22201-3834; Tel. 703-907-7600, Fax 703-907-7601

Equal Access to Software and Information (EASI), c/o AAHE, One DuPont Circle, Suite 360, Washington, DC 20036; Tel. 202-293-6440 x48; (Web site: http://www.rit.edu/~easi/). *Adaptive technology, disabilities resources*

Forum for Discussions of AAC Funding Policy: majordomo@asel.udel.edu (Leave the subject area blank; type "subscribe aac-medicaid" in the body of the message)

Forum for RESNA, USSAAC and ASHA: majordomo@asel.udel.edu (Leave the subject area blank; type "subscribe aac" in the body of the message)

Great Lakes Disability and Business Technical Assistance Center, University of Illinois at Chicago, 1640 West Roosevelt Rd., Chicago, IL 60608; Tel. 312-413-1407, 312-413-0453(TDD)

IBM National Support Center for Persons with Disabilities, PO Box 2150, Atlanta, GA 30301-2105; Tel. 800-426-2133(V), 800-284-9482(TDD); (Web site: http://www.inform.umd.EdRes./Topic/Disability) *Resource guide for persons with speech and language impairments*

International Society for Augmentative and Alternative Communication (ISAAC), PO Box 1762-Station R, Toronto, Ontario M4G 4A3, Canada; Tel. 905-737-9308, Fax 905-737-0624; (e-mail: liz_baer@mail.cepp.org); *AAC Journal, Biennial international conference*

National Council on Disability, 800 Independence Ave., SW, Suite 814, Washington, DC 20591; Tel. 202-267-3846, 202-267-3232(TDD), Fax 202-453-4240

National Easter Seal Society, 230 W. Monroe St., Ste. 1800, Chicago, IL 60606-4802; Tel. 312-726-6200(V), 312-726-4258(TDD), 800-221-6827, Fax 312-726-1494; (Web site: http://www.seals.com)

National Federation of the Blind (NFB), 1800 Johnson St., Baltimore, MD 21230; Tel. 410-659-9314, Fax 410-685-5653; (e-mail: nfb@acess.digex.net; Web site: http://www.nfb.org)

National Information Center for Children and Youth with Handicaps (NICHCY), PO Box 1492, Washington, DC 20013; Tel. 800-999-5599, 703-893-6061, 703-893-8614(TDD); (e-mail: nicd@gallux.gallaudet.edu; Web site: http://www.aed.org/nichy)

National Library Service for the Blind and Physically Handicapped, Library of Congress, 1291 Taylor St. NW, Washington, DC 20542

National Organization on Disability (NOD), 910 Sixteenth St., NW, Washington, DC 20006; Tel. 202-293-5960, 202-293-5968(TDD), Fax 202-293-7999; (Web site: http://www.nod.org)

National Parent Network on Disabilities, 1600 Prince St., #115, Alexandria, VA 22314; Tel. 703-684-6763 (V/TDD), Fax 703-836-1232

National Rehabilitation Information Center (NARIC), 8455 Colesville Rd., Suite 935, Silver Spring, MD 20910-3319; Tel. 800-346-2742(V/TDD), 301-588-9284(V/TDD), Fax 301-587-1967; *NARIC Quarterly, brochures, resource guides, free publications*

National Resource Center of Sweden, Educational Aids for Special Schools, Mariehemsv 2 902 36, Umeå, Sweden

National Special Education Alliance, Apple Office of Special Education, 20525 Mariani Ave., Cupertino, CA 95014

National Spinal Cord Injury Association, 8300 Colesville Rd., Ste. 551, Silver Spring, MD 20910; Tel. 301-588-6959, 800-962-9629, Fax 301-588-9414; (e-mail: nscia2@aol.com; Web site: http://www.spinalcord.org)

National Support Center for Persons with Disabilities, PO Box 2150, Atlanta, GA 30005

PennTech-Central Instructional Support Center, 6340 Flank Dr., Suite 600, Harrisburg, PA 17112; Tel. 800-360-7282 in PA only, 717-541-4960, Fax 717-541-4968; (Web site: http://www.cisc.k12.pa.us); *one of the first state-wide AAC resource centers*

Project ACCESS, Wayne County RESA, 33500 Van Born Rd., Wayne, MI 48184

RERC* on Adaptive Computers and Information Services, Trace Center/University of Wisconsin, Waisman Center, S-151, 1500 Highland Avenue, Madison, WI 53705; Tel. 608-262-6966(V), 608-263-5408(TDD), Fax 608-262-8848

RERC* on Assistive Technology and Environmental Intervention for Older Persons with Disabilities and **RERC on Technology Evaluation and Transfer**, State University of New York, Buffalo, Center for Assistive Technology, 515 Kimball Tower, Buffalo, NY 14214; Tel. 800-628-2281(V/TDD), Fax 716-829-3217

RERC* in Augmentative and Alternative Communication, and RERC on Rehabilitation Robotics to Enhance the Functioning of Individuals with Disabilities, University of Delaware, A.I. duPont Institute, 1600 Rockland Rd., PO Box 269, Wilmington, DE 19899; Tel. 302-651-6830, 302-651-6834(TDD), Fax 302-651-6895

RERC* on Hearing Enhancement and Assistive Devices, The Lexington Center, Inc., Research Division, 30th Avenue and 75th Street, Jackson Heights, NY 11370; Tel. 718-899-8800 x230(V/TDD), Fax 718-899-3433

RERC* on Modifications to Worksites and Educational Settings, Cerebral Palsy Research Foundation of Kansas, 2021 North Old Manor, Box 8217, Wichita, KS 67208-0217; Tel. 316-688-1888(V/TDD), Fax 316-688-5687

RERC* on Rehabilitation Technology Services in Vocational Rehabilitation, Rehabilitation Center for Rehabilitation Technology Services, South Carolina Vocational Rehabilitation, Department 1410-C, Boxton Avenue West, Columbia, SC 29170; Tel. 803-822-5362 (V/TDD), Fax 803-822-4301

RERC* at Smith-Kettlewell Eye Research Institute, 2232 Webster St., San Francisco, CA 94115; Tel. 415-561-1630, Fax 415-561-1610

RESNA (Rehabilitation Engineering and Assistive Technology Society of North America, previously the Rehabilitation Engineering Society of North America), 1700 N Moore St., Suite 1540, Arlington, VA 22209-1930; Tel. 703-524-6686(V), 703-524-6639(TDD), Fax 703-524-6630; (e-mail: natoffice@resnq.org; Web site: http://www.resna.org/resna/reshome.htm)

RESNA AAC Special Interest Group (SIG)—03

RESNA Speech Language Pathologists/Audiologists Professional Specialty Group (PSG)—06

Royal Institute of Technology, Dept. of Speech Communication and Music Acoustics, Box 70014, Stockholm, S-10044, Sweden

Social Security Administration (SSA), Office of Public Inquiries, 6401 Security Blvd., Room 4-C-5 Annex, Baltimore, MD 21235; Tel. 800-772-1213(V), 800-325-0778(TDD); (Web site: http://www.ssa.gov/); *Medicaid, Medicare, other sources of support*

Tetra Society of North America, Plaza of Nations, Suite 27, 770 Pacific Boulevard South, Vancouver, British Columbia, Canada V6B 5E7; Tel. 604-688-6464, Fax 604-688-6463

The Arc of the United States (previously Association for Retarded Children and the Association for Retarded Citizens), 500 Border St., Suite 300, PO Box 1047, Arlington, TX 76010; Tel. 817-261-6003(V), 817-227-0553; (Web site: http://www.thearc.org)

The Association for Persons with Severe Handicaps (TASH), 11201 Greenwood Ave. N, Seattle, WA 98113

Trace Research and Development Center, University of Wisconsin, S-151 Waisman Center, 1500 Highland Ave., Madison, WI 53705-2280; Tel. 608-262-6966(V); 608-263-5408(TDD); (e-mail: infor@trace.wisc.edu; Web site: http://trace.wisc.edu/)

United Cerebral Palsy Association (UCPA), 1660 L St. NW, Suite 700, Washington, DC 20036; Tel. 800-872-5827 (V/TDD), Fax 202-776-0406

---

*There were 14 RERCs (Rehabilitation Engineering Research Centers) funded by the National Institute on Disability and Rehabilitation Research (NIDRR) of the U.S. Department of Education in 1997. The seven that are most relevant to AAC are listed in this Appendix.

United States Society for Augmentative and Alternative Communication (USSAAC), PO Box 5271, Evanston, IL 60204-5271, Tel. 847-869-2122, Fax 847-869-5689; (e-mail: USSAAC@Northshore.net)

Veterans Administration (VA), (operates through regional offices which can be identified through telephone or web site); Tel. 800-827-1000(V), 800-829-4833(TDD); (Web site: http://www.va.gov)

Visually Impaired Student's Initiative ON Science (VISIONS) Laboratory, Purdue University, 1393 BRWN Box #88, West Lafayette, IN 47907; Tel. 765-496-2865; (Web site: www.chem.purdue.edu/facilities/sightlab/index. html); *Braille products, vision technology, tactile graphics*

World Health Organization (WHO), International Headquarters, CH-1211, Geneva 27, Switzerland; Tel. 41-22-791-2111, Fax 41-22-791-0746; (e-mail: postmaster@who.ch; Web site: http://www.who.org/); Regional Office for the Americas (AMRO), Pan American Health Organization (PAHO), 525 23rd Street, N.W., Washington, DC 20037; Tel. 202-974-3000(V), Fax 202-974-3663

Appendix B-4   Periodicals and Newsletters

This appendix lists refereed journals, newsletters, magazines, and directories related to AAC. Where applicable, it is indicated which newsletters are free.

ABLEDATA, 8455 Colesville Road, Suite 935, Silver Springs, MD 20910; Tel. 800-227-0216, 301-588-9284, Fax 301-587-1967

Alternatively Speaking, Augmentative Communication, Inc., 1 Surf Way, Suite 237, Monterey, CA 93940; Tel. 408-649-3050, Fax 408-646-5428; *newsletter*

Augmentative and Alternative Communication (AAC), see ISAAC address in Appendix B-3; *refereed journal, reduced rate for ISAAC members*

Augmentative and Alternative Communication Newsletter (of ASHA Div. 12), see ASHA address in Appendix B-3; *quarterly newsletter, free to Div. 12 affiliates*

Augmentative Communication News, Augmentative Communication, Inc., 1 Surf Way, Suite #215, Monterey, CA 93940; *newsletter*

The Bumpy Gazette, Repro-Tronics, Inc., 75 Carver Ave., Westwood, NJ 07675; Tel. 800-948-8453; (Web site: http://www.repro-tronics.com/)

Closing the Gap Resource Directory, PO Box 68, Henderson, MN 56044, Tel. 612-248-3294

Communicating Together, PO Box 986, Thornhill, Ontario L3T 4A5, Canada; *quarterly magazine, reduced rate for ISAAC members*

Communication Outlook, 405 Computer Center, Michigan State University, East Lansing, MI 48824-1024, *newsletter, reduced rate for ISAAC members*

Conn SENSE Bulletin, Special Education Center, Technology Lab, The University of Connecticut, U-64, Room 227, 249 Glenbrook Rd., Storrs, CT 06269-2064; Tel. 203-486-0172

The ISAAC Bulletin, see ISAAC address in Appendix B-3; *quarterly newsletter, free with membership*

REACH/Rehabilitation Engineering Associates, Tel. 800-485-5040; *newsletter*

SpeakUp!, see USSAAC address in Appendix B-3; *newsletter, free with membership*

Technology Resource Directory, Susan Mack, Exceptional Parent, 1170 Commonwealth Ave., 3rd Floor, Boston, MA 02134-9942

WorkTech, Seaside Education Associates, Inc., PO Box 6341, Lincoln Center, MA 01773; *newsletter*

DEVICES AND SOFTWARE*

This appendix contains a compilation of AAC devices and software organized according to 11 categories. The compilation is not intended to be an exhaustive listing but rather a representative sample of devices and software. Some of the devices and software are no longer commercially available (e.g., Touch Talker and Light Talker), but are included because they are still in current clinical and/or educational use. For information on how to contact product manufacturers and/or vendors, see Appendix B.

Appendix C-1 Input Devices

Alternate Keyboards/Emulators

Adaptive Firmware Card (AFC)   Don Johnston, Inc. Computer card that allows a variety of input methods for off-the-shelf software; allows custom setups; Apple IIe, IIGS.

BAT (one-handed keyboard)   Infogrip, Inc. A one-handed keyboard configured for either right- or left-handed users; seven keys can be operated for easy input of data, either by pressing single keys or "chording"; estimated learning time for use is under 10 hours; users with good finger dexterity can input up to 50 words per minute.

Breakthru Box   EKEG Electronics Co., Ltd. Allows use of membrane keyboards configured for AFC to be used with computers without AFC cards installed; also variety of input/access devices; Apple IIGS, Macintosh, IBM PC.

DADAEntry   TASH, Inc. Keyboard emulator; IBM PC.

DARCI TOO   WesTest Engineering Corp. Keyboard/mouse emulator connected between computer and user's input device; allows variety of access methods (e.g., switches, joysticks) and operating modes, such as Morse code, scanning, matrix keyboard, and DARCI code; Apple IIe, IBM PC.

Headmaster Plus   Prentke Romich Co. Keyboard emulator allowing use of one's head to move a cursor across the screen; puff switch acts as mouse button; switches can be added; on-screen keyboard software available; Macintosh, IBM PC.

Headmouse   Madenta Communications, Inc. Mouse emulator.

IBM AccessDOS   IBM Special Needs Systems. Utility to extend keyboard and mouse access on computer; allows for separate key action for multiple key sequences.

IntelliKeys   IntelliTools. Alternate keyboard that plugs directly into the computer with no need for interface; comes with six overlays; setup overlay allows adjustment of keyboard options (e.g., repeat rate and keyboard sensitivity); Apple IIGS, Macintosh, and IBM PC. An upgrade/replacement of the Unicorn keyboard.

JOUSE   Prentke Romich Co. Joystick-operated mouse, controlled with the mouth.

Ke:nx On-Board V3.0   Don Johnston, Inc. Membrane alternative board allowing adjustable sensitivities; includes Macintalk II.

Ke:nx V3.0   Don Johnston, Inc. Keyboard and mouse emulator that allows full computer access via a variety of input methods (e.g., switches, Morse code, on-screen keyboard); includes Macintalk II; Macintosh.

Key Largo   Don Johnston, Inc. Membrane keyboard that can be used with Ke:nx or AFC and other interfaces; can create and print own overlays.

Lipstick   McIntyre Computer Systems. Joystick with flexible gooseneck that enables cursor movement and selection of menu-driven items on a computer screen by using lips, chin, cheek, shoulder, arm, hand, or foot; used by individuals with little or no hand movement or control.

Mac King Keyboard; Win King Keyboard   TASH, Inc. Large-sized alternative keyboard for individuals with gross motor problems; allows adjustment of key pressures and change of key layouts; keys are slightly recessed to prevent accidental activation.

---

*Compiled by Raymond W. Quist and Lyle L. Lloyd.

Mac Mini Keyboard; Win Mini Keyboard Tash, Inc. QWERTY keyboard for persons with limited range of motion and/or better accuracy for smaller movements.

MicroKeyboard INCAP (Dallas). A keyboard designed with a very small field to facilitate use by a person with minimal strength and a highly limited range in hand/finger action.

MiniKeyboards EKEG Electronics Co., Ltd. Keyboard with same layout as the expanded keyboards, but with a much smaller field, requiring very little range of motion; auditory and visual feedback provided with each key press; Apple IIGS, Macintosh, IBM compatible.

Newton Apple. Updated version of the touch screen/pad.

Power Key for Apple and Power Key for IBM Dunamis, Inc. Allows users to operate software with a PowerPad. Can customize setups. Versions for both Apple IIe and for IBM-compatible computers; IIe version will work with AFC.

Powerpad Dunamis. 12″ × 12″ surface alternate keyboard that can be configured for communication overlays up to 144 squares; Apple IIGS, DOS, Macintosh.

Touch Window Edmark. Window attachment for monitors that permits input by touch; Apple IIGS, DOS, Macintosh.

Optical Character Recognition Devices (Visual Impairments)

An Open Book, Open Book Unbound System, and Arkenstone Reader Arkenstone, Inc. System includes a scanner and DECtalk. Storage capacity of 20,000 pages of scanned text; Braille displays and speech output; the Unbound System is only one with scanner, supporting Braille displays and voice output. Arkenstone Reader has three components that together make up a reading system for individuals with visual impairments: TrueScan recognition card, a Hewlett-Packard scanner, and scanner interface card; IBM PC.

CompuSight Workstation Complete computer workstation allowing scanning of a variety of printed materials and generating word processing documents; comes complete with adaptive aids and software.

Kurzweil Personal Reader Xerox Imaging Systems, Inc. Transportable reading system that converts text to speech; designed for individuals who are either visually impaired or have difficulty reading printed material; IBM PC.

PC Kurzweil Personal Reader Xerox Imaging Systems, Inc. Scans text and converts to speech, Braille, or word

processing; useful for individuals with visual impairments or reading difficulties.

Reading Edge Xerox Imaging Systems, Inc. Portable (24 pounds) reading machine that uses optical character recognition, a scanner, and a speech synthesizer (DECtalk); available in seven languages.

Readman Schamex Research. Twenty-pound, standalone reading machine that reads aloud one selected page at a time; uses DECtalk.

Robotron Rainbow Reading System Integrated Assistive Technologies. Standalone reading machine with scanning and DECtalk speech output.

SenSei System Safko International, Inc. Versatile device that can serve as communication device with switch access, a optical reading/scanning device with speech output for individuals with visual impairments, and environmental control.

VisionKey H.K. EyeCan, Ltd. Small and lightweight eyegaze device that mounts on a standard eyeglass frame. Through the use of reflected infrabeam lights, the user has access to a 49-key ABC chart providing the functionality of a regular keyboard.

Speech Recognition

DragonDictate for Windows/DOS Dragon Systems, Inc. Speaker adaptive voice recognition capable of 60,000 words; allows free dictation software into any text-based document and can format documents; IBM/DOS Windows.

HAL Entry System Voice Connection. Includes IntroVoice 6 hardware and software with headset microphone, modem, speaker phone, and software.

IBM Personal Dictation System IBM Independence Series Information System software. Allows operation of computer through speech; DOS.

IntroVoice V Voice Connection. A speech recognition system that can recognize 500 words with 99% accuracy; because the user learns functions, not keys, the learning time is reduced; IBM PC.

Kurzweil Voice for Windows Kurzweil Applied Intelligence. Voice-recognition system that allows the user to

run computer operations; has a 60,000-word vocabulary and a 200,000-word on-line dictionary; adapts to the user's voice during use.

Kurzweil Voice Report Kurzweil Applied Intelligence. Voice-recognition system with 40,000-word vocabulary; allows word-by-word dictation, as well as voice generation of printed documents.

Micro IntroVoice V, VI Voice Connection. A voice-recognition system of 1,000 words that can be identified with 98% accuracy; unlimited text-to-speech synthesis; IBM PC, MS-DOS.

Voice Navigator II Articulate Systems, Inc. Combined software/hardware package that allows spoken commands to execute any keyboard function; capable of learning multiple voices; can be customized to any application.

Appendix C-2   Speech Synthesizers

Accent   AICOM Corporation. IBM PC-compatible; variety of standalone and computer versions, including Toshiba.

Artic Transport Classic   Artic Technologies. External, rechargeable, battery operated; plugs into serial port; under 2 lbs.; compatible with IIe, IIGS, Macintosh, and IBM PC.

Audapter Speech System   Personal Data Systems, Inc. Alphanumeric text-to-speech conversion through ASCII text; rate adjustable to 500 words/minute; voice and pitch can be adjusted; compatible with Apple IIe, IIGS, Macintosh, IBM PC.

Clarity   Phillips. Human quality synthesizer installed in Innocomp devices, Say-It-All II Plus, Say-It-Simply Plus, and Scan-It-All; male and female voices available; can be adjusted in pitch and rate.

DECtalk PC   Digital Equipment Corporation. Voice synthesizer option card that accepts text and converts to high-quality human speech (1 user defined; 9 voices available; male, female, and child); controls for rates (120–550 words per minute), volume, pronunciation, and intonation; now an available option on a number of communication devices, such as TouchTalker, Liberator, EvalPac, Words+, and DynaVox.

DoubleTalk   RC Systems, Inc. Card contains two speech synthesizers (i.e., DoubleTalk PC1), text-to-speech compatible with RC system's Slotbuster II Doubletalk LT and LPC synthesizer built into DoubleTalk; compatible with all software written for Echo speech synthesizers.

Echo, Echo II, Echo II with Textalker   Echo Speech Corporation. Economical, varying models; plug-in text-to-speech synthesis card; female voice available on some; MC has higher quality digitized speech; available as Apple LC (Apple IIe, Apple IIC Apple IIC+, and Macintosh), or IBM PC and PC II.

IntroVoice VI   Voice Connection. Requires IBM PC-compatible computer; on board unlimited text-to-speech synthesizer.

Messenger IC   AICOM Corporation. Speech chip Ai902 requires PCMCIA Type II slot computers; includes power amplifier; compatible with Apple IIe, IIGS, Macintosh, and IBM PC.

Micro IntroVoice   Voice Connection. Input/output system requiring IBM-compatible computer of Texas Instruments; on board unlimited text-to-speech synthesizer.

MultiVoice   Institute of Applied Technology, Children's Hospital. Requires RS-232 port device; joint product of Children's Hospital and Digital Equipment Corporation; external unit 3½ lbs. including rechargeable battery; speech synthesizer with options of custom voice or one of eight others (male, female, child); compatible with IBM PC and Macintosh.

Personal Speech System   Vysion, Inc. Requires RS-232C Interface or Centronics parallel; compatible with IIe, IIGS, Commodore, Commodore 64, and IBM PC compatibles; self-contained voice synthesizer; can mix speech output with sound effects.

RealVoice (C)   ACS Technologies. Diphone-based portable, battery-powered speech Real Voice PC (B) synthesizer (male or female voice); easily attached to Epson keyboard; can use pictures with nonreaders; upgradable to EvalPac or ScanPac; also available with a small memory keyboard.

Screen Power Speech   Telesensory. Speech synthesizer coupled with a screen reading program; IBM PC.

SmarTalk   Automated Functions, Inc. Five-ounce external speech synthesizer that can operate on a battery up to 40 hours; IBM PC.

SmoothTalker   First Byte. Configured for use with a variety of computers and provided in a number of standalone, dedicated communicators (e.g., LightTalker, TouchTalker).

Sounding Board   GW Micro, Inc. Requires IBM-compatible computer; installed speech synthesizer card capable of 10 levels of volume, pitch, and speech rates and 26 tone levels.

Speak Out   GW Micro, Inc. Small, battery-powered speech synthesizer similar to Sounding Board; installed in computers and compatible with Apple IIe, IIGS, Macintosh, and IBM PC.

Symphonix 210, MC-310   Artic Technologies. Plug-in circuit card with on-board speaker; SONIX2 text-to-speech synthesizer; IBM PC and compatibles.

Appendix C-3   Assistive Communication Devices

Dedicated Communication Devices

The following lists include a variety of communication devices that are dedicated; that is, they function independently of a computer. However, many can be interfaced with a computer to use the expanded functions.

These lists have been developed from such sources as Closing the Gap (1995) and Church and Glennan (1992); they are not meant to be complete, but rather to provide useful information. Please see Hyper-AbleData

(Trace Center) and Closing the Gap for more complete listings. Letters have been assigned as follows to indicate the cost range for these devices.

A = inexpensive, below $1,000
B = inexpensive to moderate, $1,000–$3,000
C = moderate, $3,000–$5,000
D = moderate to expensive, $5,000–$7,000
E = expensive, over $7,000

Action Voice (A)   Ability Research. Records up to 19 messages; keypad; single switch/lightboard; scanning.

AlphaTalker (B)   Prentke Romich. Compatible with IBM PC, Apple IIGS, and Macintosh; 3–5 minutes speech; keyboard/headpointer/switch; Minspeak; icon prediction; auditory prompts. An upgrade/replacement of the IntroTalker.

AudioScan (B)   Detroit Institute for Children. Portable, multifunctional communication system; single switch; scanning; controls wheelchair and Windsford feeder.

DeltaTalker (C)   Prentke Romich. Replaces the TouchTalker and LightTalker, but combines their features in one unit; Minspeak and Unity application program.

DigiVox (B)   Sentient Systems Technology. Digitized speech; 4 levels of messages; messages arranged by area, picture, spelling, and message-linking; direct, visual/auditory scanning; portable; under 4 lbs.

DynaMyte (B)   Sentient Systems Technology. Lighter version of the DynaVox series.

DynaVox, DynaVox 2, DynaVox 2c (D)   Sentient Systems Technology. Touch activated, single/dual switch, mouse, joystick; DECtalk; portable; DynaCard memory cartridges contain a variety of programs; use DynaSyms; 2 and 2c have infrared ECU and computer access; 2c is a color unit.

Eval Pac with Real Voice (C); Scan Pac with Real Voice (C)   Adaptive Communication Systems Technologies. Communication device with RealVoice diphone-based speech, male or female voice; standard and alternate membrane keyboard; portable/battery; direct, lightpointer, joystick, single/dual switch; scanning; built-in printer.

FingerFoniks (A)   Words+, Inc. 1 lb, handheld; membrane keyboard with phoneme keys; synthesized and recorded speech, can be prestored.

Hawk, Black Hawk (A)   ADAMLAB. Housed in a Wolf case; 9 message areas; up to 45 seconds recording time.

Liberator (E)   Prentke Romich. Compatible with IBM PC, Apple IIGS, and Macintosh. Portable standalone or interface with computer. Keyboard, pointing, switch access; communication, environmental control, and educational activities (math, spelling, word processing); built-in printer; DECtalk; auditory feedback; icon prediction; Minspeak and Unity application program.

LightTalker (D)   Prentke Romich. Compatible with IBM PC, Apple IIGS, and TouchTalker Macintosh; portable, battery/AC adapter; keyboard, optical pointer, multiple switches; 8/32/128 locations; interfaces with computers; environmental control; Minspeak; SmoothTalker (standard) or DECtalk (additional) Scanning; TouchTalker offers above features except for scanning or switch access.

LightWRITERS (B–D)   Zygo Industries. Models vary, some with dual visual displays, internal (SL30, SL35, SL4A, SL5, or external speech output, one or two keyboards, abbreviation expansion, SL55, SL56, SL8, & SL80) and prestored programmable vocabulary, switch access, and scanning.

Lingraphica (E)   Tolfa Corporation. Multimedia communication device housed in a customized Apple laptop; uses 2000+ icons to retrieve words to assemble graphic or auditory messages.

Lynx (A)   ADAMLAB. Small; 4 message keys; single or multiple switches; visual or auditory scanning.

Macaw; Big Blue Macaw; Green Macaw; Great Green Macaw (B)   Zygo Industries. Portable; 32 keys, 4 × 8 matrix of 1.5" squares; 1–8½ minutes of digitally recorded speech; switch access; expandable keyboard; messages can be individual, string messages, link keys, multiple levels. Green and Great Green allow more programmable area and access options. Big Blue permits multiple users.

MessageMate (A)   Words+, Inc. Handheld (under 2 lbs.); analog recorded speech; direct or 1–2 switch access; 20 or 40¾-inch squares can be grouped for larger input areas; variety of scanning modes; key accept times can be varied.

Parrot (A)   Zygo Industries. Walkman sized; 32–64 minutes digitally recorded speech; up to 16 messages.

PeaceKeyper (A); Peacemaker (A)   Tiger Communication Systems, Inc. Combined 66-page picture communication binder with foldout Franklin Specialist Speaking Ace 200 battery-operated communicator with 5 × 5.5 × 1 keyboard and LCD display. Peacemaker adds the following functions: LCD; adjustable font sizes; 75-word authorable list. Optional AC adapter. Specialist adds LCD and voice output options and can override spelling errors with text-to-speech.

Pegasus (E), Pegasus Lite (E)   Words+, Inc. A compact, self-contained AAC dedicated communication device that includes a CD-ROM drive, a built-in touch window, and built-in MultiVoice (DECtalk). Contains Talking Screen for Windows and uses thousands of high-quality color symbols, including PCS, Blissymbols, CommPic, Imaginart, and Commun.I.mage. Allows user to record and playback hours of sound.

Polycom/Polytalk (B–D)   Zygo Industries. Miniature typing aid with menu-driven programs; 29 phrases retrievable with 2 keystrokes; abbreviation expansion; telephone access for hearing impaired; printer port; speech synthesizer available in variety of languages.

Say-It-All; Say-It-All II Plus (B); Say-It-All Gold (C); Say-It-Simply Plus (B); Say-It-Simply Gold (C); Scan-It-All (C); Scan-It-All Gold (C)   Innocomp. 2.25 lbs., portable, battery powered, with Clarity speech synthesizer (digital with male or female voice); keyboard; LCD, stores up to 846 words or phrases that are retrievable with 1 keystroke; interfaces with computer. Say-It-Simply Plus is 4.5 lbs., has 144 1" squares that can be reconfigured for larger input areas, accepts a keyboard overlay, and can be programmed for up to 762 words or phrases. Scan-It-All has same features but allows for a variety of scanning modes. Gold versions include DECtalk.

Scan Com-PS (B)   Med Labs, Inc. Portable, battery powered; LCD; internal speech synthesizer available in English or Spanish; 1–2 switches; visible or audible scanning; environmental control.

ScanMate4, ScanMate8, SwitchMate 8 (A)   TASH, Inc. Stores eight 8-second phrases; permits direct selection and automatic/step scanning.

SpeakEasy (A)   AbleNet, Inc. Portable, under 3 lbs., measures 8" × 6" × 3"; membrane keyboard; switch; can record up to 2 minutes of digitized speech in 12 message slots; battery and AC adapter.

Speaking Ace 200 (A)   Tiger Communication Systems, Inc. Portable; battery; compact QWERTY 5 × 5.5 × 1" keyboard; LCD; voice output, but without text-to-speech synthesizer.

Special Friend (B–C)   Shea Products. Portable or with power pac; membrane keyboard; preprogrammed phrases by categories, and user-created words/phrases can be produced in volume ranging from whisper to shout.

Steeper Communication Teaching Aid (B)   Zygo Industries. 4 × 4 matrix of 2" backlit message squares for scanning. Must be connected to the Parrot for speech output.

Switchboard (B)   Zygo Industries. Variable matrix scanning unit permitting 4 messages; direct or scanning multiswitch selection; row-column scanning.

TouchTalker (D)   Prentke Romich. Compatible with IBM PC, Apple IIGS, and Macintosh; portable, battery/AC adapter; keyboard, 8/32/128 locations; interfaces with computers; environmental control; Minspeak; Smooth-Talker (standard) or DECtalk (additional). Recently discontinued, replaced by DeltaTalker.

Type 'n Speak (B)   Blazie Engineering. Notetaker for the Braille 'n Speak that uses standard rather than Braille keyboard; built-in word processing, spell checker, and calculator with 768k of memory.

Vocal Assistant (A)   Luminaud, Inc. Portable (5 lbs.); battery; allows recording of 16 messages; single switch scanning.

VoiceMate (8)   TASH, Inc. Stores up to four 4-second phrases; direct and switch access.

VoicePal, VoicePal Plus (A)   Adapt Tech., Inc. Handheld, battery-operated recorder/playback device; up to 60 seconds and 10 messages; keypad plus T ACTION pads for input; Voice Pal Plus permits the scanning of 2, 3, 4, 10 messages.

VOIS 160, VoisShapes (C)   Phonic Ear, Inc. Apple IIe, IBM-PC; portable, battery powered; two-line VOIS 160 (C) LCD; (with P.A.L.S. software) text-to-speech synthesizer or SmoothTalker DECtalk; programming by level/location, sequencing, or abbreviation expansion; stores up to 60,000 entries on 7 levels; allows selection of words/phrases from 14,000 core vocabulary. VoisShapes uses visual motor encoding based on ASL sign parameters. These devices are no longer produced.

Walker Talker (B)   Prentke Romich. All components of the communicator are worn inside a waist belt; 1–2 minutes of digitized speech.

Wolf (Mega, Whisper) (A)   ADAMLAB. Manufactured by Texas Instruments; portable, battery-operated communicator housed in a Touch 'n Tell plastic case; variable touch-pad grid; contains 500-word user-specified vocabulary or choice of 3 overlays, user-programmable memory sections (3, each with 800 words). Whisper version has single-switch access and auditory scanning. Selections can be spoken on a private speaker for user editing before public speech.

Computer-based Communication Devices

EZ Keys/Key Wiz   Words+, Inc. Requires IBM-compatible computer; adaptable keyboard to allow single-finger operation and adjustments in key action time and repeat rate; dual word prediction; abbreviation expansion. Used with a variety of text-to-speech synthesizers (e.g., Multivoice).

Handy Speech   IBM compatible required; speech; printer; multifunctional; audioscanning; single switch; customized vocabulary; controls powered wheelchair and Windsford feeder.

Handy Speech Synthesizer   IBM compatible required; single switch; sound detection switch (JK); (Models JK & Model K) telephone interface.

Kurzweil Personal Reader   Kurzweil Reading Machine System, Xerox Imaging Kurzweil VOICE Systems. Requires IBM-compatible computer; 50,000-word vocabulary with a 200,000-word on-line vocabulary that allows word processing, spreadsheet, database, and other software through voice recognition; for visual and print-disabled individuals.

Morse Code Equalizer   Words+, Inc. Requires IBM-compatible computer; word processing and speech output; 1–2 switch Morse code input; originally designed for blind user who only had eyelid movement, but can be used by sighted or visually impaired; abbreviation expansion; instant speech; automatic capitalization of letters.

Portable Transaction   Voice Connection. IBM compatible; 500 words and text-to-speech Voice Computer (PTVC-756) synthesis voice recognition; 34 oz., 9.5 × 4 × 2.5" dimensions.

Samy System   ACS Technologies. Macintosh required, Real Voice (male, female, child); educational system; keyboard, touch screen, mouse; expanded keyboard; Navigator voice recognition; Boardmaker, Talking Pictures; scanning.

Small Talk PC   GW Micro, Inc. Battery powered; IBM compatible; 6–11 lbs., Sounding Board speech synthesizer and Vocal Eyes access software.

Speaking Dynamically   Don Johnston, Inc. Communication software program that provides communication board layouts, including speech output and text-to-speech capabilities. Programs can be cut and pasted into any configuration according to user's needs. Works in conjunction with Boardmaker; Macintosh.

Speaqualizer   American Printing House for the Blind. Requires IBM PC-compatible computer; cable-connected device that will read character's from monitor; user can control volume, rate, and other features of speech output.

Speech Thing   Covox, Inc. Requires IBM-compatible computer; device plugs into PC parallel port without interfering with applications; text-to-speech synthesis can be incorporated into software applications.

Synergy PC   Synergy. Requires Synergy Mac wheelchair mounted and powered by wheelchair battery; built-in touch screen, alternative keyboard, and environmental control; IBM-compatible or Macintosh computer.

System 2000/Versa   Words+, Inc. Requires IBM-compatible computer. All connections via single box to give total computer capability and yet have advantages of a dedicated communicator. Dynamic display of color pictographic language; 1–5 switches; joystick, trackball, touchscreen; auditory scanning available.

Talking Screen   Words+, Inc. Requires IBM-compatible computer; on-screen communication board can be created from library of graphic symbols which can be used separately or in sequence; 1–5 switches; mouse, trackball, touch pad, joystick, optical pointer or touch screen; can be used with variety of speech synthesizers (e.g., Multivoice).

Verbette Mark I and Mark II   Computer Conversations. Requires IBM-compatible computer; internal card to produce speech output with verbal operating system software; can also use interface with other speech software; Mark II is an external box that attaches to parallel port and is portable, battery operated, and can be used as an AC adapter.

Words+ Equalizer   Words+, Inc. Requires IBM-compatible computer; AAC evaluation package that simulates a variety of available AAC systems.

Appendix C-4   Word Processing Software

AppleWorks Companion   R.C. Systems. Modifies AppleWorks so it can be used by individuals with visual impairments; speech output for keys and screens; Apple IIe, Apple IIGS.

Bankstreet Writer Plus   Broderbund Software, Inc. Easy word processing package designed for children through adults that includes a 6,000-word automatic spelling feature with option to add personal vocabulary; Apple IIe, Apple IIGS, IBM compatible (DOS).

Children's Writing   Learning Company. Word processing and page design capabilities. Publishing Center allows children to create a variety of printed documents (e.g., stories, awards); Apple IIe, Apple IIGS, IBM compatible (DOS).

Collaborative Writer   Research Design Associates, Inc. Software that includes on-line word processing and is designed to teach collaborative writing, such as memos, proposals, and utilization of network services; Macintosh.

Eye Relief   SkiSoft Publishing Corp. Word processing program for individuals with visual impairments. Allows high-quality enlarged fonts with user control of spacing on the screen; PC compatibles (DOS).

Freedom Writer   World Communications. Word processing software allowing the user to select and construct sentences with words rather than letters; scanning, joystick, mouse, light pen, and cursor versions available; user can define words and phrases for a personal dictionary; IBM compatible (DOS).

IntelliTalk   IntelliTools. Simple word processing program that includes speech output during typing; works with IntelliKeys and can be used as a communication device; Apple IIe, Apple IIGS, Macintosh, IBM compatible (DOS).

KidsWord   Kidsview Software. Large-print word processing program for children (preschool through secondary); Apple.

Perfect Scribe   Arts Computer Products, Inc. WordPerfect word processing program designed for individuals with disabilities; IBM compatible (DOS).

Primary Editor Plus   IBM Eduquest. Entry-level word processor for elementary students that includes spelling checker and banner maker; IBM compatible (DOS).

ProWord Talking Word Processor   Access Unlimited. Wrap-around, large-print word processor designed for the visually impaired; direct access to key commands rather than menu display; word output uses Echo, Cricket, or Slotbuster II speech synthesizer; Apple IIe, Apple IIGS.

Write Away Institute of Applied Technology, The Children's Hospital. Combined word processing and communication program that includes speech output as user types; built-in scanning and word prediction; IBM compatible (DOS).

Write On! Humanities Affirmative. Computers to Help People, Inc. Software that uses word processing features to teach basic writing skills and focus on literature; designed for school-age and adults; Apple IIe, Apple IIGS, and IBM compatible (DOS).

Write: OutLoud 2.0 Don Johnston, Inc. Word processing program that includes speech output, spell checking and exceptional dictionary; text can be spoken in entirety or in selected segments.

Appendix C-5 Rate Enhancement Software

Audscan Words+. Auditory scanning program for individuals with visual and/or motor impairments that allows 4 levels of scanning; with use of a speech synthesizer, includes speech output with variety of voices; scanner voice can be varied; user easily can alternate between private monitoring of scanning speech through an earphone and speech output for communication; includes abbreviation expansion; included in Talking Screen.

Aurora ACS Technologies. Software program that allows individuals with severe disabilities to access computer and use accelerated typing; program includes word prediction, word guessing, automatic capitalization and punctuation, and flexibility in setting scanning and key delays; speech output available when used with a speech synthesizer; IBM compatible (DOS).

CoWriter Don Johnston Inc. Word prediction based on person's word use; e.g., recency and redundancy; includes speech output program, MacTalk II; works with most word processing programs; Macintosh.

DealWrite II Deal Communication Centre. Text writing system that uses word prediction; comes with an external switch box that accommodates up to 9 external switches; allows two switch scanning; use is facilitated by instructions on a screen menu.

EZ Keys, Key Wiz, Equalizer Words+. Keyboard assistance programs that use word prediction and EZ Keys/Key Wiz abbreviation expansion; allows use of standard software; speech output is available when used with a speech synthesizer.

Gus Abbreviations for Windows Gus Communications, Inc. Program that runs in the background and/or monitors keystrokes to accelerate typing through abbreviation expansion (letter to word or word to sentence); also allows calculation of numbers; IBM compatible (Windows).

Gus Talking Board for Windows Gus Communications, Inc. Program that combines an on-screen keyboard with word/sentence prediction and abbreviation expansion; speech output through speech synthesizer (Sound Blaster); allows male or female voice and 4 different languages (American, German, French, and Spanish).

HandiKey Microsystems Software, Inc. An alternative HandiKey Deluxe keyboard setup that allows access and scanning through use of switches (up to 5), mouse/trackball, and digitizer tablet; includes word prediction and abbreviation expansion; deluxe version can be configured for auditory scanning; IBM compatible (DOS, Windows).

HandiWord; HandiWord Deluxe Word processing software that includes a statistically weighed, memory resident word prediction program; includes a dictionary for adding specific words and abbreviation expansion that can be operated through a numeric keyboard; deluxe version includes dictionaries for English, German, French, and Spanish; IBM PC compatible (DOS, Windows).

Help U Type and Speak; Help U Type for Windows World Communications. Word processing program that provides keyboard access for individuals who use one finger or a mouth/headstick; includes word prediction and abbreviation expansion; IBM compatible (DOS, Windows).

KeyCache OMS Development. Memory resident word expansion program that includes pop-up menus of possible words as the user types; includes abbreviation expansion and automatic spacing; IBM compatible (DOS, Windows).

PRD+ Basic Edition Productivity Software International. Memory resident abbreviation expansion program that allows entry of commands, words, phrases, sentences, and paragraphs with 1–2 keystrokes; IBM compatible (DOS, Windows).

Predict-It Word processing program that uses word prediction and easy, rapid program access to grammatically correct endings of words; compatible with the Adaptive Firmware Card; Apple IIe, Apple IIGS.

Scanning WSKI II Words+. Scanning program that allows multiple input access (e.g., switch, mouse, joystick, sip/puff) and uses word predication and abbreviation expansion; can add voice output with a speech synthesizer; IBM PC compatible.

Appendix C-6   Braille and Text Enlargement Software

Artic Magnum GT   Artic Technologies. Provides text enlargement up to 8 times using standard off-the-shelf software programs; multiple split-screen display, search and read functions, bar tracking, and user definable keys; DOS, Windows.

Breakthrough to Language   Vocabulary and sentence building program that provides large-print and speech output, as well as adapted access through keyboard, AFC, and IntelliKeys; Spanish versions available; Apple IIe, IIGS, Macintosh, DOS.

Breakthrough to Writing   Program that allows user to trace letters on TouchWindow and hear a human voice produce the phonic sound of letters and words; teacher can use authoring part of program to create memory boards and on-screen lessons; large print; Apple IIe, IIGS, Macintosh, DOS.

Closeview   Apple Computer, Inc. Screen magnification utility (up to 16 times) that is included with the computer; Apple IIGS, Macintosh.

Duxbury Braille Translator for Windows (DBTWin)   Duxbury Systems, Inc. Braille translator for automatic print-to-braille conversion of standard word processor documents (Windows and Macintosh). Covers many foreign languages, mathematics, and other special topics of Braille translation.

In Focus   Program allows magnification of one line of text, and either a portion or the entire screen; uses pop-up menus and allows the programming of hot keys; DOS.

In LARGE   Berkeley Systems, Inc. Program allowing 2–16 times magnification of any portion of the computer screen; includes automatic scanning, image stretching, and the ability to change black-and-white display to white-on-black display.

Large Print DOS   Optelec USA, Inc. Natural-looking font can be enlarged up to 12 times; works with word processing, spreadsheets, games, and educational software; DOS, Windows.

MAGic   Microsystems Software Inc. Screen-magnification program that allows 2× enlargement of text and graphics for a variety of software; DOS, Windows.

Powerama   Syntha-Voice Computers, Inc. Large-print and screen review software are synchronized to permit simultaneous seeing and listening to text; commands allow interactive synchronization of visual and synthetic speech output; DOS.

Powerama Window Bridge   Syntha-Voice Computers, Inc. A screen review program for the IBM that integrates large print with synthetic speech output; allows access to both DOS and Windows environments; DOS, Windows.

Sentence Scan   Computers to Help People, Inc. Allows the entry of up to 20 words that can be displayed in large print; the user can build words and sentences by selecting letters with the use of a switch and scanning; Apple IIe, IIGS, Macintosh.

Zoom Text; Zoom Text Plus   Ai Squared. Provides 2–16 times magnification of text and graphics in common computer programs; allows zooming in on a single line, a portion of the screen, or the entire screen; complete control over both tracking and scrolling; DOS.

Appendix C-7   Adapted Access, Cause and Effect, and Motor Training Software

Keyboard Emulator and Switch/Scanning Software

AFC Custom Scans   Technology for Language and Learning. Has 15+ switch scans for cause and effect programs; Apple IIGS.

AFC Literacy Setups   Don Johnston Inc. 100+ setups for scanning, Key Largo, Morse code, AFC Access, and TouchWindow; overlays for Unicorn, Key Largo, and TouchWindow; Apple IIe, IIGS.

AFC Setups for Sharon's   Access Unlimited. Quickstart setups that allow access through 1 or more program switches or through assisted keyboard format; Apple IIe, IIGS.

Audscan   Words+. Has 4 levels of scanning for visually and motorically impaired; spelling and abbreviation expansion; DOS.

CNTRL, ALT, & SHIFT; KEY ADAPTATION   Bradley Murray, S.J. Setups of keys so that a one-finger or stick user can do key sequences (acting as if hitting keys simultaneously); DOS.

Easy Access   Apple Computer, Inc. Allows key action by individuals unable to press more than one key at a time (headstick or one finger). Sticky keys let user handle a sequence one key at a time, mouse keys use keys on calculator in place of mouse, and slow keys adjust delay times of keys; Apple IIGS, Macintosh.

EEK   OMS Development. On-screen keyboard in a Windows environment that can be activated by a cursor (mouse); MS Windows (IBM).

Expanded Keyboard Emulator   Words+. Allows the use of abbreviation, expansion, and word prediction; allows single-finger operation; five different voice outputs; interface allows connection of a variety of keyboards; DOS.

E Z Morse   Words+. Software program that works with switch input and is designed to input via single-switch or dual-switch Morse code; includes Keyboard Expander and E Z Scan.

E Z Scan   Words+. Keyboard emulator that allows input via single or dual switch; included with Keyboard Emulator and E Z Morse.

Freedom Writer   World Communications. Word processor with scanning, mouse, light pen, joystick, and cursor key access; DOS.

HandiKEY; HandiKey Deluxe   Microsystems Software Inc. Scanning/direct matrix input; word prediction and abbreviation expansion; access via keyboard, mouse, joystick, trackball, and single switch; 5-switch access optional; IBM compatible, DOS, Windows.

Handy Speech   Consultants for Communication Technology. Software for Handy Speech Communication System; direct selection and scanning; prestored sentences and text-to-speech synthesis; DOS.

Help U Key   World Communications. Alternate input allowing single key or single switch scanning; DOS.

JOKUS Single Switch Software   Don Johnston Inc. Five different topics of software with graphics operated by up to five switches, an alternate keyboard, mouse, Ke:nx, or direct selection.

Joystick Games   Technology for Language and Learning. Variety of joystick game programs to teach eye–hand coordination needed for scanning with a joystick, as well as teaching electronic wheelchair control.

KeyAbility   Meeting the Challenge, Inc. Software program that allows the user option for either Dvorak Board or standard keyboard and to DOS program key sequences so a single-finger user can operate multiple-key functions.

KeyUp   Ability Systems Corporation. DOS program allowing special key setups for individuals who have difficulty with normal key operation; allows keys to activate on upstroke, turns repeat functions of keys on and off, and allows two or more keys to be activated at once by sequential selection of single keys.

MouseKeys for Windows   World Communications. On-screen keyboard allows user to perform functions with trackball, mouse, or other mouse emulators; includes word prediction, abbreviation expansion, and auto select keys; Windows.

ProKey for DOS   CE Software, Inc. Software for single-finger/stick users; allows ProKey for Windows multiple-key strokes to be entered as separate keystrokes; versions for IBM DOS and Windows.

QuicKeys   CE Software, Inc. Software allowing series of keystrokes/commands to be entered with a single keystroke; works with Easy Access; Macintosh.

Rabbit Scanner   Exceptional Childrens' Software. Space bar, game paddle, and switch access; teaches horizontal scanning; Apple IIe.

Scanning WSKE II   Words+. Software that, with appropriate hardware interface, allows a variety of input devices and single- and multiple-switch access; provides word prediction and abbreviation expansion; IBM PC compatible, DOS.

ScreenDoors   Three on-screen keyboard layouts that allow use of various access methods (e.g., mouse, trackball); includes word prediction; Macintosh.

Sentence Scan   Computers to Help People. Single- or double-switch or keyboard access; allows programming of scanning delay.

Sight Words   UCLA Intervention Program for Handicapped Children. Keyboard or switch access; can set scanning speed.

Speech Link   Zygo Industries. Auditory scanning program with single-switch operation; DOS.

Sticky   Center for Computer Assistance to the Disabled. Allows one-finger users to handle multiple-key sequences by hitting one key at a time.

Talking Screen   Words+. Communication program that allows creation and use of symbol boards; access is by one to five switches or other keyboard emulators (e.g., mouse or optical pointer).

WikVik   Prentke Romich Co. On-screen keyboard allowing entry of text with pointing mechanisms (e.g., trackball, mouse, head-pointing devices); nineteen keyboard layouts are available and customized layouts can be arranged.

Cause and Effect Software

101 Animations   RJ Cooper and Associates. Cause and effect program that is designed so that each activation of a switch activates one of 101 animations (with accompanying sounds); Macintosh, IBM PC (Windows).

Build a Scene   RJ Cooper and Associates. Starting with a blank computer screen, the user can build a scene by adding parts with each hit of a switch; with the use of an Echo speech synthesizer, each scene part added can be accompanied with a word or sound; includes animation; shareware; Apple IIe, Apple IIGS.

Cause and Effect   Technology for Language and Learning. Eight programs used with AFC Custom Scans to teach cause and effect using games (public domain package); Apple IIe, Apple IIGS.

Cause 'n Effect   Marblesoft. Program provides four activities in which the user can start, stop, or change the action by pressing any key; can be used with Echo or Cricket speech synthesizer and a single switch, TouchWindow, or IntelliKeys; Apple IIe, Apple IIGS.

Children's Switch   RJ Cooper and Associates. Transition cause and effect program to teach associations between appropriate behavior and consequence; TouchWindow Progressions reinforce cause and effect, attending to task, following verbal directions, and responding to timed screen prompts; shareware; Apple IIe, Apple IIGS, IBM PC compatibles.

One-Switch Paintbrush   Adaptive Computers. A one-switch cause and effect program where each activation of the switch moves a cursor to draw a mosaic picture; Apple IIe, Apple IIGS.

One Switch Picasso   Bill and Richard's Software. Two volumes of drawing software designed for use with one switch; each activation of the switch allows user to color a picture.

Switch It-Change It   UCLA Intervention Program for Handicapped Children. Switch-activated program designed for children who are either very young or low functioning; colored, animated 3-D objects are presented for identification, selection, and/or matching contingent on the activation of a switch.

Switch 'n See   ACCT (Activating Children Through Technology). Program that trains cause and effect by activating a picture with accompanying music each time a switch is pressed; Apple IIe, Apple IIGS.

Switch Training Program   Assistive Device Center, School of Engineering and Computer Science. Switch training program with five scenarios involving actions; in the cause and effect mode, any switch activation causes the action; Apple IIe, Apple IIGS.

Motor Training Software

Joystick Games   Technology for Language and Learning. Program includes toddler, preschool, and elementary school age games using a joystick; reinforces skills needed for electronic operation of a wheelchair.

Joystick Trainer   RJ Cooper and Associates. Software includes nine activities for helping individuals develop gross and fine motor controls needed for electronic controlled devices and wheelchairs.

Motor Training Games   Computers to Help People. Program includes switch-controlled games (e.g., bumper cars, basketball) with large-print menus to assess motor abilities.

Motor Training Games   Don Johnston Inc. Fourteen switch games adaptable to the Adaptive Firmware Card and switch-activated communication devices.

Appendix C-8   Communication Boards/Overlay Software

Access Bliss   Blissymbolics Communication International. Dictionary of Blissymbols that allows copying of selected symbols into word processing or drawing documents; Macintosh. Specifically designed for use with Blissymbols.

Aladin   INCAP. Symbol communication program with over 1,200 symbols and speech output; can rearrange symbols into category and subcategory pages and vary color and size; IBM PC compatibles (Windows).

Boardmaker International   Mayer-Johnson Co. Program that allows the user to select, modify, and print any of 3,000 Picture Communication Symbols (PCS); allows the user to customize communication boards according to specific needs; symbols allow accompanying labels to be in English or any of nine other languages; separate versions available for Macintosh or Windows.

Gus! Mayer-Johnson Symbol Set   Gus Communications, Inc. Dictionary of 3,000 Mayer-Johnson symbols that can be used with Gus! Multimedia Systems for Windows for setting up communication displays; used with the multimedia system, it completes a full multimedia communication system with multiple pages and subcategories;

high-quality digitized/synthesized speech; available in English, French, German, and Spanish; IBM compatible (Windows).

IntelliKeys Overlay Maker   IntelliTools. Allows the creation and printing of custom overlays from a library of 300 symbols; Apple IIe, IIGS, Macintosh.

Mousing Around   Mayer-Johnson Co. Dictionary of over 3,000 Picture Communication Symbols for use with Unicorn Overlay Express for communication displays or for importing into other Apple II programs that will accept pictures; Apple IIe, Apple IIGS.

Start Talking: A Unicorn User's Keyboard   IntelliTools. Prepared setups for Talking Word Board and overlays for the Unicorn Expanded Keyboard and the Adaptive Firmware Card; variety of topics for communication activities and early learning activities; Apple IIe, Apple IIGS.

Unicorn Overlay Express   IntelliTools. Allows the creation of custom overlays for Unicorn Overlay Express, Picture the Unicorn Board; permits printout of 2, 8, or 32 square Communication Symbols layouts; Apple IIe, Apple IIGS.

Up and Running   IntelliTools. Custom overlay kits for the Unicorn Expanded Keyboard and the Adaptive Firmware Card; Apple IIe, Apple IIGS.

Up and Running for the Lightboard   Ability Research, Inc. Custom overlay for the Lightboard, Ke:nx, or Adaptive Firmware Card that provides setups and software for instantaneous use of a variety of software programs; Apple IIe, Apple IIGS, Macintosh.

Appendix C-9   Language and Cognition Software

Literacy and Language Development Software

AFC Literacy Setups   Don Johnston Inc. 100+ setups for scanning, Key Largo, Morse code, AFC Access, and TouchWindow; overlays for Unicorn, Key Largo, and TouchWindow; Apple IIe, IIGS.

Bailey's Bookhouse   Edmark Corporation. Development introduction to reading for preschool children; allows exploration of six interactive activities with questions and feedback; uses lively music and colorful graphics; Macintosh, IBM compatible (DOS).

BlissLiteracy*   Blissymbolics Communication International. Allows user to create stories using a combination of words and Blissymbols; includes mini-authoring system so instructors can create lessons; IBM PC compatibles.

BlissReader, BlissWriter*   Requires AccessBliss to be used; BlissWriter allows creation of stories with text that can be broken down to phrases associated with Blissymbols; BlissReader allows choice of having the story read aloud or using Blissymbols, words, or both; Macintosh.

Blissymbolics: Bliss Skills*   Vocational and Rehabilitation Research Institute. Drill program to assist in the learning of Blissymbols, components, and syntax; Apple IIe, Apple IIGS.

Breakthrough to Language; Breakthrough to Writing   Creative Learning, Inc. Series of programs designed to teach basic skills needed for reading and writing to preschool and elementary age children; student progresses through series with increase vocabulary and language usage and understanding; makes use of phonics and pictures; works with Echo or Cricket speech synthesizer; writing version has authoring program to allow teachers to develop memory boards and on-screen lessons; Apple IIe, IIGS, Macintosh, IBM compatible (DOS).

Bring the Classics to Life   A/V Concepts Corporation. Language/reading development program with each disk representing a complete classic novel divided into ten short chapters, including controlled vocabulary and questions to assess vocabulary learning and reading comprehension; Apple IIe, Apple IIGS.

Charlotte's Web   Sunburst Communications. Animated story for elementary children designed for users to develop vocabulary and reading comprehension through a series of questions regarding characters and events.

Cloze Clues   Continental Press. Exercises progress from grade 2 to 6 reading levels; makes use of nonfictional passages and lessons to teach contextual clues; program provides feedback and a game for reward; teachers can develop additional cloze passages.

Clozemaster   Research Design Associates, Inc. Program for generation of cloze reading passages.

CLOZE Plus   Taylor Associates. Program includes eight reading levels with exercises for learning vocabulary within context, as well structured cloze activities.

CLOZE Vocabulary and More   A/V Concepts Corporation. Program designed to build and reinforce reading comprehension and vocabulary, including word parts (e.g., prefixes and suffixes); includes cloze vocabulary.

Communication Series   Dunamis, Inc. Language development programs focusing on a wide range of communication concepts (e.g., needs, emotion, places, activities).

Edmark Reading Program   Edmark Corporation. Program for early language development and teaching beginning reading; teaches words and word endings through sequenced and repetitive sight word approach using computer spoken cues; permits teacher considerable flexibility in instructional approach.

Emerging Literacy   Technology for Language and Learning. Five-volume set of favorite stories (e.g., Three Bears, Jack and the Beanstalk) with speech output (Echo speech synthesizer). Pages can be turned with either the Open-Apple key or a switch.

HyperBliss*   Blissymbolics Communication International. Program that allows users to retrieve Blissymbols by components and can provide a prioritized list of appropriate symbols; teaching portion trains in proficient use of the symbols; scanning is available; can be operated through the keyboard or a single switch; Macintosh.

Mickey's Magic Reader   Sunburst Communications. Programs to teach reading comprehension and problem-solving skills, as well as to encourage reading for enjoyment through the use of the colorful Disney characters; visual reinforcement provided for correct answers.

Micro-Lads   Laureate Learning Systems, Inc. Language assessment and development program that teaches syntax; lessons are centered around such combinations as noun

---

* Specifically designed for use with Blissymbols.

plurals and noun-verb agreement, verb forms, etc.; French version is also available; menus allow tailoring lessons to student needs; Apple IIe, Apple IIGS, Macintosh, IBM compatible (DOS).

Muppet series   Sunburst Communications. Series of programs using Muppet characters within a game format to teach basic skills for reading and writing (e.g., letters, words, concepts); Muppet Word Books include simple words so that students can write their names and short sentences.

My Own Stories   MECC. Open-ended writing software that allows users to combine words and pictures to write about events in their lives; IBM (DOS), Macintosh.

Old MacDonald's Farm   kidTECH/SoftTouch. Song is used to teach vocabulary and sounds of animals; use of colored animation with song when child selects an animal; Macintosh.

Principles Alphabet Literacy (PALS)   IBM: Eduquest. Basic interactive reading/writing program to teach literacy skills in adolescents and adults through the use of a phonemic approach; multimedia presentations involve combinations of text, music, video, graphics, speech, and touch; combined use of computer and TV; IBM compatible (DOS).

Readable Stories   Laureate Learning Systems, Inc. Series of stories centered around a theme (e.g., birthday, puppet show) designed to increase reading comprehension in children in grades 1 to 4; includes text, graphics, speech output, and animated presentations followed by comprehension questions; Apple IIe, IIGS.

Reader Rabbit   Learning Company. Four sequenced games to train letter/word recognition, vocabulary, and memory skill; provides practice with over 200 phonetic consonant-vowel-consonant words from a typical reading curriculum; Apple IIe, Apple IIGS, Macintosh, and IBM compatible (DOS).

Read, Write, and Publish Series   Program providing students with writing ideas and practice in all phases of writing through final publication form; students can read information about characters and activities and expand on it in their writing; Apple IIe, Apple IIGS, IBM compatible (DOS).

Sticky Bear Series   Optimum Resource, Inc. Series of programs that focus on drawing, music, alphabet, numbers, reading, and language learning; Apple IIe, Apple IIGS. Selected programs also work with IBM compatible, DOS (e.g., Sticky Bear Reading), and Macintosh (e.g., Stickybear's Early Learning Activities).

Story Bliss*   Blissymbolics Communication International. Consists of two software programs: Storytime; Apple IIGS (single switch); Construction Series I; Powerpad Software; Just for Fun Creative Communicating. Collections of stories for the development of reading skills allowing a variety of input modes (e.g., switch, powerpad, TouchWindow, scanning, keyboard); Construction Series I uses Hypercard. Powerpad works with Apple IIGS. Just for Fun and Construction Series works with Macintosh.

Talking Text Library   Programs to teach preschool and elementary children having difficulty learning reading; speech output allows stories to be read aloud while specific words are highlighted; includes graphic enhancement and printing capabilities; Apple IIe, Apple IIGS, Macintosh.

Talking Text Writer   Scholastic Software. Programs (with speech output) to build reading and writing skills; language development activities through a combination of reading, writing, and listening approaches; dictionary pronounces and defines words; Apple IIe, Apple IIGS, Macintosh.

Cognitive Rehabilitation Software

Aphasia Diagnostic Reading   Technology for Language and Learning. Reading comprehension program that measures ability to match, read, and understand language (e.g., letters, words, synonyms, math); provides analysis and storage of data; treatment program consists of six lessons in various aspects of language and math use; Apple IIe, Apple IIGS, Macintosh.

Attention, Perception, and Discrimination Plus for Windows   Software to assist individuals with cognitive impairments with skills such as matching, attention, and discrimination; IBM (DOS, Windows).

Captain's Log   Brain Train, Inc. Series of programs that train individuals with cognitive impairment in attending, problem solving, conceptual skills, numeric concepts, memory, and visual/motor skills; IBM compatible (DOS).

Cognitive Drills: Set I (Visual Tasks)   Sunset Software. Eleven menu-driven programs for training attention, reaction time, memory, visual field, scanning, and discrimination; Apple IIe, Apple IIGS.

Cognitive Rehabilitation   Technology for Language and Learning. Four volumes of public domain programs to reinforce cognitive skills, memory, language, and visual motor skills; includes mind mapping, speed reading using tachistoscopic exercises, and spelling programs; Apple IIe, Apple IIGS, Macintosh.

COGREHAB   Life Science Associates. Software programs targeting Apple diagnosis and treatment of attention, perception, and memory, as well as visual scanning, problem solving, and reasoning; IIe, IBM compatibles (DOS).

---

* Specifically designed for use with Blissymbols.

Foundations I & II   Psychological Software Services, Inc. Computer programs to restore (access) cognitive rehab functions in attention, discrimination, and initiation/inhibition; Foundations II expands on the training of the first series; Apple IIe, IBM compatible (DOS).

Memory I & II   Psychological Software Services, Inc. Programs that provide memory training, including encoding, categorizing, and organizing skills; skills in these activities rely heavily on training provided in the Foundations I and II.

Appendix C-10   Telecommunication Software

ClarisWorks   Claris Corporation. Integrated software package that provides word processing, database, spreadsheet, and telecommunications functions.

Collaborative Writer   Research Design Associates. Software that includes on-line word processing and is designed to teach collaborative writing, such as memos, proposals, and utilization of network services; Macintosh.

Crosstalk for Macintosh; Crosstalk for Windows   Digital Electronics Corporation. Telecommunications packages available for either the Macintosh or IBM Windows environment; includes faxing capabilities.

Fulltalk Windows   Microflip, Inc. An answering machine with built-in speaker that includes remote access and auto detection for TDD; variety of functions include automatic redial and three dialing modes, incoming call flashing, memo message editors, date/time display, call progress indicator, and directories; Macintosh, DOS.

HandiPHONE   Microsystems Software Inc. Computer-controlled telephone communication system allowing access to incoming and outgoing calls without interrupting other software applications; DOS.

PDS Fax Talk Plus Package   Personal Data Systems, Inc. Software package including batch files for sending and printing faxes, as well as converting fax files into image files for OCR reading; works with Vocal-Eyes; IBM PC compatible (DOS).

Smartcom   Hayes Microcomputer Products, Inc. Powerful and easy-to-use telecommunications product with a reasonably large screen buffer; available in either a Macintosh or IBM Windows compatible version.

Appendix C-11   Environmental Control Software

ACS Controller   ACS Technologies. Wheelchair-mountable infrared system ACS Controller with Voice Activate that can be operated by keyboard or scanning; controls most environmental devices (e.g., lights, TV, VCR, infrared telephone) and can be interfaced (serial port) to computer; Voice Activate version includes control by one utterance commands.

Environmental Control   Consultants for Communication Technology. Allows infrared control of up to 16 switches or outlets (X-10); IBM PC.

Eyegaze Computer System   LC Technologies/Eyegaze Systems. A keyboard emulator and an environmental control device based on computerized analysis of eye focal point; computer system allows a variety of functions (word processing with printer control, text reading, speech output, and games) as well as control of appliances and telephone; IBM PC.

HAL Entry System   Voice Connection. Allows voice control of devices in the environment; IBM PC.

HECS (Hospital/Home)   Prentke Romich. System integrates with nurse call system and allows user to control devices within the room (e.g., lights, telephone, TV); backlit display with large print mounted to arm that can be adjusted as bed is raised or lowered; permits a variety of interfaces, such as sip/puff, tongue switch, or rocking lever.

Home Automation Link (H.A.L.) System   Voice Connection. Voice output control system that allows concurrent operation of environmental devices (e.g., lights, telephone, TV, appliances) with standard software; IBM PC.

MasterVoice E.C.U.   Automated Voice Systems, Inc. Voice-activated environmental control system that works up to a distance of 20 feet; controls a variety of devices (e.g., lights, TV, heating systems, telephone) as well as serving as an intrusion detection system; interfaces with a computer through RS232 port.

TEAM System   Microsystems Software, Inc. Wireless PC environmental control (e.g., lights, TV, appliances) software operating infrared and X-10 controllers with the PC computer; IBM PC.

U-Control   Words+. Provides wireless, portable (infrared) control of environmental devices (e.g., lights, TV, VCR, CD) in conjunction with Words+ software, such as EZ Keys, Talking Screen; IBM PC.

X-10 Home Automation Interface   Computer interface system that allows the user to control environmental devices from the computer, yet also use computer for other ongoing functions; system consists of eight rocker switches for immediate on/off functions of devices; Apple IIe, Macintosh, IBM PC.

POSSIBLE AAC TEAM MEMBERS AND TRADITIONAL RESPONSIBILITIES

The following list of traditional responsibilities is not intended to be exhaustive, but includes professionals and other individuals who may be members of an AAC assessment and/or intervention team. For any given AAC user, a core of individuals including the AAC user, family members, and professionals from two or three disciplines is typically active as the AAC team. Professional core members of the Purdue-GLASS AAC assessment team, for example, are an occupational therapist, a special educator, and a speech-language pathologist. Other team members are involved to a greater or lesser degree as required depending on the abilities and needs of the AAC user.

AAC User Identifies own abilities, limitations, needs, interests, and goals.

Audiologist Assesses auditory acuity, perception, and processing; assesses the effects of hearing loss on communication; assesses, selects, and trains use of assistive listening devices; assesses the acoustic characteristics of different environments; aural rehabilitation.

Case Manager/Social Worker Coordinates services; assesses counseling needs of AAC user and family; provides support throughout assessment and intervention; advocates for the rights of the AAC user and family; counsels.

Dietitian Assesses nutritional, caloric needs; recommends dietary intake.

Educational Administrator Facilitates educational opportunities; provides resources; monitors compliance with laws and regulations.

Educator Assesses current and projected educational abilities; adapts curricular materials as needed for accurate and thorough assessment of learning needs and learning potential; uses appropriate materials in the classroom.

Family Member(s)/Caregiver(s) Provides pertinent information on the AAC user's background; medical history; current abilities; limitations; interests; day-to-day communication needs; family dynamics, strength, needs; family and/or community resources; environmental characteristics.

Manufacturer's Representative Assists in obtaining and maintaining appropriate AAC technology.

Occupational Therapist (OT) Assists in evaluation of visual and motor perceptual skills; assesses most effective means of positioning and/or mounting of AAC devices; assesses motor skills; evaluates motor control for activities of daily living, including AAC; intervenes to maximize motor control for communication; selects and modifies adaptive equipment, assistive technology, and mobility aids.

Orientation and Mobility (O & M) Specialist Assesses abilities for orientation to physical environment and independent mobility; assists with assessment of how AAC devices may be interfaced with mobility equipment.

Physical Therapist (PT) Assesses motor skills; evaluates motor performance and learning; intervenes to maximize strength, endurance, flexibility, coordination, and range and resolution of movement; selects and modifies splints and braces; selects and trains use of seating and mobility aids.

Physician Assesses medical status, prognosis, constraints, and needs; manages medical and therapeutic programs; recommends assessments, therapies, and AAC devices when third party payers are involved; prescribes appropriate medications; provides information regarding effects of medications on cognition and behavior.

Psychologist Assesses cognitive abilities using standard and/or adapted procedures; assesses AAC user's and family's needs for counseling related to communication and other disabilities; counsels.

Rehabilitation Engineer Matches features and AAC user's abilities and needs to assistive technology; designs features, modification, and operation of electronic and mechanical devices; installs assistive devices.

Rehabilitation Specialist/Counselor Assesses abilities and needs; programs and implements selected AAC services.

Rehabilitation/Therapy Assistant Implements selected AAC services under the direction and supervision of a qualified professional.

Residential Manager Assesses AAC user's day-to-day communication needs, typical communicative performance, characteristics of the living environment.

Seating-Positioning Specialist   Evaluates posture, tone, and function; selects and installs seating and positioning equipment.

Special Educator   Assesses academic strengths and weaknesses; assesses impact of communication and other disabilities on education.

Speech-Language Pathologist (SLP)   Assesses receptive and expressive communication; assesses oromotor skills; assesses present and future communication abilities, needs, opportunities, and barriers; plans and implements communication intervention; evaluates and treats dysphagia.

Technical Specialist   Assesses features, operations, and maintenance of available technology; selects, installs, modifies, and trains use of software.

Trainer/Supervisor/Counselor   Assesses communication needs in the vocational setting; evaluates vocational skills and potential; trains staff.

Vision Specialist   Assesses visual acuity, perception, and processing; develops appropriate visual materials, assistive devices and/or technologies for visual impairment.

Vocational Rehabilitation Counselor   Assesses employment potential; assists in securing employment and obtaining necessary assistive technology.

GLOSSARY

AAC   See augmentative and alternative communication.

AAC-based approaches to problem behavior   Communication-based approaches that use AAC as alternative behaviors to less desirable behaviors (e.g., self-injurious behavior [SIB] and acting out).

AAC interface   A component of the AAC transmission processes of the AAC model proposed by Lloyd, Quist, and Windsor. The interface refers to the aid or device (e.g., communication board, electronic communication device, pen) used to transmit a message.

AAC service delivery   Provision of direct or consultative assessment and intervention services to individuals with little or no functional speech.

AAC system   An integrated network of aided and unaided means to represent (symbols), select, and transmit; and the strategies, techniques, skills, and devices that an individual uses to communicate. A system involves the integrated use of many components for communication; aka communication system.

AAC transmission processes   An integral part of the AAC model proposed by Lloyd, Quist, and Windsor that refers to the means to represent, means to select, and means to transmit a message. The means to represent takes place via symbols that can be selected through aided or unaided means and transmitted through aided or unaided means.

AAC user   An individual with little or no functional speech who is currently using or is a candidate for an AAC system.

AAMR   See American Association on Mental Retardation.

Abbreviation expansion   The expansion of typical or idiosyncratic abbreviations (e.g., contractions, truncations). Abbreviation expansion provides for the transmission of complete messages with a reduced number of keystrokes.

Abduction   Movement of an extremity away from the midline of the body.

ABR   See auditory brainstem response.

Abstract   A term used to describe intangible referents such as beliefs, concepts, emotions, and ideas. For graphic symbols, abstract referents are difficult to depict by pictographs and are more typically depicted by ideographs or arbitrary symbols (e.g., traditional orthography [TO]).

Accentuation   Modification of alphabet letters or other graphic symbols in an attempt to make words or symbols more closely resemble their referents; aka elaboration, embellishment.

Acceptability   Selection consideration related to how acceptable symbols or communication devices are to an AAC user, family members, caregivers, peers, and the general community.

Accessibility   (1) Ability to approach, enter, or communicate. Accessibility allows an individual with disabilities to enter a building, participate with others in an activity, gain an education, and/or communicate with others. (2) Ability to select or activate components of an AAC system (e.g., retrieve vocabulary from a communication device). The term *accessible* is often used to describe components that a person can physically manipulate, such as a computer keyboard or a switch-activated scanning system.

Acculturation   The process of modifying one's original belief system and way of being to become more like those of another culture.

Acquired disability   A disability not present at birth that usually occurs as a result of disease or injury.

Activation force   The minimal and maximal amount of force that an individual can exert using a given anatomic site.

Activity Participation Inventory (API)   An inventory that measures the level of participation for each skill/task necessary to complete an activity within an environment, comparing a target student to a peer and determining discrepancies that may exist between them. Barriers due to lack of opportunity and/or inability to access are identified. The API was developed and modified by Zangari and members of the Purdue AAC Group based, in part, on the Beukelman and Mirenda participation model and Activity/Standards Inventory.

Activity/Standards Inventory   An inventory developed by Beukelman and Mirenda that measures an AAC user's level of participation and identifies possible barriers to participation across a wide variety of activities.

AD   See Alzheimer's disease.

ADA   See Americans with Disabilities Act.

Adaptive Firmware Card (AFC)   A keyboard emulation device manufactured by Adaptive Peripherals, Inc. that allows Apple IIe or IIGS software to be operated with a variety of input methods (e.g., expanded keyboards, scanning, switches).

Adduction   Movement of an extremity toward the midline of the body.

AFC   See Adaptive Firmware Card.

Agglutination   In Amer-Ind, the process of forming new concepts by combining symbols in sequence (e.g., the symbols "taste" and "reject" are sequenced to produce "bitter").

Aggression   Behavior(s) directed toward other persons (e.g., biting, kicking, punching, scratching) or things (i.e., property destruction).

Agnosia Loss of ability to recognize. Agnosia is typically modality-specific (e.g., auditory agnosia, tactile agnosia, visual agnosia).

Aid An assistive device or interface (e.g., communication board) that augments or serves as an alternative to natural speech and/or writing.

Aided A term used to refer to communication symbols, strategies, or techniques that use something external to the body to represent, select, or transmit messages.

Aided communication Communication that uses aided symbols and some type of external aid or assistive communication device.

Aided communication techniques Communication techniques that use some type of external aid or assistive communication device.

Aided language stimulation (ALS) A technique in which communication partners combine use of AAC with natural speech. This technique has the dual purpose of augmenting spoken input to enhance an AAC user's comprehension and providing models of AAC; aka augmented input or augmented communicative input.

Aided symbol A symbol that requires an external aid or assistive communication device to display and transmit (e.g., Blissymbol, picture, Sigsymbol, synthetic speech, TO).

Air conduction testing A general term applied to audiological testing in which sound is presented to the listener via earphones.

AKA See Alphabet de Kinemes Assistes.

ALD See assistive listening device.

Alphabet de Kinemes Assistes (AKA) A hand-cued system designed by Wouts.

Alphabet encoding The process of language formulation based on the systematic organization of information/messages for storage and retrieval using letters (e.g., fingerspelling, TO); aka letter encoding.

Alphanumeric encoding The process of language formulation based on the systematic organization of information/messages for storage and retrieval using letters and numbers (e.g., G-3 may represent the third message in the greeting category—Good Morning).

ALS See aided language stimulation and amyotrophic lateral sclerosis.

Alternative communication A communication approach that is a substitute for (or alternative to) natural speech and/or writing.

Alternative input devices Devices that enable access to technology through alternatives to direct selection (e.g., single or multiple switches, expanded keyboards).

Alternative keyboard A hardware device that replaces the standard keyboard. It can be reconfigured to meet the needs of the user (e.g., IntelliKeys, Unicorn Keyboard).

Alzheimer's disease (AD) The most common cause of primary, degenerative dementia. Stage I is characterized by deterioration of recent memory, disorientation, mood disturbances, and difficulty in dealing with day-to-day tasks. Stage II involves rapid intellectual deterioration and symptoms resembling aphasia, apraxia, and agnosia. In stage III, a person is highly demented and bed-bound.

Amblyopia Visual impairment in the absence of apparent disease.

American Association on Mental Retardation (AAMR) An interdisciplinary professional association of administrators, educators, occupational therapists, physical therapists, psychologists, speech-language pathologists, social workers, and others concerned with mental retardation (cognitive impairment) and developmental disabilities. There are several professional divisions. Of particular relevance to AAC is the Communication Disorders Division.

American Sign Language (ASL) The natural sign language used by the Deaf community in the United States and parts of Canada.

American Speech-Language-Hearing Association (ASHA) A major professional organization for audiologists, speech-language pathologists, speech and hearing scientists, and others interested in human communication and human communication disorders. Of particular relevance to AAC is the AAC Special Interest Division (SID 12).

Americans with Disabilities Act (ADA) Public Law 101-336, passed in 1990, prohibiting discrimination in hiring individuals with disabilities and mandating modification of the work environment to accommodate individuals with disabilities.

Amer-Ind An unaided set of gestures based on the gestures that the North American Indian tribes used for intertribal communication.

Amyotrophic lateral sclerosis (ALS) A progressive, degenerative neurological disease of unknown etiology that affects motor neurons of the brain and spinal cord resulting eventually in total loss of muscle function and death; often referred to as Lou Gehrig's disease.

Analog A continuous representation, in real time, of light or sound waves.

Anterior In front.

Anterior superior iliac spines (ASIS) Front (anterior), upper (superior), protrusions (spines) of the ilium (upper part of the bony pelvis above the hip joint); commonly called "the hip bones."

Aphasia Impairment in the comprehension and formulation of language symbols resulting from damage to certain areas of the brain. Aphasia is frequently caused by focal brain lesions in the cortical and subcortical areas of the left hemisphere as a result of hemorrhage or thromboembolic clots. Deficits are demonstrated in aspects of communication (e.g., comprehension, speaking/signing, reading, writing) either singly or in combination.

API See Activity Participation Inventory.

Apraxia Disorder of motor planning caused by damage to the motor control areas of the brain; inability to execute volitional movements. Limb apraxia and apraxia of speech are characterized by difficulty sequencing and coordinating movements in the absence of paralysis or weakness of muscles, usually resulting in highly inconsistent performance.

Arbitrary   A term used to describe symbols that bear little or no discernible relationship to their referents. The meanings of arbitrary symbols must be learned.

ARC   See Association for Retarded Children.

Arousal   Alertness, which is necessary to interact with the environment. The reticular formation in the brain stem is particularly important for normal wakefulness.

Articulation   The production of speech sounds through movement of the structures of the vocal tract (e.g., tongue, teeth, lips, and throat) and the production of manual signs (with the parameters location, movement, handshape, orientation).

Artificial larynx   A device that uses pulmonary airflow directed through the stoma to produce speech; used by individuals who have had their larynx surgically removed. See also electrolarynx.

Artificial sign system   A pedagogical tool for signed communication within the Deaf community (e.g., manually coded sign).

ASHA   See American Speech-Language-Hearing Association.

ASIS   See anterior superior iliac spines.

ASL   See American Sign Language.

Assertiveness   An attribute of the means to transmit that allows the AAC user to influence interactions by initiating a request or interrupting a partner, warding off interruptions from others, or protesting something.

Assessment   A process whereby data is collected and information is gathered to make intervention and/or management decisions.

Assistive communication device   Any electronic or non-electronic device that assists an individual in communication.

Assistive listening device (ALD)   An amplification device that improves the signal-to-noise ratio so that the important sound source is delivered to the ear at an advantage over background noise.

Assistive technology (AT)   (1) Any technology used to enable individuals to perform tasks that are difficult or impossible due to disabilities. (2) The field or area of development and provision of assistive technology.

Assistive technology device   "Any item, piece of equipment, or product system, whether acquired commercially off the shelf, modified, or customized, that is used to increase, maintain, or improve the functional capabilities of individuals with disabilities" (PL 100-407, 1988 [Tech Act]; modified for PL 101-476, 1990 [IDEA], by substituting the word children for individuals).

Assistive technology service   "Any service that directly assists an individual with a disability in the selection, acquisition, or use of assistive technology devices" (PL 100-407; modified for PL 101-476, 1990 [IDEA], by substituting the words a child for an individual).

Association for Retarded Children (ARC)   A parent organization founded in 1950 that played a role in identifying children with cognitive impairments considered to be good candidates for AAC services. The organization was instrumental in securing educational opportunities and paving the way for the provision of special services in the public schools. It was renamed the Association for Retarded Citizens and recently renamed again The Arc.

Astigmatism   An irregular curvature of the front surface of the eye's cornea resulting in an aspherical surface and blurred vision.

Asymmetrical   A characteristic of manual signs and gestures in which both hands describe different motor pathways on or in relation to the body of the signer. Asymmetrical signs generally pose a higher degree of difficulty than symmetrical signs and gestures.

AT   See assistive technology.

Athetosis   A type of cerebral palsy characterized by repetitive, involuntary movements.

Attention   Concentration or direction of the mind to objects or people in the environment.

Audiogram   The graph onto which the results of an audiometric evaluation are charted to indicate ability to hear pure tones at each of the test frequencies.

Auditory brainstem response (ABR)   A noninvasive procedure that measures electrical responses along the auditory pathway at the level of the brainstem; aka auditory evoked response (AER), brainstem response (BSR) and brainstem auditory evoked response (BSAER).

Auditory scanning   A message-selection technique in which names of items can be heard through earphones or in free field. The user interrupts the scan to make a selection.

Aug com   A shortened term not widely used. See augmentative and alternative communication (AAC).

Augmentative and alternative communication (AAC)   (1) The supplementation or replacement of natural speech and/or writing using aided and/or unaided symbols. Blissymbols, pictographs, Sigsymbols, tangible symbols, and electronically produced speech are examples of aided symbols. Manual signs, gestures, and fingerspelling are examples of unaided symbols. The use of aided symbols requires a transmission device, whereas the use of unaided symbols requires only the body. (2) The field or area of clinical/educational practice to improve the communication skills of individuals with little or no functional speech.

Augmentative communication   A communication approach that augments or serves as an addition to natural speech and/or writing. The term is used correctly when some natural speech and/or writing is present.

Augmented input   See aided language stimulation.

Augmented-input communicator   An individual whose communication partners use AAC in addition to natural speech.

Authoring programs   Computer programs (software) that enable individuals to construct programs for specific uses (e.g., interactive lessons, multimedia presentations).

Autism   Pervasive developmental disorder marked by severe interruption of social interaction. Individuals with autism are often described as being severely withdrawn, being rigidly dependent on routine, avoiding social contact, and showing repetitive, stereotypic behaviors.

Autistic leading   A nonlinguistic form of requesting in which individuals take communication partners by the wrist, lead them to a desired object, and then place their hands on objects. Autistic leading is sometimes perceived as socially unacceptable behavior.

Automatic linear scanning   A message-selection technique in which the movement of the cursor is automatic and continuous according to a preset pattern. The user activates a switch to stop the cursor and make a selection; aka automatic scanning.

Automatic-reinforcement-motivated problem behavior   Problem behavior that may be maintained by sensory consequences (e.g., auditory, tactile, visual) provided automatically by engaging in the behavior; aka sensory-consequences-motivated problem behavior.

Automatic scanning   See automatic linear scanning.

Averaged activation   Switch activation set for a specified duration or pressure to reduce false hits; aka filtered activation.

Baseline data   The natural level of occurrence of a behavior before intervention. The results of an intervention or program can be judged against the baseline.

Basic-choice communicator   An individual who requires maximal assistance from communication partners to make basic choices often as a result of persisting global aphasia and severe neurological impairment.

Basic rebus   An aided set of graphic symbols composed of pictographs and some ideographs and relational symbols; aka simple rebus.

Beam/light sensor   A method of direct selection that uses a light beam and light sensor for environmental control and making selections on communication displays.

Behavior chain interruption technique   Technique that uses a predictable routine to increase early developing intentional communication. An established sequence is interrupted, and the learner is expected to indicate that the sequence should be continued.

Bicultural   Simultaneously belonging to two cultural groups.

Bilateral   Referring to both sides of the body, as in bilateral hearing impairment.

Bilingual   Having command of two languages. Bilingualism is balanced when an individual has equal competence in both languages. If competence in one language exceeds the other, there is dominance. The term describes educational systems in which two languages are used to foster general development and language acquisition. Bilingualism is often used in the education of immigrant children whose home language is different from the dominant community language.

Binary code   A code system based on the representation of things by combinations of two symbols, such as one and zero, true and false, and the presence and absence of voltage; aka binary logic.

Binary logic   See binary code.

Bit   Term for binary digit; a single digit (1 or 0) representing the basic unit of information used in computers.

Blissymbolics   An aided system of graphic symbols originally designed to enhance international communication. Blissymbols are composed of a finite set of meaning-based elements, some iconic and some opaque, which can be combined according to generative rules and logic to create a virtually unlimited vocabulary.

Block grants   Federal monies provided to the states with no mandates or restrictions as to how they should be spent.

Block/group scanning   A message-selection technique in which a block/group of items is initially selected (e.g., $\frac{1}{2}$, $\frac{1}{4}$, $\frac{1}{8}$ of the display), and then progressively smaller blocks/groups are selected until the target item is selected; aka group-item scanning, multidimensional scanning.

Bone conduction testing   A general term applied to audiological testing in which sound is presented to the listener via a vibrator coupled to the skull.

Borel-Maisonny   A French hand-coding alphabet system designed by Suzanne Borel-Maisonny to provide psychomotor support for children with learning disabilities learning to read.

Bottom-up strategy   A cognitive style of processing linguistic or nonlinguistic information which typically begins by identifying low-level elements (e.g., sounds, printed letters, strokes in a picture) and discovering how they relate to each other in terms of order, spatial, and temporal configuration in higher level structures (e.g., words, pictures) and, eventually, in still higher structures (e.g., sentences, discourse). The strategy starts with identifying simple, basic elements and moves to identifying and understanding complex, more meaningful wholes.

British Sign Language (BSL)   The natural sign language used by the Deaf community in Britain.

Bubble-jet printer   A nonimpact printer that forms characters on paper when heated bubbles of ink burst.

Byte   Eight bits; the number of bits needed to store a single alphanumeric character in a computer.

CAI   See computer-assisted instruction.

CAMA   See Communication Aid Manufacturers Association.

Case conference committee   A committee typically composed of family members/caregivers, general education teacher, special education teacher, speech-language pathologist, school psychometrist, and occupational and physical therapists for the purpose of identifying abilities and needs of an AAC user.

Cataract   An abnormality of the eye characterized by opacity of the lens.

Cathode-ray tube (CRT)   A display device (e.g., computer monitor) in which streams of electrons are projected onto light-sensitive material to create a visible image.

Causality   A sensorimotor scheme having to do with the ability to search for a source behind a problem.

Cause and effect   A relationship between two events such that one is the cause of the other (e.g., flipping a switch causes a light to turn on).

CBI See community-based instruction and computer-based instruction.

CD-ROM See compact disk read-only memory.

CEC See Council for Exceptional Children.

Central processing unit (CPU) The "brain" of the computer (microchips) that processes information, executes software commands, and coordinates actions with the hardware.

Cerebral palsy A central nervous system disorder affecting motor control occurring at or about the time of birth, prior to the achievement of muscular coordination.

Cerebrovascular accident (CVA) An interruption of blood supply to brain tissue; aka stroke.

Cerumen A waxlike substance in the external ear canal.

Cervical spinal cord injury Injury at the cervical level of the spinal cord (segments C1 through C8) frequently resulting in paresis or paralysis of upper limbs in addition to lower limbs.

CGA See color graphics adapter.

Chart-based encoding Encoding that involves the use of a chart to which a sender can refer while sending messages. The chart can be used by a receiver to decode messages, eliminating the need to memorize codes.

Circular scanning A message-selection technique in which a selector (e.g., clock hand) moves in a clockwise or counterclockwise direction to point to items or messages displayed in a circular format.

Cleft palate An opening in the hard and/or soft palate(s) caused by failure of the embryonic palatal elements to fuse.

Coding (1) The systematic organization of information/messages for storage and retrieval. (2) A code/system of signals (e.g., eye-blink codes).

Cognition Awareness and ability to understand and process information.

Cognitive effort The level of complexity and intensity of cognitive processes required to complete a task.

Cognitive load The amount of cognitive processing imposed by a task, activity, or event.

Collaboration Sharing information and expertise to generate plans, programs, and solutions to problems.

Collaborative consultation Consultation that involves interaction among team members with diverse backgrounds and expertise to generate solutions to problems; most closely associated with transdisciplinary service delivery.

Collaborative learning A method of learning that involves participation in small diverse groups. Students exchange information and use the contributions of individual group members to complete a learning task; aka cooperative learning.

Collaborative teamwork model A model of transdisciplinary service delivery in which collaboration takes place among team members.

Color coding The use of color as a basis for the systematic organization of information/messages for storage and retrieval; used in color encoding.

Color graphics adapter (CGA) A color monitor allowing a 320×200 dpi (dots per inch) display in four colors.

Communication The transmission or exchange of thoughts and information from one individual to another, whatever the means (e.g., speech, manual sign, gestures, TO, or other graphic symbols). Communication may be linguistic or nonlinguistic.

Communication Aid Manufacturers Association (CAMA) An organization of manufacturers of assistive communication devices, specialized AAC materials, and software. The chair of the organization rotates. CAMA currently uses the services of a professional meeting planner: James F. Neal Conferences, Inc.

Communication-based approaches to problem behavior Approaches that involve the assessment of the communication functions of problem behavior and the teaching of alternative behaviors that serve the same communication function and replace the problem behavior.

Communication board A low technology communication device that displays aided symbols (e.g., Blissymbols, pictures).

Communication contexts See communication environments.

Communication environments The physical and social environments of the message sender and receiver during communication. The communication environments or contexts are affected by factors of the transmission environments (transmission/signal channels) such as distance between communication partners, noise level, and variations in lighting; aka communication contexts.

Communication system See AAC system.

Communicative competence The ability to communicate functionally and adequately in most or all situations. In AAC, this includes linguistic, operational, social, and strategic competence.

Communicative mastery The ability to communicate in most or all situations at the highest skill level; seldom achieved even by native speakers of a language.

Community-based instruction (CBI) An approach to special education and rehabilitation in which functional, daily living goals are met in the actual context in which skills are required (e.g., various public and community settings); aka community-referenced instruction.

Community language The vernacular language used by the largest group in a community. Mastery of and access to the community language is a critical factor for participation in the economic and cultural life of the community.

Community-referenced instruction See community-based instruction (CBI).

Compact disk read-only memory (CD-ROM) A disk with optical storage of up to 800 MB of data that can be read and copied, but not modified or deleted.

Complexity The physical complexity of a graphic symbol or manual sign (e.g., the number of strokes, semantic elements). The degree to which the figure of a graphic symbol stands out from its background may also be an indicator of complexity. Complexity of manual signs is influenced by handshape difficulty, number of different movements, and type of movements.

Complex rebus   See expanded rebus.

Components   Elements or parts of a whole. The means to represent, select, and transmit a message are the major components of an AAC system.

Comprehension   The process whereby the meaning of language is understood.

Comprehensive capability profiling   Gathering maximal information about an individual in various areas to develop a comprehensive profile of abilities and disabilities.

Comprehensive communicator   An individual with aphasia who is typically able to augment limited spoken language with graphic and manual symbols to communicate in a variety of communication contexts.

Computer-assisted instruction (CAI)   A method of instruction that includes the use of the computer.

Computer-based communication system   A computer system that uses specifically developed software and input modes to enhance communication.

Computer-based instruction (CBI)   A method of instruction involving computer systems where the students learn through word processing, database spreadsheets, and/or graphic design programs.

Computerized visual input communication (C-VIC) system   A computer system containing a lexicon of linear-sequenced iconographic symbols that are accessed using a mouse. Researchers observe whether individuals with severe aphasia can access, manipulate, and combine visual icons specific to the grammatical structures of this system.

Conceptual encoding   The process of language formulation based on the systematic organization of information/messages for storage and retrieval according to an individual's association of meanings with symbols.

Concrete   A term used to describe tangible referents such as people, places, and objects. For graphic symbols, pictographs depict concrete referents more easily than abstract referents.

Conductive hearing impairment   A hearing loss caused by impairment or loss of function in outer and/or middle ear structures.

Congenital disability   A disability present at birth usually as a result of disease or injury.

Consultant   One who provides "expert" information to another.

Consultee   One who receives "expert" information from a consultant and often implements programs based on this information.

Consumer   See AAC user. A family member of an AAC user may also be referred to as a consumer.

Continuum of services   The range of services and programs available to individuals with AAC needs.

Contoured seats   Chairs and other seats with surfaces that are curved to approximate the shape of the body.

Contracture   Tightening of soft tissues around a joint that results in restricted joint movement.

Controlled-situation communicator   An individual who may have persistant Broca's, Wernicke's, or global aphasia who does not typically initiate communication and who needs a great degree of assistance to engage in routine conversational exchanges.

Conventionality   In AAC, the acceptance of a symbol as a representation of a specific referent or group of referents and its use by a group.

Cooperative learning   See collaborative learning.

Core vocabulary   Words and/or messages with universal utility across individuals; includes commonly used structure words.

Cosmesis   The aesthetic quality (as defined by the user and others) of symbols and communication devices.

Cotreatment   Service delivery in which professionals from more than one discipline provide treatment at the same time (e.g., an occupational therapist [OT] works alongside a speech-language pathologist to facilitate communication for an AAC user during lunch).

Council for Exceptional Children (CEC)   A national association dedicated to improving services for exceptional individuals (e.g., gifted individuals, individuals with cognitive impairments, emotional disturbances, learning disabilities, and physical impairments). Membership includes professionals in special education and related fields, parents, and individuals with disabilities. CEC divisions of particular relevance to AAC include the Division for Children's Communication Development (DCCD), Division for Culturally and Linguistically Diverse Exceptional Learners (DDEL), Division on Mental Retardation and Developmental Disabilities (MRDD), Division for Physical and Health Disabilities (DPHD), and Technology and Media Division (TAM).

Coverage vocabulary   A limited number of words and/or messages that enable an individual to communicate on a wide range of topics.

CPU   See central processing unit.

Criteria-based assessment   Assessment designed to determine whether skills are sufficient to support particular AAC strategies and techniques based on predetermined criteria.

Criteria-based profiling   Judging an individual's abilities against a set of criteria considered essential to that area of investigation.

Cross-modal   Use of more than one mode (e.g., use of speech and manual signs as in manually coded English [MCE]).

CRT   See cathode-ray tube.

Cued Speech   An unaided symbol system developed in the 1960s by Orin Cornett to be used as a visual aid synchronously with speech articulation to disambiguate visual information in speechreading (lipreading).

Cued systems   Communication systems in which symbols represent partial phonemic or phonologic information.

Cues   Naturally occurring stimuli in the environment that may prompt a response (e.g., the sight and/or smell of a cookie may cause an individual to ask for it).

Cultural background   An individual's background set of beliefs, values, traditions, behaviors, language institutions, technologies, and survival systems that relate to an individual's life experience.

Culture   The total of beliefs, values, traditions, behaviors, and communication patterns shared by members of a community learned as a function of social membership.

Custom contoured seats   Chairs and other seats with surfaces customized to conform to the shape of an individual.

CVA   See cerebrovascular accident.

C-VIC system   See computerized visual input communication system.

Daily routine diary   A tool for identifying vocabulary needed for communication and participation in daily routines. Words, phrases, and sentences that an AAC user needs to engage in activities are recorded.

Daisywheel printer   An impact printer that forms letters with character spokes (very close together) that press through an inked ribbon. Because dots are much closer together than those produced with a dot matrix printer, the letters are of higher quality.

Danish Mouth-Hand System   A Danish system for visually disambiguating the patterns of the moving mouth, lips, cheeks, and face during speech to make speechreading more accurate.

Day clock   A clock face onto which activities of an AAC user's daily routine are entered to display information about an individual's typical schedule.

Decoding   The cognitive process of interpreting a sender's message (i.e., converting the sender's symbols into the message).

DECtalk™   Digital Equipment Corporation's synthetic speech that results from a combination of text-to-speech synthesis and digitization. It includes a variety of voices (e.g., Beautiful Betty, Kit the Kid, Perfect Paul).

Dedicated communication device   A device specifically designed to be used for communication but that may also interface to a computer, printer, and an environmental control unit (ECU) (e.g., DynaVox 2c, Liberator, MessageMate, Pegasus).

Degree of ambiguity   A measure related to the number of concepts that one encodes for a single symbol. The more meanings for a single symbol, the greater its ambiguity.

Dementia   An acquired progressive deterioration of cognitive function.

Deposition   A statement taken under oath to be used as testimony in a due process hearing or a court of law.

Desktop   Area on the monitor screen of a computer where hard drive, trash, and disk icons usually appear.

Developmental apraxia   Developmental disorder of speech production, usually marked by unintelligible speech in the absence of paralysis, dysarthria, or other obvious organic impairment.

Developmental disability   A disability that is present prior to adolescence/adulthood that affects particular areas of development such as cognition, communication, motor, and social-emotional. See acquired disability.

Developmental period   The period from birth to approximately 18 years of age.

Developmental vocabulary   Vocabulary that an individual is learning but may not yet be able to recognize or read.

Dialogue method   A method for selecting vocabulary that considers age and cognitive appropriateness, colloquialism, vocabulary richness, reusability, and intelligibility of synthesized speech.

Digital   Storage of data in binary code.

Digitized speech   Speech that is electronically produced when the human voice is recorded and digitized.

Diplopia   Double vision.

Directed scanning   A message-selection technique in which the movement of a cursor is directed by a switch (e.g., joystick) that controls movement in four or more directions.

Direct methods   Methods such as the use of antecedent-behavior-consequence charts, scatterplot analyses, and direct observations that identify natural covariation between problem behavior and environmental events occurring prior and subsequent to problem behavior.

Direct selection   A message-selection technique in which an AAC user indicates choices on a display using a body part or prosthesis interfaced with a body part (e.g., touching with a finger, gazing with the eyes, touching with a stylus).

Disability   The limitation to engage in activities or perform skills due to an impairment (e.g., a motor impairment might cause a walking disability).

Display   The housing of aided AAC symbols (e.g., communication book, board, wallet, computer overlay).

Display-based encoding   Encoding that involves the use of a display with a control device that allows the AAC user to send a message without the need to memorize a code or refer to a chart.

Display permanence   A symbol-selection consideration that refers to aided symbols that can be mounted on a communication device external to the body.

Disruptive behavior   Behavior that disrupts instruction (e.g., falling on the floor, manipulating lights in the classroom).

Dopamine   Neurotransmitter released by basal ganglia neurons (brain cells). Deficiency causes Parkinson's disease.

Dot matrix printer   An impact printer that forms patterns of tiny dots to create characters on a page when pressed through an inked ribbon.

Down syndrome   A congenital condition (Trisomy 21) that typically results in cognitive impairment.

Dual sensory impairment (DSI)   Impairment of both hearing and vision.

Durability   The ability of symbols and communication devices to withstand the rigors of daily use.

Dvorak keyboard   A keyboard that, unlike a standard typewriter keyboard, has the most frequently occurring letters arranged in the "home" or middle row where they may be most accessible.

Dynamic A term used to describe (1) symbols in which movement or change is necessary to understand meaning (e.g., most manual signs) and (2) symbols that are animated on the display of a device (e.g., DynaSyms).

Dynamic display A visual display in which (1) graphic symbols are arranged by categories and selection results in the display of a new array of symbols and in which (2) graphic symbols are animated on the display.

DynaSyms Graphic symbols developed by Faith Carlson and used on DynaVox devices.

Dysarthria Motor impairment in the production of speech due to damage to the central and/or peripheral nervous systems, causing a disturbance in any or all of the processes of speech (articulation, phonation, prosody, resonance, respiration). Paralysis, weakness, and lack of coordination of muscles involved in speech production are characteristic of dysarthria.

Dysphagia A term related to a disorder in the preparation, movement, and/or swallowing of food.

Echolalia Speech that is a parrotlike echoing of words spoken by others.

Ecological inventory A tool for gathering information for identifying vocabulary needs through systematic task analyses of routines and activities; similar to an environmental inventory.

ECU See environmental control unit.

Education for All Handicapped Children Act (EHA) Public Law 94-142 enacted in 1975 to ensure a free, appropriate public education (FAPE) for all children with disabilities.

EGA See enhanced graphics adapter.

EHA See Education for All Handicapped Children Act.

Elaboration See accentuation.

Electrolarynx A type of battery-operated artificial larynx that generates sound. When the device is placed against the throat or in the mouth, sound is transmitted into the oral-pharyngeal cavity, which can be modified into phonemes for speech by movement of the articulators.

Electronic scanning A message-selection technique that uses an electronic device to select an item from a display.

Embedded skills Specific behaviors or abilities that occur within the context of a larger, more encompassing activity.

Embellishment See accentuation.

Emulator A device that simulates the action of another device (e.g., a mouse simulates the function of a keyboard when it is used to select letters from a screen).

Encoding Formulation of language. In AAC, encoding refers to the systematic organization of information/messages for storage and retrieval and the process by which signals/symbols are used to express messages.

Endogenous feedback Feedback originating from within the organism. Proprioceptive feedback is a form of endogenous feedback for humans.

Endurance Ability to sustain an activity (e.g., sustain muscle forces necessary to direct select).

Enhanced graphics adapter (EGA) A high quality color monitor that allows a 640×360 dpi (dots per inch) display in 16 colors.

Enhancement The provision of visual cues to clarify the meaning of graphic symbols. Enhancements are usually faded so that individuals learn the meaning of original (unenhanced) symbols.

Environmental control unit (ECU) An electronic device that allows the user to exercise control over objects in the environment (e.g., fan, lights, television).

Environmental inventory A tool for gathering information for identifying vocabulary needs related to the interests and activities of individuals; similar to an ecological inventory.

Error analysis The process of examining incorrect responses to gain insight into an individual's use of ineffective strategies and/or productions.

Errorless learning Learning in which few or no errors are made. The clinician/educator uses procedures such as stimulus shaping, fading, and most-to-least prompting so that the learner has minimal opportunity for errors. If the learner begins to reach toward an incorrect symbol, for example, the clinician/educator may provide a physical prompt directing the learner to a correct symbol.

Escape-motivated problem behavior Problem behavior that may be used to terminate, postpone, or escape demands.

Esotropia The movement of something turning inward (e.g., an eyeball).

Ethics Principles relating to morals; containing precepts of morality.

ETRAN A transparent board with the center cut out that enables an AAC user to sit across from a communication partner and send a message by gazing at symbols (i.e., eye transfer).

Evaluation The process of assessing abilities and using formal and informal procedures to determine the nature, extent, and impact of a problem.

Existing communicative repertoire Receptive skills (e.g., understanding symbols and functions) and expressive skills (e.g., producing symbols and functions) that an individual has already learned.

Exogenous feedback Feedback originating from outside the organism. In communication, head nods and other signals that indicate the listener understands the sender's message are forms of exogenous feedback.

Exotropia The movement of something turning outward (e.g., an eyeball).

Expanded abbreviation See abbreviation expansion.

Expanded keyboard A keyboard with touch-sensitive membrane switches (cells) that can be reconfigured to different sizes to meet the needs of individuals with severe motor disabilities (e.g., Unicorn Keyboard).

Expanded rebus An aided system of graphic symbols that includes pictographs and/or ideographs combined with alphabet letters to represent referents. It also includes pictures with names that rhyme with referents or sound the same as intended words (e.g., picture of wood for *would*); aka complex rebus.

Expansion capability   The capability of a set of symbols to be expanded beyond the initial lexicon through the use of well-defined rules and logic for expansion. This variable differentiates symbol sets from symbol systems.

Ex parte communication   Undisclosed communication between the judge/impartial hearing officer (IHO) and one of the two parties involved in a legal action. This type of communication is considered illegal and applies to hearings as well as civil and criminal cases.

Experiential background   The sum knowledge an individual possesses from all previous experiences.

Expert consultation   Consultation services of fixed duration in which a professional provides assessment and intervention information, but does not implement programs. Program recommendations are implemented by the consultee. No set procedures for follow-up exist.

Expressive vocabulary   In AAC, words and messages that are available to an AAC user to express to a communication partner.

Extended keyboard   A keyboard that has function keys in addition to the keys of a standard keyboard.

Extension   The straightening of a joint, increasing the joint angle.

Extrapyramidal   A term that refers to the descending nerve tracts that are not part of the pyramids of the medulla.

Eye-blink codes   Codes made up of agreed-upon sequences of eye blinks that can be used to send messages. Each set of eye blinks has a specific meaning.

Eye gaze   The act of looking toward a specific location, symbol, or thing (sometimes referred to as eye pointing, an inappropriate term because of the inability of eyes to point).

Eye pointing   Technically incorrect term. See eye gaze.

Facilitated communication (FC)   An intervention technique that provides physical and emotional support to individuals with severe communication disabilities to facilitate written expression via an alphabet board or keyboard. The efficacy of FC as a legitimate technique has not received widespread support in the field of AAC. Professional organizations (AAMR, American Psychological Association [APA], ASHA) have passed resolutions questioning the validity of this technique.

Fading   The gradual reduction in the strength, frequency, and/or duration of prompts that assist an individual to produce a response. When fading is accomplished, an individual produces a response without prompts.

FAPE   See free, appropriate public education.

FC   See facilitated communication.

Feature matching   A process in which an AAC user's current and projected needs are matched to features of AAC symbols and devices. Because no AAC symbol set/system or device may have all of the desired features, selections that have the most desirable features for an AAC user's needs are made to achieve "goodness of fit".

Feedback   Information conveyed to a communicator, whether from within the communicator's body (internal/endogenous) or from the environment or communication partner (external/exogenous), which helps the communicator adjust communication output.

Figure   The part of a graphic symbol that conveys the important information that carries the meaning of the symbol. See ground.

Filtered activation   See averaged activation.

Fingerspelling   Using a manual alphabet to communicate. Letters are formed by hand configurations and put together to spell words.

Fitzgerald Key   An organizational structure originally designed for teaching language to individuals with hearing impairments. In AAC, symbols on a communication board are arranged from left to right in subject-verb-object order.

Flexion   Bending a joint, reducing the joint angle.

Force   (1) Strength or power exerted on an object (pressure). (2) Intensity of effect. See activation force.

Free, appropriate public education (FAPE)   Special education and related services provided at public expense under public supervision that meet the standards of the state education agency (SEA) and IDEA and the needs of individuals with disabilities.

French Sign Language (FSL)   The natural sign language used by the Deaf community in France.

Fringe vocabulary   Words and/or messages specific to an individual AAC user's situations, interests, and needs.

FSL   See French Sign Language.

Full inclusion   The inclusion of individuals with disabilities into all aspects of general educational programming.

Functional analysis   The experimental manipulation of environmental aspects that represent the hypothesized functions of a variety of behaviors including problem behavior.

Functional assessment   The full range of strategies and procedures used (1) to develop and test hypotheses regarding antecedents and consequences that control behaviors including problem behavior and (2) to determine abilities in real-life situations.

Functional communication   Communication that allows an individual to express basic needs and desires, transfer information, establish social closeness, and demonstrate social etiquette. Individuals who fail to develop functional communication are typically limited in their independence and may exhibit learned helplessness.

Functional equivalence   The relationship of an alternative behavior to a problem behavior.

Functional gain   The gain that can be directly attributed to the addition of a new approach or device (e.g., the gain resulting from adding technology to an individual's AAC system).

Funded mandates   Legislation requiring specific functions, services, and/or activities for which funds are provided. Although the term is typically applied to federal mandates, it could also apply to state mandates. See unfunded mandates.

Funding Financial support for an item or activity (e.g., funding the purchase of an AAC device and services).

Funding coordinator The member of the service delivery team charged with the responsibility of guiding the efforts of seeking and obtaining funding.

Generalization The transfer of a learned behavior to a novel situation. Generalization may be across people, settings, or stimuli.

Generally understood gestures A set of gestures used with and by persons with severe cognitive disabilities.

Gestuno An unaided set of manual signs selected by a committee from the World Federation of the Deaf to facilitate communication among users of different sign languages.

Gesture A body movement or series of coordinated body movements to represent an object, idea, action, or relationship without the linguistic constraints of manual signs. Gestures play an important role in early prelinguistic communication and the transition to linguistic communication.

Gesture dictionary A personalized inventory of gestures used by a given individual for receptive and/or expressive communication.

Gigabyte A thousand megabytes (1,073,741,824 bytes). See megabyte.

Glaucoma An eye disease characterized by increased intraoccular pressure.

Global aphasia A neurological condition that results in extensive impairment in all areas of speech-language (i.e., naming, comprehension, repetition, reading, and writing).

Gloss A printed word that accompanies a graphic symbol.

Glossectomy Surgical removal of all or part of the tongue.

Grammar The structures of a language. The grammar of any language is a limited set of basic elements (phonemes) and the rules that govern the creation of meaningful combinations (words) and strings (sentences). A central part of the grammar is the lexicon.

Grapheme The visual shape or letter of a language.

Grapheme-phoneme correspondence The correspondence between the visual shape or letter (grapheme) and the sound that the letter represents (phoneme).

Graphic A term used to describe visual displays (e.g., drawings, logos, paintings, photographs, printed words, other markings).

Graphic symbol A visual symbol that represents a referent to convey meaning (e.g., Blissymbol, line drawing, Sigsymbol).

Graphic tablet A device with a touch-sensitive surface that accepts drawing and inputs it to a computer.

Graphic user interface (GUI) A computer-operated system that depicts information in graphic form on a screen, allowing the user to perform tasks by manipulating pictures representing programs, files, etc.

Grapho-phonic elements The graphemes (letters) used in TO and the grapheme-phoneme correspondences they represent.

Ground Contextual information of a graphic symbol that may enhance the meaning of the symbol. If there is poor discrimination between figure and ground, however, the ground may detract from interpreting the meaning of the symbol. See figure.

Group-item scanning See block/group scanning.

GUI See graphic user interface.

Hand alphabet Unaided symbols that consist of hand configurations representing the letters of the alphabet. Several hand alphabets are in use throughout the world. These alphabets usually represent the TO of the spoken language. They also include numbers; aka manual alphabet.

Hand configuration See handshape.

Hand-cued speech A system that provides information crucial to the identification of phonemes that appear the same on the lips. For example /p/, /b/, and /m/ would be cued by different handshapes.

Hand-cued systems See hand-cued speech.

Handicap The impact of a disability on an individual's role in society. The term *handicap* should be avoided unless the author intends to convey that there is a negative impact on the individual's role in society.

Handshape One of the basic parameters of manual signs along with location and movement. A manual sign typically uses a limited set of between 25 and 50 handshapes; aka hand configuration.

Haptic Use of the sense of touch to perceive (e.g., an object) via active exploration (as opposed to tactile, which is passive).

HeadMaster Plus™ A device manufactured by Prentke Romich Company that emulates a mouse to control a cursor on the screen of an Apple IIGS, Macintosh, or IBM. A computer is used with a software program called Screen Keys, which places an image of the computer keyboard on the screen. The Headmaster Plus allows the user to input through a two-step process of moving the head-mounted light beam to move the cursor, and sucking and/or puffing a pneumatic switch to click on the choice.

Head pointer An adaptive device affixed to the head (e.g., with a band or helmet) to be used for direct selection.

Hearing impairment A deficiency of hearing caused by a sensorineural and/or conductive loss.

Hearing threshold level (HTL) A decibel level of sound at which an individual responds to 50% of the pure tones.

Hemianopia (hemianopsia) Loss of one-half of the visual field.

High technology Technology that uses a computer chip or integrated circuit. A communication device that has speech and/or print output, programming and editing capabilities.

HTL See hearing threshold level.

Hyperopia Farsightedness.

Hypotheses development Identifying possible functional relationships between a problem behavior and naturally occurring environmental events.

Hypotheses testing   The testing of hypotheses developed from direct and/or indirect methods through a functional analysis.

IC   See integrated circuit.

Icon   A picture or symbol that represents a referent.

Iconic   A term used to describe symbols that readily depict referents or some easily identifiable aspect of referents (e.g., iconic symbols).

Iconic encoding   Misnomer for conceptual/semantic encoding.

Iconicity   A term that refers to the visual relationship between a symbol (e.g., manual sign or graphic symbol) and its referent. Iconicity is frequently considered in terms of transparency and translucency.

Icon prediction   A feature of Minspeak that allows the user to retrieve stored messages more quickly and with less cognitive effort because the series of icons associated with the first icon selected is lighted.

IDEA   See Individuals with Disabilities Education Act.

Ideograph   A graphic representation that suggests the idea of the referent it represents, but does not depict the referent directly. Ideographs are typically used to depict more abstract referents.

Idiosyncratic   Specific to an individual (e.g., idiosyncratic gestures or signs).

Idiosyncratic gestures   Gestures that have developed within an individual's repertoire of gestural symbols for referents and meanings. These remain idiosyncratic as long as they have not become conventional (i.e., as long as they have not yet been accepted and used by others).

IEP   See individualized education program.

IHO   See impartial or independent hearing officer.

Imageability   The ability of a word to elicit a visual image of the referent.

Imitation   The sensorimotor scheme having to do with the ability to copy behavior.

Impairment   The absence or deficiency of a specific structure or function. In most usages, the specific nature of the impairment should be identified (e.g., rather than saying that an individual has an impairment, one should state that the individual has a motor impairment).

Impartial or independent hearing officer (IHO)   As applied to special education, an individual who is trained in special education law and is appointed to conduct special education hearings.

Inclusion   A philosophy of educating children who have disabilities in the same setting with children who do not.

Indirect methods   Rating scales, structured interviews, and qualitative interviews. These indirect methods are typically completed by or with partners who are familiar with the particular individual.

Individualized education program (IEP)   An educational program designed by an IEP team to meet the special needs of a child.

Individuals with Disabilities Education Act (IDEA)   Public Law 101-476 enacted in 1990, which modified the Education for All Handicapped Children Act (EHA) (PL 94-142, 1975). Modifications include substituting the term *disability* for *handicapped*, adding assistive technology for individuals with disabilities, adding specific disabilities to be covered (e.g., autism and brain injury), and extending services to preschoolers.

Informant   An individual who provides information about a topic or individual.

Informational consultation   Consultation services in which a consultant provides information to a consultee that meets the needs of a targeted AAC user, but is broad enough so that the principles may be applied to similar AAC users; most closely associated with interdisciplinary service delivery.

Infrared rays (IR)   Light rays outside of the human visual range that are digitally coded to activate remote controlled devices.

Inkjet printer   A nonimpact printer that uses sprayed ink to form characters on a page.

Input   Transmission of data into a computer. Examples of input devices include keyboards and scanners.

Integrate   To make someone or something become a part of a larger whole (e.g., mainstreamed society, a general education program, a work environment).

Integrated circuit (IC)   An electronic circuit in which all components are formed on a single piece of semiconductor material, usually silicon.

Integrated environments   Settings where an individual with disabilities functions alongside peers without disabilities.

Integrated objectives   Objectives that target meaningful communication used in natural contexts and in important activities for the individual.

Integrated therapy   An approach to service delivery in which intervention uses an individual's daily experiences as both a context and focus.

Intelligibility   The ability of a symbol to be recognized and understood without cues or explanations.

Interdisciplinary team model   One of several models for team assessment and intervention in which members share information with one another to influence decision making. Assessment and intervention may, however, be carried out independently of other team members.

Interface   (1) Surfaces or devices that come together. Computer devices are interfaced through the use of cables that allow the transmission of data from the output port of one computer to the input port of another computer. (2) The connection of the AAC user to the means of transmission and other devices. The AAC user may interface with the environment through unaided means (e.g., signs, gestures) or aided means (e.g., materials, devices).

International   (1) Having global aspects or characteristics or at least being multinational in nature. (2) Symbols that are generally understood across cultures (e.g., mathematical symbols).

International Society for Augmentative and Alternative Communication (ISAAC)   An organization devoted to encouraging scholarship, promoting research, and improving service delivery in the field of AAC.

Intervention   The provision of services designed to improve communication so that an individual can interact more effectively and participate more fully in activities of choice.

Inverse scanning   A message-selection technique in which switch activation begins scanning and scanning continues while switch closure is maintained. Switch release stops the scanning and selects an item.

Invisible unaided symbols   Unaided symbols that cannot be monitored visually during production. Although speech is obviously an invisible unaided symbol, the term is more frequently used to refer to manual signs or gestures that are made outside of the visual field of the sender/producer (e.g., pointing to one's own ear).

IR   See infrared rays.

ISAAC   See International Society for Augmentative and Alternative Communication.

Joystick   An input device used to control the movement of an object on a screen. A joystick can be used for directed scanning.

Ke:nx®   Keyboard emulation system marketed by Don Johnston Incorporated. Ke:nx allows options for single switch scanning, Morse code, alternate keyboard, and synthesized speech.

Keyboard emulator   Any device that simulates the input functions of the keyboard (e.g., IntelliKeys, mouse, Unicorn Keyboard™).

Key symbols   (1) A set of graphic symbols used in functional communication that may be idiosyncratic. (2) The group of semantic elements from which a virtually unlimited number of Blissymbols are created.

Key word signing   The use of manual signs to represent key words (e.g., nouns and verbs) as they are spoken. In Britain, this is called signs supporting English.

Kyphosis   Increased forward bending or curvature of the spine.

Language   A system of symbols (e.g., manual signs, words) that can be used for a communicative function (e.g., expressing feelings, transferring information).

Language content   The semantics or meaning of language, as well as the rules for linking meaning with the units of language (i.e., semantic relations).

Language form   The elements of language consisting of its sounds and sound system (i.e., phonology), its units (i.e., morphology), and its structures (i.e., syntax).

Language use   The pragmatics of language having to do with an understanding of and ability to use the social exchange dimension of communication.

Laryngectomy   Surgical removal of all or part of the larynx.

Laser printer   A nonimpact printer in which characters are formed on a page by heating dried ink that has been electrically charged on a rotating drum.

Lateral   To the side.

Law of best fit   Use the device, system, or approach that provides a maximal match of features to the needs and characteristics of the user.

Law of minimal energy   Use the device, system, or approach that requires the least amount of energy or effort.

Law of minimal interference   Use the device, system, or approach that avoids other competing or conflicting tasks or processes (e.g., the use of a device, system, or approach should not interfere with any task or process, nor should the task or process interfere with the use of the device, system, or approach).

Law of minimal learning   Use the device, system, or approach that requires the least amount of learning.

Law of parsimony   Use the simplest device, system, or approach possible.

Law of practicality and use   Use the device, system, or approach that is most appropriate for the environment in which it will be used and that is consistent with available resources. This law also implies conforming with all the other laws (e.g., best fit, minimal energy, minimal interference, minimal learning, and parsimony).

LCD   See liquid crystal display.

LEA   See local education agency.

Least restrictive environment (LRE)   (1) A legal mandate that all children with disabilities be educated with children without disabilities and that special classes, separate schooling, or removal of children from the general educational environment occurs only when the nature or severity of the disability is such that general education classes with the use of supplementary aids and services cannot be achieved satisfactorily. Children should be afforded opportunities for education, work, living, and recreation that are as near as possible to those afforded individuals without disabilities. (2) Environment in which a child is least restricted and has greatest access to educational opportunities.

LED   See light-emitting diode.

Letter category encoding   The process of language formulation based on the systematic organization of information/messages for storage and retrieval by using letters to represent categories.

Letter coding/encoding   See alphabet encoding.

Level of abstraction   The amount of detail that is provided in the object or event being depicted in a symbol (the figure as opposed to the ground). The less detail presented, the greater the level of abstraction, and vice versa.

Levodopa   A drug for individuals with Parkinson's disease that replaces dopamine, a substance in the neurotransmitter system facilitating volitional movements.

Lexical prediction   See word prediction.

Lexicon   A collection of manual signs and/or vocabulary words.

Lexigrams   An aided graphic set of symbols composed of combinations of nine basic design elements originally developed for language research with the chimpanzee Lana at Yerkes Regional Primate Center.

License   Legal status granted to an individual to engage in a defined professional practice that provides legal penalties for violations in that practice.

Light-emitting diode (LED)   Electronic component of a communication device that gives off light, enabling a viewer to read a visual display.

Linear scanning   A message selection technique in which items are scanned individually in a specific sequence (e.g., as on circular or row display).

Linguistic communication   Signed, spoken, or written communication that uses linguistic symbols according to the combination rules (i.e., syntax) of a naturally developed language (e.g., sign languages, spoken languages).

Linguistic competence   Competence that consists of (1) knowledge of the rules of syntax, semantics, and phonology necessary to produce and understand an unlimited number of grammatical utterances of a language, and (2) mastery of an AAC system's symbols and symbol arrangements, leading to the ability to use the system to accomplish linguistic exchanges.

Liquid crystal display (LCD)   A type of flat-panel display in which liquid crystals placed between two glass sheets give positive and negative polarity emitting light as a result of changes in electrical charge (e.g., as on notebook computers).

Literate   Descriptive term for an individual who has learned to read, write, and spell.

LLC   See logical letter coding.

Local education agency (LEA)   A public agency authorized or required to provide free, appropriate public education for children with disabilities.

Localization   The systematic use of points in space in manual signing for referencing. In sign languages, localization is one of the major syntactical mechanisms.

Location   One of the basic parameters of manual signs along with movement and handshape. Location defines the area on or near the signer's body where a sign is made.

Locus ceruleus   A bluish gray nucleus in the floor of the fourth ventricle of the brain responsible for the generation of the neurotransmitter norepinephrine.

Logic   The inherent conformity of a symbol system to rules allowing the creation of new symbols (expansion capability) that are consistent with symbols already existing in the system.

Logical letter coding (LLC or LOLEC)   A systematic organization of information/messages for storage and retrieval that is based on the use of letters and letter combinations that have meaning for the user (e.g., HM could be the code for the message "Help me"); aka salient letter encoding.

Logograph   A letter, character, or other graphic symbol used to represent a word.

LOLEC   See logical letter coding.

Low technology   Any electronic or nonelectronic device that does not use a computer chip or integrated circuit.

LRE   See least restrictive environment.

Macula   Central retina of the eye.

Makaton   An instructional program arranged in nine stages for teaching a preselected vocabulary of approximately 350 manual signs from British Sign Language.

Mandated funding   See funded mandates.

Mand-model procedure   A procedure used for promoting expressive communication that involves a sequence of steps: gaining the learner's attention, producing a mand (i.e., request or command), pausing to allow for a response, and modeling the correct response if necessary.

Manual alphabet   See hand alphabet.

Manually coded English   See manually coded language.

Manually coded language   An unaided communication system that uses manual signs to represent successive elements of a spoken language. Typically, manual signs are used as labels for whole words, but they can also be used for part words such as suffixes (e.g., -ed, -ing) or prefixes (e.g., a-, un-). Manually coded languages differ in the degree to which they represent all the elements of a spoken language. For teaching purposes, where the accurate representation of the spoken language is important, more strict systems such as Signed English and Signing Exact English are sometimes preferred. On the other hand, for communication purposes, so-called key word signing is often preferred, especially with hearing individuals who have cognitive impairments.

Manual signs   Unaided symbols that can be applied to either a natural sign language (e.g., ASL) or used as a code for a spoken language (e.g., Signed English or Signing Exact English). This involves the simultaneous use of manual signs and speech, either when each word is signed or when only key words are signed (e.g., key word signing, manually coded English, signs supporting English).

Means-ends relationships   The sensorimotor scheme involving the understanding that problem solving has both a problem solving process (i.e., means), and a solution or problem solving goal (i.e., ends).

Means to represent   One of the transmission processes of an AAC model that refers to the symbols (aided and unaided) used to encode a message for communication.

Means to select   One of the transmission processes of an AAC model that refers to the manner in which the user makes symbol choices. The means to select can be aided (e.g., direct selection with a head pointer) or unaided (e.g., direct selection with a finger).

Means to transmit   One of the transmission processes of an AAC model that refers to the manner in which a user transmits a message. The means to transmit can be aided (e.g., a communication board) or unaided (e.g., direct transmission).

Medicaid   A government-sponsored health program for individuals who qualify on the basis of financial hardship.

Medicare   A government-sponsored health program for individuals 65 years and older.

Medium frequency (MF)   Radio waves that are of midfrequency range, typically 300 KHz to 3 MHz.

Megabyte   A million bytes (1,048,576 bytes); sometimes referred to as a meg.

Membrane board   A hard contact type of keyboard in which each key contains a foam rubber dome that, when pressed, completes an electrical circuit to activate the controller chip.

Memory The amount of data that can be stored, either in RAM or on a floppy or hard disk.

Memory-based encoding The process of language formulation in which a storage and retrieval organizational scheme is committed to memory (i.e., not a chart-based system).

Message A communication that has a purpose and conveys meaning (e.g., expressing an opinion, making a request).

Message prediction A precoded graphic symbol system that allows the user to retrieve encoded messages more quickly and with less effort because the specific symbol series associated with the first graphic symbol selected is lighted (e.g., Minspeak).

Metalinguistic ability The ability to consciously reflect on the form and functions of language separate from its use in context. In typical development, these abilities are presumed to develop in tandem with language itself.

Method (1) An orderly or systematic way of doing something; (2) A predetermined procedure.

MF See medium frequency.

Microcultures Social organizations resulting from associations of individuals with common factors such as age, education, gender, health, occupation, and socioeconomic status.

Mime An elaborate form of gesturing. The user of mime typically assumes a role and enacts sequences of gestures.

Mini Keyboard A small keyboard that has keys arranged closely together so that they can be activated by individuals with a limited range of motion.

Minimal pair Two lexical items (e.g., words, manual signs, pictures) that differ only in one of the constituting elements (e.g., *cave* and *gave*).

Minspeak™ A system of encoding and organizing messages for storage and retrieval based on the use of pictures (i.e., icons) that have multiple meanings.

Mixed hearing impairment A hearing loss with both conductive and sensorineural components.

Modality The particular channel through which information is transmitted or received.

Mode A particular way of communication (e.g., oral mode, manual-motor mode, ocular-motor mode).

Model A graphic representation of a structured theory/principle designed to organize and serve as a pattern. Some taxonomies serve as models.

Modeling Presenting a target behavior for an individual to imitate.

Modified orthography Orthography that has been accentuated or enhanced so that a word bears some resemblance to its referent.

Molded seats See custom contoured seats.

Molding See physical guidance.

Morse code An international system that combines dots and dashes that can be input through switches to communication devices and output as letters, punctuation, and numbers.

Motor control Initiation and execution of movement.

Motor encoding A storage/retrieval organization scheme based on motor patterns.

Mouse An input device that allows selection of items on the screen. The pointer or cursor on the screen moves in accordance with the mouse as it is dragged across a surface.

Mouse emulator Any device that simulates the input functions of the standard mouse (e.g., Headmouse™).

Mouth-Hand System See Danish Mouth-Hand System.

Mouthstick An adaptive device (i.e., stick) that is held in the mouth and used to point to a desired object/picture/word from an array of choices.

Movement One of the basic parameters of manual signs along with location and handshape.

MS See multiple sclerosis.

Multicultural Simultaneously belonging to two or more cultural groups.

Multidimensional scanning See block/group scanning.

Multidisciplinary team model One of several models for team assessment and intervention in which members of different professions or disciplines function relatively independently of one another.

Multimodal Use of more than one mode, channel, or form (e.g., auditory, visual, tactile).

Multimodal approach An intervention approach that uses more than one mode of communication (e.g., use of residual speech, gestures, manual signs, graphic symbols).

Multimodal communication The use of more than one mode, channel, or form to communicate (e.g., use of residual speech, gestures, manual signs, graphic symbols).

Multiple sclerosis (MS) Disease of the central and/or peripheral nervous system characterized by loss of the fatty sheaths (i.e., myelin) that surround the nerve fibers resulting in a variety of symptoms such as double vision, loss or reduction of sensation, tingling in the extremities, dizziness, and dysarthria. MS is common in young adults and is characterized by remissions and relapses.

Muscle stiffness Abnormal muscle contraction or lack of extensibility, often caused by spasticity and/or simultaneous contraction of muscles on both sides of a joint. Muscles may also lack sufficient stiffness to the extent that they appear floppy.

Muscle weakness Reduced force production, which can be of either muscle or nerve origin.

Musculoskeletal The muscles and skeleton, and their relationships.

Myelin sheath A sheath of fatty substance that surrounds and insulates the axons of nerve cells.

Myopia Nearsightedness.

National Institute on Disability and Rehabilitation Research (NIDRR) A federal agency within the office of Special Education Programs and Rehabilitation Services of the U.S. Department of Education. NIDRR funds the state Tech Act projects, Rehabilitation Engineering Research Centers (RERCs), and other projects related to AAC and AT.

Natural contexts   The settings and activities in which an individual would function on a regular basis if not engaged in an intervention program (e.g., community, home, work).

Needs assessment   An assessment of the communication needs of an AAC user. A specific list of mandatory and/or desirable needs is usually generated, and AAC technologies that can support these needs are sought.

Negative reinforcement   Removal of an aversive or undesirable consequence, resulting in an increase in a desired behavior.

Neurogenic degenerative diseases   Neurologically-based diseases that cause deterioration as the disease progresses.

Neuromuscular   The nerves and muscles, and their relationships.

Neuromusculoskeletal   The nerves, muscles, and skeleton, and their relationships.

Neurotransmitters   Any substance that helps in the transmission of nerve impulses between two neurons or between a nerve and a muscle.

NIDRR   See National Institute on Disability and Rehabilitation Research.

Nonlinguistic communication   Vocal, graphic, or gestural communication that uses symbols that, in general, are not part of a linguistic system such as speech or a natural sign language. Nonlinguistic communication includes some vocalizations (e.g., those that express pleasure, discomfort, pain), line drawings, and gestures.

Nonliterate   Descriptive term for an individual who has had the time and opportunity to learn to read and/or write but has not yet accomplished the skill.

Nonmanual components   Significant elements of manual signs that are not expressed by features of the hands or arms. Nonmanual components are mostly facial or bodily expressive elements used in a systematic way (e.g., raising the eyebrows to mark a question).

Nonoral   (1) Literally, without speech, voice, or oral production. (2) Term previously used to describe AAC.

Nonspeech   (1) Literally, without spoken words. (2) Term previously used to describe AAC.

Nonverbal   An ambiguous term that technically means without language. It is generally used to describe types of evaluation tools that, using spatial and motor tasks with gestural instructions, purport to measure the *nonverbal* intelligence of individuals who have difficulty comprehending or producing the spoken language of their present community (e.g., individuals with hearing impairments, individuals with brain damage, nonnative speakers). It is occasionally used to describe individuals with little or no functional speech, as in "The child was nonverbal." In this text, the term *nonverbal* is only used to describe communication or tasks; it is not used to describe individuals with little or no functional speech.

Nonvocal   See nonoral.

Norm-referenced test   Any test that is commercially prepared to be administered to large groups of individuals to compare the performance of any one individual against the scores obtained by the normative sample.

Number encoding   See numeric encoding.

Numeric encoding   The process of language formulation based on the systematic organization of information/messages for storage and retrieval using numbers and number combinations; aka number encoding.

Nystagmus   Involuntary rapid movement of the eye.

O & M specialist   See orientation and mobility specialist.

Object concept   The sensorimotor scheme having to do with the ability to apply appropriate behaviors to act on objects, as influenced by their perceptual properties.

Object permanence   The sensorimotor scheme having to do with a knowledge that objects exist when they are not perceptible.

Objects   Objects used for symbolic representation (i.e., real objects, parts of objects, and/or miniature objects). See tangible symbols.

Occupational therapist (OT)   A professional who works with individuals with disabilities to establish or reestablish life functions (e.g., fine motor function, wheelchair transfers, mobility).

OCR   See optical character recognition.

OM   See otitis media.

Onset–rime   The syllable segment preceding the vowel of the syllable (onset), and the vowel segment and any subsequent phonemic elements (rime). Thus, in the syllable /see/, "s" constitutes the onset, and "ee" forms the syllable rime; in /seat/, "s" is the onset, and "eat" is the rime; finally, in /street/, "str" is the onset, and "eet" is the rime.

Opaque   A term used to describe symbols that have little to no visual resemblance to their referents (e.g., opaque symbols).

Opaqueness   A term used to describe the absence of iconicity in which symbols have little to no visual resemblance to their referents.

Operational competence   The ability to efficiently and independently operate an AAC system.

Optical character recognition (OCR)   The process by which visual information (e.g., print) is digitized for computer storage and retrieval.

Optical input   The transmission of visual data into a computer.

Optical scanning   Scanning with a device to input visual information (e.g., graphic symbols) into a computer.

Orientation   A parameter of manual signs related to the direction the palms and fingers are facing (e.g., to the front, to the left, upward). Orientation is sometimes considered to be a minor parameter of manual signs because it gives additional information about another parameter (handshape).

Orientation and mobility (O & M) specialist   A professional who assists individuals with low vision to learn mobility skills.

Orthography   Written language.

Orthotics   Devices that support weak or ineffective joints or muscles (e.g., brace, shoe insert, splint).

OT   See occupational therapist.

Otitis media (OM)   Inflammation of the middle ear.

Output   (1) Transmission of data from a computer. Output devices include monitors and printers. (2) The product of aided high technology AAC systems, including voice output and/or print.

Paget Gorman Sign System (PGSS)   An entirely artificial sign system developed in Britain designed to represent the English language.

Parallel port   A port that allows the transmission of data eight bits at a time. Parallel ports transmit data much faster than serial ports.

Parkinson's disease   A neurological disease usually resulting from arteriosclerotic changes in the basal ganglia characterized by rhythmic tremors of the limbs, slowness and stiffness of voluntary movement, rigid facial expression, and stooped posture.

Participation model   An assessment and intervention model based on functional participation of an AAC user compared with peers of the same chronological age proposed by Beukelman and Mirenda, based on previously published approaches.

Partner-assisted scanning   A message-selection technique in which the scanning is provided by another person who presents items through spoken, tactile, and/or visual means.

PAS   See personal amplification system.

Pause time   Time during which a communication partner pauses without giving additional prompts in anticipation of a response. See time delay.

PCS   See Picture Communication Symbols.

Pedigogical sign systems   See artificial sign systems.

Perceptual distinctness   The degree to which symbols can be easily discriminated from each other or are perceived as appearing distinctly different.

Perlocutionary behaviors   Behaviors that are not intentional but may be assigned an intention by the listener (e.g., a listener may conclude that an infant cries to express hunger).

Personal amplification system (PAS)   A hardware amplification system consisting of a body-worn amplifier and headphones for an individual with hearing impairment.

PGSS   See Paget Gorman Sign System.

Phoneme   A speech sound.

Phoneme analysis   An operation of dividing up a spoken syllable or word into individual phonemes; aka phoneme segmenting.

Phoneme blending   An operation of producing a complete syllable or word on hearing the spoken individual phonemes; also known as phoneme synthesis.

Phoneme segmenting   See phoneme analysis.

Phoneme synthesis   See phoneme blending.

Phonemics   (1) The study of phonological segments of speech sounds. (2) Of or relating to the smallest category of speech sound, or the smallest unit that distinguishes one utterance from another (e.g., /p/ vs. /b/).

Phonetics   The study of the description and classification of speech sounds; of or relating to the actual or variant production of a phoneme (e.g., aspirated vs. unaspirated /p/).

Phonics   (1) Of or relating to the sounds of speech. (2) A method of teaching reading by demonstrating the relationship of letters to sounds.

Phonologic awareness   The ability to consciously reflect on the sound system of a language, to manipulate phonemic structure, and to recognize similarities and differences in phonemic properties.

Phonology   The study of the sound components of language: segments, suprasegmentals, syllables, and phonotactics.

Physical effort   The physical effort (calories of energy expended) required to perform a response.

Physical guidance   The provision of physical assistance to move an individual through desired motor behaviors; aka molding.

Physical therapist (PT)   A professional who works to restore gross motor functions in individuals who have muscular or neurological dysfunction.

PICSYMS   A graphic symbol system of pictographs and ideographs developed by Faith Carlson.

Pictogram   See pictograph.

Pictograph   A symbol that depicts a concrete or abstract referent that is easily depicted by simple pictures or line drawings; aka pictogram.

Picture Communication Symbols (PCS)   A large set of aided symbols composed primarily of simple line drawings with words printed above them.

Piezoelectric crystal switch (P switch)   Switch activated by eye movements registered by electrodes.

Pixel   A tiny dot of light representing bits of graphic information on a computer screen. A greater number of pixels results in a better quality image on the screen.

Planar seats   Chairs and other seats with flat or nearly flat surfaces.

Plasma display   A type of visual output display dependent on emission of gases.

Play audiometry   The measurement of auditory acuity in which responses are made through play (e.g., a young child may drop a block in a box after hearing the auditory signal).

Pointing   Indicating objects, persons, or events in the immediate environment. Pointing is typically done with the index finger, but can also be done with another finger, a head movement, shoulder movement, or movement or position of any other body part. Pointing may exceed indication of the direct environment when objects or persons serve as symbols (e.g., when pointing to the refrigerator means "drink").

Port   Receptacle on the back of the central processing unit of a computer that permits the plugging in of input and output devices. There are two types of ports, serial and parallel.

Portability   A selection consideration that refers to the ease or difficulty that an AAC user experiences in transporting symbols or communication devices.

Positioning Placing and maintaining a person in a sitting, sidelying, standing, prone, or other postural alignment.

Posterior Behind.

Postural control Regulation of the body's position in space for stability and orientation.

Pragmatics The use of language in communicative contexts. It relates to how the message is communicated rather than the content.

Predictive profiling A type of criteria-based profiling. As an individual's abilities are judged against a set of standards considered essential to a skill area, a prognosis or prediction is made about the individual's potential for certain performances.

Preliterate Descriptive term for an individual who has not yet learned to read, write, and spell, but appears to have the cognitive skills to do so if given the opportunity.

Presbyopia The gradual decrease in visual accommodation related to aging.

Problem behavior Behaviors such as aggression, autistic leading, disruption, self-injurious behavior, tantrums, and unconventional verbal behavior.

Progressive supranuclear palsy (PSP) A sporadic degenerative condition characterized chiefly by failure of vertical eye movements. Postural impairment and general motor decline are observed as the disease progresses.

Projectability A selection consideration that refers to the degree to which a message can be transmitted over a distance using symbols or a communication device.

Prompts The stimuli and other forms of assistance given to help an individual produce a desired response or behavior. Prompts may be partial or full. They may be verbal (spoken, signed, written), gestural, physical, and/or visual.

Prone Lying face down (on the stomach).

Pronominal reference Reference to someone or something by using a pronoun.

Proprioception Sensation that occurs during movement that keeps the nervous system appraised of body status.

Prosthesis An artificial device, often mechanical or electrical, used to replace a missing part or assist a defective part of the body (e.g., electrolarynx, eyeglasses, hearing aid, VOCA).

Protoreading Reading-like behavior in which children turn the pages of a book and engage in oral storytelling.

PSP See progressive supranuclear palsy.

P switch See piezoelectric crystal switch.

PT See physical therapist.

Ptosis Drooping of the upper eyelid.

Pyramidal A term that refers to the nerve tracts that are part of the pyramids (cone-shaped structures) of the medulla.

QWERTY keyboard A keyboard similar to the traditional typewriter keyboard in which the QWERTY letters are arranged from the left along the top row of keys.

Radio frequency (RF) Signals transmitted through the air that are within the same general range as radio broadcasts (e.g., 300 KHz to 3 MHz for AM; 30 to 300 MHz for FM; and 300 to 3000 MHz for UHF).

RAM See random-access memory.

Ranchos Los Amigos Scale of Cognitive Functioning Scale that outlines eight progressive stages of recovery in individuals with traumatic brain injury.

Random-access memory (RAM) The temporary or working memory in the computer that allows access by the CPU. Information in this memory is lost when the computer is turned off.

Range of motion The maximal distance across which an individual can move a body part.

Raphe nuclei neurons Neural cells located along the midline of the brainstem (i.e., medulla) connected to neural fibers that generate the neurotransmitters serotonin, noradrenaline, and dopamine.

Reaction time The time from the onset of a stimulus to a response.

Read-only memory (ROM) The permanent memory of a computer. Data in ROM can only be read, not modified. It is not lost when the computer is turned off.

Rebus Latin word for *thing*. A representation of syllables or words by pictures with names that sound the same as the intended syllables or words. See basic rebus and expanded rebus.

Recasting Restating an individual's utterance by expanding, reordering, or omitting lexical/structural information.

Receiver The person in a communication dyad who receives the message.

Receptive vocabulary Words and messages that are received and understood by a listener.

Recline The position of a chair when the back is lowered or raised altering the seat-to-back angle.

Referent An object, person, place, abstract idea, or other entity that is represented by a symbol.

Rehabilitation Act Public Law 93-112, enacted in 1973, authorizing rehabilitation programs and services; includes Section 504, which prohibits discrimination on the basis of disability by recipients of federal financial assistance.

Rehabilitation engineer An engineer who specializes in designing, adapting, and/or constructing equipment for individuals with disabilities.

Reliability The extent to which performance on an evaluation or test is consistent across items (i.e., internal consistency), forms (i.e., alternate reliability), and time (i.e., test-retest reliability).

Repetition rate See response repetition.

Representational range A selection consideration referring to the breadth of thought that symbols allow the user to express. A wide representational range implies that the user can express both concrete and abstract thoughts.

Reproducibility A selection consideration that refers to how conducive symbols are to rapid duplication or creation, either by hand or photocopying.

Required specificity of the means to represent Minimal specificity necessary in a symbol to convey meaning. As a guiding principle, regardless of the type of means to represent, symbols should be sufficiently generic to allow the user to communicate in a large range of contexts while being sufficiently specific to minimize the communicative burden on the partner.

RESNA Official name for the Rehabilitation Engineering and Assistive Technology Society of North America, formerly known as the Rehabilitation Engineering Society of North America. It is an interdisciplinary organization including such areas as audiology, occupational therapy, orthotics, physical therapy, prosthetics, rehabilitation engineering, special education, and speech-language pathology. It is organized with professional specialty groups (PSGs) that are discipline specific, and a large number of relevant special-interest groups (SIGs) including AAC, Computer Applications, and Special Education.

Resolution The detail and clarity of an image of a visual/graphics display. (2) Reduction to a simpler form.

Resolution of motion The minimal movement an individual can reliably and accurately execute.

Response efficiency The efficiency of an alternative behavior in relation to the problem behavior. Three variables affect the efficiency of response: physical effort, schedule of reinforcement, and time delay. An alternative behavior must be more efficient than the problem behavior for it to replace the problem behavior.

Response repetition The average number of responses made during a specified time period.

Response repetition rate See response repetition.

Retinopathy Changes in the retina, usually associated with systemic disease.

RF See radio frequency.

Rime The syllable vowel and subsequent phonemic elements. See onset–rime.

Role release The sharing of information and function across members of a transdisciplinary team. Role release grows out of continuous staff development.

ROM See read-only memory.

Row-column scanning A message-selection technique in which selections are offered by scanning down rows until the user interrupts the scan. Selections are then offered by scanning across the columns in the selected row.

Salient letter encoding Term used by Beukelman and Mirenda for using the initial letters of salient content words as a code for a message; aka logical letter coding.

Sanction Public acknowledgment of wrongdoing (often published in professional journals). The sanctioned person may or may not be expelled from membership in an organization, but there is no legal punishment (e.g., imprisonment).

Scanning A message-selection technique in which items are presented sequentially for an individual who cannot use direct selection (e.g., automatic scanning, partner-assisted scanning).

Schedule of reinforcement The number of appropriate communicative responses required to obtain the requested consequence.

Scoliosis Sideways (i.e., lateral) deviation of the spine with or without rotation or deformity of the vertebrae.

Screening Part of an evaluation process whereby individuals are sorted into two groups; those who need follow-up (i.e., evaluation) and those who do not.

Scripting Breaking an activity down into small steps and recording the words and expressions needed to participate in the activity.

SEA See state education agency.

Seating Devices and their components that assist people in maintaining a sitting position. Seating includes ordinary seats (e.g., office chairs and couches) and specialized seats designed for individuals with disabilities (e.g., Rifton Chair).

Selection considerations Empirically tested or clinically conceived variables that allow educators/clinicians to make sound decisions regarding the selection of appropriate symbols or communication devices for an individual with a severe communication disability.

Self-injurious behavior (SIB) Behavior that causes injury to self (e.g., headbanging, pica, rumination, self-biting, self-slapping, vomiting).

Self-stimulating behavior See stereotypic behavior.

Semantic compaction The encoding system used in Minspeak in which many associations are made with each icon.

Semantic encoding The process of language formulation based on the systematic organization of information/messages for storage and retrieval according to an individual's association of meanings with symbols. Minspeak is an example of a widely used semantic encoding system.

Semantics The meaning system of a language.

Semiphonetic spelling Spelling in which some aspect of the sound representation of a letter is incorporated. The phonetic information may derive from the name of the letter rather than the phoneme it represents (e.g., *you are* may be written *U R*).

Sender The person in a communication dyad who sends the message.

Sensorineural hearing impairment A hearing loss caused by damage to inner ear structures, including the cochlea and/or auditory nerve.

Sensory-consequences-motivated problem behavior See automatic-reinforcement-motivated problem behavior.

Serial port A port that allows the transmission of one bit of information at a time.

Set A collection or finite number of symbols with no rules or logic governing expansion.

Severe aphasia A neurological condition that results in extensive impairment in at least one area of speech-language.

Shaping A training technique based on behaviorism, which initially accepts a response that only grossly approximates the desired response. Gradually, an individual must produce more and more accurate responses until the desired response is produced.

SIB See self-injurious behavior.

Signal channel   See transmission environment.

Sign language   (1) The visual language used by many deaf individuals (e.g., ASL). It is not a universal language and is different from the spoken language of a country/culture. This term should not be used if one is referring to the simultaneous use of both speech and manual signs. (2) A language using manual signs that is developed in a natural way within Deaf communities (on the basis of natural language skills). Sign language most probably evolved quickly (within one single generation of users) from an iconic gestural level through conventionalization to a linguistic level with decreased iconicity.

Sign-linked symbols   Symbols that illustrate how a manual sign is produced or that realistically or schematically depict some aspect of manual sign production (e.g., some Sigsymbols).

Signs supporting English   British term for key word signing.

Sigsymbols   A graphic symbol system of pictographs, ideographs, and sign-linked symbols that is primarily composed of graphic representations of manual signs from British or American Sign Language.

Simple rebus   See basic rebus.

Simultaneous communication   The simultaneous use of two modes of communication. Typically, a manually coded language (e.g., Signed English) is used at the same time as spoken language. The manual signs and spoken words parallel each other synchronously.

Simultaneous method   The use of simultaneous communication, often manual signing and speaking.

Size   A quantitative amount proportionally measured.

SLP   See speech-language pathologist.

Social-attention-motivated problem behavior   Problem behavior that may be used to elicit or request attention. The behavior may be reinforced by giving social attention.

Social competence   The ability to appropriately use the pragmatic aspects of communication such as when to talk and what to talk about.

Social Security Act   Public Law 74-271, passed in 1935, to ensure basic retirement income for all individuals who had worked for a designated minimal number of quarters (i.e., $\frac{1}{4}$ year periods). The act was amended to provide income for children of deceased individuals and individuals who became unable to work.

Software   Programs that include commands written in computer language (e.g., DOS, BASIC) that instruct the computer to perform specific functions (e.g., word processing, database, statistics). The programs typically are stored on separate floppy disks or CD-ROMs that are run on a floppy disk drive, a CD-ROM drive, or a hard disk drive.

Spatial relationships   The sensorimotor scheme having to do with an ability to understand the dimensionality of objects.

Special educator   A professional who works with children who have a variety of special needs related to cognitive, motor, psychological, and/or sensory impairments.

Specific-need communicators   Individuals who may have any of the classic types of aphasia who need communication support in specific situations.

Speech   The human or electronic production of spoken language. Speech is considered to be vocal, although not all vocalizations are speech.

Speech impairment   An impairment in the production of speech due to the absence or deficiency of a specific structure or physiological function.

Speech-language pathologist (SLP)   A professional who is licensed to work with individuals who have a variety of communication disorders (e.g., aphasia, dysarthria, stuttering).

Speech reception threshold (SRT)   The level at which 50% of spoken words that have syllables of equal stress (e.g., baseball) are correctly identified.

Speech recognition   The process of matching voice or speech input of an individual with prestored, digitally recorded patterns, allowing the execution of computer commands by voice or speech; aka voice recognition.

Speech synthesis   Computer generation of speech by phonetic and mathematical rules and algorithms for the parameters of the speech signal. It is highly flexible and can use text-to-speech to produce virtually any typed message. There is a wide range of quality depending on the rules/algorithms stored in the computer memory. In general, the intelligibility of synthesized speech is not as high as digitized speech.

Speed   Rapidity of movement.

State education agency   The government agency responsible for monitoring and enforcing all policies related to education.

Static   A term used to describe symbols in which movement or change is not necessary to understand meaning (e.g., most aided symbols).

Step linear scanning   See step scanning.

Step scanning   A message-selection technique in which each switch closure results in the movement of a cursor through a preset selection pattern, one step at a time. This procedure involves repeated switch activation and is often fatiguing; aka step linear scanning.

Stereotypic behavior   Repetitive behavior (e.g., incessant rocking back and forth, repetitively moving fingers in front of eyes, flapping hands in the air); aka self-stimulating behavior.

Stereotypic movement   Limited variety of movement options that results in use of the same or similar patterns of movement to accomplish different motor tasks.

Stimulus shaping   The process of gradually adding items to an array to increase the discriminative demands of the learner.

Strategic competence   The ability to use compensatory strategies to communicate effectively within the restrictions imposed by AAC systems.

Strategy   (1) A plan of action. (2) A process that involves the implementation of assessment and intervention.

Strength   Muscular force that produces movement or stability at a joint.

Stroke   See cerebrovascular accident (CVA).

SubASIS bar   A rigid padded bar secured below the anterior superior iliac spine (ASIS) that is used to maintain the position of the pelvis in the seated position.

Substantia nigra   A layer of gray substance in the midbrain containing deeply pigmented nerve cells related to motor function.

Supine   Lying face up (on the back).

Supported employment   An approach to employing a person with a disability in which human, technological, and other supports are provided in an effort to achieve competitive employment in a community setting.

Switch   Component of an AAC system that serves as an interface with a communication device allowing a user to make selections by scanning.

Symbol   (1) Something used to stand for or represent another thing or concept (e.g., real object, picture, line drawing, word). (2) In communication, anything used to represent thought (e.g., acoustic symbols via speech, letters of the alphabet via writing). AAC symbols can be acoustic, graphic, manual, and/or tactile. A symbol may be classified as aided or unaided, static or dynamic, and iconic or opaque. Symbols may also be taxonomically grouped as sets or systems. In some countries (e.g., United Kingdom) the AAC professional jargon limits the use of symbol to refer only to graphic symbols.

Symbol collection   A combination of symbol sets and systems that facilitates multimodal communication.

Symbol complexity   See complexity.

Symbol set   A defined number (i.e., closed set) of symbols. It can be expanded, but it does not have clearly defined rules or logic for expansion.

Symbol system   Symbols designed to work together for maximum communication. It includes generative rules or logic for the development of additional symbols.

Symmetrical   A characteristic of gestures or manual signs where both hands perform mirror-image movement patterns. Symmetrical gestures and manual signs are generally easier to learn than asymmetrical patterns in young children and individuals with cognitive and/or developmental disabilities.

Syntax   The structural or grammatical aspects of a language.

Syntax-morphology   The syntax of a language and the rules for modifying words to reflect grammatical purposes and for generating sentences.

Synthesized speech   Speech that is artificially produced (e.g., by electronic means) rather than by the human vocal tract. See speech synthesis.

System   (1) An integrated group of components that work as a unit or whole. (2) As related to symbols, having generative rules or logic. (3) In the broader context of AAC, the use of a variety of means to represent, select, and transmit.

System efficiency   The relationship between symbols or activations and the number of messages they convey. The fewer the number of symbols or activations required to generate the most messages, the higher the system efficiency.

Systems consultation   Consultation that involves the consultant providing assessment, prescribing intervention, and evaluating intervention effectiveness as a consultee carries out programs. Set procedures of consultant follow-up should exist; most closely associated with interdisciplinary service delivery.

Tactile   Use of the sense of touch to perceive (e.g., a texture) via passive stimulation of the skin (as opposed to haptic, which is active).

Tadoma method   A vibrotactile method in which a user places a hand on a speaker's jaw and lips to perceive breath from the nose, movements of the lips, and vibrations from the throat.

Tangible consequences   Positive reinforcement given by individuals' obtaining or maintaining access to tangibles (e.g., toys, food, activities).

Tangible-consequences-motivated problem behavior   Problem behavior that is positively reinforced by individuals' obtaining or maintaining access to tangibles (e.g., toys, food, activities).

Tangible symbols   An aided set of objects, parts of objects, miniature objects, or textures that may be accessed by tactile or haptic means.

Tantrums   Problem behavior that involves prolonged screaming and crying.

Task analysis   The process of breaking activities or teaching/learning tasks into the smallest steps and arranging them in sequence.

Taxonomy   Science of classification including laws and principles.

TBI   See traumatic brain injury.

TC   See total communication and total communication approach.

Technique   An approach or method of performance used for service delivery.

Technology   (1) Application of science to industrial use. (2) Science of mechanical and industrial arts. (3) A term that refers to devices used to perform industrial, mechanical, and other functions (e.g., use of orthotics and prostheses) in assistive technology and communication devices in AAC.

Technology-Related Assistance for Individuals with Disabilities Act (Tech Act)   Public Law 100-407, passed in 1988, (Public Law 103-218, passed in 1994, providing amendments/extension) encouraging states to develop programs for increasing awareness, training, and availability of technology for individuals with disabilities.

Text-to-speech synthesis   The creation of artificial speech by typing letters on a keyboard (or emulator). It involves the retrieval and arrangement of stored phonemes according to a prescribed set of phonetic and mathematical rules and algorithms.

Textured symbols A specific type of tangible symbol which uses different textures to represent various referents.

The Arc See Association for Retarded Children (ARC).

Thermal printer An early type of printer that uses heat sensitive paper that accepts a liquid ink spray.

Tilt in space A feature of a seat that permits it to be tipped back, upright, or forward without altering the seat-to-back angle.

Timed activation Switch activation that is set for a specified time.

Time-delay (1) The time during which a communication partner waits for an initiation or response from an AAC user without providing additional prompts; aka pause time. (2) A teaching strategy that involves pairing a known stimulus that has meaning for an individual with a new stimulus. The new stimulus is presented prior to the old one, and the time span is gradually increased until the individual responds to the new stimulus. (3) The time between the presentation of the discriminative stimulus for a target response and delivery of the reinforcer for that response.

TO See traditional orthography.

Tokyo Reed An artificial larynx that produces speech, consisting of a trumpetlike mouthpiece, a metal cavity containing a tightly stretched rubber strip, and a rubber or plastic tube that is inserted into the mouth. The mouthpiece is placed directly on the stoma, and pulmonary air causes the rubber strip to vibrate. The resulting sound is passed into the oral cavity through the tube and speech is produced by the movement of the articulators.

Top-down strategy A cognitive style of processing linguistic or nonlinguistic information in which an individual starts with a contextual or global concept and relationship of elements, and then proceeds to more basic low-level structures and elements. This strategy is generally predictive and sets forward hypotheses.

Topographical dissimilarity The difference between manual signs as they are reflected in distance of place of articulation on or near the body; a physical characteristic of manual signing that distinguishes the shared features between symbols. See minimal pair.

Total communication (TC) A philosophy developed in the 1960s in the field of deafness stressing the importance of communication (and language development) regardless of the modes or methods. It embraced the use of the most appropriate communication modes or methods for the individual. Although it was originally developed as a philosophy, some refer to it as a communication method.

Total communication (TC) approach An intervention approach that emphasizes language and communication development without regard to sensory system or communication modes. It usually implies the pairing of speech and manual sign.

Touch screen A transparent device/interface that can be attached to a monitor that allows input by touching areas on the screen.

Tracheotomy A surgical procedure involving cutting into the trachea through the outer skin to alleviate breathing difficulties.

Trackball An input device that allows selection of items on the screen. The pointer or cursor on the screen moves in accordance with the trackball, located on the surface of the device, as it is rotated by the hand.

Trackpad An input device that allows selection of items on a computer screen. The pointer or cursor on the screen moves in accordance with the movement of a finger along a touch sensitive pad.

Traditional orthography (TO) An aided system of alphabet letters (or characters) that are used to encode the language of the community in written form (e.g., the 26 letters of the English alphabet).

Transdisciplinary team model One of several models for team assessment and intervention in which members jointly engage in decision making. Transdisciplinary teams are based on maximum collaboration and interaction among team members who are expected to cross boundaries and release roles to share knowledge and responsibility.

Transition services The process and/or delivery of services involved in individuals passing from home to school, school to school, school to work, and so forth.

Translucency An aspect of iconicity in which the visual relationship between a symbol and its referent is such that a symbol's meaning is not readily understood (i.e., guessable). The visual relationship generally becomes recognized or understood when symbol and referent appear together.

Translucent A term used to describe symbols that are not readily understood (i.e., guessable) without knowing the referents. Translucent symbols are generally recognizable once the referents are known.

Transmission The sending of a message to a communication partner. In AAC, transmission can be accomplished through a variety of means (e.g., visual/gestural, voice output, print output).

Transmission environment A component of an AAC model that describes the media in which communication symbols are sent and received (e.g., air, light waves, vibration); aka signal channel, transmission/signal channel.

Transmission processes The means of communicating a message using AAC, including the means to represent (symbols), means to select symbols, and means to transmit symbols.

Transmission/signal channel See transmission environment.

Transparency An aspect of iconicity in which the visual relationship between a symbol and its referent is such that a symbol's meaning is readily understood (i.e., guessable) even when the referent is not present.

Transparent A term used to describe symbols that are readily understood (i.e., guessable) because of their visual relationship to their referents.

Traumatic brain injury (TBI) Physical damage to the brain or nervous system caused by bruises, lacerations, penetrations, or shearing as a result of any number of sudden physical injuries. An injury that does not involve penetration or laceration may be called a closed head injury.

Tympanogram A graphic representation of how the immittance of the middle-ear system is altered in response to air pressure variation in the ear canal.

Ultra high frequency (UHF) Radio waves in the ultra high frequency range, typically 300 MHz to 3,000 MHz.

Unaided A term used to refer to communication symbols, strategies, or techniques that use only the body or parts of the body to represent, select, or transmit information.

Unaided communication Communication using unaided symbols and only parts of the body without any aids or devices (e.g., facial expression, gesture, manual sign, natural speech).

Unaided symbol A symbol that requires only the human body to produce (e.g., ASL, gesture, manual sign, natural speech).

Unconventional verbal behavior Verbal behavior not typically used for effective communication (e.g., immediate echolalia, delayed echolalia, perseverative speech, incessant questioning).

Unfunded mandates Legislation requiring specific functions, services, and/or activities for which no funds are provided. Although the term is typically applied to federal mandates, it could also apply to state mandates. See funded mandates.

Unicorn Keyboard™ An expanded membrane keyboard that allows a variety of configurations of pressure-sensitive areas to meet a user's needs (e.g., size, location, pressure, delay time). It can be used with a variety of computers interfaced through a device such as an Adaptive Firmware Card or Ke:nx®.

Unidisciplinary model One of several models for assessment and intervention in which only one discipline is involved.

Unilateral Referring to one side of the body (e.g., unilateral hearing loss).

United States Society for Augmentative and Alternative Communication (USSAAC) A national chapter of the International Society for Augmentative and Alternative Communication (ISAAC). USSAAC is an interdisciplinary society for the advancement of research and services in AAC.

Verbal A term that technically means the use of words (i.e., linguistic or synonymous for language). It is occasionally used to mean "with speech." In this text, it is only used to mean language or linguistic.

Versatility Ability to perform in a variety of ways for different purposes (e.g., a hand has more ways of moving and can be used for more purposes than a foot or an eye).

Very high frequency (VHF) Radio waves in the very high frequency range, typically 30 MHz to 300 MHz.

VGA See video graphic adapter.

VHF See very high frequency.

VIC system See visual input communication system.

Video graphics adapter (VGA) High-quality color monitor typically in use today, allowing display of 256 colors with pixel arrangements with 640×480 dpi (regular VGA) and more.

Visible unaided symbol Unaided symbols that can be visually monitored by the user during production. Most gestures and manual signs are at least partially visible to the signer.

Visual impairment Impairment in the ability to see and/or process visual information due to the absence or deficiency of a specific structure or physiological function.

Visual input communication (VIC) system A system that uses visual symbols that has been used in intervention with individuals with severe and global aphasia.

Visual-motor encoding A storage and retrieval organization system based on visual representations that relate to motor components of manual signs or gestures that represent meaning.

Visual reinforcement audiometry (VRA) The measurement of auditory acuity in which a loud tone is presented (usually in a sound-treated booth) followed by activation of a light, video display, and/or movement of a mechanical toy. The audiologist notes when an individual looks toward a reinforcer in anticipation that it will be activated.

Visual scanning A message-selection technique in which symbols are presented visually.

VOCA See voice output communication aid.

Vocal Voice or oral production of sounds that may or may not be speech sounds (e.g., cries, moans, sighs).

Vocational rehabilitation The retraining of individuals who have injuries/disabilities so they can return to work.

Voice output communication aid (VOCA) An assistive communication device that provides synthetic and/or digitized speech.

Voice recognition See speech recognition.

VRA See visual reinforcement audiometry.

Word prediction (1) An encoded word retrieval system that facilitates and increases word retrieval by selecting high frequency words based on the initial letter selected. (2) A software that minimizes keystrokes by presenting the user with a menu of numbered or lettered choices based on input letters; it may be organized by frequency of use or user's conceptual pattern; aka lexical prediction.

Yes/no headshakes A means of communication in which one communication partner answers yes/no questions by headshakes.

Zero reject principle Principle stating that all children are eligible to participate in the educational process without having to meet any specified criteria.

REFERENCES

Acredolo, L., & Goodwyn, S. (1990). Sign language in babies: The significance of symbolic gesturing for understanding language development. In R. Vasta (Ed.), *Annals of child development*. London: Jessica Kingsley Publishers.

Adamovich, B. B., Henderson, J. A., & Auerbach, S. (1985). *Cognitive rehabilitation of closed head injured patients: A dynamic approach*. Boston: College-Hill Press.

Adams, M. J. (1990). *Beginning to read: Thinking and learning about print*. Cambridge, MA: MIT Press.

Adams, M. R. (1966). Communication aids for the person with amyotrophic lateral sclerosis. *Journal of Speech and Hearing Disorders, 31*, 274–275.

Adamson, L. B., & Dunbar, B. (1991). Communication development of young children with tracheostomies. *Augmentative and Alternative Communication, 7*, 275–283.

Adamson, L. B., Romski, M. A., Deffebach, K., & Sevcik, R. (1992). Symbol vocabulary and the focus of conversations: Augmenting language development for youth with mental retardation. *Journal of Speech and Hearing Research, 35*, 1333–1343.

Adaptive Communication Systems. (1988). *ACS manual 4.1* (pp. 5–17). Pittsburgh, PA: Author.

Adler, S. (1993). *Multicultural communication skills in the classroom*. Boston: Allyn & Bacon.

Ahlgren, I., & Bergman, B. (Ed.). (1980). *Stockholm—79 Papers from the first international symposium on sign language research*. Leksand, Sweden: The Swedish National Association of the Deaf.

Ahlgren, I., Bergman, B., & Brennan, M. (Eds.). (1994). *Papers from the fifth international symposium on sign language research. Volume I: Perspectives on sign language structure. Volume II: Perspectives on sign language use*. Durham, England: International Sign Linguistics Association and Deaf Studies Research Unit, University of Durham.

Ahlgren, I., & Hyltenstam, K. (Eds.). (1994). *Bilingualism in deaf education*. Hamburg, Germany: Signum.

Aitchison, C., Easty, D. L., & Jancar, J. (1990). Eye abnormalities in the mentally handicapped. *Journal of Mental Deficiency Research, 34*, 41–48.

Albano, M., Fox, B., York, J., & York, R. (1981). Educational teams for students with severe and multiple handicaps. In R. York, W. K. Schofield, D. J. Ryndak, & B. Rainforth (Eds.), *Organizing and implementing services for students with severe and multiple handicaps* (pp. 23–34). Springfield, IL: Illinois Department of Education.

Alcorn, S. (1932). The Tadoma method. *Volta Review, 34*, 195–198.

Alegria, J., Leybaert, J., Charlier, B., & Hage, C. (1992). On the origin of phonological representations in the deaf: Hearing lips and hands. In J. Alegria, D. Holender, J. Junça de Morais, & M. Radeau (Eds.), *Analytic approaches to human cognition* (pp. 107–132). Amsterdam: North Holland.

Alexander, M. P., & Loverso, F. (1992). Specific treatment for global aphasia. *Clinical Aphasiology, 21*, 277–289.

Alexander, P. K. (1990). The effects of brain damage on visual functioning in children. *Journal of Visual Impairment and Blindness, 84*, 372–376.

Alexander, R., & Bigge, J. (1982). Facilitation of language and speech. In J. L. Bigge (Ed.), *Teaching individuals with physical and multiple handicaps* (2nd ed.). Columbus, OH: Merrill Publishing Company.

Alexander, R., Boehme, R., & Cupps, B. (1993). *Normal development of functional motor skills: The first year of life*. Tucson, AZ: Therapy Skill Builders.

Alexis v. Harwich Public Schools. EHLR 509:306 (MA SEA, 1988).

Allaire, J. H., Gressard, R. P., Blackman, J. A., & Hostler, S. L. (1991). Children with severe speech impairments: Caregiver survey of AAC use. *Augmentative and Alternative Communication, 7*, 248–255.

Allen, D. A., Rapin, I., & Wiznitzer, M. (1988). Communication disorders of preschool children: The physician's responsibility. *Developmental and Behavioral Pediatrics, 9*, 164–169.

Allen, R. M., & Collins, M. G. (1955). Suggestions for the adaptive administration of intelligence tests for those with cerebral palsy. *Cerebral Palsy Review, 16*, 11–14.

Alpert, C. L., Kaiser, A. P., Hemmeter, M. L., & Ostrosky, M. (1987, November). *Training adults to use environmental arrangement strategies to prompt language*. Paper presented at the annual meeting of the Division of Early Childhood, Council on Exceptional Children, Denver, CO.

Alpiner, J. G., & McCarthy, P. A. (Eds.). (1993). *Rehabilitative audiology: Children and adults* (3rd ed.). Baltimore: Williams & Wilkins.

Altman, M. (1977). *Visual imagery as a facilitator of paired-associate learning with aphasic adults*. Unpublished master's thesis, Hunter College, City University of New York, NY.

Amend, S. (1987). *Research report regarding Visual Phonics to the Sertoma Foundation*. Edina, MN: International Communication Learning Institute.

American Speech-Language-Hearing Association. (1988). The role of speech-language pathologists in the identification, diagnosis, and treatment of individuals with cognitive-communication impairments. *Asha, 30,* 79.

American Speech-Language-Hearing Association. (1989). Competencies for speech-language pathologists providing services in augmentative communication. *Asha, 31,* 107–110.

American Speech-Language-Hearing Association. (1991). Position statements, guidelines, reports. *Asha, 33* (Suppl. 5).

American Speech-Language-Hearing Association. (1992). Guidelines, position statements, reports. *Asha, 34* (Suppl. 7).

American Speech-Language-Hearing Association. (1994). Code of ethics: Issues in ethics. *Asha, 36* (Suppl. 13), 1–27.

American Speech-Language-Hearing Association. (1995). Position statement on facilitated communication. *Asha, 37* (Suppl. 14), 22.

Amstrong, D. (1983). Iconicity, arbitrariness and duality of patterning in signed and spoken language: Perspective on language evolution. *Sign Language Studies, 38,* 51–83.

Anderson, N. B., & Battle, D. E. (1993). Cultural diversity in the development of language. In D. E. Battle (Ed.), *Communication disorders in multicultural populations* (pp. 158–185). Boston: Andover Medical Publishers.

Anderson, R., Miles, M., & Matheny, P. (1963). *Communicative evaluation chart.* Cambridge, MA: Educators Publishing Service.

Anderson, R., Wilson, P., & Fielding, L. (1988). Growth in reading and how children spend their time outside of school. *Reading Research Quarterly, 23,* 285–303.

Anderson, S. R., & Spradlin, J. E. (1980). The generalized effects of productive labeling training involving comment object classes. *Journal of the Association for the Severely Handicapped, 5,* 143–157.

Anthony, D. (1966). *Signing essential English.* Unpublished manuscript, Eastern Michigan University, Ypsilanti, MI.

Anthony, D. (1971). *Seeing essential English.* Anaheim, CA: Educational Services Division, Anaheim Union High School District.

Anthony, D. (1974). *The seeing essential English manual.* Greeley, CO: The University of Northern Colorado Bookstore.

Apffel, J., Kelleher, J., Lilly, M., & Richardson, R. (1975). Developmental reading for moderately retarded children. *Education and Training of the Mentally Retarded, 10,* 229–236.

Aram, D. M., Ekelman, B. L., & Nation, J. E. (1984). Preschoolers with language disorders: Ten years later. *Journal of Speech and Hearing Research, 27,* 232–244.

Arkell, C. (1982). Functional curriculum development for multiply involved hearing-impaired students. *The Volta Review, 84,* 198–208.

Arnason, B. G. W. (1982). Multiple sclerosis: Current concepts and management. *Hospital Practice, 17,* 81–89.

Arthur, G. (1952). *The Arthur adaptation of the Leiter international performance scale.* Chicago: Stoelting.

Arthur, M. (1989). Augmentative communication systems for learners with severe disabilities: Towards effective assessment and placement practices. *Australia and New Zealand Journal of Developmental Disabilities, 15*(2), 119–125.

Asher, P., & Schonell, F. (1950). A survey of 400 cases of cerebral palsy in childhood. *Archives of Disease in Childhood, 25,* 360–379.

Atkinson, J. (1989). New test of vision screening and assessment in infants and young children. In J. H. French, S. Harel, & P. Casaer (Eds.), *Child neurology and developmental disabilities. RE:view, 25,* 57–66.

Atwater, S. W. (1991). Should the normal developmental sequence be used as a theoretical model in pediatric physical therapy? In M. J. Lister (Ed.), *Contemporary management of motor control problems: Proceedings of the II STEP conference* (pp. 89–93). Alexandria, VA: Foundation for Physical Therapy.

Automotive Safety for Children Program at Riley Hospital for Children. (1993). *Special care for transporting special kids: Getting children with special needs to and from school safely: A manual for school transportation professionals.* Indianapolis, IN: Riley Hospital for Children.

Baer, D. M., Wolf, M. M., & Risley, T. R. (1968). Current dimensions of applied behavior analysis. *Journal of Applied Behavior Analysis, 1,* 91–97.

Bailey, B. R., & Head, D. N. (1993). Providing O & M services to children and youth with severe multiple disabilities. *RE:view, 25,* 57–66.

Bailey, D. B. (1989). Assessment and its importance in early intervention. In D. B. Bailey & M. Wolery (Eds.), *Assessing infants and preschoolers with handicaps* (pp. 1–21). Columbus, OH: Merrill.

Bailey, D. B., & Rouse, T. L. (1989). Procedural consideration in assessing infants and preschoolers with handicaps. In D. B. Bailey & M. Wolery (Eds.), *Assessing infants and preschoolers with handicaps* (pp. 47–63). Columbus, OH: Merrill.

Bailey, D. B., & Wolery, M. (Eds.). (1989). *Assessing infants and preschoolers with handicaps.* Columbus, OH: Merrill.

Bailey, J. S., & Pyles, D. A. M. (1989). Behavioral diagnostics. In E. Cipani (Ed.), *The treatment of severe behavior disorders* (pp. 85–110). Washington, DC: American Association on Mental Retardation.

Bailey, R. W. (1989). *Human performance engineering.* Englewood Cliffs, NJ: Prentice Hall.

Baken, R. J. (1987). *Clinical measurement of speech and voice.* Boston: College-Hill Press.

Baker, B. (1982). Minspeak: A semantic compaction system that makes self-expression easier for communicatively disabled individuals. *Byte, 7,* 186–202.

Baker, B. (1986). *How to establish a core vocabulary through the dialogue method and how to write dialogue.* Unpublished manuscript, Pittsburgh, PA.

Baker, B. (1987). Semantic compaction for subsentence vocabulary units compared to other encoding and prediction systems. *RESNA '87: Proceedings of the 10th annual conference* (pp. 118–120). Washington, DC: RESNA.

Baker, B. R. (1997). Vocabulary selection: Historical trends. In *The 6th symposium on literacy and disabilities* (pp. 7–9). Durham, NC.

Baker, C. (1978). How does "Sim-Com" fit into a bilingual approach to education? In F. Caccamise & D. Hicks (Eds.), *American Sign Language in a bilingual, bicultural context* (pp. 13–26). Coronado, CA: National Symposium on Sign Language Research and Teaching.

Baker, C., & Cokely, D. (1980). *American Sign Language: A teacher resource text on grammar and culture.* Silver Spring, MD: T. J. Publishers.

Baker, L., & Cantwell, D. P. (1982). Developmental, social, and behavioral characteristics of speech and language disordered children. *Child Psychiatry and Human Development, 12,* 195–206.

Baldwin, D. S., Jeffries, G. W., Jones, V. H., Thorp, E. K., & Walsh, S. A. (1992). Collaborative systems design for Part H of IDEA. *Infants and Young Children, 5,* 12–20.

Balick, S., Spiegel, D., & Greene, G. (1976). Mime in language therapy and clinician training. *Archives of Physical Medicine and Rehabilitation, 57,* 35–38.

Ball, E. (1993). Assessing phoneme awareness. *Language, Speech, and Hearing Services in Schools, 24,* 130–139.

Bane, M. C., & Birch, E. E. (1992). Forced-choice preferential looking and visual evoked potential acuities of visually impaired children. *Journal of Visual Impairment & Blindness, 86,* 21–24.

Bangs, T., & Dodson, S. (1979). *Birth to three developmental scales.* Hingham, MA: Teaching Resources.

Bannatyne, A. (1968). *Psycholinguistic color system: A reading, writing, spelling, and language program.* Urbana, IL: Learning Systems Press.

Barron, R. W., Golden, J. O., Seldon, D. M., Tait, C. R., Marmurek, H. H. C., & Haines, L. P. (1992). Teaching prereading skills with a talking computer. *Reading and Writing: An Interdisciplinary Journal, 4,* 179–204.

Barsch, R., & Rudell, B. (1962). A study of reading development among 77 children with cerebral palsy. *Cerebral Palsy Review, 23*(2), 3–12.

Basil, C., & Ruiz, R. (1985). *Sistemas de communicación no vocal: Para niños con disminuciones físicas* (Nonvocal communication systems for children with physical handicaps). Madrid, Spain: Los Libros de Fundesco.

Bates, E., Camaioni, L., & Volterra, V. (1975). The acquisition of performatives prior to speech. *Merrill Palmer Quarterly, 21,* 205–226.

Batshaw, M. L., & Perret, Y. M. (1986). *Children with handicaps* (2nd ed.). Baltimore: Paul H. Brookes Publishing.

Batshaw, M. L., & Perret, Y. M. (1992). *Children with handicaps: A medical primer* (3rd ed.). Baltimore: Paul H. Brookes Publishing.

Batstone, S., & Harris, G. (1990). *Questions regarding the functional vision of people with multiple disabilities with reference to communication needs.* Victoria, British Columbia: Arbitrus Society for Children.

Battison, R. (1978). *Lexical borrowing in American Sign Language.* Silver Spring, MD: Linstok Press.

Battle, D. E. (Ed.). (1993). *Communication disorders in multicultural populations.* Boston: Andover Medical Publishers.

Bauman, R. A., Shull, R. L., & Brownstein, A. J. (1975). Time allocation on concurrent schedules with asymmetrical response requirements. *Journal of the Experimental Analysis of Behavior, 24,* 53–57.

Baumgart, D., Johnson, J., & Helmstetter, E. (1990). *Augmentative and alternative communication systems for persons with moderate and severe disabilities.* Baltimore: Paul H. Brookes Publishing.

Bayles, K. (1982). Language function in senile dementia. *Brain and Language, 19,* 98–114.

Bayles, K., & Kaszniak, A. (1987). *Communication and cognition in normal aging and dementia.* Boston: Little Brown.

Bayley, N. (1969). *Bayley scale of infant development.* New York: Psychological Corporation.

BCI Catalog. (1995). Toronto: Blissymbolics Communication International.

Beare, P. L., Severson, S. J., Lynch, E. C., & Schneider, D. (1992). Small agency conversion to community-based employment: Overcoming the barriers. *Journal of the Association for Persons with Severe Handicaps, 17,* 170–178.

Beatties, P. M. (1993). Federal policies that clarify the right to technology in special education. *A.T. Quarterly, 4*(3), 3, 8.

Beaulac, D. A., Pehringer, J. L., & Shough, L. F. (1989). Assistive listening devices: Available options. *Seminars in Hearing, 10*(1), 11–30.

Beck, J., Broers, J., Hogue, E., Shipstead, J., & Knowleton, E. (1994). Strategies for functional community-based instruction and inclusion for children with mental retardation. *Teaching Exceptional Children, 26*(2), 44–48.

Beevers, R., & Hallinan, P. (1990). Talking word processors and text editing for visually impaired children: A pilot case study. *Journal of Visual Impairment & Blindness, 84,* 552–555.

Begab, M. J. (1977). Closing session address: Some priorities for research in mental retardation. In P. Mittler (Ed.), *Research to practice in MR-volume 1: Core and prevention* (pp. A21–A30). Baltimore: University Park Press.

Behrmann, M. M., Jones, J. K., & Wilders, M. L. (1989). Technology intervention for very young children with disabilities. *Infants and Young Children, 1,* 66–77.

Bellugi, U., & Klima, E. (1976). Two faces of sign: Iconic and abstract. In S. R. Harnad (Ed.), *Origins and evolution of language and speech* (Vol. 280, pp. 514–538). New York: Annals of the New York Academy of Sciences.

Bellugi, U., Poizner, H., & Klima, E. S. (1983). Brain organization for language: Clues from sign aphasia. *Human Neurobiology, 2,* 155–170.

Benedict, H. (1979). Early lexical development: Comprehension and production. *Journal of Child Language, 6,* 183–200.

Bennet, T. L. (Ed.). (1992). *The neuropsychology of epilepsy.* New York: Plenum Press.

Bergen, A. F., Presperin, J., & Tallman, T. (1990). *Positioning for function: Wheelchairs and other assistive technologies*. Valhalla, NY: Valhalla Rehabilitation Publications.

Berger, K. (1967). The most common words used in conversations. *Journal of Communication Disorders, 1*, 201–214.

Berko, R. M., Wolvin, A. D., & Wolvin, D. R. (1977). *Communicating: A social and career focus*. Boston: Houghton Mifflin.

Berliss, J., Borden, P., & Vanderheiden, G. (1989). *Trace resource book: Assistive technologies for communication, control, and computer access*. Madison, WI: Trace Research and Development Center.

Berninger, V. W., & Gans, B. M. (1986a). Assessing word processing capability of the nonvocal, nonwriting. *Augmentative and Alternative Communication, 2*, 56–63.

Berninger, V. W., & Gans, B. M. (1986b). Language profiles in nonspeaking individuals of normal intelligence with severe cerebral palsy. *Augmentative and Alternative Communication, 2*, 45–50.

Bernstein, D. K., & Tiegerman, E. (1993). *Language and communication disorders in children*. New York: Merrill Publishing Company.

Bertoni, B., Stoffel, A. M., & Weniger, D. (1991). Communicating with pictographs: A graphic approach to the improvement of communicative interactions. *Aphasiology, 5*, 341–353.

Bess, F. H., & Humes, L. E. (1990). *Audiology: The fundamentals*. Baltimore, MD: Williams & Wilkins.

Bess, F. H., & Sinclair, J. S. (1985). Amplification systems used in education. In J. Katz (Ed.), *Handbook of clinical audiology* (3rd ed., pp. 970–985). Baltimore: Williams & Wilkins.

Beukelman, D. R. (1995, September). *Messaging and vocabulary selection*. Presentation at the Fifth Biennial State of the Art Conference on Augmentative and Alternative Communication and Crossroads Conference on Communicative Disorders, Purdue University, West Lafayette, IN.

Beukelman, D. R., & Ansel, B. M. (1995). Research priorities in augmentative and alternative communication. *Augmentative and Alternative Communication, 11*, 131–134.

Beukelman, D. R., Calculator, S., Fried-Oken, M., Light, J., Lloyd, L., Romski, M. A., & Yorkston, K. (1989, November). *Augmentative and alternative communication research issues and needs*. Special research symposium presented at the Conference of the American Speech-Language-Hearing Association, New Orleans, LA.

Beukelman, D. R., & Garrett, K. (1988). Augmentative and alternative communication for adults with acquired severe communication disorders. *Augmentative and Alternative Communication, 4*, 104–121.

Beukelman, D. R., Jones, R. S., & Rowan, M. (1989). Frequency of word usage by nondisabled peers in integrated preschool classrooms. *Augmentative and Alternative Communication, 5*, 243–248.

Beukelman, D. R., Kraft, G., & Freal, J. (1985). Expressive communication disorders in persons with multiple scle-rosis: A survey. *Archives of Physical Medicine and Rehabilitation, 66*, 675–677.

Beukelman, D. R., McGinnis, J., & Morrow, D. (1991). Vocabulary selection in augmentative and alternative communication. *Augmentative and Alternative Communication, 7*, 171–185.

Beukelman, D. R., & Mirenda, P. (1988). Communication options for persons who cannot speak: Assessment and evaluation. In C. A. Coston (Ed.), *Proceedings of the national planners conference on assistive device service delivery* (pp. 151–165). Washington, D.C.: RESNA and the Association for the Advancement of Rehabilitation Technology.

Beukelman, D. R., & Mirenda, P. (1992). *Augmentative and alternative communication: Management of severe communication disorders in children and adults*. Baltimore: Paul H. Brookes Publishing.

Beukelman, D. R., & Yorkston, K. (1977). A communication system for the severely dysarthric speaker with an intact language system. *Journal of Speech and Hearing Disorders, 42*, 265–270.

Beukelman, D. R., & Yorkston, K. (1985). *Frequency of letter occurrence in the communication samples of augmented communicators*. Unpublished manuscript, University of Washington, Seattle.

Beukelman, D. R., & Yorkston, K. (1989). Augmentative and alternative communication application for persons with severe acquired communication disorders: An introduction. *Augmentative and Alternative Communication, 5*, 42–48.

Beukelman, D. R., Yorkston, K., & Dowden, P. (1985). *Communication augmentation: A casebook of clinical management*. Austin, TX: Pro-Ed.

Beukelman, D. R., Yorkston, K. M., Poblete, M., & Naranjo, C. (1984). Frequency of word occurrence in communication samples produced by adult communication aid users. *Journal of Speech and Hearing Disorders, 49*, 360–367.

Bigelow, A. (1990). Relationship between the development of language and thought in young blind children. *Journal of Visual Impairment & Blindness, 84*, 414–419.

Bigge, J. L. (1982). *Teaching individuals with multiple disabilities* (2nd ed.). Columbus, OH: Charles E. Merrill.

Bihm, E. M., Kienlen, T. L., Ness, M. E., & Poindexter, A. R. (1991). Factor structure of the Motivation Assessment Scale for persons with mental retardation. *Psychological Reports, 68*, 1235–1238.

Bijou, S. W., Peterson, R. F., & Ault, M. H. (1968). A method to integrate descriptive and experimental field studies at the level of data and empirical concepts. *Journal of Applied Behavior Analysis, 1*, 175–191.

Biklen, D. (1990). Communication unbound: Autism and praxis. *Harvard Educational Review, 60*, 291–314.

Biklen, D., Morton, M. W., Gold, D., Berrigan, C., & Swaminathan, S. (1992). Facilitated communication: Implications for individuals with autism. *Topics in Language Disorders, 12*(4), 1–28.

Birch, E. E., & Bane, M. C. (1991). Forced-choice preferential looking acuity of children with cortical visual impairment. *Developmental Medicine and Child Neurology, 33,* 722–729.

Bird, F., Dores, P. A., Moniz, D., & Robinson, J. (1989). Reducing severe aggressive and self-injurious behaviors with functional communication training: Direct, collateral and generalized results. *American Journal on Mental Retardation, 94,* 37–48.

Bishop, D. (1985). Spelling ability in congenital dysarthria: Evidence against articulatory coding in translating between phonemes and graphemes. *Cognitive Neuropsychology, 2,* 229–251.

Bishop, D. (1988). Language development in children with abnormal structure or function of the speech apparatus. In D. Bishop & K. Mogford (Eds.), *Language development in exceptional circumstances* (pp. 220–238). Edinburgh, Scotland: Churchill Livingstone.

Bishop, D., Byers-Brown, B., & Robson, J. (1990). The relationship between phoneme discrimination, speech production, and language comprehension in cerebral palsied individuals. *Journal of Speech and Hearing Research, 33,* 210–219.

Bishop, D., & Mogford, K. (1993). *Language development in exceptional circumstances.* Hillsdale, NJ: Lawrence Erlbaum Associates.

Bishop, D., & Robson, J. (1989). Accurate non-word spelling despite congenital inability to speak: Phoneme-grapheme conversion does not require subvocal articulation. *British Journal of Psychology, 80,* 1–13.

Bishop, K., Rankin, J., & Mirenda, P. (1994). Impact of graphic symbol use on reading acquisition. *Augmentative and Alternative Communication, 10,* 113–125.

Bishop, V. (1988). Making choices in functional vision evaluation: "Hoodles, needles, and haystacks." *Journal of Visual Impairment & Blindness, 82,* 94–99.

Blachman, B. A. (1991). Early intervention for children's reading problems: Clinical applications of the research in phonological awareness. *Topics in Language Disorders, 12*(1), 51–65.

Blackstone, S. (1986). *Augmentative communication: An introduction.* Rockville, MD: American Speech-Language-Hearing Association.

Blackstone, S. (1988). Vocabulary selection: Current practices and a glimpse at the future. *Augmentative Communication News, 1*(5), 1–3, 5.

Blackstone, S. (1989). *Augmentative Communication News, 2*(1).

Blackstone, S. (1990). Assistive technology in classrooms: Beyond communication devices. *Augmentative Communication News, 3*(6), 1–4.

Blackstone, S. (1993a). Designing displays: Hints and examples. *Augmentative Communication News, 6*(1), 4–6.

Blackstone, S. (1993b). Examining the cost factors in low tech devices. *Augmentative Communication News, 6*(1), 7.

Blackstone, S. (1993c). Low-tech communication displays: Are we considering everything? *Augmentative Communication News, 6*(1), 1–3.

Blackstone, S. (1993d). Results of ANC survey. *Augmentative Communication News, 6*(4), 4–5.

Blackstone, S. (1994). The purpose of AAC assessment. *Augmentative Communication News, 7*(1), 2–3.

Blackstone, S., & Cassatt-James, E. L. (1988). Augmentative communication. In N. J. Lass, L. V. McReynolds, & J. L. Northern (Eds.), *Handbook of speech-language pathology and audiology* (pp. 986–1013). Toronto: B. C. Decker.

Blackstone, S., & Painter, M. (1985). Speech problems in multihandicapped children. In J. Darby (Ed.), *Speech and language evaluation in neurology: Childhood disorders* (pp. 225–226). Orlando, FL: Grune & Stratton.

Blake, R., Field, B., Foster, C., Platt, F., & Wertz, P. (1991). Effect of FM auditory trainers on attending behaviors of learning-disabled children. *Language, Speech, and Hearing Services in Schools, 22,* 111–114.

Blau, A. F. (1983). Vocabulary selection in augmentative communication: Where do we begin? In H. Winitz (Ed.), *Treating language disorders: For clinicians by clinicians.* Baltimore: University Park Press.

Blau, A. F. (1986). The development of literacy skills for severely speech- and writing-impaired children. In S. Blackstone (Ed.), *Augmentative communication: An introduction* (pp. 293–299). Rockville, MD: American Speech-Language-Hearing Association.

Bligh, S., & Kupperman, P. (1993). Evaluation procedure for determining the source of communication in facilitated communication accepted in a court case. *Journal of Autism and Developmental Disorders, 23,* 553–557.

Blischak, D. (1993, April). *AAC assessment.* Presentation at Howard University, Washington, DC.

Blischak, D. M. (1994). Phonological awareness: Implications for individuals with little or no functional speech. *Augmentative and Alternative Communication, 10,* 245–254.

Blischak, D. M. (1995). Thomas the writer: Case study of a child with severe physical, speech, and visual impairments. *Language, Speech, and Hearing Services in Schools, 26,* 11–20.

Blischak, D. M., & Lloyd, L. L. (1996). Multimodal augmentative and alternative communication. *Augmentative and Alternative Communication, 12,* 37–46.

Blischak, D. M., & McDaniel, M. A. (1995). Effects of picture size and placement on memory for written words. *Journal of Speech and Hearing Research, 38,* 1–7.

Bliss, C. (1949). *Semantography.* Sydney, Australia: Semantography Publications.

Bliss, C. (1965). *Semantography* (2nd ed.). Sydney, Australia: Semantography Publications.

Blissymbolics Communication Institute. (1984). *Picture your Blissymbols.* Toronto: Author.

Bloom, L., & Lahey, M. (1978). *Language development and language disorders.* New York: John Wiley & Sons.

Bloomberg, K. (1984). *The comparative translucency of initial lexical items represented by five graphic symbol systems.* Unpublished master's thesis, Purdue University, West Lafayette, IN.

Bloomberg, K. (1985). *Comics: Computer pictographs for communication.* Presentation on behalf of the Victorian Symbol Standardization Committee at the Australian Group on Severe Communication Impairment Study Day, Melbourne, Australia.

Bloomberg, K., Karlan, G. R., & Lloyd, L. L. (1990). The comparative translucency of initial lexical items represented by five graphic symbol systems. *Journal of Speech and Hearing Research, 33,* 717–725.

Blyden, A. E. (1989). Survival word acquisition in mentally retarded adolescents with multihandicaps: Effects of color-revised stimulus materials. *Journal of Special Education, 22,* 493–501.

Board of Education of Hendrick Hudson Central School District v. Rowley, 458 U.S. 176 102 S Ct. 3034, 73 L.Ed.2nd 690 [5 Ed.Law Rep [34]] (1982).

Board of Education of the City School District of New York City, 21 IDELR 265 (N.Y. SEA, 1994).

Bodine, C., & Beukelman, D. R. (1991). Prediction of future speech performance among potential users of AAC systems: A survey. *Augmentative and Alternative Communication, 7,* 100–111.

Boller, F., Mizutani, T., Roessmann, U., & Gambetti, P. (1980). Parkinson disease, dementia and Alzheimer disease: Clinicopathological correlations. *Annals of Neurology, 7,* 329–335.

Bolton, S. O., & Dashiell, S. E. (1984). *INteraction CHecklist for augmentative communication: INCH.* Bisbee, AZ: Imaginart.

Bonvillian, J., & Miller, A. (1995). Everything old is new again: Observations from the nineteenth century about sign communication training with mentally retarded children. *Sign Language Studies, 88,* 245–254.

Bonvillian, J., Orlansky, M., Novack, L., & Folven, R. (1983). Early sign language acquisition and cognitive development. In D. Rogers & J. Sloboda (Eds.), *The acquisition of symbolic skills* (pp. 207–214). New York: Plenum Press.

Bonvillian, J., Orlansky, M., Novack, L., Folven, R., & Holley-Wilcox, P. (1985). Language, cognitive, and cherological development: The first steps in sign language acquisition. In W. Stokoe & V. Volterra (Eds.), *SLR'85: Sign Language Research* (pp. 10–22). Silver Spring, MD: Linstok Press (& Rome: Instituto di Psicologia, CNR).

Boole, G. (1854). *An investigation of the laws of thought on which are founded the mathematical theories of logic and probabilities.* London: Walton & Maberly.

Boothroyd, A. (1990). Impact of technology on the management of deafness. *The Volta Review, 92*(4), 74–82.

Borden, G. J., & Harris, K. S. (1984). *Speech science primer: Physiology, acoustics, and perception of speech.* Baltimore: Williams & Wilkins.

Borel-Maisonny, S. (1960). *Langage oral et écrit. (Spoken and written language), Vols 1 & 2.* Neuchatel, France: Delachaux et Niestlé.

Bornstein, H. (1973). A description of some current sign systems designed to represent English. *American Annals of the Deaf, 118,* 454–463.

Bornstein, H. (1974). Signed English: A manual approach to English language development. *Journal of Speech and Hearing Disorders, 39,* 330–343.

Bornstein, H., Hamilton, L., Saulnier, K., & Roy, H. (1975). *The Signed English dictionary for preschool and elementary levels.* Washington, DC: Gallaudet College Press.

Bornstein, H., & Jordan, I. K. (1984). *Functional signs: A new approach from simple to complex.* Baltimore: University Park Press.

Bornstein, H., Kannapell, B., Saulnier, K., Hamilton, L., & Roy, H. (1973). *Basic preschool Signed English dictionary.* Washington, DC: Gallaudet College Press.

Bornstein, H., & Saulnier, K. (1984). *The Signed English starter.* Washington, DC: Gallaudet College Press.

Bornstein, H., Saulnier, L., & Hamilton, L. (1983). *The comprehensive Signed English dictionary.* Washington, DC: Gallaudet University Press.

Bos, H. (1990). Person and location marking in Sign Language of the Netherlands: Some implications of a spatially expressed syntactic system. In S. Prillwitz & T. Vollhaber (Eds.), *Current trends in European sign language research: Proceedings of the 3rd European congress on sign language research* (pp. 221–246). Hamburg, Germany: Signum Press.

Bos, H. (1993). Agreement and prodrop in Sign Language of the Netherlands. In F. Drijkoningen & K. Hengeveld (Eds.), *Linguistics in the Netherlands* (pp. 37–48). Amsterdam: John Benjamins Publishing Company.

Bourgeois, M. (1990). Enhancing conversational skills in patients with Alzheimer's disease using a prosthetic memory aid. *Journal of Applied Behavior Analysis, 23,* 31–64.

Bourgeois, M. (1991). Communication treatment for adults with dementia. *Journal of Speech and Hearing Research, 34,* 831–844.

Bourgeois, M. (1992). Evaluating memory wallets in conversations with patients with dementia. *Journal of Speech and Hearing Research, 35,* 1344–1357.

Bourgeois, M. (1993). Effects of memory aids on the dyadic conversations of individuals with dementia. *Journal of Applied Behavior Analysis, 26,* 77–87.

Bowerman, M. (1981). Language development. In H. C. Triandis & A. Heron (Eds.), *Handbook of cross-cultural psychology: Developmental psychology* (Vol. 4, pp. 93–186). Boston: Allyn & Bacon.

Bowlby, C. (1993). *Therapeutic activities with persons disabled by Alzheimer's disease and related disorders.* Gaithersburg, MD: Aspen Publications.

Boyd, L. H., Boyd, W. L., & Vanderheiden, G. C. (1990). The graphical user interface: Crisis, danger, and opportunity. *Journal of Visual Impairment & Blindness, 84,* 496–502.

Boyes-Braem, P. (1973). *A study of the acquisition of the DEZ in American Sign Language.* Unpublished paper, Salk Institute, La Jolla, CA.

Boyes-Braem, P. (1982). *Features of the handshape in American Sign Language.* Unpublished doctoral dissertation, University of California at Berkeley.

Bradley, L., & Bryant, P. (1983). Categorizing sounds and learning to read: A causal connection. *Nature, 30,* 419–421.

Bradley, L., & Bryant, P. (1985). *Rhyme and reason in reading and spelling.* Ann Arbor, MI: University of Michigan Press.

Bradley, N. S. (1994). Motor control: Developmental aspects of motor control in skill acquisition. In S. K. Campbell (Ed.), *Physical therapy for children* (pp. 39–77). Philadelphia: W. B. Saunders.

Brady, N. C., & Saunders, K. J. (1991). Considerations in the effective teaching of object-to-symbol matching. *Augmentative and Alternative Communication, 7,* 112–116.

Brady-Dobson, G. (1982). *Brady-Dobson Alternative Communication (B-DAC).* Elmira, OR: Author.

Bragman, R. (1989). Integrating technology into a student's IEP. *NICHCY News Digest, 13,* 8–9, 11, 13.

Braithwaite, D. O. (1991). Viewing persons with disabilities as a culture. In L. A. Samovar & R. E. Porter (Eds.), *Intercultural communication: A reader* (pp. 136–150). Belmont, CA: Wadsworth.

Brereton, B. (1978a). Can a symbol system help children with impaired hearing? *The Australian Teacher of the Deaf, 19,* 42–46.

Brereton, B. (1978b). *Sounds and symbols: The big dictionary.* Mosman, Australia: The Spastic Centre of New South Wales.

Brereton, B., Burnett, L., & Ivimey, M. (1979a). *Sounds and symbols: Further stages.* Mosman, Australia: The Spastic Centre of New South Wales.

Brereton, B., Burnett, L., & Ivimey, M. (1979b). *Sounds and symbols: Stage I.* Mosman, Australia: The Spastic Centre of New South Wales.

Brereton, B., Burnett, L., & Ivimey, M. (1979c). *Sounds and symbols: The everyday dictionary.* Mosman, Australia: The Spastic Centre of New South Wales.

Briggs, T. R. (1983). *An investigation of the efficiency and effectiveness of three nonvocal communication systems with severely handicapped students.* Unpublished doctoral dissertation, Georgia State University, Atlanta.

Bristow, D. (1993, February). *The dream and reality of the Americans with Disabilities Act: Focus on people with multiple disabilities.* Paper presented at the Convention of the Illinois Speech-Language-Hearing Association, Chicago.

Brookner, S. P., & Murphy, N. O. (1975). The use of a total communication approach with a nondeaf child: A case study. *Language, Speech, and Hearing Services in Schools, 6,* 131–137.

Browder, D. M., & Lalli, J. S. (1991). Review of research on sight word instruction. *Research in Developmental Disabilities, 12,* 203–228.

Brown v. Topeka Board of Education, 347 U.S. 483 (1954).

Brown, C. (1954). *My left foot.* London: Secker and Warburg.

Brown, C. W., Perry, D. F., & Kruland, S. (1994). Funding policies that affect children: What every early interventionist should know. *Infants and Young Children, 6*(4), 1–12.

Brown, L., Branston, M., Hamre-Nietupski, S., Pumpian, I., Certo, N., & Bruenewald, L. (1979). A strategy for developing chronological age appropriate and functional curricular content for severely handicapped adolescents and young adults. *Journal of Special Education, 13,* 81–90.

Brown, R. (1977). Why are signed languages easier to learn than spoken languages? In W. C. Stokoe (Ed.), *National symposium on sign language research and teaching* (pp. 9–24). Chicago: National Association of the Deaf.

Brown, R. (1978). Why are signed languages easier to learn than spoken languages?—Part Two. *Bulletin of the American Academy of Arts and Sciences, 32*(3), 25–44.

Brown, S. (1994, June). *Students who use assistive technology: Science gets ahead of the law.* Paper presented at the Annual RESNA Convention, Nashville.

Bryen, D. N., Goldman, A. S., & Quinslisk-Gill, S. (1988). Sign language with students with severe/profound mental retardation: How effective is it? *Education and Training in Mental Retardation, 23,* 129–137.

Bryen, D. N., & Joyce, D. G. (1986). Sign language and the severely handicapped. *The Journal of Special Education, 20,* 183–194.

Bryen, D. N., McGinley, V. (1991). Sign language input to community residents with mental retardation. *Education and Training in Mental Retardation, 26,* 207–213.

Buck, D. (1993). Interest on lawyer account (IOLA) fund. *A.T. Quarterly, 4*(1), 3.

Bull, G. L., Cochran, P. S., & Snell, M. E. (1994). Beyond CAI: Computers, language, and persons with mental retardation. In *Severe communication disorders—Intervention strategies: Topics in language disorders series.* Gaithersburg, MD: Aspen Publishers.

Bullis, M., & Otos, M. (1988). Characteristics of programs for children with deaf-blindness: Results of a national survey. *Journal of the Association for Persons with Severe Handicaps, 13,* 110–115.

Bulwer, J. B. (1644). *The natural language of the hand.* London: R. Whitaker.

Burd, L., Hammes, K., Bornhoeft, D., & Fisher, W. (1988). A North Dakota prevalence study of nonverbal school-age children. *Language, Speech, and Hearing Services in Schools, 19,* 371–383.

Burkhart, L. J. (1993). *Total augmentative communication in the early childhood classroom.* Eldersburg, MD: Author.

Burroughs, J., Albritton, E., Eaton, B., & Montague, J. (1990). A comparative study of language delayed preschool children's ability to recall symbols from two symbol systems. *Augmentative and Alternative Communication, 6,* 202–206.

Burrows, N. L., & Lloyd, L. L. (1972). Programming considerations for the deaf-retarded. *Report of the proceedings of the 45th meeting of the convention of American in-*

structors of the deaf. Washington, DC: U.S. Government Printing Office.

Burt, D. B., Loveland, D. A., & Lewis, K. R. (1992). Depression and the onset of dementia in adults with mental retardation. *American Journal on Mental Retardation, 96,* 502–511.

Butler, C. (1989). High tech tots: Technology for mobility, manipulation, communication, and learning in early childhood. *Infants and Young Children, 1,* 66–73.

Butler, C. (1991). Augmentative mobility: Why do it? *Physical Medicine and Rehabilitation Clinics of North America, 2,* 801–815.

Butterworth, J., Jr., & Strauch, J. D. (1994). The relationship between social competence and success in the competitive work place for persons with mental retardation. *Education and Training in Mental Retardation and Developmental Disabilities, 29,* 118–132.

Button, C. (1993). Reauthorized Rehabilitation Act increases access to assistive technology. *A.T. Quarterly, 4*(1), 1, 4–6, 11.

Buzolich, M. J. (1988). Creative funding for services. In S. Blackstone, E. L. Cassatt-James, & D. M. Bruskin (Eds.), *Augmentative communication: Implementation strategies* (pp. 8.23–8.27). Rockville, MD: American Speech-Language-Hearing Association.

Buzolich, M. J., King, J. S., & Baroody, S. M. (1991). Acquisition of the commenting function among systems users. *Augmentative and Alternative Communication, 7,* 88–99.

Buzolich, M. J., & Wiemann, J. M. (1988). Turn taking in atypical conversations: The case of the speaker/augmented-communicator dyad. *Journal of Speech and Hearing Research, 31,* 3–18.

Byers, V. W., & Bristow, D. C. (1990). Audiologic evaluation of nonspeaking, physically challenged populations. *Ear and Hearing, 11,* 382–386.

Bzoch, K. R., & League, R. (1970). *Receptive-expressive emergent language scale.* Baltimore: University Park Press.

Calculator, S. N. (1988a). Exploring the language of adults with mental retardation. In S. N. Calculator & J. L. Bedrosian (Eds.), *Communication assessment and intervention for adults with mental retardation* (pp. 95–105). Boston: College-Hill Press.

Calculator, S. N. (1988b). Promoting the acquisition and generalization of conversational skills by individuals with severe disabilities. *Augmentative and Alternative Communication, 4,* 94–103.

Calculator, S. N., & Bedrosian, J. L. (Eds.). (1988). *Communication assessment and intervention for adults with mental retardation.* Boston: Little Brown.

Calculator, S. N., & Jorgensen, C. M. (1991). Integrating AAC instruction into regular education settings: Expounding on best practices. *Augmentative and Alternative Communication, 7,* 204–214.

Caldwell, B. M., & Bradley, R. H. (1972). *Home observation and measurement of the environment inventory.* Little Rock, AR: Center for Child Development and Education, University of Arkansas at Little Rock.

Campbell, A., & Lloyd, L. L. (1986, May). *Graphic symbols and symbol systems: What research and clinical practice tell us.* Paper presented at the Conference of the American Association on Mental Deficiency, Denver, CO.

Campbell, D., Draper, R., & Crutchley, E. (1991). The Milan systemic approach to family therapy. In A. S. Burman & D. P. Kniskern (Eds.), *Handbook of family therapy* (pp. 325–362). New York: Brunner/Mazel.

Campbell, P. (1989). Dysfunction in posture and movement in individuals with profound disabilities: Issues and practices. In F. Brown & D. H. Lehr (Eds.), *Persons with profound disabilities: Issues and practices* (pp. 163–189). Baltimore: Paul H. Brookes Publishing.

Campbell, S. K. (1991). Central nervous system dysfunction in children. In S. K. Campbell (Ed.), *Pediatric neurologic physical therapy* (2nd ed., pp. 1–17). New York: Churchill Livingstone.

Campbell-Taylor, I. (1995). Motor speech changes. In R. Lubinski (Ed.), *Dementia and communication* (pp. 70–82). San Diego, CA: Singular Publishing Group.

Campos, J. J., & Bertenthal, B. I. (1987). Locomotion and psychological development in infancy. In K. M. Jaffe (Ed.), *Childhood powered mobility: Developmental, technical and clinical perspectives: Proceedings of the RESNA First Northwest Regional Conference* (pp. 11–42). Washington, DC: RESNA.

Canale, M. (1983). From communicative competence to communicative language pedagogy. In J. C. Richards & R. W. Schmidt (Eds.), *Language and communication* (pp. 2–27). White Plains, NY: Longman.

Cannezzio, L. (1977). *The effects of visual coding, word frequency and word imageability on aphasic's word-matching abilities.* Unpublished master's thesis, Hunter College, City University of New York, NY.

Cannito, M. P., Hayashi, M. M., & Ulatowska, H. K. (1988). Discourse in normal and pathologic aging: Background and assessment strategies. *Seminars in Speech and Language, 9,* 117–134.

Cantwell, D. P., Baker, L., & Mattison, R. E. (1980). Psychiatric disorders in children with speech and language retardation. *Archives of General Psychiatry, 37,* 423–426.

Caplan, A. L., Callahan, D., & Maas, J. (1987). Ethical and policy issues in rehabilitation medicine. *A Hastings Center report: Special supplement* (pp. 1–19). Briarcliff, NY: The Hastings Center.

Caprici, O., Iverson, J., Pizzuto, E., & Volterra, V. (1996). Gestures and words during the transition to two-word speech. *Journal of Child Language, 23*(3), 645–673.

Capute, A. J., & Accardo, P. J. (1991). A neurodevelopmental perspective on the continuum of developmental disabilities. In A. J. Capute & P. J. Accardo (Eds.), *Developmental disabilities in infancy and childhood* (pp. 7–41). Baltimore: Paul H. Brookes Publishing.

Carlsen, W. R., Galluzze, K. E., Forman, L. F., & Cavlieri, T. A. (1994). Comprehensive geriatric assessment: Applications for community-residing, elderly people with mental retardation/developmental disabilities. *Mental Retardation, 32,* 334–340.

Carlson, F. (1981). A format for selecting vocabulary for the nonspeaking child. *Language, Speech, and Hearing Services in Schools, 12,* 240–245.

Carlson, F. (1982). *Prattle and play.* Omaha: University of Nebraska Medical Center.

Carlson, F. (1985). *Picsyms categorical dictionary.* Lawrence, KS: Baggeboda Press.

Carlson, F. (1987). Communication strategies for infants. In E. T. McDonald (Ed.), *Treating cerebral palsy* (pp. 191–207). Austin, TX: PRO-ED.

Carlson, F., & James, C. A. (1980). *Picsyms system and symbol system.* Unpublished paper, Meyer Children's Rehabilitation Institute of the University of Nebraska Medical Center, Lincoln.

Carlson, F., & Kovarik, A. M. (1985, November). *Developmental comprehension of PICSYMS, an augmentative communication symbol system.* Paper presented at the Annual Convention of the American Speech-Language-Hearing Association, Washington, DC.

Carlson, S. J., & Ramsey, C. (1994). Assistive technology. In S. K. Campbell (Ed.), *Physical therapy for children* (pp. 621–650). Philadelphia: W. B. Saunders.

Carr, E. G. (1988). Functional equivalence as a means of response generalization. In R. H. Horner, G. Dunlap, & R. L. Koegel (Eds.), *Generalization and maintenance: Life style changes in applied settings* (pp. 221–241). Baltimore: Paul H. Brookes Publishing.

Carr, E. G., & Durand, V. M. (1985a). The social-communicative basis of severe behavior problems in children. In S. Reiss & R. R. Bootzin (Eds.), *Theoretical issues in behavior therapy* (pp. 219–254). New York: Academic Press.

Carr, E. G., & Durand, V. M. (1985b). Reducing behavior problems through functional communication training. *Journal of Applied Behavior Analysis, 18,* 111–126.

Carr, E. G., & Kemp, D. C. (1989). Functional equivalence of autistic leading and communicative pointing: Analysis and treatment. *Journal of Autism and Developmental Disorders, 19,* 561–578.

Carr, E. G., & Kologinsky, E. (1983). Acquisition of sign language by autistic children II: Spontaneity and generalization effects. *Journal of Applied Behavior Analysis, 16,* 297–314.

Carr, E. G., Levin, L., McConnachie, G., Carlson, J. I., Kemp, D. C., & Smith, C. E. (1994). *Communication-based intervention for problem behavior: A user's guide for producing positive change.* Baltimore: Paul H. Brookes Publishing.

Carrier, Jr., J. K. (1974). Application of functional analysis to a non-speech response mode to teaching language. In L. V. McReynolds (Ed.), *Developing systematic procedures for training children's language* (ASHA Monograph No. 18a, pp. 47–95). Rockville, MD: American Speech-Language-Hearing Association.

Carrier, J. K., Jr. (1976). Application of a nonspeech language system with the severely language handicapped. In L. L. Lloyd (Ed.), *Communication assessment and intervention strategies* (pp. 523–547). Baltimore: University Park Press.

Carrier, Jr., J. K., & Peak, T. (1975). *Program manual for Non-SLIP (Non-speech language initiation program).* Lawrence, KS: H & H Enterprises.

Cassatt-James, E. L. (1989). *Funding for communication devices.* Pittsburgh: Adaptive Communication Systems.

Cassette Books. (1992). *National library service for the blind and physically handicapped.* Washington, DC: The Library of Congress.

Catlett, C. (1989). Constructing a competitive proposal. *Asha, 18,* 70–72.

Catts, H. W. (1989). Phonological processing deficits and reading disabilities. In A. Kamhi & H. Catts (Eds.), *Reading disabilities: A developmental language perspective* (pp. 101–132). Boston: College-Hill Press.

Catts, H. W. (1991). Facilitating phonological awareness: Role of speech-language pathologists. *Language, Speech, and Hearing Services in Schools, 22,* 196–203.

Catts, H., & Kamhi, A. (1986). The linguistic bases of reading disorders: Implications for the speech-language pathologist. *Language, Speech, and Hearing Services in Schools, 17,* 329–341.

Cauley, K. M., Golinkoff, R. M., Hirsh-Pasek, K., & Gordon, L. (1989). Revealing hidden competencies: A new method for studying language comprehension in children with motoric impairment. *American Journal on Mental Retardation, 94,* 53–63.

Caulfield, M. B., Fischel, J., DeBaryshe, B. D., & Whitehurst, G. J. (1989). Behavioral correlates of developmental expressive language disorders. *Journal of Abnormal Child Psychology, 17,* 187–201.

Cermak, L. S., & Tarlow, S. (1978). Aphasic and amnestic patients' verbal vs. nonverbal retentive abilities. *Cortex, 14,* 32–40.

Chalifoux, L. M. (1991). Macular degeneration: An overview. *Journal of Visual Impairment & Blindness, 85,* 249–252.

Chapman, B. L. M. (1982). Computer assisted teaching of communication to handicapped users project. In *Research unit handbook.* Research Unit, School of Education, University of Bristol, England.

Chapman, R., & Miller, J. (1980). Analyzing language and communication in the child. In R. L. Schiefelbusch (Ed.), *Nonspeech language and communication: Acquisition and intervention* (pp. 159–196). Baltimore: University Park Press.

Chaves, T., & Solar, J. (1974). Pedro Ponce de Leon: First teacher of the deaf. *Sign Language Studies, 5,* 48–63.

Chen, D., & Smith, J. (1992). Developing orientation and mobility skills in students who are multihandicapped and visually impaired. *RE:view, 24,* 133–139.

Chen, L. Y. (1968). "Talking hand" for aphasic patients. *Geriatrics, 23,* 145–148.

Child with a Disability, Case No. 94-15. 21 IDELAR 749 (CT SEA, 1994).

Chomsky, N. (1965). *Aspects of the theory of syntax.* Cambridge, MA: MIT Press.

Christopoulous, C., & Bonvillian, J. D. (1985). Sign language, pantomime, and gestural processing in aphasic persons: A review. *Journal of Communication Disorders, 18,* 1–20.

Church, G., & Glennan, S. (1992). *The handbook of assistive technology.* San Diego, CA: Singular Publishing Group.

Clark, C. R. (1977). *Research report #107: A comparative study of young children's ease of learning words represented in the graphic systems of Rebus, Bliss, Carrier-Peak, and traditional orthography.* Unpublished manuscript, Research, Development and Demonstration Center in Education of Handicapped Children, Minneapolis, MN.

Clark, C. R. (1981). Learning words using traditional orthography and the symbols of Rebus, Bliss, and Carrier. *Journal of Speech and Hearing Disorders, 46,* 191–196.

Clark, C. R. (1984). A close look at the standard Rebus system and Blissymbolics. *Journal of the Association for Persons with Severe Handicaps, 9,* 37–48.

Clark, C. R., Davies, C. O., & Woodcock, R. W. (1974). *Standard Rebus glossary.* Circle Pines, MN: American Guidance Service.

Clark, C. R., Moores, D. F., & Woodcock, R. W. (1975). *The Minnesota Early Language Development Sequence (MELDS).* Research, Development and Demonstration Center in Education of Handicapped Children, University of Minnesota, Minneapolis.

Clark, C. R., & Woodcock, R. W. (1976). Graphic systems of communication. In L. L. Lloyd (Ed.), *Communication assessment and intervention strategies* (pp. 549–605). Baltimore: University Park Press.

Clark, D. A. (1980). Neonates and infants at risk for hearing and speech-language disorders. *Topics in Language Disorders, 10*(1), 1–12.

Clark, J. E. (1983). Intelligibility comparisons for two synthetic and one natural speech source. *Journal of Phonetics, 11,* 37–49.

Clark, L., & Witte, K. (1995). Nature and efficacy of communication management in Alzheimer's disease. In R. Lubinski (Ed.), *Dementia and communication* (pp. 238–254). San Diego, CA: Singular Publishing Group.

Clark, R. (1980). *Guidelines for NU-VUE-CUE.* Bowling Green, IN: Author.

Clark, R. (1984, April). *Verbal eyes verbalize.* A presentation at the Council for Exceptional Children Convention, Washington, DC.

Clay, M. M. (1975). *What did I write?* Aukland, New Zealand: Heinemann Educational Books Limited.

Clay, M. M. (1991). *Becoming literate.* Portsmouth, NH: Heinemann Educational Books Limited.

Clement, M. (1961). Morse code method of communication for the severely handicapped cerebral palsied child. *Cerebral Palsy Review, 22,* 15–16.

Cleveland (OH) v. Public School District. EHLR 353-307 (OCR, 1988).

Closing the Gap (1955, February/March). *Resource Directory.* Henderson, MN: Closing the Gap, Inc.

Coelho, C. (1982). *An investigation of sign acquisition and use by severe chronic aphasic subjects.* Unpublished doctoral dissertation, University of Connecticut, Storrs, CT.

Coelho, C., & Duffy, R. J. (1987). The relationship of the acquisition of manual signs to severity of aphasia: A training study. *Brain and Language, 31,* 328–345.

Coerts, J. A. (1992). *Nonmanual grammatical markers: An analysis of interrogatives, negations and topicalisations in Sign Language of the Netherlands.* Doctoral dissertation, University of Amsterdam: University of Amsterdam Press.

Cohen, C. (1986). Funding high tech. *NICHCY News Digest, 10,* 14–16.

Cohen, C. (1994, June). *P.L. 103-218: Technology Related Assistance for Individuals with Disabilities Act: Amendments for 1994.* Paper presented at the Annual RESNA Convention, Nashville.

Cohen, C. G., & Palin, M. W. (1986). Speech syntheses and speech recognition devices. In M. L. Grossfeld & C. A. Grossfeld (Eds.), *Microcomputer application in rehabilitation of communication disorders* (pp. 183–211). Rockville, MD: Aspen.

Coleman, C. I., Cook, A. M., & Meyers, L. S. (1980). Assessing non-oral clients for assistive technology devices. *Journal of Speech and Hearing Disorders, 45,* 515–526.

Coleman, C. I., & Meyers, L. (1991). Computer recognition of the speech of adults with cerebral palsy and dysarthria. *Augmentative and Alternative Communication, 7,* 34–43.

Coleman, P. P. (1992). Literacy lost: A qualitative analysis of the early literacy experiences of preschool children with severe speech and physical impairments (Doctoral dissertation, University of North Carolina at Chapel Hill, 1991). *Dissertation Abstracts International, 53,* 119A.

Collier, B. (1991). Report on the ISAAC developing countries seminar. *Augmentative and Alternative Communication, 7,* 138–146.

Collins, D. W. (1974). Patient initiated light operated telecontrol (PILOT). In K. Copeland (Ed.), *Aids for the severely handicapped* (pp. 31–41). New York: Grune & Stratton.

Collins, T. (1994). Effect of position on caregivers' expectations of the communicative competence of students with profound multiple disabilities. *Pediatric Physical Therapy, 6,* 211 (Abstract).

Compton, C. L. (Ed). (1989). *Seminars in Hearing, 10*(1), 104–120.

Conners, F. A. (1992). Reading instruction for students with moderate mental retardation: Review and analysis of research. *American Journal on Mental Retardation, 96,* 577–597.

Conti, R. V., & Jenkins-Odorisio, C. (Eds.). (1993). *Proceedings of the first annual Pittsburgh employment conference for augmented communicators.* Pittsburgh, PA: SHOUT Press.

Conti, R. V., & Jenkins-Odorisio, C. (Eds.). (1994). *Proceedings of the second annual Pittsburgh employment conference for augmented communicators. Pittsburgh, PA: SHOUT Press.

Conti-Ramsden, G. (1990). Maternal recasts and other contingent replies to language-impaired children. *Journal of Speech and Hearing Disorders, 55*, 262–274.

Cook, A. M., & Hussey, S. M. (1995). *Assistive technologies: Principles and practice.* St. Louis, MO: Mosby.

Cooper, F. S., Delattre, P. C., Liberman, A. M., Borst, J. M., & Gertsman, L. J. (1952). Some experiments on the perception of synthetic speech sounds. *Journal of the Acoustical Society of America, 24*, 597–606.

Cooper, R., & Fuller, D. R. (1994). Differences in preschool children's learning of black-on-white versus white-on-black graphic symbols. Unpublished manuscript, University of Arkansas at Little Rock/University of Arkansas for Medical Sciences, Little Rock.

Copeland, K. (Ed.). (1974). *Aids for the severely handicapped.* New York: Grune & Stratton.

Corina, D. P., Poizner, H., Bellugi, U., Feinberg, T., Dowd, D., & O'Grady-Batch, L. (1992). Dissociation between linguistic and nonlinguistic gestural systems: A case for compositionality. *Brain and Language, 43*, 414–447.

Cornell, T. (1988). Characteristics of effective occupational literacy programs. *Journal of Reading, 31*(7), 654–656.

Cornett, O. (1967). Cued speech. *American Annals of the Deaf, 112*, 3–13.

Corson, D. (1989). Adolescent lexical differences in Australia and England by social group. *Journal of Educational Research, 82*, 146–157.

Costello, J. M., & Shane, H. C. (1994, November). *Augmentative communication assessment and the feature matching process.* Presentation at the Annual Convention of the American Speech-Language-Hearing Association, New Orleans, LA.

Council for Exceptional Children. (1991). *Code of ethics of the Council for Exceptional Children.* Reston, VA: Author.

Cox, R. M., Alexander, G. C., & Rivera, I. M. (1991). Comparison of objective and subjective measures of speech intelligibility in elderly hearing-impaired listeners. *Journal of Speech and Hearing Research, 34*, 904–915.

Crain, S. K. (1988). Metacognition and the teaching of reading. *Journal of Reading, 31*(7), 682–685.

Crandell, C. C., & Roeser, R. J. (1993). Incidence of excessive impacted cerumen in individuals with mental retardation: A longitudinal investigation. *American Journal on Mental Retardation, 97*, 568–574.

Crawford, J., Brockel, B., Schauss, S., & Miltenberger, R. G. (1992). A comparison of methods for the functional assessment of stereotyped behavior in persons with mental retardation. *Journal of the Association for Persons with Severe Handicaps, 17*, 77–86.

Creech, R. (1992). *Reflections from a unicorn.* Greenville, NC: RC Publishing.

Creedon, M. P. (Ed.). (1975). *Appropriate behavior through communications: A new program in simultaneous language.* Chicago: Developmental Institute, Humana Hospital.

Creer-Berti, D. E. (1993). *Diana: A woman of courage, a child of mischief!* Rockford, IL: Author.

Cregan, A. (1980a). *Sigsymbols* [Videotape]. Watford, England: Chiltern Consortium.

Cregan, A. (1980b). *Sigsymbols: A nonvocal aid to communication and language development.* Long study submitted in partial fulfillment of the Advanced Diploma in Education of Children with Special Needs, Cambridge Institute of Education, Cambridge, England.

Cregan, A. (1982). *Sigsymbol dictionary.* Hatfield, Herts, England: Author.

Cregan, A. (1993). Sigsymbol system in a multimodal approach to speech elicitation: Classroom project involving an adolescent with severe mental retardation. *Augmentative and Alternative Communication, 9*, 146–160.

Cregan, A., & Lloyd, L. L. (1984, October). *Sigsymbols: Graphic symbols conceptually linked with manual signs.* Paper presented at the Third International Conference on Augmentative and Alternative Communication, International Society for Augmentative and Alternative Communication, Cambridge, MA.

Cregan, A., & Lloyd, L. L. (1990). *Sigsymbols: American edition.* Wauconda, IL: Don Johnston Incorporated.

Cress, C., & French, G. J. (1994). The relationship between cognitive load measurements and estimates of computer input control skills. *Assistive Technology, 6*, 54–66.

Cress, C., & Goltz, C. (1989). Cognitive factors affecting accessibility of computers and electronic devices. In *Proceedings of the 12th annual RESNA conference* (pp. 25–26). Washington, DC: RESNA.

Cress, P. J., Spellman, C. R., DeBriere, T. J., Sizemore, A. C., Northam, J. K., & Johnson, J. L. (1981). Vision screening for persons with severe handicaps. *Journal of the Association for the Severely Handicapped, 6*, 41–50.

Crew, J. E., & Frey, W. D. (1993). Family concerns and older people who are blind. *Journal of Visual Impairment & Blindness, 87*, 6–11.

Crossley, R. (1992). Lending a hand: A personal account of the development of facilitated communication training. *American Journal of Speech-Language Pathology, 1*(3), 15–18.

Crystal, D., & Craig, E. (1978). Contrived sign language. In I. M. Schlesinger & L. Namir (Eds.), *Sign language of the deaf* (pp. 141–168). New York: Academic Press.

Cudahy, E. (1988). *Introduction to instrumentation in speech and hearing.* Baltimore: Williams & Wilkins.

Culp, D. M., & Carlisle, M. (1988). *Partners in augmentative training: A resource guide for interaction facilitation training for children.* Tucson, AZ: Communication Skill Builders.

Cumley, G., & Jones, R. (1992). Persons with primary speech, language and motor impairments. In D. R. Beukelman & P. Mirenda (Eds.), *Augmentative and alternative communication: Management of severe communication disorders in children and adults* (pp. 229–254). Baltimore: Paul H. Brookes Publishing.

Cummins, J. (1986). Empowering minority students: A framework for intervention. *Harvard Educational Review, 56,* 18–36.

Cummins, R. A., & Prior, M. P. (1992). Autism and assisted communication: A response to Biklen. *Harvard Educational Review, 62,* 228–298.

Damiano, D. L., Kelly, L. E., & Vaughn, C. L. (1995). Effects of quadriceps femoris muscle strengthening on crouch gait in children with spastic diplegia. *Physical Therapy, 75,* 658–667.

Daniloff, J. K., Noll, J. D., Fristoe, M., & Lloyd, L. L. (1982). Gesture recognition in patients with aphasia. *Journal of Speech and Hearing Disorders, 47,* 43–49.

Daniloff, J., & Vergara, D. (1984). Comparison between the motoric constraints for Amer-Ind and ASL sign formation. *Journal of Speech and Hearing Research, 27,* 76–88.

Darley, F., Aronson, A., & Brown, J. (1975). *Motor speech disorders.* Philadelphia: W. B. Saunders.

Davis School District. 18 IDELR 696 (UT.SEA, 1992).

Davis, J. M., Elfenbein, J., Schum, R., & Bentler, R. A. (1986). Effects of mild and moderate hearing impairments on language, educational, and psychosocial behavior of children. *Journal of Speech and Hearing Disorders, 51,* 53–62.

Day, R. M., Johnson, W. L., & Schussler, N. G. (1986). Determining the communicative properties of self-injury: Research, assessment, and treatment implications. In K. D. Gadow (Ed.), *Advances in learning and behavioral disabilities* (Vol. 5, pp. 117–139). Greenwich, CT: JAI Press.

Day, R. M., Rea, J. A., Schussler, N. G., Larsen, S. E., & Johnson, W. L. (1988). A functionally based approach to the treatment of self-injurious behavior. *Behavior Modification, 12,* 565–589.

Dechant, E. V. (1991). *Understanding and teaching reading: An interactive model.* Hillsdale, NJ: Lawrence Erlbaum Associates.

Deich, R. F., & Hodges, P. M. (1977). *Language without speech.* New York: Brunner/Mazel.

Dekker, R., & Koole, F. D. (1992). Visually impaired children's visual characteristics and intelligence. *Developmental Medicine & Child Neurology, 34,* 123–133.

DeLattre, P. C., Liberman, A. M., & Cooper, F. S. (1955). Acoustic loci and transitional cues for consonants. *Journal of the Acoustical Society of America, 27,* 769–773.

Demasco, P. (1994). Human factors consideration in the design of language interfaces in AAC. *Assistive Technology, 6,* 10–25.

Demasco, P., Mineo, B., Gray, J., & Bender, R. (1994). The design and development of a computer based system for assessing and training two-dimensional language representation. In *Proceedings of the RESNA '94 annual conference.* Arlington, VA: Resna Press.

Denckla, M., & Rundel, R. (1976). Naming of object-drawings by dyslexic and other learning disabled children. *Brain and Language, 3,* 1–15.

Dennis, R., Reichle, J., Williams, W., & Vogelsberg, R. T. (1982). Motor factors influencing the selection of vocabulary for sign production programs. *Journal of the Association for the Severely Handicapped, 7,* 20–32.

Denton, D. M. (1970). Remarks in support of total communication. In *Communication symposium.* Frederick, MD: Maryland School for the Deaf.

DeRenzi, E. (1968). Non-verbal memory and hemispheric site of lesion. *Neuropsychologia, 6,* 181–189.

DeRenzi, E., & Lucchelli, F. (1993). The fuzzy boundaries of apperceptive agnosia. *Cortex, 29,* 187–215.

DeRenzi, E., & Vignolo, L. A. (1962). The token test: A sensitive test to detect receptive disturbances in aphasics. *Brain, 85,* 665–678.

DeRuyter, F., & Donoghue, K. (1989). Communication and traumatic brain injury: A case study. *Augmentative and Alternative Communication, 5,* 49–54.

DeRuyter, F., & Kennedy, M. (1991). Augmentative communication following traumatic brain injury. In D. Beukelman & K. Yorkston (Eds.), *Communication disorders following traumatic brain injury: Management of cognitive, language, and motor impairments* (pp. 317–365). Austin, TX: Pro-Ed.

DeRuyter, F., & Lafontaine, L. (1987). The nonspeaking brain injured: A clinical and demographic database report. *Augmentative and Alternative Communication, 3,* 18–25.

Devereux, K., & van Oosterom, J. (1984). *Learning with rebuses.* Stratford-Upon-Avon, UK: National Council for Special Education (Developing Horizons in Special Education Series, No. 8).

Dixon, H. N. (1890). *Simplification of the letters of the alphabet and methods of teaching deaf-mutes to speak* (J. P. Bonet, Trans.). Harrogate, England: Farrar. (Original work published in 1620).

Dixon, L. S. (1981). A functional analysis of photo-object matching skills of severely retarded adolescents. *Journal of Applied Behavior Analysis, 14,* 465–478.

Doherty, J. E. (1985). The effects of sign characteristics on sign acquisition and retention: An integrative review of the literature. *Augmentative and Alternative Communication, 1,* 108–121.

Doherty, J. E. (1986). The effects of translucency and handshape difficulty on sign acquisition by preschool children. (Doctoral dissertation, Purdue University, West Lafayette, IN, 1985). *Dissertation Abstracts International, 46,* 3317A.

Doherty, J. E., Daniloff, J., & Lloyd, L. L. (1985). The effect of categorical representation on Amer-Ind transparency. *Augmentative and Alternative Communication, 1,* 10–16.

Donnellan, A. M., Mirenda, P. L., Mesaros, R. A., & Fassbender, L. L. (1984). Analyzing the communicative functions of aberrant behavior. *Journal of the Association for Persons with Severe Handicaps, 9,* 201–212.

Donovan, W. (1981). Spinal cord injury. In W. Stolov & M. Clowers (Eds.), *Handbook of severe disability* (pp. 55–64). Washington, DC: U.S. Government Printing Office.

Dorman, C. (1985). Classification of reading disability in a case of congenital brain damage. *Neuropsychologia, 23,* 393–402.

Doss, L. S. (1988). *The effects of communication instruction on food stealing in adults with developmental disabilities.* Unpublished doctoral dissertation, University of Minnesota, Minneapolis.

Doss, L. S., Locke, P. A., Johnston, S. S., Reichle, J., Sigafoos, J., Charpentier, P. J., & Foster, D. J. (1991). Initial comparison of the efficiency of a variety of AAC systems for ordering meals in fast food restaurants. *Augmentative and Alternative Communication, 7,* 256–265.

Doss, L. S., & Reichle, J. (1989). Establishing communicative alternatives to the emission of socially motivated excess behavior: A review. *Journal of the Association for Persons with Severe Handicaps, 14,* 101–112.

Doss, L. S., & Reichle, J. (1991a). Replacing excess behavior with an initial communicative repertoire. In J. Reichle, J. York, & J. Sigafoos (Eds.), *Implementing augmentative and alternative communication: Strategies for learners with severe disabilities* (pp. 215–237). Baltimore: Paul H. Brookes Publishing.

Doss, L. S., & Reichle, J. (1991b). Using graphic organization aids to promote independent functioning. In J. Reichle, J. York, & J. Sigafoos (Eds.), *Implementing augmentative and alternative communication: Strategies for learners with severe disabilities* (pp. 275–288). Baltimore: Paul H. Brookes Publishing.

Downing, J. (1963). *The Downing readers.* London: Initial Teaching Publication.

Downing, J. (1970). Cautionary comments on some American i.t.a. reports. *Educational Research, 13,* 70–72.

Downing, J., & Eichinger, J. (1990). Instructional strategies for learners with dual sensory impairments in integrated settings. *Journal of the Association for Persons with Severe Handicaps, 15,* 98–105.

Downing, J., & Jones, B. (1966). Some problems of evaluating i.t.a.: A second experiment. *Educational Research, 8,* 100–114.

Downs, M. P. (1994). The case for detection and intervention at birth. *Seminars in Hearing, 15*(2), 75–84.

Drolet, C. (1982). *Unipix: Universal language of pictures.* Los Angeles: Imaginart Press.

DuBose, R. F. (1983). Working with sensorily impaired children. In S. G. Garwood (Ed.), *Educating young handicapped children: A developmental approach* (2nd ed., pp. 235–276). Rockville, MD: Aspen Publishing.

Dudley, H., Reisz, R. R., & Watkins, S. S. A. (1939). A synthetic speaker. *Journal of the Franklin Institute, 227,* 739–764.

Duffy, R. J., & Duffy, J. R. (1981). Three studies of deficits in pantomime expression and pantomime recognition in aphasia. *Journal of Speech and Hearing Research, 24,* 97–111.

Duffy, R. J., & Duffy, J. R., & Pearson, R. L. (1975). Impairment of pantomime recognition in aphasics. *Journal of Speech and Hearing Research, 18,* 115–132.

Duker, P., & Remington, B. (1991). Manual sign-based communication for individuals with severe or profound mental handicap. In B. Remington (Ed.), *The challenge of severe mental handicap* (pp. 167–187). London: John Wiley & Sons.

Duncan, J. L., & Silverman, F. H. (1977). Impacts of learning American Indian Sign Language on mentally retarded children: A preliminary report. *Perceptual and Motor Skills, 44,* 1138.

Dunham, J. K. (1989). The transparency of manual signs in a linguistic and an environmental nonlinguistic context. *Augmentative and Alternative Communication, 5,* 214–225.

Dunn, L., & Dunn, L. (1981). *Peabody picture vocabulary test: Revised.* Circle Pines, MN: American Guidance Service.

Dunn, M. L. (1982). *Pre-sign language motor skills.* Tucson, AZ: Communication Skill Builders.

Dunst, C. J., & Lowe, L. W. (1986). From reflex to symbol: Describing, explaining, and fostering communicative competence. *Augmentative and Alternative Communication, 2,* 11–18.

Durand, V. M. (1990). *Severe behavior problems: A functional communication training approach.* New York: Guilford Press.

Durand, V. M. (1993). Functional communication training using assistive devices: Effects on challenging behavior and affect. *Augmentative and Alternative Communication, 9,* 168–176.

Durand, V. M., & Berotti, D. (1991). Treating behavior problems with communication. *Asha, 33,* 37–39.

Durand, V. M., Berotti, D., & Weiner, J. (1993). Functional communication training: Factors affecting effectiveness, generalization, and maintenance. In J. Reichle & D. P. Wacker (Eds.), *Communicative alternatives to challenging behavior: Integrating functional assessment and intervention strategies* (pp. 317–340). Baltimore: Paul H. Brookes Publishing.

Durand, V. M., & Carr, E. G. (1991). Functional communication training to reduce challenging behavior: Maintenance and application in new settings. *Journal of Applied Behavior Analysis, 24,* 251–264.

Durand, V. M., & Crimmins, D. B. (1988). Identifying the variables maintaining self-injurious behavior. *Journal of Autism and Developmental Disorders, 189,* 99–117.

Durand, V. M., & Crimmins, D. B. (1992). *The Motivation Assessment Scale (MAS) administration guide.* Topeka, KS: Moinaco & Associates.

Durand, V. M., & Kishi, G. (1987). Reducing severe behavior problems among persons with dual sensory impairments: An evaluation of a technical assistance model. *Journal of the Association for Persons with Severe Handicaps, 12,* 2–10.

Dworkin, J. P. (1991). *Motor speech disorders: Treatment guide for apraxia and dysarthria.* St. Louis, MO: Mosby-Yearbook.

Dyer, K., Dunlap, G., & Winterling, V. (1990). Effects of choice making on the serious problem behaviors of students with severe handicaps. *Journal of Applied Behavior Analysis, 23,* 515–524.

D'Zamko, M. E., & Hampton, I. (1985). Personnel preparation for multihandicapped hearing-impaired students: A review of the literature. *American Annals of the Deaf, 130,* 9–14.

Eagleson, H. M., Vaughn, G. R., & Knudson, A. B. (1970). Hand signals for dysphasia. *Archives of Physical Medicine and Rehabilitation, 51,* 111–113.

Earl, C. (1972). *Don't say a word! The picture language book.* London: Charles Knight & Company, Ltd.

Eberlin, M., McConnachie, G., Ibel, S., & Volpe, L. (1993). Facilitated communication: A failure to replicate the phenomenon. *Journal of Autism and Developmental Disorders, 23,* 507–530.

Ecklund, S., & Reichle, J. (1987). A comparison of normal children's ability to recall symbols from two logographic systems. *Language, Speech, and Hearing Services in Schools, 18,* 34–40.

Edman, P. (1991). Relief Bliss: A low tech technique. *Communicating Together, 9,* 21–22.

Edwards, A. D. N. (1991). *Speech synthesis: Technology for disabled people.* London: Paul Chapman Publishing.

Egan, J. P. (1948). Articulation testing methods. *Laryngoscope, 58,* 955–991.

Ehri, L. (1989). The development of spelling knowledge and its role in reading acquisition and reading disability. *Journal of Learning Disabilities, 22,* 356–365.

Ehri, L. (1991). The development of reading and spelling in children: An overview. In M. Snowling & M. Thomson (Eds.), *Dyslexia: Integrating theory and practice* (pp. 63–79). London: Whurr Publishers Ltd.

Elder, P. S., & Bergman, J. S. (1978). Visual symbol communication instruction with nonverbal multiply-handicapped individuals. *Mental Retardation, 16,* 107–112.

Eldon (MO) v. R-I School District. ELHR 352:144 (OCR, 1986).

Ellis, N. (1981). Visual and name coding in dyslexic children. *Psychological Research, 43,* 201–219.

Ellis, N. (1991). Spelling and sound in learning to read. In M. Snowling & M. Thomson (Eds.), *Dyslexia: Integrating theory and practice* (pp. 80–94). London: Whurr Publishers Ltd.

Ellis, N. (1993). *Reading, writing and dyslexia: A cognitive analysis* (2nd ed.). Hove, England: Lawrence Erlbaum Associates.

Ellsworth, S., & Kotkin, R. (1975). If only Jimmy could speak. *Hearing and Speech Action, 43,* 6–10.

Emerick, L. (1969). *The parent interview.* Danville, IL: Interstate Printers and Publishers.

Emery, A., & Holloway, S. (1982). Familial motor neuron disease. In L. Rowland (Ed.), *Human motor neuron diseases.* New York: Raven Press.

Emery, D. B. (1986). Linguistic decrement in normal aging. *Language and Communication, 6,* 47–74.

Enders, A. (1989). *Funding for assistive technology and related services: An annotated bibliography.* Washington, DC: Rehabilitation Engineering Center.

Enders, A., & Hall, M. (1990). *Assistive technology sourcebook.* Washington, DC: RESNA Press.

Engberg-Pedersen, E. (1986). The use of space with verbs in Danish Sign Language. In B. Tervoort (Ed.), *Signs of life: Proceedings of the second European congress on sign language research* (pp. 32–41). Amsterdam: University of Amsterdam.

Engberg-Pedersen, E. (1993). *Space in Danish Sign Language: The semantics and morphosyntax of the use of space in a visual language.* Hamburg, Germany: Signum Press.

English, K. M. (1995). *Educational audiology across the lifespan.* Baltimore: Paul H. Brookes Publishing.

Enstrom, D. H. (1992). The communication resource center: A New Jersey AAC service delivery model. *Augmentative and Alternative Communication, 8,* 234–242.

Erhardt, R. P. (1987). Visual function in the student with multiple handicaps: An integrative transdisciplinary model for assessment and intervention. *Education of the Visually Impaired, 19,* 87–98.

Erhardt, R. P. (1990). *Developmental visual dysfunction.* Tucson, AZ: Therapy Skill Builders.

Ericksen, K. (1979). *Communication skills for the human services.* Reston, VA: Reston Publishing Company.

Erickson, J. G., & Iglesias, A. (1986). Assessment of communication disorders in non-English proficient children. In O. L. Taylor (Ed.), *Nature of communication disorders in culturally and linguistically diverse populations* (Chap. 7, pp. 181–217). San Diego, CA: College-Hill Press.

Erin, J. N. (1986). Frequencies and types of questions in the language of visually impaired children. *Journal of Visual Impairment and Blindness, 80,* 670–674.

Evans, L. (1982). *Total communication: Structure and strategy.* Washington, DC: Gallaudet College Press.

Fairbanks, G. (1954). Systematic research in experimental phonetics: 1. A theory of the speech mechanism as a servomechanism. *Journal of Speech and Hearing Disorders, 19,* 133–139.

Falvey, M. A. (1986). *Community-based curriculum.* Baltimore: Paul H. Brookes Publishing.

Fant, G. (1960). *Acoustic theory of speech production.* The Hague, The Netherlands: Mouton.

Fant, G. (1969). Distinctive features and phonetic dimensions. *STL-OPSR, 2–3.*

Fawcett, G. F., & Clibbens, J. S. (1983). The acquisition of signs by the mentally handicapped. *British Journal of Disorders of Communication, 18,* 13–22.

Fay, W. H., & Schuler, A. L. (1980). *Emerging language in autistic children.* Baltimore: University Park Press.

Feallock, B. (1958). Communication for the non-vocal individual. *American Journal of Occupational Therapy, 12,* 60.

Fee, V. E., & Matson, J. L. (1991). Definition, classification, and taxonomy. In J. K. Luiselli, J. L. Matson, & N. N. Singh (Eds.), *Self-injurious behavior: Analysis, assess-*

ment, and treatment (pp. 3–20). New York: Springer Verlag.

Ferguson, D. L. (1994). Is communication really the point? Some thoughts on interventions and membership. *Mental Retardation, 32*, 7–18.

Ferster, C. B. (1965). Classification of behavioral pathology. In L. Krasner & L. P. Ullmann (Eds.). *Research in behavior modification* (pp. 6–26). New York: Holt, Rinehart, & Winston.

Fevlado (1983). *Woord en gebaar (Word and sign)*. Ghent, Belgium: Fevlado.

Field, S., LeRoy, B., & Rivera, S. (1994). Meeting functional curriculum needs in middle school and general education classrooms. *Teaching Exceptional Children, 26*(2), 40–43.

Finnie, N. (1977). *Handling the young cerebral palsied child at home* (2nd ed.). New York: Dutton.

Fischer, S. D. (1994). Review of D. McNeill's *Hand and mind. Language, 70*, 345–350.

Fischer, S., & Gough, B. (1978). Verbs in American Sign Language. *Sign Language Studies, 18*, 17–48.

Fischer, S., Metz, D., Brown, P., & Caccamise, F. (1991). The effects of bimodal communication on the intelligibility of sign and speech. In P. Siple & S. Fischer (Eds.), *Theoretical issues in sign language research. Vol 2: Psychology* (pp. 135–147). Chicago: University of Chicago Press.

Fischer, S., & Siple, P. (Eds.). (1990). *Theoretical issues in sign language research*. Chicago: University of Chicago Press.

Fisher, W., Piazza, C., Cataldo, M., Harrell, R., Jefferson, G., & Conner, R. (1993). Functional communication training with and without extinction and punishment. *Journal of Applied Behavior Analysis, 26*, 23–36.

Fishman, I. R. (1987). *Electronic communication aids: Selection and use*. San Diego, CA: College-Hill Press.

Fitch-West, J. (1983). Heightening visual imagery: A new approach to aphasia therapy. In E. Perecman (Ed.), *Cognitive processing in the right hemisphere* (pp. 215–228). New York: Academic Press.

Fletcher, H. (1929). *Speech and hearing*. New York: Van Nostrand.

Flynn, P. T. (1978). Effective clinical interviewing. *Language, Speech, and Hearing Services in Schools, 9*, 265–271.

Foley, B. E. (1989). *Phonological recoding and congenital dysarthria*. Unpublished doctoral dissertation, University of Massachusetts, Amherst, MA.

Foley, B. E. (1993). The development of literacy in individuals with severe congenital speech and motor impairments. *Topics in Language Disorders, 13*(2), 16–32.

Folven, R. J., & Bonvillian, J. (1991). The transition from non-referential to referential language in children acquiring American Sign Language. *Developmental Psychology, 27*, 806–816.

Forchhammer, G. (1903). *On Nodvendigheden of Sikra Meddelesmidler Dovstumme under Ervisingen*. Copenhagen: J. Frimodts, Fortag. (Text of English translation: *The need of a sure means of communication in the instruction of the deaf*. London: Royal National Institute for the Deaf Library.)

Ford, A., Schnorr, R., Meyer, L., Davern, L., Black, J., & Dempsey, P. (1989). *The Syracuse community-referenced curriculum guide for students with moderate and severe disabilities*. Baltimore: Paul H. Brookes Publishing.

Forester, A. D. (1988). Learning to read and write at 26. *Journal of Reading, 31*(7), 604–613.

Foster, R., Giddan, J. J., & Stark, J. (1973). *Assessment of children's language comprehension*. Palo Alto, CA: Consulting Psychologists Press.

Fourcin, A. J. (1975). Language development in the absence of expressive speech. In E. Lenneberg & E. Lenneberg (Eds.), *Foundations of language development: Vol. 1: A multidisciplinary approach* (pp. 263–268). New York: Academic Press.

Francis, W., Nail, B., & Lloyd, L. (1990, November). *Mentally retarded adults' perception of emotions represented by pictographic symbols*. Paper presented at the annual convention of the American Speech-Language-Hearing Association, Seattle.

Franklin, K. (1992). A.T.: Progress made and promises to be kept. *A.T. Quarterly, 3*(1), 9–11.

Franklin, K. (1993). Characteristics of consumer-responsive Tech Act projects defined at institute. *A.T. Quarterly, 4*(2), 7–8.

Frasca, J., Blumbergs, P. C., Henschke, P., & Burns, R. J. (1991). A clinical and pathological study of progressive supranuclear palsy. *Clinical and Experimental Neurology, 28*, 79–89.

Frassinelli, L., Superior, K., & Meyers, J. (1993). A consultation model for speech and language intervention. *Asha, 35*, 25–30.

Frattali, C. M., Thompson, C. K., Holland, A. L., Wohl, C. B., and Ferketic, M. M. (1995). *Functional assessment of communication skills for adults*. Rockville, MD: American Speech-Language-Hearing Association.

Fredericks, H. D. B., & Baldwin, V. L. (1987). Individuals with sensory impairments: Who are they? How are they educated? In L. Goetz, D. Guess, & K. Stremel-Campbell (Eds.), *Innovative program design for individuals with dual sensory impairments* (pp. 3–12). Baltimore: Paul H. Brookes Publishing.

French, J. L. (1964). *Pictorial test of intelligence*. Boston: Houghton Mifflin Company.

French, N. R., & Steinberg, J. C. (1947). Factors governing the intelligibility of speech sounds. *Journal of the Acoustical Society of America, 19*, 90–119.

Friedman, L. (1975). Space, time and person reference in American Sign Language. *Language, 51*, 940–961.

Fried-Oken, M. (1992). The AAC assessment cube for adults with severe communication disabilities. *Communication Outlook, 14*(1), 14–18.

Fried-Oken, M., Howard, J. M., & Stewart, S. R. (1991). Feedback on AAC intervention from adults who are temporarily unable to speak. *Augmentative and Alternative Communication, 7*, 43–50.

Fried-Oken, M., & More, L. (1992). An initial vocabulary for nonspeaking preschool children based on developmental and environmental language sources. *Augmentative and Alternative Communication, 8,* 41–56.

Fried-Oken, M., & Tarry, E. (1985). Development of an auditory scanning communication system with multiple voice output for severely disabled users. In C. Brubaker (Ed.), *Proceedings of the eighth annual conference on rehabilitation technology.* Washington, DC: RESNA.

Friel-Patti, S. (1990). Otitis media with effusion and the development of language: A review of the evidence. *Topics in Language Disorders, 11*(1), 11–22.

Friel-Patti, S. (1994). Commitment to theory. *American Journal of Speech-Language Pathology: A Journal of Clinical Practice, 3*(2), 30–34.

Fristoe, M., & Lloyd, L. L. (1977a). Manual communication for the retarded and others with severe communication impairment. *Mental Retardation, 15,* 18–21.

Fristoe, M., & Lloyd, L. L. (1977b, March). *The use of manual communication with the retarded.* Paper presented at the 10th Annual Gatlinburg Conference on Research in Mental Retardation and Developmental Disabilities, Gatlinburg, TN.

Fristoe, M., & Lloyd, L. L. (1979a). Nonspeech communication. In N. R. Ellis (Ed.), *Handbook of mental deficiency: Psychological theory and research* (2nd ed., pp. 401–430). New York: Lawrence Erlbaum Associates.

Fristoe, M., & Lloyd, L. L. (1979b). Signs used in manual communication training with persons having severe communication impairments. *AAESPH Review, 4,* 364–373.

Fristoe, M., & Lloyd, L. L. (1980). Planning an initial expressive sign lexicon for persons with severe communication impairment. *Journal of Speech and Hearing Disorders, 45,* 170–180.

Fristoe, M., Lloyd, L. L., & Wilbur, R. B. (1977). Non-speech communication: Systems and symbols. *Asha, 19,* 541–542. (Abstract)

Fromm, D., & Holland, A. (1989). Functional communication in Alzheimer's disease. *Journal of Speech and Hearing Disorders, 54,* 535–540.

Fry, E. (1964). A diacritical marking system to aid beginning reading instruction. *Elementary Engineering, 41,* 526–529.

Fuchs, L., & Fuchs, D. (1984). Teaching beginning reading skills: A unique approach. *Teaching Exceptional Children, 17,* 48–53.

Fuller, D. R. (1988). Effects of translucency and complexity on the associative learning of Blissymbols by cognitively normal children and adults. (Doctoral dissertation, Purdue University, West Lafayette, IN, 1987). *Dissertation Abstracts International, 49,* 710B.

Fuller, D. R., & Lloyd, L. L. (1987). A study of physical and semantic characteristics of a graphic symbol system as predictors of perceived complexity. *Augmentative and Alternative Communication, 3,* 26–35.

Fuller, D. R., & Lloyd, L. L. (1991). Toward a common usage of iconicity terminology. *Augmentative and Alternative Communication, 7,* 215–220.

Fuller, D. R., & Lloyd, L. L. (1992). Effects of physical configuration on the paired-associate learning of Blissymbols by preschool children with normal cognitive abilities. *Journal of Speech and Hearing Research, 35,* 1376–1383.

Fuller, D. R., Lloyd, L. L., & Schlosser, R. W. (1991, October). *Symbol selection considerations: An integrative review.* Paper presented at the 1991 Think Tank Symposium, Purdue University, West Lafayette, IN.

Fuller, D. R., Lloyd, L. L., & Schlosser, R. W. (1992). Further development of an augmentative and alternative communication symbol taxonomy. *Augmentative and Alternative Communication, 8,* 67–74.

Fuller, D. R., Lloyd, L. L., & Schlosser, R. W. (1997). What do we know about graphic AAC symbols, and what do we still need to know about them? *Theoretical and methodological issues in augmentative and alternative communication: Proceedings of the fourth ISAAC research symposium, Vancouver, Canada, August 11–12, 1996.* Vasteras, Sweden: Malardalen University Press.

Fuller, D. R., Schlosser, R. W., & Lloyd, L. L. (1994). Aided symbol selection considerations: An integrative review. Unpublished manuscript, University of Arkansas at Little Rock.

Fuller, D. R., & Stratton, M. M. (1991). Representativeness versus translucency: Different theoretical backgrounds, but are they really different concepts? A position paper. *Augmentative and Alternative Communication, 7,* 51–58.

Fulwiler, R., & Fouts, R. (1976). Acquisition of American Sign Language by a noncommunicating autistic child. *Journal of Autism and Childhood Schizophrenia, 6,* 43–51.

Funk, T. A. (1988). Character analysis through courtroom drama. *Journal of Reading, 31,* 680–681.

Funnell, E., & Allpert, A. (1989). Symbolically speaking: Communication with Blissymbols in aphasia. *Aphasiology, 3,* 279–300.

Furth, H. G. (1961). A psychologist's view on the slow learning deaf child. In *Report of the proceedings of the 40th meeting of the Convention of American Instructors of the Deaf* (pp. 189–196). Washington, DC: U.S. Government Printing Office.

Gainotti, G., & Lemmo, M. A. (1976). Comprehension of symbolic gestures in aphasia. *Brain and Language, 3,* 451–460.

Gainotti, G., Silveri, M. C., & Sena, E. (1989). Pictorial memory in patients with right, left and diffuse brain damage. *Journal of Neurolinguistics, 4,* 479–495.

Galda, L., Cullinan, B., & Strickland, D. (1993). *Language, literacy and the child.* London: Harcourt Brace Jovanovich College Publishers.

Gallivan-Fenlon, A. (1994). "Their senior year": Family and service provider perspectives on the transition from school to adult life for young adults with disabilities.

Journal of the Association for Persons with Severe Handicaps, 19, 11–23.

Galyas, K. (1987, August). *Applications of microcomputer technology and/or voice output issues and development.* Paper presented at the Biennial Thinktank, Purdue University, West Lafayette, IN.

Galyas, K., Fant, G., & Hunnicut, S. (1993). *Voice output communication aids.* Vällingby, Sweden: Handikappinstitutet.

Gans, D., & Gans, K. D. (1993). Development of a hearing test protocol for profoundly involved multi-handicapped children. *Ear and Hearing, 14,* 128–140.

Gardner, H., Zurif, E., Berry, T., & Baker, E. (1976). Visual communication in aphasia. *Neuropsychologia, 14,* 275–292.

Gardner, M. F. (1979). *Expressive one-word picture vocabulary test.* Novato, CA: Academic Therapy Publications.

Gardner, R., & Gardner, B. (1969). Teaching sign language to a chimpanzee. *Science, 165,* 664–672.

Gardner, R., & Gardner, B. (1979). Teaching sign language to a chimpanzee. In R. L. Schiefelbusch & J. H. Hollis (Eds.), *Language intervention from ape to child* (pp. 171–204). Baltimore: University Park Press. (Reprinted from *Science, 165,* 1969, 664–672.)

Garretson, M. D. (1976). Total communication. In D. R. Frizina (Ed.), *A bicentennial monograph on hearing impairment: Trends in the USA* (pp. 88–95). Washington, DC: Alexander Graham Bell Association for the Deaf.

Garrett, K., & Beukelman, D. R. (1992). Augmentative communication approaches for persons with severe aphasia. In K. M. Yorkston (Ed.), *Augmentative communication in the medical setting* (pp. 245–338). Tucson, AZ: Communication Skill Builders.

Garrett, K., Beukelman, D. R., & Low-Morrow, D. (1989). A comprehensive augmentative communication system for an adult with Broca's aphasia. *Augmentative and Alternative Communication, 5,* 55–61.

Garrett, K., Schutz-Muehling, L., & Morrow, D. (1990). Low level head injury: A novel AAC approach. *Augmentative and Alternative Communication, 6,* 124. (Abstract)

Garrett, R., Andrews, P., Olsson, C., & Seeger, B. (1990). Development of a computer-based expert system for the selection of assistive communication devices. In J. P. Presperin (Ed.) *RESNA 1990, Proceedings of the 13th Annual Conference: Capitalizing on Technology* (pp. 348–349). Washington, DC: RESNA.

Garrett, S. (1986). A case study in tactile Blissymbols. *Communicating Together, 4,* 16.

Gartner, A., & Lipsky, D. (1987). Beyond special education: Toward a quality system for all students. *Harvard Educational Review, 57,* 367–395.

Gdowski, B. S., Sanger, D. D., & Decker, T. N. (1986). Otitis media: Effect on a child's learning. *Academic Therapy, 21,* 283–291.

Gee, P., & Mounty, J. (1991). Nativization, variability, and style shifting in the sign language development of deaf children of hearing parents. In P. Siple & S. Fischer

(Eds.), *Theoretical issues in sign language research. Vol 2: Psychology* (pp. 65–83). Chicago: University of Chicago Press.

Gelatt, J. P. (1989). Obtaining grant funding: Ten steps to success. *Asha, 31,* 67–69.

Gellhaus, M. M., & Olson, M. R. (1993). Using color and contrast to modify the educational environment of visually impaired students with multiple disabilities. *Journal of Visual Impairment and Blindness, 87,* 19–20.

Gentry, R. (1982). An analysis of the developmental spellings in Gnys at wrk. *The Reading Teacher, 36,* 192–200.

Gerber, S., & Kraat, A. (1992). Use of a developmental model of language acquisition: Application to children using AAC systems. *Augmentative and Alternative Communication, 8,* 19–32.

Geruschat, D. R. (1992). Using the acuity card procedure to assess visual acuity in children with severe and multiple impairments. *Journal of Visual Impairment & Blindness, 86,* 25–27.

Geschwind, N. (1965). Disconnection syndromes in animal and man. *Brain, 88,* 237–294.

Gethen, M. (1981). *Communicaid.* Cheltenham, Gloucestershire, England: Author.

Giangreco, M. F. (1990). Making related service decisions for students with severe disabilities: Roles, criteria, and authority. *Journal of the Association for Persons with Severe Handicaps, 13*(1), 22–31.

Giangreco, M. F., Cloninger, C. J., Mueller, P. H., Yuan, S., & Ashworth, S. (1991). Perspectives of parents whose children have dual sensory impairments. *Journal of the Association for Persons with Severe Handicaps, 16,* 14–24.

Giangreco, M. F., York, J., & Rainforth, B. (1989). Providing related service to learners with severe handicaps in educational settings: Pursuing the least restrictive option. *Pediatric Physical Therapy, 1,* 55–63.

Gibson, E. J. (1969). *Principles of perceptual learning and development.* New York: Appleton-Century-Crofts.

Gibson, J. J. (1966). *The senses considered as perceptual systems.* Boston: Houghton Mifflin.

Gibson, N. (1990a). Collaborative consultation: A model of service delivery (Part 1). *Communicating Together, 8*(2), 7–8.

Gibson, N. (1990b). Collaborative consultation: A model of service delivery (Part 2). *Communicating Together, 8*(3), 17–18.

Gill, N. B. R. (1985). Introducing Blissymbols in Brazil. *Communicating Together, 3,* 18–19.

Gillam, R. B., & Johnston, J. R. (1992). Spoken and written relationships in language/learning-impaired and normally achieving school-age children. *Journal of Speech and Hearing Research, 35,* 1303–1315.

Ginsberg, I. A., & White, T. P. (1985). Otologic considerations in audiology. In J. Katz (Ed.), *Handbook of clinical audiology* (3rd ed., pp. 15–38). Baltimore: Williams & Wilkins.

Gitlis, K. R. (1975, November). *Rationale and precedents for the use of simultaneous communication as an alter-*

nate system of communication for nonverbal children. Paper presented at the 50th Annual Convention of the American Speech and Hearing Association, Washington, DC.

Gitterman, M. R., & Sies, L. F. (1992). Nonbiological determinants of the organization of language in the brain: A comment on Hu, Qiou, and Zhong. *Brain and Language, 43,* 162–165.

Glaser, B. G., & Strauss, A. L. (1967). *The discovery of grounded theory: Strategies for qualitative research.* New York: Aldine DeGruyter.

Glass, A. V., Gazzaniga, M. S., & Premack, D. (1973). Artificial language training in global aphasics. *Neuropsychologia, 11,* 95–103.

Glennen, S. L. (1989). Guidelines for customizing communication aids for children. In *Proceedings of the fourth annual Minspeak conference,* St. Louis.

Glennen, S. L., & Calculator, S. N. (1985). Training functional communication board use: A pragmatic approach. *Augmentative and Alternative Communication, 1,* 134–142.

Goddard, C. (1977). Application of symbols with deaf children. *Blissymbolics Communication Institute Newsletter, No. 3.* Toronto, Canada: Blissymbolics Communication Institute.

Goetz, L., Gee, K., & Sailor, W. (1983). Cross modal transfer of stimulus control: Preparing students with severe multiple disabilities for audiologic assessment. *Journal of the Association for Persons with Severe Handicaps, 10,* 21–30.

Goetz, L., Gee, K., & Sailor, W. (1985). Using a behavior chain interruption strategy to teach communication skills to students with severe disabilities. *Journal of the Association for Persons with Severe Handicaps, 10,* 21–30.

Goetz, L., Guess, D., & Stremel-Campbell, K. (1987). *Innovative program design for individuals with dual sensory impairments.* Baltimore: Paul H. Brookes Publishing.

Goldberg, H. R., & Fenton, J. (1960). *Aphonic communication for those with cerebral palsy: Guide for the development and use of a conversation board.* New York: United Cerebral Palsy of New York State.

Goldin-Meadow, S., & Morford, M. (1985). Gesture in early child language: Studies of deaf and hearing children. *Merrill-Palmer Quarterly, 31,* 145–176.

Goldin-Meadow, S., & Mylander, C. (1990). Beyond the input given: The child's role in the acquisition of language. *Language, 66,* 323–355.

Goldman, R., & Lynch, M. (1971). *Goldman-Lynch sounds and symbols developmental kit.* Circle Pines, MN: American Guidance Service.

Goldsmith, T. (1994). Levels of care. In *Managing managed care: A practical guide for audiologists and speech-language pathologists* (Working draft). Rockville, MD: American-Speech-Language-Hearing Association.

Goldstein, H., & Cameron, H. (1952). New method of communication for the aphasic patient. *Arizona Medicine, 8,* 17–21.

Goldstein, L. H., Canavan, A. G. M., & Polkey, C. E. (1988). Verbal and abstract designs paired associate learning after unilateral temporal lobectomy. *Cortex, 24,* 41–52.

Golinker, L. (1992). Funding assistive technology. *Rehabilitation Management, 5,* 129–133.

Golinker, L. (1994, October). *Augmentative communication device funding: Recent developments and future predictions.* Paper presented at the Second Annual Pittsburgh Employment Conference, Pittsburgh.

Goodenough-Trepagnier, C. (1981, June). *Representation of language for nonvocal communication.* Paper presented at the AACP&T-NEMC meeting on Advances in Technical Aids for Children with Physical Disabilities, Tufts University, Medford, MA.

Goodenough-Trepagnier, C. (1995). Visual analogue communication: An avenue of investigation and rehabilitation of severe aphasia. *Aphasiology, 9,* 321–341.

Goodenough-Trepagnier, C. (1994). Design goals for augmentative communication. *Assistive Technology, 6,* 3–9.

Goodenough-Trepagnier, C., & Prather, P. (1981). Communication systems for the nonvocal based on frequent phoneme sequences. *Journal of Speech and Hearing Research, 24,* 322–329.

Goodenough-Trepagnier, C., Tarry, E., & Prather, P. (1982). Derivation of an efficient nonvocal communication system. *Human Factors, 24,* 163–172.

Goodglass, H., & Kaplan, E. (1983). *Boston diagnostic examination for aphasia.* Philadelphia: Lea & Febiger.

Goodman, K. S. (1986). *What's whole in whole language: A parent-teacher guide.* Portsmouth, NH: Heinemann Educational Books Limited.

Goossens', C. A. (1984). The relative iconicity and learnability of verb referents differentially represented as manual signs, Blissymbolics, and Rebus symbols: An investigation with moderately retarded individuals. (Doctoral dissertation, Purdue University, 1983). *Dissertation Abstracts International, 45,* 809A.

Goossens', C. A. (1989). Aided communication intervention before assessment: A case study of a child with cerebral palsy. *Augmentative and Alternative Communication, 5,* 14–26.

Goossens', C. A., & Crain, S. (1986). *Augmentative communication: Intervention resource.* Wauconda, IL: Don Johnston Incorporated.

Goossens', C. A., & Crain, S. (1987). Overview of nonelectronic eye-gaze communication techniques. *Augmentative and Alternative Communication, 3,* 77–89.

Goossens', C. A., & Crain, S. (1992). *Utilizing switch interfaces with children who are severely physically challenged.* Austin, TX: Pro-Ed.

Goossens', C., Crain, S., & Elder, P. (1992). *Engineering the preschool environment for interactive, symbolic communication.* Birmingham, AL: Southeast Augmentative Communication Publications.

Gorga, D. (1989). Occupational therapy treatment practices with infants in early intervention. *American Journal of Occupational Therapy, 43,* 733.

Goswami, U. (1994). Reading by analogy: Theoretical and practical perspectives. In C. Hulme & M. Snowling (Eds.), *Reading development and dyslexia* (pp. 18–30). London: Whurr Publishers Limited.

Goswami, U., & Bryant, P. (1990). *Phonological skills and learning to read.* East Sussex, England: Lawrence Erlbaum Associates.

Granlund, M. (1993). *Communicative competence in persons with profound mental retardation.* Uppsala, Sweden: Acta Universitatis Upsaliensis.

Gravel, J. S. (1994). Auditory integration training: Placing the burden of proof. *American Journal of Speech-Language Pathology: A Journal of Clinical Practice, 3*(2), 25–29.

Gray, H. (1988). *Key points for funding of augmentative devices.* Pittsburgh: Adaptive Communication Systems, Inc.

Green, G. (1994). The quality of evidence. In H. C. Shane (Ed.), *Facilitated communication: The clinical and social phenomenon* (pp. 157–225). San Diego, CA: Singular Publishing Group.

Greenwood County School District #52. 19 IDELR 355 (S.C. SEA, 1992).

Griffith, P. L. (1979). *The influence of iconicity and phonological similarity on sign learning in mentally retarded persons.* Unpublished doctoral dissertation, Kent State University, Kent, OH.

Griffith, P. L., & Robinson, J. H. (1980). Influence of iconicity and phonological similarity on sign learning by mentally retarded children. *American Journal of Mental Deficiency, 85*, 291–298.

Groce, N. E., & Zola, I. K. (1993). Multiculturalism, chronic illness, and disability. *Pediatrics, 91*, 1048–1055.

Grove, N. (1990). Developing intelligible signs with learning disabled students: A review of the literature and an assessment procedure. *British Journal of Disorders of Communication, 25*, 265–293.

Grove, N., & Dockrell, J. (1994, April). *Multi-sign utterances—strings or necklaces? Analysing the linguistic skills of signers with learning disabilities.* Presentation at the Symposium on Developing Language and Communication Skills for Nonspeaking Children at the 23rd International Congress of Applied Psychology, Madrid.

Grove, N., & Walker, M. (1990). The Makaton vocabulary: Using manual signs and graphic symbols to develop interpersonal communication. *Augmentative and Alternative Communication, 6*, 15–28.

Gualtieri, C. (1988). Pharmacotherapy and the neurobehavioral sequelae of traumatic brain injury. *Brain Injury, 2*, 101–129.

Guerette, P., & Sumi, E. (1994). Integrating control of multiple assistive devices: A retrospective review. *Assistive Technology, 6*, 67–76.

Guess, D., Benson, H., & Siegel-Causey, E. (1985). Concepts and issues related to choice-making and autonomy among persons with severe disabilities. *Journal of the Association for Persons with Severe Handicaps, 10*, 79–86.

Guess, D., Roberts, S., Siegel-Causey, E., Ault, M., Guy, B., & Thompson, B. (1993). Analysis of behavior state conditions and associated environmental variables among students with profound handicaps. *American Journal on Mental Retardation, 97*, 634–653.

Guess, D., Sailor, W., & Baer, D. M. (1976). *Functional speech and language training for the severely handicapped.* Lawrence, KS: H & H Enterprises.

Gustason, G. (1990). Signing Exact English. In H. Bornstein (Ed.), *Manual communication: Implications for education* (pp. 108–127). Washington, DC: Gallaudet University Press.

Gustason, G., Pfetzing, D., & Zawolkow, E. (1980). *Signing exact English* (3rd ed.). Los Alamitos, CA: Modern Signs Press.

Hagen, C., & Malkmus, D. (1979, November). *Intervention strategies for language disorders secondary to head trauma.* Presentation at the Annual Convention of the American Speech-Language-Hearing Association, Atlanta.

Hall, A., Orel-Bixler, D., & Haegerstrom-Portnoy, G. (1991). Special visual assessment techniques for multiple handicapped persons. *Journal of Visual Impairment & Blindness, 85*, 23–29.

Hall, S., & Conn, T. (1972). Current trends in services for the deaf retarded in schools for the deaf and residential facilities for the mentally retarded. In *Report of the proceedings of the 46th meeting of the Convention of American Instructors of the Deaf.* Washington, DC: U.S. Government Printing Office.

Hall, S., & Talkington, L. (1970). Evaluation of a manual approach to programming for deaf retarded. *American Journal on Mental Deficiency, 75*, 378–380.

Hamilton, B. L., & Snell, M. E. (1993). Using the milieu approach to increase spontaneous communication book use across environments by an adolescent with autism. *Augmentative and Alternative Communication, 9*, 259–272.

Hammond, M. (1992). Funding in Utah. ED 3589609.

Hamre-Nietupski, S., Fullerton, P., Holz, K., Ryan-Flottum, M., Stoll, A., & Brown, L. (1977). Curricular strategies for teaching selected nonverbal communication skills to nonverbal and verbal severely handicapped students. In L. Brown, J. Nietupski, S. Lyon, S. Hamre-Nietupski, T. Crowner, & L. Gruenewald (Eds.), *Curricular strategies for teaching nonverbal communication, functional object use, problem solving, and mealtime skills to severely handicapped students* (Vol III, Part I). Madison, WI: University of Wisconsin-Madison and Madison Metropolitan School District.

Hamre-Nietupski, S., Nietupski, J., & Rathe, T. (1985). Letting the data do the talking: Selecting the appropriate nonverbal communication system for severely handicapped students. *Teaching Exceptional Children, 18*, 131–133.

Haney, C. (1995, April). *Environmental inventory: Creating a vocabulary pool.* Presentation at the AAC & AT Workshops by Purdue University and Porter County Education Interlocal, Indianapolis.

Hanson, M. J. (1992). Ethnic, cultural, and language diversity in intervention settings. In E. W. Lynch & M. J. Hanson (Eds.), *Developing cross-cultural competence: A guide for working with young children and their families* (pp. 3–19). Baltimore: Paul H. Brookes Publishing.

Hanson, M. J., & Hanline, M. F. (1985). An analysis of response-contingent learning experience of young children. *Journal of the Association for Persons with Severe Handicaps, 15,* 211–230.

Hanson, V. L. (1991). Phonological processing without sound. In S. A. Brady & D. P. Shankweiler (Eds.), *Phonological processes in literacy* (pp. 153–161). Hillsdale, NJ: Lawrence Erlbaum Associates.

Hanson, V. L., & Fowler, C. A. (1987). Phonological coding in word reading: Evidence from hearing and deaf readers. *Memory & Cognition, 15,* 199–207.

Hardick, E., & Davis, J. (1986). *Rehabilitative audiology for adults and children.* New York: Wiley & Sons.

Haring, T. G., Neetz, J. A., Lovinger, L., Peck, C., & Semmel, M. I. (1987). Effects of four modified incidental teaching procedures to create opportunities for communication. *Journal of the Association for Persons with Severe Handicaps, 12,* 218–227.

Harris, O. (1995, March). *AAC intervention and maintenance with African-Americans.* Presentation at the Workshop on Multicultural Issues in Augmentative and Alternative Communication, Howard University, Washington, DC.

Harris-Vanderheiden, D. (1976). Blissymbols and the mentally retarded. In G. Vanderheiden & K. Grilley (Eds.), *Nonvocal communication techniques and aids for the severely physically handicapped.* Austin, TX: Pro-Ed.

Harry, B. (1992). *Cultural diversity, families, and the special-education system.* New York: Teachers College Press.

Harry, B., Allen, N., & McLaughlin, M. (1995). Communication versus compliance: African-American parents' involvement in special education. *Exceptional Children, 61,* 364–377.

Harste, J., Woodward, V., & Burke, C. (1984). *Language stories and literacy lessons.* Portsmouth, NH : Heinemann.

Hart, B. (1980). Pragmatics: How language is used. *Analysis and Intervention in Developmental Disabilities, 2,* 3–20.

Hayden, D. A. (1994). Differential diagnosis of motor speech dysfunction in children. *Clinics in Communication Disorders, 4*(2), 119–141.

Hayes, A. W. (Ed.). (1985). *Toxicology of the eye, ear, and other special senses.* New York: Raven Press.

Haywood, H. C., & Switzky, H. N. (1986). The malleability of intelligence: Cognitive processes as a function of polygenic-experimental interactions. *School Psychology Review, 15,* 245–255.

Hazenkamp, J., & Huebner, K. M. (1989). *Program planning and evaluation for blind and visually impaired students.* New York: American Foundation for the Blind.

Healy, S. (1994). The use of a synthetic speech output communication aid with a youth having severe developmental disability. In K. Linfoot (Ed.), *Communication strategies for people with developmental disabilities: Issues from theory and practice* (pp. 156–176). Baltimore: Paul H. Brookes Publishing.

Hebbeler, K., Smith, B., & Black, T. (1991). Federal early childhood special education policy: A model for the improvement of services for children with disabilities. *Exceptional Children, 58,* 104–112.

Hegde, M. N. (1985). *Treatment procedures in communicative disorders.* San Diego, CA: College-Hill Press.

Hehner, B. (1980). *Blissymbols for use.* Toronto, Ontario: Blissymbolics Communication International.

Helfman, E., (1992). *On being Sarah.* Morton Grove, IL: A. Whitman.

Helm-Estabrooks, N., Fitzpatrick, P., & Barresi, B. (1982). Visual action therapy for global aphasia. *Journal of Speech and Hearing Disorders, 47,* 385–389.

Helm-Estabrooks, N., Ramsberger, G., Morgan, A., & Nicholas, M. (1989). *Boston assessment of severe aphasia.* Chicago: Riverside Publishing.

Henegar, M. E., & Cornett, R. D. (1971). *Cued speech handbook for parents.* Washington, DC: Gallaudet College.

Heriza, C. B. (1991). Implications of a dynamical systems approach to understanding infant kicking behavior. In *Movement science* (pp. 214–227). Alexandria, VA: American Physical Therapy Association.

Hern, S., Lammers, J., & Fuller, D. R. (1994). The effects of translucency, complexity, and other variables on the acquisition of Blissymbols by institutionalized individuals with mental retardation. Unpublished manuscript, University of Arkansas at Little Rock/University of Arkansas for Medical Sciences.

Hernandez, R. D. (1994). Reducing bias in the assessment of culturally and linguistically diverse populations. *Journal of Educational Issues of Language Minority Students, 14,* 269–300.

Herrmann, M., Reichle, T., Lucius-Hoene, G., Wallesch, C. W., & Johannsen-Horbach, H. (1988). Nonverbal communication as a compensatory strategy for severely nonfluent aphasics: A quantitative approach. *Brain and Language, 33,* 41–54.

Hetzroni, O. E., & Harris, O. L. (1996). Cultural aspects in the development of AAC users. *Augmentative and Alternative Communication, 12,* 52–58.

Higginbotham, D. J. (1992). Evaluation of keystroke savings across five assistive communication technologies. *Augmentative and Alternative Communication, 8,* 258–272.

Hipskind, N. M., & Nerbonne, P. (1970). The most common words used in conversations: Western Massachusetts. *Journal of Communication Disorders, 3,* 47–58.

Hirdes, J. P., Ellis-Hale, K., & Hirdes, B. P. (1993). Prevalence and policy implications of communication disabilities among adults. *Augmentative and Alternative Communication, 9,* 273–280.

Hirsh, I. J. (1952). *The measurement of hearing.* New York: McGraw-Hill.

Hiskey, M. S. (1966). *Hiskey-Nebraska test of learning aptitude*. Lincoln, NE: Author.

Hjelmquist, E., Sandberg, A. D., & Hedelin, L. (1994). Linguistics, AAC, and metalinguistics in communicatively handicapped adolescents. *Augmentative and Alternative Communication, 10*, 169–183.

Hodge, M. M. (1994). Assessment of children with developmental apraxia of speech: A rationale. *Clinics in Communication Disorders, 4*(2), 91–101.

Hodge, M. M., & Hancock, H. R. (1994). Assessment of children with developmental apraxia of speech: A procedure. *Clinics in Communication Disorders, 4*(2), 102–118.

Hodges, P. M., & Schwethelm, B. (1984). A comparison of the effectiveness of graphic symbol and manual sign training with profoundly retarded children. *Applied Psycholinguistics, 5*, 223–253.

Hodgson, W. R. (1985). Testing infants and young children. In J. Katz (Ed.), *Handbook of clinical audiology* (3rd ed., pp. 642–663). Baltimore: Williams & Wilkins.

Hodson, B. W., & Paden, E. P. (1991). *Assessment of phonological processes: Revised*. Austin, TX: Pro-Ed.

Hoffmeister, R., & Farmer, A. (1972). The development of manual sign language in mentally retarded deaf individuals. *Journal of Rehabilitation of the Deaf, 6*, 19–26.

Hofstetter, H. W. (1991). Efficacy of low vision services for visually impaired children. *Journal of Visual Impairment & Blindness, 85*, 20–22.

Hogg, J., & Sebba, J. (1987). *Profound retardation and multiple impairment: Vol 1: Development and learning*. Rockville, MD: Aspen Publishers.

Holland, A. L. (1975). Language therapy for children: Some thoughts on context and content. *Journal of Speech and Hearing Disorders, 40*, 514–523.

Holland, A. L. (1980). *Communicative abilities in daily living*. Austin, TX: Pro-Ed.

Holm, A. (1972). The Danish mouth-hand system. *The Teacher of the Deaf, 70*, 486–490.

Holvoet, J. F., & Helmstetter, E. (1989). *Medical problems of students with special needs: A guide for educators*. Boston: College-Hill Press.

Honsinger, M. (1989). Midcourse intervention in multiple sclerosis: An inpatient model. *Augmentative and Alternative Communication, 5*, 71–73.

Hoogeveen, F. R., Smeets, P. M., & Lancioni, G. E. (1989). Teaching moderately mentally retarded children basic reading skills. *Research in Developmental Disabilities, 10*, 1–18.

Hooper, J., Connell, T. M., & Flett, P. J. (1987). Blissymbols and manual signs: A multimodal approach to intervention in a case of multiple disability. *Augmentative and Alternative Communication, 3*, 67–76.

Hooper, J., & Lloyd, L. L. (1986). An investigation of the effect of element explanation on the ability of preschool children to learn Blissymbols. Unpublished manuscript, Purdue University, West Lafayette, IN.

Hoover, J., Reichle, J., Van Tasell, D., & Cole, D. (1987). The intelligibility of synthesized speech: Echo II versus Votrax. *Journal of Speech and Hearing Research, 30*, 425–431.

Horak, F. B. (1991). Assumptions underlying motor control for neurologic rehabilitation. In M. J. Lister (Ed.), *Contemporary management of motor control problems: Proceedings of the II STEP conference* (pp. 11–27). Alexandria, VA: Foundation for Physical Therapy.

Horner, R. H. (1994). Functional assessment: Contributions and future directions. *Journal of Applied Behavior Analysis, 27*, 401–404.

Horner, R. H., & Budd, G. M. (1985). Acquisition of manual sign use: Collateral reduction of maladaptive behavior and factors limiting generalization. *Education and Training of the Mentally Retarded, 20*, 39–47.

Horner, R. H., & Day, H. M. (1991). The effects of response efficiency on functionally equivalent competing behaviors. *Journal of Applied Behavior Analysis, 24*, 719–732.

Horner, R. H., Sprague, J. R., O'Brien, M., & Heathfield, L. (1990). The role of response efficiency in the reduction of problem behaviors through functional equivalence training: A case study. *Journal of the Association for Persons with Severe Handicaps, 15*, 91–97.

Hornykiewicz, O., & Kish, S. J. (1986). Biochemical pathophysiology of Parkinson's disease. *Advances in Neurology, 45*, 84–107.

Horvat, M. (1987). Effects of a progressive resistance training program on an individual with spastic cerebral palsy. *American Corrective Therapy Journal, 41*, 7–11.

Huer, M. B. (1994, November). *Diversity now: Multicultural issues in AAC*. A miniseminar at the Annual Convention of the American Speech-Language-Hearing Association, New Orleans.

Huer, M. B., & Lloyd, L. L. (1988a). Parents' perspectives of AAC users. *Exceptional Parent, 18*(4), 32–33.

Huer, M. B., & Lloyd, L. L. (1988b). Perspectives of AAC users. *Communication Outlook, 9*(3), 10–18.

Huer, M. B., & Lloyd, L. L. (1990). AAC users' perspectives on augmentative and alternative communication. *Augmentative and Alternative Communication, 6*, 242–249.

Hughes, M. J. (1979). Sequencing of visual and auditory stimuli in teaching words and Blissymbols to the mentally retarded. *Australian Journal of Mental Retardation, 5*, 298–302.

Hughes-Wheatland, R. (1989). *Translucency, body contact and production complexity: Effects on the acquisition of American Sign Language signs by aphasic adults*. Unpublished doctoral dissertation, City University of New York, NY.

Hull, R. H. (Ed.). (1992). *Aural rehabilitation* (2nd ed.). San Diego: Singular Publishing Group.

Hulme, J. B., Poor, R., Schulein, M., & Pezzino, J. (1983). Perceived behavioral changes observed with adaptive seating devices and training programs for multihandicapped, developmentally disabled individuals. *Physical Therapy, 63*, 204–208.

Hundertmark, L. H. (1985). Evaluating the adult with cerebral palsy for specialized adaptive seating. *Physical Therapy*, *65*, 209–212.

Hunt, P., Alwell, M., & Goetz, L. (1988). Acquisition of conversational skills and the reduction of inappropriate social interaction behaviors. *Journal of the Association for Persons with Severe Handicaps*, *13*, 20–27.

Hunt, P., Alwell, M., & Goetz, L. (1991). Interacting with peers through conversation turntaking with a communication book adaptation. *Augmentative and Alternative Communication*, *7*, 117–126.

Hunt, P., Alwell, M., Goetz, L., & Sailor, W. (1990). Generalized effects of conversation skill training. *Journal of the Association for Persons with Severe Handicaps*, *15*, 250–260.

Huntress, L. M., Lee, L., Creaghead, N. A., Wheeler, D. D., & Braverman, K. M. (1990). Aphasic subjects' comprehension of synthetic and natural speech. *Journal of Speech and Hearing Disorders*, *55*, 21–27.

Hurlbut, B., Iwata, B., & Green, J. (1982). Nonvocal language acquisition in adolescents with severe physical disabilities: Blissymbol versus iconic stimulus formats. *Journal of Applied Behavior Analysis*, *15*, 241–258.

Hussey, I. (1991). Beginning AAC in Zimbabwe. *Communicating Together*, *9*, 19–20.

Hux, K., Rankin, D. R., Beukelman, D. R., & Hahn, D. (1993). Alternative procedure to evaluate semantic classification. *Augmentative and Alternative Communication*, *9*, 119–125.

Hymes, D. (1971). Competence and performance in linguistic theory. In R. Huxley & E. Ingram (Eds.), *Language acquisition: Models and methods* (pp. 3–28). London: Academic Press.

Iacono, T. (1992). Individual language learning styles and augmentative and alternative communication. *Augmentative and Alternative Communication*, *8*, 33–40.

Iacono, T., Mirenda, P., & Beukelman, D. (1993). Comparison of unimodal and multimodal AAC techniques for children with intellectual disabilities. *Augmentative and Alternative Communication*, *9*, 83–94.

Idol, L., Paolucci-Whitcomb, P., & Nevin, A. (1986). *Collaborative consultation*. Rockville, MD: Aspen Publishers.

Illinois Assistive Technology Project. (1991). *Basic skills in assistive technology handbook*. Springfield, IL: Author.

International Communication Learning Institute. (1986). *Introducing Visual Phonics* [Videotape]. Edina, MN: Author.

Irving Independent School District v. Tatro. 468 U.S.883, 104 S. Ct. 3371, 82 L.Ed.2nd 664 [18 Ed.Law Rep.[138]] (1984).

Itard, J. M. (1801). Mémoire sur les premier développements de Victor de l' Aveyron (1801). In L. Malson (Ed.), *Les enfants sauvages (1964)*. Paris: Union Générale d' Editions.

Iwata, B. A., Dorsey, M. F., Slifer, K. J., Bauman, K. E., & Richman, G. S. (1982). Toward a functional analysis of self-injury. *Analysis and Intervention in Developmental Disabilities*, *2*, 3–20.

Iwata, B. A., Vollmer, T. R., & Zarcone, J. R. (1990). The experimental (functional) analysis of behavior disorders: Methodology, applications, and limitations. In A. C. Repp & N. N. Singh (Eds.), *Perspectives on the use of nonaversive and aversive interventions for persons with developmental disabilities* (pp. 301–330). Sycamore, IL: Sycamore Publishing Company.

Jacobson, J. T., & Hyde, M. L. (1985). An introduction to auditory evoked potentials. In J. Katz (Ed.), *Handbook of clinical audiology* (3rd ed., pp. 496–533). Baltimore: Williams & Wilkins.

Jacobson, J. W., Sutton, M. S., & Janicki, M. P. (1985). Demography and characteristics of aging and aged mentally retarded persons. In M. P. Janicki and H. M. Wisniewski (Eds.), *Aging and developmental disabilities* (pp. 115–141). Baltimore: Paul H. Brookes Publishing.

Jaffe, K. M. (Ed.) (1987). Childhood powered mobility: Developmental, technical and clinical perspectives. In *Proceedings of the RESNA first northwest regional conference*. Washington, DC: RESNA.

James, W. C. (1963). Mentally retarded deaf children in a California state hospital. In *Report of the proceedings of the International Congress on Education of the Deaf and the 41st meeting of the Convention of American Instructors of the Deaf* (pp. 573–577). Washington, DC: U.S. Government Printing Office.

Jan, J. E., & Groenveld, M. (1993). Visual behaviors and adaptations associated with cortical and ocular impairments in children. *Journal of Visual Impairment & Blindness*, *87*, 101–105.

Jeffree, D. (1981). A bridge between pictures and print. *Special Education Forward Trends*, *8*, 28–31.

Jenkins, J. J. (1986). Cognitive development in children with recurrent otitis media: Where do we stand? In J. F. Kavanagh (Ed.), *Otitis media and child development* (pp. 211–221). Parkton, MD: York Press.

Jinks, A., & Sinteff, B. (1994). Consumer response to AAC devices: Acquisition, training, use, and satisfaction. *Augmentative and Alternative Communication*, *10*, 184–190.

Joffee, E., & Rikhye, C. H. (1991). Orientation and mobility for students with severe visual and multiple impairments: A new perspective. *Journal of Visual Impairment & Blindness*, *85*, 211–216.

Johannsen-Horbach, H., Cegla, B., Mager, U., Schempp, B., & Wallesch, C. W. (1985). Treatment of chronic global aphasia with a nonverbal communication system. *Brain and Language*, *24*, 74–82.

Johnson, L. J., Pugach, M. C., & Himmitte, D. J. (1988). Barriers to effective special education consultation. *Remedial and Special Education*, *9*(6), 41–47.

Johnson, R. (1981). *The Picture Communication Symbols*. Solana Beach, CA: Mayer-Johnson Co.

Johnson, R. (1985). *The Picture Communication Symbols—Book II*. Solana Beach, CA: Mayer-Johnson Co.

Johnson, R. (1992). *The Picture Communication Symbols—Book III*. Solana Beach, CA: Mayer-Johnson Co.

Johnson, R. E., Liddell, S. K., & Erting, C. J. (1989). *Unlocking the curriculum: Principles for achieving access in deaf education.* Washington, DC: Gallaudet University Press.

Johnston, S. S., & Reichle, J. (1993). Designing and implementing interventions to decrease challenging behavior. *Language, Speech, and Hearing Services in Schools, 24,* 225–235.

Johnston, T. (1991). Spatial syntax and spatial semantics in the inflection of signs for the marking of person and location in Auslan. *International Journal of Sign Linguistics, 2,* 29–62.

Joint Committee for Meeting the Communication Needs of Persons with Severe Disabilities. (1992). Guidelines for meeting the communication needs of persons with severe disabilities. *Asha, 34*(Suppl. 7), 1.

Jones, J. (1979). A rebus system of non-fade visual language. *Child Care, Health, and Development, 5,* 1–7.

Jones, K. R. (1972). Rebus materials in pre-school playgroups. In *Teachers' research groups journal.* Bristol, England: Research Unit, School of Education, University of Bristol.

Jones, K. R. (1976). The development of pre-reading procedures based upon the reading of Rebus materials. In A. Cashdan (Ed.), *The content of reading.* London: Ward Look Educational.

Jones, K. R., & Cregan, A. (1986). *Sign and symbol communication for mentally handicapped people.* London: Croom Helm.

Jones, M., Dayton, G., Bernstein, L., Strommen, E., Osborne, M., & Watanabe, K. (1966). Pilot study of reading problems in cerebral palsied adults. *Developmental Medicine and Child Neurology, 8,* 417–427.

Jones, S., Jolleff, N., McConachie, H., & Wisbeach, A. (1990). A model for assessment of children for augmentative communication systems. *Child Language Teaching and Therapy, 6*(3), 305–321.

Jones-Gotman, M. (1979). Incidental learning of image-mediated or pronounced words after right temporal lobectomy. *Cortex, 15,* 187–197.

Jones-Gotman, M. (1986). Memory for designs: The hippocampal contribution. *Neuropsychologia, 24,* 193–203.

Jones-Gotman, M., & Milner, B. (1978). Right temporal lobe contribution to image-mediated verbal learning. *Neuropsychologia, 16,* 61–71.

Jonker, V., & Heim, M. (1992, August). *A communication program for nonspeaking children and their partners.* Presentation at the Fifth Biennial Conference of the International Society for Augmentative and Alternative Communication, Philadelphia.

Jordan, E., Gustason, G., & Rosen, R. (1976). Current communication trends and programs for the deaf. *American Annals of the Deaf, 121,* 527–532.

Jorm A., & Share, D. (1983). Phonological recoding and reading acquisition. *Applied Psycholinguistics, 4,* 103–147.

Julnes, R. E., & Brown, S. E. (1993). Commentary: The legal mandate to provide assistive technology in special education programming. *Education Law Report, 82,* 737–748.

Kaiser, A. P. (1993). Functional language. In M. E. Snell (Ed.), *Instruction of students with severe disabilities* (4th ed., pp. 347–379). New York: Merrill Publishing Company.

Kaiser, A. P. (1994). Parent-implemented language intervention: An environmental system perspective. In A. P. Kaiser & D. B. Gray (Eds.), *Enhancing children's communication: Research foundation for intervention* (Vol. 2, pp. 63–84). Baltimore: Paul H. Brookes Publishing.

Kaiser, A. P., & Gray, D. B. (1994). *Enhancing children's communication: Research foundation for intervention* (Vol. 2). Baltimore: Paul H. Brookes Publishing.

Kalsbeek, W., McLauren, R., Harris, B., & Miller, J. (1981). The national head and spinal cord injury survey: Major findings. *Journal of Neurosurgery, 53,* 519–531.

Kangas, K. A., & Allen, G. D. (1990). Intelligibility of synthetic speech for normal-hearing and hearing-impaired listeners. *Journal of Speech and Hearing Disorders, 55,* 751–755.

Kangas, K. A., & Lloyd, L. L. (1985). Selection of specific unaided augmentative and alternative communication approaches. In D. E. Yoder & R. D. Kent (Eds.), *Decision making in speech-language pathology* (pp. 82–83). Toronto, Canada: B. C. Decker, Inc.

Kangas, K. A., & Lloyd, L. L. (1988). Early cognitive skills as prerequisites to augmentative and alternative communication use: What are we waiting for? *Augmentative and Alternative Communication, 4,* 211–221.

Kantor, R. (1980). The acquisition of classifiers in American Sign Language. *Sign Language Studies, 26,* 193–208.

Kaplan, H., Gladstone, V. S., & Lloyd, L. L. (1993). *Audiometric interpretation* (2nd ed.). Boston: Allyn & Bacon.

Karlan, G. R., & Lloyd, L. L. (1983). Considerations in the planning of communication intervention: Selecting a lexicon. *Journal of the Association for Persons with Severe Handicaps, 8,* 13–25.

Karp, A. (1983). Aural rehabilitation strategies for the visually and hearing impaired patient. *Journal of the Academy of Rehabilitative Audiology, 16,* 23–32.

Katayama, M., & Tamas, L. B. (1987). Saccadic eye-movements of children with cerebral palsy. *Developmental Medicine and Child Neurology, 29,* 36–39.

Kates, B., & McNaughton S. (1975). *The first application of Blissymbolics as a communication medium for nonspeaking children: History and development, 1971–1974.* Don Mills, Ontario: Easter Seals Communication Institute.

Kaufman, A. S., & Kaufman, N. L. (1983). *Kaufman assessment battery for children: Interpretive manual.* Circle Pines, MN: American Guidance Service.

Kearney, C. A. (1994). Interrater reliability of the Motivation Assessment Scale: Another closer look. *Journal of the Association for Persons with Severe Handicaps, 2,* 139–142.

Keenan, J. E., & Barnhart, K. S. (1993). Development of yes/no systems in individuals with severe traumatic brain injuries. *Augmentative and Alternative Communication,* *9,* 184–190.

Kekelis, L., & Anderson, E. (1984). Family communication styles and language development. *Journal of Visual Impairment & Blindness, 78,* 54–65.

Kelford-Smith, A., Thurston, S., Light, J., Parnes, P., & O'Keefe, B. (1989). The form and use of written communication produced by physically disabled individuals using microcomputers. *Augmentative and Alternative Communication, 5,* 115–124.

Kelley, P., Davidson, R., & Sanspree, M. J. (1993). Vision and orientation and mobility consultation for children with severe multiple disabilities. *Journal of Visual Impairment & Blindness, 87,* 7–9.

Kelsch, J. E. (1979). *Amer-Ind recognition in patients with aphasia.* Unpublished master's thesis, Purdue University, West Lafayette, IN.

Kent, R. D. (1994). *Reference manual for communicative sciences and disorders.* Austin, TX: Pro-Ed.

Kertesz, A. (1982). *Western aphasia battery.* New York: Grune & Stratton.

Kiernan, C. C., & Jones, M. (1985). The heuristic programme: A combined use of sign and symbols with severely mentally retarded autistic children. *Australian Journal of Human Communication, 13,* 153–168.

Kiernan, C. C., Reid, B., & Jones, L. (1982). *Signs and symbols: A review of literature and survey of the use of nonvocal communication.* London: Heinemann Educational Books.

Kimble, S. L. (1975, November). *A language teaching technique with totally nonverbal, severely mentally retarded adolescents.* Paper presented at the 50th Annual Convention of the American Speech and Hearing Association, Washington, DC.

Kimura, D. (1990). How special is language? *Sign Language Studies, 66,* 79–84.

King, C. M., & Quigley, S. P. (1985). *Reading and deafness.* San Diego, CA: College-Hill Press.

King-DeBaun, P. (1990). *Storytime: Stories, symbols and emergent literacy activities for young, special needs children.* Acworth, GA: Author.

Kinkoph, S., Fulton, J., & Oliver, K. (1994). *Computers: A visual encyclopedia.* Indianapolis, IN: Alpha Books.

Kinney, P., Oullette, T., & Wolery, M. (1989). Screening and assessing sensory functioning. In D. B. Bailey and M. Wolery (Eds.), *Assessing infants and preschoolers with handicaps* (pp. 144–164). Columbus, OH: Merrill Publishing Company.

Kirstein, I. (1981). *Oakland picture dictionary.* Wauconda, IL: Don Johnston Incorporated.

Kirstein, I., & Bernstein, C. (1981). *Oakland schools picture dictionary.* Pontiac, MI: Oakland Schools Communication Enhancement Center.

Kladde, A. G. (1974). Nonoral communication techniques: Project summary No. 1, 1967. In B. Vicker (Ed.), *Nonoral communication system project 1964/1973* (pp. 57–104). Iowa City, IA: University of Iowa Campus Stores.

Kleinmuntz, D. N., & Schkade, D. A. (1993). Information displays and decision processes. *Psychological Science, 4,* 221–227.

Klima, R., & Bellugi, U. (1979). *The signs of language.* Cambridge, MA: Harvard University Press.

Klin, A. (1993). Auditory brainstem responses in autism: Brainstem dysfunction or peripheral hearing loss? *Journal of Autism and Developmental Disorders, 23,* 15–35.

Koegel, R. L., & Koegel, L. K. (1989). Community-referenced research on self-stimulation. In E. Cipani (Ed.), *The treatment of severe behavior disorders* (pp. 129–150). Washington, DC: AAMR Monographs.

Koehler, L., Lloyd, L., & Swanson, L. (1992). Metalinguistic features of manual communication that facilitate literacy. *Augmentative and Alternative Communication, 8,* 144. (Abstract)

Koehler, L., Lloyd, L., & Swanson, L. (1994). Visual similarity between manual and printed alphabet letters. *Augmentative and Alternative Communication, 10,* 87–94.

Koenen, L. (1993). Interview with Susan Fischer about nuances in sign language. *NRC Handelsblad,* p. 3.

Koenen, L., Bloem, T., & Janssen, R. (1993). *Gebarentaal: De Taal van doven in Nederland. (Sign language: The language of deaf people in the Netherlands).* Amsterdam: Nijgh & van Ditmar.

Koester, H. H., & Levine, S. P. (1994). Learning and performance of able-bodied individuals using scanning systems with and without word prediction. *Assistive Technology, 6,* 42–53.

Kohl, F. L. (1981). The effects of motor requirements on the acquisition of manual sign responses by severely handicapped students. *American Journal of Mental Deficiency, 85,* 396–403.

Koke, S., & Neilson, J. (1987). *The effects of auditory feedback on the spelling of nonspeaking physically disabled individuals.* Unpublished master's thesis, University of Toronto.

Konstantareas, M. M., Oxman, J., & Webster, C. D. (1978). Iconicity: Effects on the acquisition of sign language by autistic and other severely dysfunctional children. In P. Siple (Ed.), *Understanding language through sign language research* (pp. 213–237). New York: Academic Press.

Konstantareas, M., Oxman, J., Webster, C., Fischer, H., & Miller, K. (1975). *A five-week simultaneous communication programme for severely dysfunctional children: Outcomes and implications for future research.* Toronto: Clarke Institute of Psychiatry.

Kopchick, G., & Lloyd, L. L. (1976). Total communication programming for the severely language impaired: A 24-hour approach. In L. L. Lloyd (Ed.), *Communication assessment and intervention strategies* (pp. 501–521). Baltimore: University Park Press.

Koppenhaver, D. A. (1991). *A descriptive analysis of classroom literacy instruction provided to children with severe speech and physical impairments.* Unpublished doctoral dissertation, University of North Carolina, Chapel Hill, NC.

Koppenhaver, D. A. (1992, March). *Literacy issues related to AAC intervention.* Invited paper submitted as written testimony to the National Institute on Disability and Rehabilitation Research Concensus Validation Conference on Augmentative and Alternative Communication, Arlington, VA.

Koppenhaver, D. A., Coleman, P. P., Kalman, S. L., & Yoder, D. E. (1991). The implications of emergent literacy research for children with developmental disabilities. *American Journal of Speech-Language Pathology, 1*(1), 38–44.

Koppenhaver, D. A., Evans, D., & Yoder, D. E. (1991). Childhood reading and writing experiences of literate adults with severe speech and motor impairments. *Augmentative and Alternative Communication, 7,* 20–33.

Koppenhaver, D. A., Pierce, P. L., Steelman, J. D., & Yoder, D. E. (1994). Contexts of early literacy intervention for children with developmental disabilities. In M. E. Fey, J. Windsor, & S. F. Warren (Eds.), *Language intervention in the early school years* (pp. 241–274). Baltimore: Paul H. Brookes Publishing.

Koppenhaver, D. A., & Yoder, D. E. (1992a). Literacy issues in persons with severe speech and physical impairments. In R. Gaylord-Ross (Ed.), *Issues and research in special education* (Vol 2., pp. 156–201). New York: Teachers College Press.

Koppenhaver, D. A., & Yoder, D. E. (1992b). Literacy learning of children with severe speech and physical impairments in school settings. *Seminars in Speech and Language, 12,* 143–153.

Koppenhaver, D. A., & Yoder, D. E. (1993). Classroom literacy instruction for children with severe speech and physical impairments (SSPI): What is and what might be. *Topics in Language Disorders, 13*(2), 1–15.

Koul, R. (1994). *The effects of graphic symbol iconicity and complexity on the acquisition of Blissymbols by individuals with aphasia and individuals with right hemisphere brain damage.* Unpublished doctoral dissertation, Purdue University, West Lafayette, IN.

Koul, R. K., & Allen, G. D. (1993). Intelligibility and speech interference thresholds of high quality speech synthesizers in the presence of interfering speech. *Journal of Speech and Hearing Research, 36,* 790–798.

Koul, R. K., & Cooper, R. (in press). Identification and production of graphic symbols by individuals with aphasia: Efficacy of a software application. *Augmentative and Alternative Communication.*

Koul, R. K., & Lloyd, L. L. (1994a). Acquisition of graphic symbols by individuals with aphasia. *Asha, 36,* 142. (Abstract)

Koul, R. K., & Lloyd, L. L. (1994b). Survey of professional preparation in augmentative and alternative communication in speech-language pathology and special education programs. *American Journal of Speech-Language Pathology, 3*(3), 13–22.

Koul, R., & Lloyd, L. L. (in press). Comparison of graphic symbol learning in individuals with aphasia and right hemisphere brain damage. *Brain and Language.*

Kozleski, E. B. (1991). Expectant delay procedure for teaching requests. *Augmentative and Alternative Communication, 7,* 11–19.

Kraat, A. (1985). *Communication interaction between aided and natural speakers: A state of the art report.* Toronto, Canada: Canadian Rehabilitation Council for the Disabled.

Kraat, A. (1986). Developing intervention goals. In S. W. Blackstone (Ed.), *Augmentative communication: An introduction* (pp. 197–266). Rockville, MD: American Speech-Language-Hearing Association.

Kraat, A. (1990). Augmentative and alternative communication: Does it have a future in aphasia rehabilitation? *Aphasiology, 4,* 321–338.

Kraat, A. (1993). ISAAC's voices grow louder and stronger. *The ISAAC Bulletin, 29,* 10–11.

Kraat, A., & Sitver-Kogut, M. (1991). *Features of portable communication devices.* Wilmington, DE: E. I. du Pont Institute, Applied Science and Engineering Laboratory, University of Delaware.

Kramer, L. C., Sullivan, R. F., & Hirsch, L. M. (1979). *Audiologic evaluation and aural rehabilitation of the deaf-blind adult.* Sands Point, NY: Helen Keller National Center for Deaf-Blind Youths and Adults.

Kuntz, J. B. (1975). A nonvocal communication program for severely retarded children. (Doctoral dissertation, Kansas State University, 1974). *Dissertation Abstracts International, 36,* 219A.

Kyle, J. G., & Woll, B. (1985). *Sign language: The study of deaf people and their language.* Cambridge, MA: Cambridge University Press.

Kynette, D., & Kemper, S. (1986). Aging and the loss of grammatical forms: A cross-sectional study of language performance. *Language and Communication, 6,* 65–72.

Ladtkow, M., & Culp, D. (1992). Augmentative communication with traumatic brain injury. In K. Yorkston (Ed.), *Augmentative communication in the medical setting* (pp. 139–244). Tucson, AZ: Communication Skill Builders.

Lafontaine, L. M., & DeRuyter, F. (1987). The nonspeaking cerebral-palsied: A clinical and demographic database report. *Augmentative and Alternative Communication, 3,* 153–162.

Lahey, M. (1988). *Language disorders and language development.* New York: Macmillan Publishing Company.

Lahey, M., & Bloom, L. (1977). Planning a first lexicon: Which words to teach first. *Journal of Speech and Hearing Disorders, 42,* 340–350.

Lahm, E., & Elting, S. (1989). Technology: Becoming an informed consumer. *NICHCY News Digest, 13,* 1–3, 12–13.

Lalli, J. S., & Browder, D. M. (1993). Comparison of sight word training procedures with validation of the most practical procedure in teaching reading for daily living. *Research in Developmental Disabilities, 14,* 107–127.

Lalli, J. S., Casey, S., & Kates, K. (1995). Reducing escape behavior and increasing task completion with functional communication training, extinction, and response chaining. *Journal of Applied Behavior Analysis, 28,* 261–268.

Lalli, J. S., & Goh, H.-L. (1993). Naturalistic observations in community settings. In J. Reichle & D. P. Wacker (Eds.), *Communicative alternatives to challenging behavior: Integrating functional assessment and intervention strategies* (pp. 11–40). Baltimore: Paul H. Brookes Publishing.

Landesman-Dwyer, S., & Sackett, G. P. (1978). Behavioral changes in nonambulatory, profoundly mentally retarded individuals. In C. E. Meyers (Ed.), *Quality of life in severely and profoundly mentally retarded people: Research foundations for improvement* (pp. 55–144). Washington, DC: American Association on Mental Deficiency.

Landman, C., & Schaeffler, C. (1986). Object communication boards. *Communication Outlook, 8,* 7–8.

Lane, H. (1984). *When the mind hears: A history of the deaf.* New York: Random House.

Lane, V. W., & Samples, J. M. (1981). Facilitating communication skills in adult aphasics: Application of Blissymbolics in a group setting. *Journal of Communication Disorders, 14,* 157–167.

Langdon, H. W., & Cheng, L. L. (1992). *Hispanic children and adults with communication disorders: Assessment and intervention.* Gaithersburg, MD: Aspen.

Langley, M. B. (1989). Assessing infant cognitive development. In D. B. Bailey & M. Wolery (Eds.), *Assessing infants and preschoolers with handicaps* (pp. 249–274). Columbus, OH: Merrill Publishing Company.

LaPointe, L. L. (1994). Neurogenic disorders of communication. In F. D. Minifie (Ed.), *Introduction to communication sciences and disorders* (pp. 351–397). San Diego, CA: Singular Publishing Group.

Laraway, L. A. (1985). Auditory selective attention in cerebralpalsied individuals. *Language, Speech, and Hearing Services in Schools, 16,* 260–265.

Larin, H. M. (1994). Motor learning: Theories and strategies for the practitioner. In S. K. Campbell (Ed.), *Physical therapy for children* (pp. 157–181). Philadelphia: W. B. Saunders.

Larson, V. L., & McKinley, N. L. (1987). *Communication assessment and intervention strategies for adolescents.* Eau Claire, WI: Thinking Publications.

Lasker, J. (1980). *Nick joins in.* Chicago: Albert Whitman & Company.

Lawrence, M., Lovie-Kitchin, J., & Brohier, W. G. (1992). Low vision: A working paper for the World Health Organization. *Journal of Visual Impairment & Blindness, 86,* 7–9.

Lazzaro, J. J. (1993). *Adaptive technologies for learning and work environments.* Chicago: American Library Association.

Lee, K., & Thomas, D. (1990). *Control of computer-based technology for people with physical disabilities: An assessment manual.* Toronto: University of Toronto Press.

Lees, A. J. (1985). Parkinson's disease and dementia. *Lancet, 1,* 43–44.

Lehr, E. (1990). *Psychological management of traumatic brain injuries in children.* Rockville, MD: Aspen Publishers.

Leibeis, S., & Leibeis, R. F. (1975). The use of signed communication with the normal-hearing, nonverbal mentally retarded. *Bureau Memorandum* (Wisconsin Department of Public Instruction), *17*(1), 28–30.

Leiter, R. G. (1959). *Leiter adult intelligence scale.* Chicago: Stoelting Company.

Lennox, D. B., & Miltenberger, R. G. (1989). Conducting a functional assessment of problem behavior in applied settings. *Journal of the Association for Persons with Severe Handicaps, 14,* 304–311.

Leonhart, W., & Maharaj, S. (1979). A comparison of initial recognition and rate of acquisition of Pictogram Ideogram Communication (PIC) and Bliss symbols with institutionalized severely retarded adults. Unpublished manuscript.

Leshin, G. J. (1961). The slow-learning deaf child. In *Report of the proceedings of the 40th meeting of the Convention of the American Instructors of the Deaf* (pp. 197–203). Washington, DC: U.S. Government Printing Office.

Letter to Anonymous. 18 IDELR 627 (OSEP, 1991).

Letter to Anonymous. 18 IDELR 1037 (OSEP, 1992).

Letter to Anonymous. 21 IDELR 745 (OSEP, 1994).

Letter to Anonymous. 21 IDELR 1057 (OSEP, 1994).

Letter to Cohen. 19 IDELR 278 (OSEP, 1992).

Letter to Goodman. 16 EHLR 1317 (OSEP, 1990).

Letter to Lambert. 18 IDELR 1039 (OSEP, 1991).

Letter to Moore. 20 IDELR 1213 (OSEP, 1993).

Letter to Seiler. 20 IDELR 1216 (OSEP, 1993).

Levelt, W. J. (1993). *Speaking: From intention to articulation.* Cambridge, MA: MIT Press.

Levelt, W. J. (1994, October). What can a theory of normal speaking contribute to AAC? In *Proceedings of the 6th biennial conference of the International Society for Augmentative and Alternative Communication.* Maastricht, The Netherlands: ISAAC.

Levett, L. M. (1971). A method of communication for nonspeaking severely sub-normal children: Trial results. *British Journal of Disorders of Communication, 6,* 125–128.

Levine, S. P., Gauger, J. R. D., Bowers, L. D., & Khan, K. J. (1986). A comparison of mouthstick and Morse code text inputs. *Augmentative and Alternative Communication, 2,* 51–55.

Levinson, R. (Ed.). (1967). *A Plato reader.* Boston: Houghton-Mifflin.

Liberman, I. Y., & Liberman, A. M. (1990). Whole language vs. code emphasis: Underlying assumptions and their implications for reading instruction. *Annals of Dyslexia, 40,* 51–76.

Liberoff, M. (1992). *Comunicación augmentativa. PCP programa de comunicación pictográfico.* Buenos Aires: Marymar.

Licklider, J. C. R., & Miller, G. A. (1951). The perception of speech. In S. S. Stevens (Ed.), *Handbook of experimental psychology* (pp. 1040–1074). New York: Wiley.

Liddell, S. (1980). *American Sign Language syntax.* The Hague, The Netherlands: Mouton.

Liebman, M., & Tadmor, R. (1991). *Neuroanatomy made easy and understandable* (4th ed.). Rockville, MD: Aspen Publishers.

Lieven, E. V. M., Pine, J. M., & Barnes, H. D. (1992). Individual differences in early vocabulary development: Redefining the referential-expressive distinction. *Journal of Child Language, 19,* 287–310.

Light, J. (1988). Interaction involving individuals using augmentative and alternative communication systems: State of the art and future directions. *Augmentative and Alternative Communication, 4,* 66–82.

Light, J. (1989). Toward a definition of communicative competence for individuals using augmentative and alternative communication systems. *Augmentative and Alternative Communication, 5,* 137–144.

Light, J., Beesly, M., & Collier, B. (1988). Transition through multiple augmentative and alternative communication systems: A three-year case study of a head injured adolescent. *Augmentative and Alternative Communication, 4,* 2–14.

Light, J., Collier, B., & Parnes, P. (1985a). Communicative interaction between young nonspeaking physically disabled children and their primary caregivers: Part I—Discourse patterns. *Augmentative and Alternative Communication, 1,* 74–83.

Light, J., Collier, B., & Parnes, P. (1985b). Communicative interaction between young nonspeaking physically disabled children and their primary caregivers: Part II—Communicative function. *Augmentative and Alternative Communication, 1,* 98–107.

Light, J., & Kelford-Smith, A. (1993). Home literacy experiences of preschoolers who use AAC systems and of their nondisabled peers. *Augmentative and Alternative Communication, 9,* 10–25.

Light, J., & Lindsay, P. (1991). Cognitive science and augmentative and alternative communication. *Augmentative and Alternative Communication, 7,* 186–203.

Light, J., Lindsay, P., Siegel, L., & Parnes, P. (1990). The effects of message encoding techniques on recall by literate adults using AAC systems. *Augmentative and Alternative Communication, 6,* 184–201.

Light, J., & McNaughton, D. (1993). Literacy and augmentative and alternative communication (AAC): The expectations and priorities of parents and teachers. *Topics in Language Disorders, 13*(2), 33–46.

Lindsey, J. D. (1987). *Computers and exceptional individuals.* Columbus, OH: Merrill Publishing Company.

Lindsey, J. D. (1993). *Computers and exceptional individuals.* Austin, TX: Pro-Ed.

Ling, D. (1984). Early total communication intervention: An introduction. In D. Ling (Ed.), *Early intervention for hear-ing-impaired children: Total communication options.* San Diego, CA: College-Hill Press.

Linville, S. E. (1977). Signed English: A language teaching technique with totally nonverbal severely mentally retarded adolescents. *Language, Speech and Hearing Services in Schools, 8,* 170–175.

Livingston, S. (1983). Levels of development in the language of deaf children: ASL grammatical processes, SE structures, and semantic features. *Sign Language Studies, 40,* 193–286.

Llewellyn-Jones, M. (1983). Signed reading project: Computer programme. Unpublished report, Arnold Derrymount School, Nottingham, England.

Llewellyn-Jones, M. (1984). Computer program: HANDS. Unpublished progress report, Arnold Derrymount School, Nottingham, England.

Lloyd, L. L. (1980). Unaided nonspeech communication for severely handicapped individuals: An extensive bibliography. *Education and Training of the Mentally Retarded, 15,* 15–34.

Lloyd, L. L. (1986). Editorial. *Augmentative and Alternative Communication, 2,* 67–68.

Lloyd, L. L. (1989). Editorial. *Augmentative and Alternative Communication, 5,* 83.

Lloyd, L. L. (1993). Editorial. *Augmentative and Alternative Communication, 9,* 227–228.

Lloyd, L. L., & Belfiore, P. J. (1994). The academic infrastructure needed to encourage scholarship on employment for the AAC community. In R. V. Conti & C. Jenkins-Odorisio (Eds.), *Proceedings of the 2nd annual Pittsburgh employment conference for augmented communicators* (pp. 109–118). Pittsburgh, PA: SHOUT Press.

Lloyd, L. L., & Blischak, D. M. (1989). AAC from A to Z. Unpublished manuscript, Purdue University, West Lafayette, IN.

Lloyd, L. L., & Blischak, D. M. (1992). AAC terminology policy and issues update. *Augmentative and Alternative Communication, 8,* 104–109.

Lloyd, L. L., & Cox, B. P. (1972). Programming for the audiologic aspects of mental retardation. *Mental Retardation, 10*(2), 22–26.

Lloyd, L. L., & Daniloff, J. K. (1983). Issues in using Amer-Ind code with retarded persons. In T. Gallagher & C. Prutting (Eds.), *Pragmatic issues: Assessment and intervention.* Houston, TX: College-Hill Press.

Lloyd, L. L., & Doherty, J. (1983). The influence of production mode on recall of signs in normal adult subjects. *Journal of Speech and Hearing Research, 26,* 595–600.

Lloyd, L. L., & Fuller, D. R. (1986). Toward an augmentative and alternative communication symbol taxonomy: A proposed superordinate classification. *Augmentative and Alternative Communication, 2,* 165–171.

Lloyd, L. L., & Fuller, D. R. (1990). The role of iconicity in augmentative and alternative communication symbol learning. In W. I. Fraser (Ed.), *Key issues in mental retardation research* (pp. 295–306). London: Routledge.

Lloyd, L. L., & Kangas, K. A. (1988). Unaided augmentative and alternative communication: General considerations. In D. E. Yoder & R. D. Kent (Eds.), *Decision making in speech-language pathology* (pp. 78–81). Toronto: B. C. Decker.

Lloyd, L. L., & Kangas, K. A. (1994). Augmentative and alternative communication. In G. H. Shames, E. H. Wiig, & W. A. Secord (Eds.), *Human communication disorders* (4th ed.) (pp. 606–657). New York: Merrill/Macmillan Publishing.

Lloyd, L. L., & Karlan, G. R. (1983, August). Nonspeech communication symbol selection considerations. *Proceedings of the XIX congress of the International Association of Logopaedics and Phoniatrics* (Vol. III, pp. 1155–1160). Edinburgh, Scotland: University of Edinburgh.

Lloyd, L. L., & Karlan, G. R. (1984). Nonspeech communication symbols and systems: Where have we been and where are we going? *Journal of Mental Deficiency Research, 28,* 3–20.

Lloyd, L. L., & Kiernan, C. (1984, June). Graphic symbols: An overview. *Proceedings of the second international conference on rehabilitation engineering (ICRE-II): Special sessions* (pp. 34–37). (Combined with the 7th Annual RESNA Conference), Ottawa, Canada.

Lloyd, L. L., Quist, R. W., & Windsor, J. (1990). A proposed augmentative and alternative communication model. *Augmentative and Alternative Communication, 6,* 172–183.

Lloyd, L. L., Romski, M. A., Beukelman, D. R., & Higginbotham, D. J. (1993, November). *Research issues in augmentative and alternative communication.* Special research symposium presented at the Conference of the American Speech-Language-Hearing Association, Anaheim, CA.

Lloyd, L. L., & Soto, G. (1994). Augmentative and alternative communication. In T. Husen & T. N. Poslethwaite (Eds.), *The international encyclopedia of education* (2nd ed). New York: Pergamon Press.

Lloyd, L. L., Spradlin, J., & Reid, M. (1968). An operant audiometric procedure for difficult-to-test patients. *Journal of Speech and Hearing Disorders, 33,* 236–245.

Locke, P. A., & Mirenda, P. (1988). A computer-supported communication approach for a nonspeaking child with severe visual and cognitive impairments: A case study. *Augmentative and Alternative Communication, 4,* 15–22.

Locke, P. A., & Mirenda, P. (1992). Roles and responsibilities of special education teachers serving on teams delivering AAC services. *Augmentative and Alternative Communication, 8,* 200–214.

Loeding, B. L., Zangari, C., & Lloyd, L. L. (1990). A "working party" approach to planning in-service training in manual signs for an entire public school staff. *Augmentative and Alternative Communication, 6,* 38–49.

Logan, J. S., Greene, B. G., & Pisoni, D. B. (1989). Segmental intelligibility of synthetic speech produced by rule. *Journal of the Acoustical Society of America, 86,* 566–581.

Logemann, J. A., Fisher, H. B., Boshes, B., & Blonsky, E. R. (1978). Frequency and co-occurrence of vocal tract dysfunctions in the speech of a large sample of Parkinson's patients. *Journal of Speech and Hearing Disorders, 43,* 47–57.

Loncke, F. (1990). *Modaliteitsinvloed op taalstructuur en taalverwerving in gebarencommunicatie (Modality influence on language structure and language acquisition in sign communication).* Unpublished doctoral dissertation, University of Brussels, Brussels, Belgium.

Loncke, F., Boyes-Braem, P., & Lebrun, Y. (Eds.). (1984). *Recent research on European sign languages.* Lisse: Swets & Zeitlinger.

Loncke, F., De Vos, C., Lyssens, H., Nijs, M., Smet, L., Sagaert, S., & Verpoest, G. (1993). Handen reiken: het gebruik van SMOG in Vlaanderen. (Reaching hands: The use of the SMOG sign communication system in Flanders.) *Communicatie Drieluik, 5*(4), 2–7.

Loncke, F., Feron, A., & Quertinmont, S. (1992, October). *Les effets d' un système de support phonémique manuel.* Paper presented at the International Conference on Audiophonology, Besançon, France.

Loncke, F., Vander Beken, K., & Lloyd, L. L. (1997). Toward a theoretical model of symbol processing and use. In E. Bjorck-Akesson & P. Lindsay (Eds.), *Theoretical and methodological issues in augmentative and alternative communication: Proceedings of the fourth ISAAC Research Symposium, Vancouver, Canada, August 11–12, 1996.* Vasteras, Sweden: Malardalen University Press.

Lorrett, L. (1969). A method of communication for non-speaking severely subnormal children. *British Journal of Disorders of Communication, 4,* 64–66.

Lovaas, I., Calori, L., & Jada, J. (1989). The nature of behavioral treatment and research with a young autistic person. In C. Gillberg (Ed.), *Diagnosis and treatment of autism* (pp. 285–305). New York: Plenum Press.

Lovaas, I., Newsom, C., & Hickman, C. (1987). Self-stimulatory behavior and perceptual reinforcement. *Journal of Applied Behavior Analysis, 20,* 45–68.

Love, R. J., & Webb, W. G. (1992). *Neurology for the speech-language pathologist* (2nd ed.). Boston: Butterworth-Heinemann.

Lucas, C. (Ed.). (1990). *Sign language research: Theoretical issues.* Washington, DC: Gallaudet University Press.

Luftig, R. L., & Bersani, H. A., Jr. (1985). An investigation of two variables influencing Blissymbol learnability with non handicapped adults. *Augmentative and Alternative Communication, 1,* 32–37.

Luftig, R. L., & Lloyd, L. L. (1981). Manual sign translucency and referential concreteness in the learning of signs. *Sign Language Studies, 30,* 49–60.

Lundberg, I., Frost, J., & Petersen O. (1988). Effects of an extensive program for stimulating phonological awareness in preschool children. *Reading Research Quarterly, 23*(3), 263–284.

Lundberg, I., Olofsson A., & Wall, S. (1980). Reading and spelling skills in the first school years predicted from phonemic awareness skills in kindergarten. *Scandinavian Journal of Psychology, 21,* 159–173.

Lundman, M. (1978). *Technical aids for the speech-impaired: An international survey on research and development projects.* Stockholm: The Swedish Institute for the Handicapped.

Lynch, E. W. (1992). From culture shock to cultural learning. In E. W. Lynch & M. Hanson (Eds.), *Developing cross-cultural competence: A guide for working with young children and their families* (Chap. 2, pp. 19–59). Baltimore: Paul H. Brookes Publishing.

Lynch, E. W., & Hanson, M. (1992). *Developing cross-cultural competence: A guide for working with young children and their families.* Baltimore: Paul H. Brookes Publishing.

Lynch, M. (1990). Tactile speech indicator: Adaptive telephone device for deaf-blind clients. *Journal of Visual Impairment & Blindness, 84,* 21–22.

Lyon, S., & Lyon, G. (1980). Team functioning and staff development: A role release approach to providing integrated educational services for severely handicapped students. *Journal of the Association for the Severely Handicapped, 5,* 250–263.

Lytton, R. (1994). Augmentative communication as a medical necessity. *Augmentative and Alternative Communication: Newsletter of Special Interest Division 12, 3*(1), 6–8.

Lytton, R. (1995). USSAAC adopts code of ethics for AAC service providers. *USSAAC Newsletter, 7*(1), 10.

MacDonald, J. E. (1978). *Environmental language inventory program.* Columbus, OH: Merrill Publishing Company.

Mace, F. C., Lalli, J. S., & Shea, M. C. (1992). Functional analysis of self-injury. In J. Luiselli, J. Matson, & N. Singh (Eds.), *Assessment, analysis, and treatment of self-injury* (pp. 122–152). New York: Springer-Verlag.

Mace, F. C., & Roberts, M. L. (1993). Factors affecting selection of behavioral interventions. In J. Reichle & D. P. Wacker (Eds.), *Communicative alternatives to challenging behavior: Integrating functional assessment and intervention strategies* (pp. 113–133). Baltimore: Paul H. Brookes Publishing.

Macht, J. (1971). Operant measurement of subjective visual acuity in nonverbal children. *Journal of Applied Behavior Analysis, 4,* 23–36.

MacNeela, J. C. (1987a). An overview of therapeutic positioning for multiply-handicapped persons, including augmentative communication users. In S. M. Attermeier (Ed.), *Augmentative communication: Clinical issues* (pp. 39–60). New York: Haworth Press.

MacNeela, J. C. (1987b). An overview of therapeutic positioning for multiply-handicapped persons, including augmentative communication users. *Physical and Occupational Therapy in Pediatrics, 7,* 39–60.

Maeder, C. (1994). *Espace, temps et relations temporologiques chez le sujet sourd (Spatial, temporal, and temperological notions in deaf subjects).* Unpublished doctoral dissertation, University of Nancy II, France.

Maeder, C., & Loncke, F. (1996). Spatial, temporal and temperological notions in French Sign Language: Comparative study of deaf and hearing subjects. *Sign Language Studies, 90,* 38–51.

Magnússon, J. (1990). Experience with the ISBLISS symbolic processing system as a written communication aid. *Augmentative and Alternative Communication, 6,* 129.

Maharaj, S. C. (1980). *Pictogram ideogram communication.* Saskatoon, Saskatchewan: The Pictogram Centre, Saskatchewan Association of Rehabilitation Centres.

Mailing, R. G., & Clarkson, D. C. (1963). Electronic controls for the tetraplegic (POSSUM). *Paraplegia, 1,* 162–174.

Mallery-Ruganis, D., & Fischer, S. (1991). Characteristics that contribute to effective simultaneous communication. *American Annals of the Deaf, 136*(3), 401–408.

Mallory, B. L., Nichols, R. W., Charlton, J., & Marfo, K. (1993). *Traditional and changing views of disability in developing countries: Causes, consequences, cautions.* University of New Hampshire: IEEIR.

Malone, J. (1962). The larger aspects of spelling reform. *Elementary English, 39,* 435–445.

Mandel, M. (1977). Iconic devices in American Sign Language. In L. Friedman (Ed.), *On the other hand: New perspectives in American Sign Language* (pp. 57–108). New York: Academic Press.

Mangan, K. (1963). A state program of services for the mentally retarded deaf child. In *Report of the proceedings of the international congress on education of the deaf and the 41st meeting of the Convention of American Instructors of the Deaf* (pp. 565–568). Washington, DC: U.S. Government Printing Office.

Mann, W. C., Hurren, D., Karuza, K., & Bentley, D. W. (1993). Needs of home-based older visually impaired persons for assistive devices. *Journal of Visual Impairment & Blindness, 87,* 106–110.

Marko, K. (1967). Symbol accentuation: Applications to classroom instruction of retardates. *Proceedings of the first congress of the International Association for the Scientific Study of Mental Deficiency* (pp. 773–775). IASSMD.

Markowicz, A., & Reeb, Jr., K. G. (1988). *An overview of Medicaid reimbursement for rehabilitation equipment in the United States.* Washington, DC: Rehabilitation Engineering Center.

Marmor, G., and Petitto, L. (1979). Simultaneous communication in the classroom: How well is English represented? *Sign Language Studies, 23,* 99–136.

Marshall, P. (1990). Augmentative communication: The call of one's life. *Communicating Together, 8*(2), 5–6.

Marvin, C. A., Beukelman, D. R., & Bilyeu, D. (1994). Vocabulary-use patterns in preschool children: Effects of context and time sampling. *Augmentative and Alternative Communication, 10,* 224–236.

Matas, J., Mathy-Laikko, P., Beukelman, D. R., & Legresley, K. (1985). Identifying the nonspeaking population: A demographic study. *Augmentative and Alternative Communication, 1,* 17–31.

Matey, C., & Kretschmer, R. (1985). A comparison of mother speech to Down's syndrome, hearing impaired, and normal hearing children. *Volta Review, 87*(4), 205–214.

Mathews, M. (1966). *Teaching to read, historically considered.* Chicago: University of Chicago Press.

Mathy-Laikko, P., Iacono, T., Ratcliff, A., Villarruel, F., Yoder, D., & Vanderheiden, G. (1989). Teaching a child with multiple disabilities to use a tactile augmentative communication device. *Augmentative and Alternative Communication, 5,* 249–256.

Mathy-Laikko, P., Ratcliff, A. E., Villarruel, F., & Yoder, D. E. (1988). Augmentative communication systems. In M. Bullis & G. Fielding (Eds.), *Communication development in young children with deaf-blindness: Literature review* (pp. 205–241). Monmouth, OR: Communication Skills Center for Young Children with Deaf-Blindness.

Maxwell, M., Bernstein, M. E., & Mear, K. M. (1991). Bimodal language production. In P. Siple & S. Fischer (Eds.), *Theoretical issues in sign language research. Vol 2: Psychology* (pp. 171–190). Chicago: University of Chicago Press.

Mayberry, R. (1976). If a chimp can learn sign language, surely my nonverbal client can, too. *Asha, 18,* 223–228.

Maynard School District. 20 IDELR 394 (Ark.SEA, 1993).

McCarthy, D. (1972). *Manual for the McCarthy scales of children's abilities.* New York: The Psychological Corporation.

McCaughrin, W. B., Ellis, W. K., Rusch, F. R., & Heal, L. W. (1993). Cost-effectiveness of supported employment. *Mental Retardation, 31,* 41–48.

McCormick, L. (1990a). Bases for language and communication development. In L. McCormick and R. L. Schiefelbusch (Eds.), *Early language intervention: An introduction* (2nd ed.). New York: Macmillan Publishing.

McCormick, L. (1990b). Child characteristics that affect learning. In L. McCormick & R. L. Schiefelbusch (Eds.), *Early language intervention: An introduction* (2nd ed., pp. 144–179). New York: Macmillan Publishing.

McCormick, L., & Schiefelbusch, R. (Eds.). (1990). *Early language intervention: An introduction* (2nd ed.). New York: Macmillan Publishing.

McCormick, L., & Shane, H. (1990). Communication systems options for students who are nonspeaking. In L. McCormick and R. L. Schiefelbusch (Eds.), *Early language intervention: An introduction* (2nd ed.). New York: Macmillan Publishing.

McCubbin, J. A., & Shasby, G. B. (1985). Effects of isokinetic exercise on adolescents with cerebral palsy. *Adapted Physical Activity Quarterly, 2,* 56–64.

McDaniel, M. A., Blischak, D. M., & Einstein, G. O. (1995). Understanding the special mnemonic characteristics of fairy tales. In C. A. Weaver III, S. Mannes, & C. R. Fletcher (Eds.), *Discourse comprehension: Essays in honor of Walter Kintsch* (pp. 157–175). Hillsdale, NJ: Lawrence Ehrlbaum.

McEwen, I. R. (1992). Assistive positioning as a control parameter of social-communicative interactions between students with profound multiple disabilities and classroom staff. *Physical Therapy, 72,* 634–647.

McEwen, I. R. (1994). Mental retardation. In S. K. Campbell (Ed.), *Physical therapy for children* (pp. 457–488). Philadelphia: W. B. Saunders.

McEwen, I. R., & Karlan, G. R. (1989). Assessment of effects of position on communication board access by individuals with cerebral palsy. *Augmentative and Alternative Communication, 5,* 235–242.

McEwen, I. R., & Lloyd, L. L. (1990a). Positioning students with cerebral palsy to use augmentative and alternative communication. *Language, Speech, and Hearing Services in Schools, 21,* 15–21.

McEwen, I. R., & Lloyd, L. L. (1990b). Some considerations about the motor requirements for manual signs. *Augmentative and Alternative Communication, 6,* 207–216.

McGinnis, J. S., & Beukelman, D. R. (1989). Vocabulary requirements for writing activities for the academically mainstreamed student with disabilities. *Augmentative and Alternative Communication, 5,* 183–191.

McGregor, G., Young, J., Gerak, J., Thomas, B., & Vogelsberg, R. T. (1992). Increasing functional use of an assistive communication device by a student with severe disabilities. *Augmentative and Alternative Communication, 8,* 243–250.

McLean, J. E., Snyder-McLean, L., Rowland, C., Jacobs, P., & Stremel-Campbell, K. (1985). *Generic skills assessment inventory: Experimental edition.* Parsons, KS: University of Kansas, Bureau of Child Research.

McLean, L. K., & McLean, J. E. (1974). A language training program for nonverbal autistic children. *Journal of Speech and Hearing Disorders, 39,* 186–194.

McLoughlin, J. A., & Lewis, R. B. (1986). *Assessing special students* (2nd ed.). Columbus, OH: Merrill Publishing Company.

McNairn, P., & Smith, Y. (1996, March). *AAC feature match software.* Paper presented at CSUN Conference, Los Angeles, CA. (Software copyright by Doug Dodgen & Associates.)

McNamara, A., Galvin, R., McNaughton, S., Lindsay, P., Dowling, J., Guy, T., Harrington, K., Marshall, P., & Millin, N. (1994). BlissNet-Two: Using computer mediated communications (CMC) to resource the communicatively impaired population. (Abstract) In *Proceedings of the sixth biennial conference of the International Society for Augmentative and Alternative Communication* (pp. 354–355). Maastricht, The Netherlands: ISAAC.

McNaughton, D., & Light, J. (1989). Teaching facilitators to support the communication skills of an adult with severe cognitive disabilities: A case study. *Augmentative and Alternative Communication, 5,* 35–41.

McNaughton, D., & Tawney, J. (1993). Comparison of two spelling instruction techniques for adults who use augmentative and alternative communication. *Augmentative and Alternative Communication, 9,* 72–82.

McNaughton, S. (1976). Blissymbols: An alternate symbol system for the non-verbal pre-reading child. In G. C. Vanderheiden & K. Grilley (Eds.), *Non-vocal communication techniques and aids for the severely physically handicapped* (pp. 85–104). Baltimore: University Park Press.

McNaughton, S. (Ed.). (1985). *Communicating with Blissymbolics.* Toronto, Canada: Blissymbolics Communication Institute.

McNaughton, S. (1990). Gaining the most from AAC's growing years. *Augmentative and Alternative Communication, 6,* 2–14.

McNaughton, S. (1993). Graphic representation systems and literacy learning. *Topics in Language Disorders, 13*(2), 58–76.

McNaughton, S., & Kates, B. (1974, May). *Visual symbols: Communication system for the pre-reading physically handicapped child.* Paper presented at the Annual Meeting of the American Association on Mental Deficiency, Toronto.

McNaughton, S., & Kates, B. (1980). The application of Blissymbolics. In R. L. Schiefelbusch (Ed.), *Nonspeech language and communication: Analysis and intervention* (pp. 303–321). Baltimore: University Park Press.

McNaughton, S., & Lindsay, P. (1995). Approaching literacy with AAC graphics. *Augmentative and Alternative Communication, 11,* 212–218.

McNaughton, S., & Warrick A. (1984). Picture your Blissymbols. *The Canadian Journal of Mental Retardation, 34,* 1–9.

McNeil, M. R., & Prescott, T. E. (1978). *Revised token test.* Baltimore, MD: University Park Press.

McNeill, D. (1985). So you think gestures are nonverbal? *Psychological Review, 92*(3), 350–371.

McNeill, D. (1993). The circle from gesture to sign. In M. Marshark & M. D. Clark (Eds.), *Psychological perspectives on deafness* (pp. 153–183). Hillsdale, NJ: Lawrence Erlbaum Associates.

McReynolds, L. V. (1988). Articulation disorders of unknown etiology. In N. J. Lass, L. R. McReynolds, J. L. Northern, & D. E. Yoder (Eds.), *Handbook of speech-language pathology and audiology* (pp. 419–441). Philadelphia: B. C. Decker, Inc.

McWilliams, B. J., Morris, H. L., & Shelton, R. L. (Eds.). (1990). *Cleft palate speech* (2nd ed.). Philadelphia: B. C. Decker, Inc.

Meador, D. M., Rumbaugh, D. M., Tribble, M., & Thompson, S. (1984). Facilitating visual discrimination learning of moderately and severely mentally retarded children through illumination of stimuli. *American Journal of Mental Deficiency, 89,* 313–316.

Medelsohn, S. (1990). *State sales tax and assistive technology: Securing exemptions for sensory, communication, and mobility aids.* Washington, DC: Rehabilitation Engineering Center.

Menyuk, P., Chesnick, M., Liergergott, J., Korngold, B., D'Agostino, R., & Belanger, A. (1991). Predicting reading problems in at-risk children. *Journal of Speech and Hearing Research, 34,* 893–903.

Miedaner, J. A. (1990). The effects of sitting positions on trunk extension for children with motor impairment. *Pediatric Physical Therapy, 2,* 11–14.

Miller, A. (1967). Symbol accentuation: Outgrowth of theory and experiment. In E. Meshorer (Chair), *A new approach to language development with retardates.* Symposium presented at the First International Congress on the Scientific Study of Mental Deficiency, Montpellier, France.

Miller, A. (1968). *Symbol accentuation—A new approach to reading.* Santa Ana, CA: Doubleday Multimedia.

Miller, A., & Miller, E. (1968). Symbol accentuation: The perceptual transfer of meaning from spoken to printed words. *American Journal of Mental Deficiency, 73,* 202–208.

Miller, A., & Miller, E. (1971). Symbol accentuation, single-track functioning and early reading. *American Journal of Mental Deficiency, 76,* 110–117.

Miller, A., & Miller, E. (1973). Cognitive-developmental training with elevated boards and sign language. *Journal of Autism and Childhood Schizophrenia, 3,* 65–68.

Miller, G. A. (1951). *Language and communication.* New York: McGraw-Hill.

Miller, G. A., Heise, G., & Lichten, W. (1951). The intelligibility of speech as a function of the context of the test materials. *Journal of Experimental Psychology, 41,* 329–335.

Millikan, C. C. (1997). Symbol systems and vocabulary selection strategies. In S. L. Glennen & D. C. DeCoste (Eds.), *Handbook of augmentative and alternative communication* (pp. 97–148). San Diego, CA: Singular Publishing.

Mills v. Board of Education. District of Columbia. 348 F. Supp. 886 (D.D.C. 1972).

Mineo, B. (Ed.). (1990). *Augmentative and alternative communication in the next decade: Visions conference proceedings.* Wilmington, DE: E. I. du Pont Institute, University of Delaware.

Minuchin, S. (1974). *Families and family therapy.* Cambridge, MA: Harvard University Press.

Mirenda, P. (1985). Designing pictorial communication systems for physically able-bodied students with severe handicaps. *Augmentative and Alternative Communication, 1,* 58–64.

Mirenda, P. (1993). AAC: Bonding the uncertain mosaic. *Augmentative and Alternative Communication, 9,* 3–9.

Mirenda, P., & Beukelman, D. R. (1990). A comparison of intelligibility among natural speech and seven speech synthesizers with listeners from three age groups. *Augmentative and Alternative Communication, 6,* 61–68.

Mirenda, P., & Datillo, J. (1987). Instructional techniques in alternative communication for students with severe intellectual handicaps. *Augmentative and Alternative Communication, 3,* 143–152.

Mirenda, P., Iacono, T., & Williams, R. (1990). Communication options for persons with severe and profound disabilities: State of the art and future directions. *Journal of the*

Association for Persons with Severe Handicaps, *15*, 3–21.

Mirenda, P., & Locke, P. (1989). A comparison of symbol transparency in nonspeaking persons with intellectual disabilities. *Journal of Speech and Hearing Disorders*, *54*, 131–140.

Mirenda, P., & Mathy-Laikko, P. (1989). Augmentative and alternative communication applications for persons with severe congenital communication disorders: An introduction. *Augmentative and Alternative Communication*, *5*, 3–13.

Mirenda, P., & Santogrossi, J. (1985). A prompt-free strategy to teach pictorial communication system use. *Augmentative and Alternative Communication*, *1*, 143–150.

Mital, M. A., Belkin, S. C., & Sullivan, M. A. (1976). An approach to head, neck, and trunk stabilization and control in cerebral palsy by use of the Milwaukee brace. *Developmental Medicine and Child Neurology*, *18*, 198–203.

Mitiguy, J. S., Thompson, G., & Wasco, J. (1990). *Understanding brain injury*. Lynn, MA: New Medico Head Injury System.

Mizuko, M. I. (1987). Transparency and ease of learning symbols represented by Blissymbols, PCS, and Picsyms. *Augmentative and Alternative Communication*, *3*, 129–136.

Mizuko, M. I., & Reichle, J. (1989). Transparency and recall of symbols among intellectually handicapped adults. *Journal of Speech and Hearing Disorders*, *54*, 627–633.

Mizuko, M. I., Reichle, J., Ratcliff, A., & Esser, J. (1994). Effects of selection techniques and array sizes on short-term visual memory. *Augmentative and Alternative Communication*, *10*, 237–244.

Moe, A. J., Hopkins, C. J., & Rush, R. T. (1982). *The vocabulary of first-grade children*. Springfield, IL: Charles C. Thomas Publishing.

Moeller, M. P., Osberger, M. J., & Morford, J. A. (1987). Speech-language assessment and intervention with preschool hearing impaired children. In J. G. Alpiner & P. A. McCarthy (Eds.), *Rehabilitative audiology: Children and adults* (pp. 163–187). Baltimore: Williams & Wilkins.

Moersch, M. (1977). Training the deaf-blind. *The American Journal of Occupational Therapy*, *3*, 425–431.

Moore, K. (1993). House holds hearing on reauthorization of the Tech Act. *A.T. Quarterly*, *4*(2), 1, 5.

Moores, D. (1978). *Educating the deaf*. Boston: Houghton Mifflin.

Morris, D., Collett, P., Marsh, P., & O'Shaughnessy, M. (1979). *Gestures: Their origins and distribution*. New York: Stein & Day.

Morris, M. (1993a). Early intervention (Part H) final regs include assistive technology. *A.T. Quarterly*, *4*(3), 5–7.

Morris, M. (1993b). National assistive technology funding study. *A.T. Quarterly*, *4*(2), 6, 8.

Morris, M., & Williams, R. R. (1992). A.T. systems change strategies for increasing funding access. *A.T. Quarterly*, *3*(1), 7.

Morris, S. A. S. (1986). *Transparency of two representational systems: Picsyms and Picture Communication Symbols*. Unpublished master's thesis, Western Carolina University.

Morrissey, M. (1986). Irish Sign System (L.A.M.H.) for individuals with mental handicap: An investigation of iconicity and guessability. In B. T. Tervoort (Ed.), *Signs of life: Proceedings of the second European congress on sign language research* (pp. 111–115). Amsterdam: Dutch Foundation for the Deaf and Hearing Impaired Child.

Morrow, D., Mirenda, P., Beukelman, D. R., & Yorkston, K. (1993). Vocabulary selection for augmentative communication systems: A comparison of three techniques. *American Journal of Speech-Language Pathology*, *2*(2), 19–30.

Morse, J. L. (1987). Assessment procedures for people with mental retardation: The dilemma and suggested adaptive procedures. In S. N. Calculator & J. L. Bedrosian (Eds.), *Communication assessment and intervention for adults with mental retardation* (pp. 109–128). Boston: College-Hill Press.

Morse, M. T. (1990). Cortical visual impairment in young children with multiple disabilities. *Journal of Visual Impairment & Blindness*, *84*, 200–203.

Morse, M. T. (1992). Augmenting assessment procedure for children with severe multiple handicaps and sensory impairments. *Journal of Visual Impairment & Blindness*, *86*, 73–77.

Mountcastle, V. B. (1978). An organizing principle for cerebral function: The unit module and the distributed system. In G. M. Edelman & V. B. Mountcastle (Eds.), *The mindful brain: Cortical organization and the group-selective theory of higher brain function* (pp. 7–50). Cambridge, MA: MIT Press.

Mounty, J. L. (1986). *Nativization and input in the language development of two deaf children of hearing parents*. Unpublished doctoral dissertation, Boston University.

Muma, J. (1978). *Language handbook: Concepts, assessment, intervention*. Englewood Cliffs, NJ: Prentice-Hall.

Murphy, J., Markova, I., Moodie, E., Scott, J., & Boa, S. (1995). Augmentative and alternative communication systems used by people with cerebral palsy in Scotland: Demographic survey. *Augmentative and Alternative Communication*, *11*, 26–36.

Murray-Branch, J., Udavari-Solner, A., & Bailey, B. (1991). Textured communication systems for individuals with severe intellectual and dual sensory impairments. *Language, Speech, and Hearing Services in Schools*, *22*, 260–268.

Musselwhite, C. R. (1982). *A comparison of three symbolic communication systems*. Unpublished doctoral dissertation, West Virginia University, Morgantown.

Musselwhite, C. R. (1985). *Songbook: Signs and symbols for children*. Wauconda, IL: Don Johnston Incorporated.

Musselwhite, C. R. (1986). *Adaptive play for special needs children: Strategies to enhance communication and learning*. San Diego, CA: College-Hill Press.

Musselwhite, C. R. (1992, August). *Emergent literacy using devices*. Presentation at the Fifth Biennial Conference of the International Society for Augmentative and Alternative Communication, Philadelphia.

Musselwhite, C. R., & St. Louis, K. W. (1988). *Communication programming for persons with severe handicaps: Vocal and augmentative strategies* (2nd ed.). San Diego, CA: College-Hill Press.

Musselwhite, C. R., & Ruscello, D. (1984). Transparency of three communication symbol systems. *Journal of Speech and Hearing Research, 27,* 436–443.

Myhr, U., & von Wendt, L. (1991). Improvement of functional sitting position for children with cerebral palsy. *Developmental Medicine and Child Neurology, 33,* 246–256.

Mylander, C., & Goldin-Meadow, S. (1991). Home sign systems in deaf children: The development of morphology without a conventional model. In P. Siple & S. Fischer (Eds.), *Theoretical issues in sign language research. Vol 2: Psychology* (pp. 41–63). Chicago: University of Chicago Press.

Naeser, M. A., Palumbo, C. L., Baker, E. H., & Nicholas, M. L. (1994). CT scan lesion site analysis in severe aphasia: Relationship to no recovery of speech and treatment with the nonverbal computer-assisted visual communication program (C-VIC). *Seminars in Speech and Language, 15,* 53–70.

Nagi, S. Z. (1991). Disability concepts revisited: Implications for prevention. In A. Pope & A. Tarlou (Eds.), *Disability in America: Toward a national agenda for prevention* (pp. 309–327). Washington, DC: National Academy Press.

Nagy, W. E., & Anderson, R. C. (1984). How many words are there in printed school English? *Reading Research Quarterly, 19,* 304–330.

Nagy, W. E., Herman, P. A., & Anderson, R. C. (1985). Learning words from context. *Reading Research Quarterly, 20,* 233–253.

Nail-Chiwetalu, B. J. (1992). The influence of symbol and learner factors on the learnability of Blissymbols by students with mental retardation. (Doctoral dissertation, Purdue University, 1991). *Dissertation Abstracts International, 53,* 1125A.

National Institute of Disability and Rehabilitation Research. (1991). National pediatric trauma registry: A progress report. *Rehabilitation Update,* 4–5.

National Joint Committee for the Communicative Needs of Persons with Severe Disabilities. (1992). Guidelines for meeting the communication needs of persons with severe disabilities. *Asha, 34* (March, Supp. 7), 1–8.

National Stroke Association (1991). The scope of stroke. *Clinical Updates, 1,* 1–3.

Nelson, K. (1973). Structure and strategy in learning to talk. *Monographs of the Society for Research into Child Development, 38* (Serial No. 149), 1–135.

Nelson, K. (1989). Strategies for a first language teaching. In M. L. Rice & R. L. Schiefelbusch (Eds.), *The teachability of language* (pp. 263–310). Baltimore: Paul H. Brookes Publishing.

Nelson, K., & Dimitrova, E. (1993). Severe visual impairment in the United States and in each state, 1990. *Journal of Visual Impairment & Blindness, 87,* 80–83.

Nelson, K., Loncke, F., & Camarata, S. (1993). Implications of research on deaf and hearing children's language learning. In M. Marshark & M. D. Clark (Eds.), *Psychological perspectives on deafness* (pp. 123–151). Hillsdale, NJ: Lawrence Erlbaum Associates.

Nelson, L. B., Ehrlick, S., Calhoun, J. H., Matteucci, T., & Finnegan, L. P. (1987). Occurrence of strabismus in infants born to drug-dependent women. *American Journal of Diseases of Childhood, 141,* 175–178.

Nelson, N. W. (1990). Curriculum-based language assessment and intervention. *Language, Speech and Hearing Services in Schools, 21,* 170–184.

Nelson, N. W. (1992). Performance is the prize: Language competence and performance among AAC users. *Augmentative and Alternative Communication, 8,* 3–18.

Newell, A. F. (1974). The talking brooch: A communication aid. In K. Copeland (Ed.), *Aids for the severely handicapped.* London: Sector Publishing.

Newell, A. F., Arnott, J. L., Booth, L., Beattie, W., Brophy, B., & Ricketts, I. W. (1992). Effect of the "PAL" word prediction system on the quality and quantity of text generation. *Augmentative and Alternative Communication, 8,* 304–311.

Newport, E. L., & Meier, R. (1985). The acquisition of American Sign Language. In D. I. Slobin (Ed.), *The cross-linguistic study of language acquisition. Vol. 1: The data* (pp. 881–938). Hillsdale, NJ: Lawrence Erlbaum Associates.

Newton, J. T., & Sturmey, A. P. (1991). The Motivation Assessment Scale: Inter-rater reliability and internal consistency in a British sample. *Journal of Mental Deficiency Research, 35,* 472–474.

Nicholas, M., Obler, L. K., Albert, M. L., & Helm-Estabrooks, N. (1985). Empty speech in Alzheimer's disease and fluent aphasia. *Journal of Speech and Hearing Research, 28,* 405–410.

Nickse, R. S, Speicher, A. M., & Buchek, P. C. (1988). An intergenerational adult literacy project: A family intervention/prevention model. *Journal of Reading, 31*(7), 634–642.

Nielsen, J., Homma, A., & Biorn-Henriksen, T. (1977). Follow-up 15 years after a gerontopsychiatric prevalence study. *Journal of Gerontology, 32,* 554–561.

Nietupski, J., & Hamre-Nietupski, S. (1979). Teaching auxiliary communication skills to severely handicapped students. *AAESPH Review, 4,* 107–124.

Nigam, R., & Karlan, G. R. (1994, November). *Cultural validation of Picture Communication Symbols set for Asian-Indian children.* Poster session presented at the Annual Convention of the American Speech-Language-Hearing Association, New Orleans.

Nishikawa, L. K. (1980). *Blissymbolics as an augmentative communication tool for adults with expressive aphasia.*

Unpublished master's thesis, Loma Linda University, Loma Linda, CA.

Niswander, P. S. (1987). Audiometric assessment and management. In L. Goetz, D. Guess, & K. Stremel-Campbell (Eds.), *Innovative program design for individuals with dual sensory impairments* (pp. 99–126). Baltimore: Paul H. Brookes Publishing.

Nolan, C. (1987). *Under the eye of the clock: The life story of Christopher Nolan.* New York: St. Martin's Press.

Noonan, M. J., & McCormick, L. (1993). Early intervention perspectives, policies, and practices. In M. J. Noonan & L. McCormick (Eds.), *Early intervention in natural environments: Methods and procedures* (pp. 1–24). Pacific Grove, CA: Brooks/Cole Publishing.

Noonan, M. J., & Siegel-Causey, E. (1990). Special needs of students with severe handicaps. In L. McCormick & R. L. Schiefelbusch (Eds.), *Early language intervention: An introduction* (2nd ed.). New York: Macmillan Publishing.

Northern, J. L., & Downs, M. P. (1991). *Hearing in children* (4th ed.). Baltimore: Williams & Wilkins.

Northup, J., Wacker, D., Sasso, G., Steege, M., Cigrand, K., Cook, J., & DeRaad, A. (1991). A brief functional analysis of aggressive and alternative behavior in an outclinic setting. *Journal of Applied Behavior Analysis, 24,* 509–522.

Norton, S., Schultz, M., Reed, C., Braida, L., Durlach, N., Rabinowitz, W., & Chomsky, C. (1977). Analytic study of the Tadoma method: Background and preliminary results. *Journal of Speech and Hearing Research, 20,* 574–595.

Noyes, J. M., & Frankish, C. R. (1992). Speech recognition technology for individuals with disabilities. *Augmentative and Alternative Communication, 8,* 297–303.

Nwaobi, O. M. (1986). Effects of body orientation in space on tonic muscle activity of patients with cerebral palsy. *Developmental Medicine and Child Neurology, 28,* 41–44.

Nwaobi, O. M. (1987). Seating orientations and upper extremity function in children with cerebral palsy. *Physical Therapy, 67,* 1209–1212.

Nwaobi, O. M., & Smith, P. D. (1986). Effect of adaptive seating on pulmonary function of children with cerebral palsy. *Developmental Medicine and Child Neurology, 28,* 351–354.

Nye, P. W., & Gaitenby, J. H. (1974). The intelligibility of synthetic monosyllabic words in short, syntactically normal sentences. *Status Report on Speech Research, 37–38,* 169–190.

O'dell, C. D., Harshaw, K., & Boothe, R. G. (1993). Vision screening of individuals with severe or profound mental retardation. *Mental Retardation, 31,* 154–160.

Offir, C. W. (1976). Visual speech: Their fingers do the talking. *Psychology Today, 10*(1), 72–78.

O'Keefe, B. M., & Dattilo, J. (1992). Teaching the response-recode form to adults with mental retardation using AAC systems. *Augmentative and Alternative Communication, 8,* 224–233.

Olmos-Lau, N., Ginsberg, M., & Geller, J. (1977). Aphasia in multiple sclerosis. *Neurology, 27,* 623–626.

Olney, S. J., & Wright, M. J. (1994). Cerebral palsy. In S. K. Campbell (Ed.), *Physical therapy for children* (pp. 489–523). Philadelphia: W. B. Saunders.

Olofsson, A. (1988). Phonemic awareness and the use of computer speech in reading remediation: Theoretical background. *Fonetiks, 1*(5), 15–27.

Olofsson, A., & Lundberg, I. (1983). Can phonemic awareness be trained in kindergarten? *Scandinavian Journal of Psychology, 24,* 35–44.

O'Neill, R. E., Horner, R. H., Albin, R. W., Storey, K., & Sprague, J. R. (1990). *Functional analysis of problem behavior: A practical assessment guide.* Sycamore, IL: Sycamore Publishing.

O'Neill, R. E., & Reichle, J. (1993). Addressing socially motivated challenging behavior by establishing communicative alternatives: Basics of a general-case approach. In J. Reichle & D. P. Wacker (Eds.), *Communicative alternatives to challenging behavior: Integrating functional assessment and intervention strategies* (pp. 205–235). Baltimore: Paul H. Brookes Publishing.

Ontario Crippled Children's Centre. (1971). *Ontario Crippled Children's Centre symbol communication programme: Year end report.* Toronto: Author.

Orcutt, D. (1984). *The Worldsign symbolbook.* Winlaw, British Columbia: Worldsign Communication Society.

Orcutt, D. (1985). Worldsign update. *Communicating Together, 3,* 24–25.

Orcutt, D. (1987). *The Worldsign exposition.* Winlaw, British Columbia: Worldsign Communication Society.

Orelove, F. P., & Sobsey, D. (Eds.). (1996). *Educating children with multiple disabilities: A transdisciplinary approach* (3rd ed.). Baltimore: Paul H. Brookes Publishing.

Orlansky, M. D., & Bonvillian, J. D. (1984). The role of iconicity in early sign language acquisition. *Journal of Speech and Hearing Disorders, 49,* 287–292.

Osberger, M. J. (1990). Audition. *The Volta Review, 92*(4), 34–53.

Ostrosky, M. M., Kaiser, A. P., & Odom, S. L. (1993). Facilitating children's social-communicative interactions through the use of peer-mediated intervention. In A. P. Kaiser & D. B. Gray (Eds.), *Enhancing children's communication: Research foundation for intervention* (Vol. 2, pp. 159–185). Baltimore: Paul H. Brookes Publishing.

Owens, R. E., Jr., & House, L. I. (1984). Decision-making processes in augmentative communication. *Journal of Speech and Hearing Disorders, 49,* 18–25.

Padden, C. (1988). *Interaction of morphology and syntax in American Sign Language.* London: Garland Publishing, Inc.

Padden, C., & Humphries, T. (1988). *Deaf in America.* Cambridge, MA: Harvard University Press.

Padula, W. V., & Shapiro, J. B. (1993). Head injury and the post-trauma vision syndrome. *RE:view, 24,* 153–158.

Paget, K. D. (1989). Assessment of cognitive skills in the preschool-aged child. In D. B. Bailey & M. Wolery (Eds.), *Assessing infants and preschoolers with handicaps.* Columbus, OH: Merrill Publishing.

Paget, R. (1951). *The new sign language*. London: The Wellcome Foundation.

Paget, R., & Gorman, P. (1968). *A systematic sign language*. London: Royal National Institute for the Deaf.

Paget, R., Gorman, P., & Paget, G. (1971). *An introduction to the Paget-Gorman Sign System with examples*. Reading, England: Association for Experiment in Deaf Education Publications Committee.

Paget, R., Gorman, P., & Paget, G. (1976). *The Paget Gorman Sign System (6th ed.)*. London: Association for Experiment in Deaf Education.

Paivio, A. (1969). Concrete image and verbal memory codes. *Journal of Experimental Psychology, 80*, 279–283.

Paivio, A. (1986). *Mental representations: A dual-coding approach*. New York: Oxford University Press.

Papandropoulou, I., & Sinclair, H. (1974). What is a word? Experimental study of children's ideas and grammar. *Human Development, 17*, 241–258.

Paradis, M., Hagiwara, H., & Hildebrandt, N. (1985). *Neurolinguistic aspects of the Japanese writing system*. Orlando, FL: Academic Press.

Parette, H. P., Hofmann, A., & VanBiervliet, A. (1994). The professional's role in obtaining funding for assistive technology for infants and toddlers with disabilities. *Teaching Exceptional Children, 26*, 22–28.

Parette, H. P., Hourcade, J. J., & VanBiervliet, A. (1993). Selection of appropriate technology for children with disabilities. *Teaching Exceptional Children, 25*, 18–22.

Parkel, D. A., White, R. A., & Warner, H. (1977). Implications of the Yerkes technology for mentally retarded human subjects. In D. M. Rumbaugh (Ed.), *Language learning by a chimpanzee: The LANA Project*. New York: Academic Press.

Parker, L. G. (1987). Educational programming. In E. McDonald (Ed.), *Treating cerebral palsy: For clinicians by clinicians*. Austin, TX: Pro-Ed.

Parnwell, E. (1977). *Oxford English picture dictionary*. Oxford, England: Oxford University Press.

Pasadena Independent School District. 21 IDELR 482 (TX SEA, 1994).

Pecyna, P. (1988). Rebus symbol communication training with a severely handicapped preschool child: A case study. *Language, Speech, and Hearing Services in Schools, 19*, 128–143.

Pennington, G., Karlan, G. R., & Lloyd, L. L. (1986). Considerations in the selection of sign systems and initial lexica. In D. Ellis (Ed.), *Sensory handicaps among mentally handicapped people* (pp. 383–407). Beckenham, England: Croom Helm, Ltd. Publishers.

Pennsylvania Association for Retarded Citizens (PARC) v. the Commonwealth of Pennsylvania. 334 F. Supp. 1257 (E.D. Pa 1971).

Pennsylvania Association for Retarded Citizens (PARC) v. Commonwealth of Pennsylvania. 343 F. Supp. 279 (E.D. Pa 1972).

Penrod, J. P. (1985). Speech discrimination testing. In J. Katz (Ed.), *Handbook of clinical audiology* (3rd ed., pp. 235–255). Baltimore: Williams & Wilkins.

Périer, O. (1987). L'enfant à audition déficiente: Aspects médicaux, éducatifs, sociologiques et psychologiques. *Acta Oto-Rhino-Laryngologica Belgica, 41*, 125–420.

Perron, J. V. (1965). Typewriter control for an aphasic quadriplegic patient. *Canadian Medical Association Journal, 92*, 557–559.

Pester, E. J., Petrosko, J. M., & Poppe, K. J. (1994). Optimizing size and spacing for introducing blind adults to the Braille code. *RE:view, 26*, 15–22.

Peters-Johnson, C. (1994). Action: School services. *Language, Speech and Hearing Services in Schools, 25*, 201–207.

Peterson, G. E., & Barney, H. L. (1952). Control methods used in a study of the vowels. *Journal of the Acoustical Society of America, 24*, 175–184.

Peterson, M., LeRoy, B., Field, S., & Wood, P. (1992). Community-referenced learning in inclusive schools. In S. Stainback & W. Stainback (Eds.), *Curriculum considerations in inclusive classrooms* (pp. 207–227). Baltimore: Paul H. Brookes Publishing.

Petitto, L. (1983). *From gesture to symbol: The acquisition of personal pronouns in American Sign Language*. Unpublished doctoral dissertation, Harvard University.

Petitto, L. A. (1994). Are signed languages "real" languages? Evidence from American Sign Language and Langue des Signes Québécoise. *Signpost, 7*, 173–182.

Petitto, L. A., & Marentette, P. (1991). Babbling in the manual mode: Evidence for the ontogeny of language. *Science, 251*, 1483–1496.

Phillippi, J. W. (1988). Matching literacy to job training: Some applications from military programs. *Journal of Reading, 31*(7), 658–666.

Phillips, V., & McCullough, L. (1990). Consultation-based programming: Instituting the collaborative ethic in schools. *Exceptional Children, 22*, 291–304.

Piché, L., & Reichle, J. (1991). Teaching scanning selection techniques. In J. Reichle, J. York, & J. Sigafoos (Eds.), *Implementing augmentative and alternative communication: Strategies for learners with severe disabilities* (pp. 257–274). Baltimore: Paul H. Brookes Publishing.

Pierce, P. L., & McWilliam, P. J. (1993). Emerging literacy and children with severe speech and physical impairments (SSPI): Issues and possible intervention strategies. *Topics in Language Disorders, 13*(2), 47–57.

Pinker, S. (1994). *The language instinct: The new science of language and mind*. London: Allan Lane.

Pisoni, D. B., & Koen, E. (1982). Some comparisons of intelligibility of synthetic and natural speech at different signal-to-noise ratios. *Journal of the Acoustical Society of America, 71*, S94.

Pizzuto, E. (1986). The verb system of Italian Sign Language. In B. Tervoort (Ed.), *Signs of life: Proceedings of the second European congress on sign language research* (pp. 17–31). Amsterdam: University of Amsterdam.

Plato (348 B.C./1960). *The laws* (A. E. Taylor, Trans.). London: J. M. Dent.

Poizner, H., Bellugi, V., & Iragui, V. (1984). Apraxia and aphasia in a visuo-gestural language. *American Journal of Physiology, 246,* R868–R833.

Poizner, H., Klima, E., & Bellugi, U. (1990). *What the hands reveal about the brain.* Cambridge, MA: MIT Press.

Polzer, K. R., Wankoff, L. L., & Wollner, S. G. (1979, April). *The acquisition of arbitrary and iconic signs: Imitation vs. comprehension.* Paper presented at New York State Speech and Hearing Association, Ellenville, NY.

Ponchillia, S. V. (1993). Complications of diabetes and their implication for service providers. *Journal of Visual Impairment & Blindness, 87,* 354–358.

Porch, B. E. (1981). *Porch index of communicative ability* (3rd ed.). Palo Alto, CA: Consulting Psychologists Press.

Porter, P., Carter, S., Goolsby, E., Martin, N., Reed, M., Stowers, S., & Wurth, B. (1985). *Prerequisites to the use of augmentative communication.* Chapel Hill, NC: Division for Disorders of Development and Learning.

Poser, C. M. (1984). *The diagnosis of multiple sclerosis.* New York: Thieme-Stratton.

Post, K., & Crawford, J. E. (1992, March). *Funding issues and strategies with regard to augmentative and alternative communication.* Paper presented at the Illinois State Speech-Language-Hearing Convention, Chicago.

Potenski, D. H. (1993). Use of blacklight as visual for people with profound mental and multiple handicaps. *Mental Retardation, 31,* 111–115.

Potter, R. K. (1945). Visible patterns of sound. *Science, 102,* 463–470.

Potter, R. K., Kopp, G. A., & Green, H. C. (1947). *Visible speech.* New York: Van Nostrand.

Potter, R. K. & Peterson, G. E. (1948). The representation of vowels and their movements: *Journal of the Acoustical Society of America, 20,* 528–535.

Pratt, F. (1939). *Secret and urgent: The story of codes and ciphers.* New York: Blue Ribbon Books.

Premack, D. (1970). A functional analysis of language. *Journal of the Experimental Analysis of Behavior, 14,* 107–125.

Premack, D. (1971a). Language in chimpanzees? *Science, 172,* 808–822.

Premack, D. (1971b). On the assessment of language competence in the chimpanzee. *Behavior of Non-human Primates, 4,* 198–228.

Premack, D., & Premack, A. J. (1974). Teaching visual language to apes and language-deficient persons. In R. L. Schiefelbusch & L. L. Lloyd (Eds.), *Language perspectives: Acquisition, retardation, and intervention* (pp. 347–376). Baltimore: University Park Press.

Prentice, J. (1994). You too can get a job—A first-person perspective. *Communication Outlook, 16*(2), 5–9.

Prentke Romich Company. (1989). *How to obtain funding for augmentative communication devices.* Wooster, OH: Author.

Prillwitz, S., & Vollhaber, T. (Eds.). (1990). *Current trends in European sign language research: Papers of the third European congress on sign language research.* Hamburg, Germany: Signum Press.

Prinz, P., Nelson, K., Loncke, F., Geysels, G., & Willems, C. (1993). A multimodality and multimedia approach to language, discourse, and literacy development. In B. Elsendoorn & F. Coninx (Eds.), *Interactive learning technology for the deaf* (pp. 55–70). Berlin, Germany: Springer Verlag.

Prinz, P. M., & Shaw, N. (1981, November). *Communication development by speech and sign in mentally retarded individuals.* Paper presented at the 56th Annual Convention of the American Speech-Language-Hearing Association, Los Angeles.

Prizant, B. M., & Rydell, P. J. (1993). Assessment and intervention considerations for unconventional verbal behavior. In J. Reichle & D. P. Wacker (Eds.), *Communicative alternatives to challenging behavior: Integrating functional assessment and intervention strategies* (pp. 263–297). Baltimore: Paul H. Brookes Publishing.

Project ACTT. (1993). *Funding technology for young children.* Macomb, IL: Western Illinois University.

Public Law 88-164. (1963). *Mental retardation facilities and community mental health centers construction act of 1963.* Washington, DC: U.S. Congress.

Public Law 89-10. (1965). *Elementary and secondary education act of 1965.* Washington, DC: U.S. Congress.

Public Law 89-97. (1965). *Social Security act of 1965.* Washington, DC: U.S. Congress.

Public Law 89-313. (1965). *Elementary and secondary education amendments of 1965 for children with handicaps.* Washington, DC: U.S. Congress.

Public Law 89-750. (1966). *Elementary and secondary education amendments.* Washington, DC: U.S. Congress.

Public Law 90-170. (1967). *Mental retardation amendments of 1967.* Washington, DC: U.S. Congress.

Public Law 90-247. (1967). *Elementary and secondary education amendments of 1967.* Washington, DC: U.S. Congress.

Public Law 91-230. (1969). *Elementary, secondary, and other education amendments of 1969.* Washington, DC: U.S. Congress.

Public Law 91-517. (1970). *Developmental disabilities services and facilities construction amendments of 1970.* Washington, DC: U.S. Congress.

Public Law 93-112. (1973). *Rehabilitation act of 1973.* Washington, DC: U.S. Congress.

Public Law 94-103. (1975). *Developmentally disabled assistance and bill of rights act amendments of 1975.* Washington, DC: U.S. Congress.

Public Law 94-142. (1975). *Education for all handicapped children act of 1975.* Washington, DC: U.S. Congress.

Public Law 98-199. (1983). *Education for all handicapped act amendments of 1983.* Washington, DC: U.S. Congress.

Public Law 98-524. (1984). *Carl D. Perkins vocational education act of 1984.* Washington, DC: U.S. Congress.

Public Law 98-527. (1984). *Developmental disabilities act of 1984.* Washington, DC: U.S. Congress.

Public Law 99-457. (1986). *Education of the handicapped act amendments of 1986.* Washington, DC: U.S. Congress.

Public Law 100-146. (1987). *Developmental disabilities assistance and bill of rights act amendments of 1987.* Washington, DC: U.S. Congress.

Public Law 100-407. (1988). *Technology-related assistance for individuals with disabilities act of 1988.* Washington, DC: U.S. Congress.

Public Law 101-336. (1990). *Americans with disabilities act of 1990.* Washington, DC: U.S. Congress.

Public Law 101-392. (1990). *Carl D. Perkins vocational and applied technology act amendments of 1990.* Washington, DC: U.S. Congress.

Public Law 101-476. (1990). *Individuals with disabilities education act (IDEA) of 1990.* Washington, DC: U.S. Congress.

Public Law 102-119. (1991). *Individuals with disabilities education act amendments of 1991.* Washington, DC: U.S. Congress.

Public Law 102-569. (1992). *Rehabilitation act amendments of 1992.* Washington, DC: U.S. Congress.

Public Law 103-218. (1994). *Technology-related assistance for individuals with disabilities amendments of 1994.* Washington, DC: U.S. Congress.

Public Law 105-17. (1997). *Individuals with disabilities education act reauthorization amendments of 1997.* Washington, DC: U.S. Congress.

Pumfrey, P. D., & Reason R. (1991). *Specific learning difficulties: Challenges and responses.* Berks, England: NFER-Nelson.

Quertinmont, S., & Loncke, F. (Ed.). (1989). *Etudes europeennes en langue des signes. (European studies in sign languages).* Brussels, Belgium: Edirsa.

Quertinmont, S., Loncke, F., & Ferreyra, P. (1991). Caractéristiques linguistiques de la langue des signes des enfants sourds à l' école: La question des signeurs de naissance. *Revue Québécoise de Linguistique Théorique et Appliquée, 10*(1), 123–140.

Quist, R. W., & Blischak, D. (1992). Assistive communication devices: Call for specifications. *Augmentative and Alternative Communication, 8,* 312–317.

Quist, R. W., & Lloyd, L. L. (1990, May). *A comparison of two teaching approaches as they relate to the learning of Blissymbols by cognitively impaired individuals: A preliminary report.* Paper presented at the Annual Meeting of the American Association on Mental Retardation, Atlanta.

Raghavendra, P., & Fristoe, M. (1990). "A spinach with a V on it": What 3-year-olds see in standard and enhanced Blissymbolics. *Journal of Speech and Hearing Disorders, 55,* 149–159.

Raghavendra, P., Rosengren, E., & Hunnicutt, S. (1994). An investigation of two speech recognition systems with dysarthric speech as input. *Proceedings of the sixth biennial conference of the International Society for Augmentative and Alternative Communication* (pp. 479–481), Maastricht, the Netherlands.

Rainforth, B. (1982). Biobehavioral state and orienting: Implications for educating profoundly retarded students. *Journal of the Association of the Severely Handicapped, 6,* 33–37.

Rainforth, B., & York, J. (1987). Positioning and handling. In F. P. Orelove & D. Sobsey (Eds.), *Educating children with multiple disabilities: A transdisciplinary approach* (pp. 67–101). Baltimore: Paul H. Brookes Publishing.

Rainforth, B., York, J., & Macdonald, C. (1992). *Collaborative teams for students with severe disabilities: Integrating therapy and educational services.* Baltimore: Paul H. Brookes Publishing.

Rankin, J., Harwood, K., & Mirenda, P. (1994). Influence of graphic symbol use on reading comprehension. *Augmentative and Alternative Communication, 10,* 269–281.

Rao, P., & Horner, J. (1979). Gesture as a deblocking modality in a severe aphasic patient. In R. Brookshire (Ed.), *Clinical aphasiology* (pp. 180–187). Minneapolis: MN: BRK Publishers.

Rao, S. (1994). Introducing a communication board for child-to-child conversations. *Communication Outlook, 16*(2), 10–12.

Ratcliff, A. (1987). *A comparison of two message selection techniques used in augmentative communication systems by normal children with differing cognitive styles.* Unpublished doctoral dissertation, University of Wisconsin, Madison.

Ratcliff, A. (1994). Comparison of relative demands implicated in direct selection and scanning: Consideration from normal children. *Augmentative and Alternative Communication, 10,* 67–74.

Ratcliff, A., & Beukelman, D. (1995). Preprofessional preparation in augmentative and alternative communication: State-of-the-art report. *Augmentative and Alternative Communication, 11,* 61–73.

Reason, R. (1990). Reconciling different approaches to intervention. In P. Pumfrey & C. Elliott (Eds.), *Children's reading, spelling and writing difficulties.* Lewes, England: Falmer Press.

Records, N. L., & Tomblin, J. B. (1994). Clinical decision-making: Describing the decision rules of practicing speech-language pathologists. *Journal of Speech and Hearing Research, 37,* 144–156.

Reeb, Jr., K. H. (1985). *Procurement of durable medical equipment under the Medicare Part B program.* Washington, DC: Rehabilitation Engineering Center.

Reeb, Jr., K. H. (1989). *Assistive financing for assistive devices: Loan guarantees for purchase of products by persons with disabilities.* Washington, DC: Rehabilitation Engineering Center.

Reeb, Jr., K. H., & Stripling, T. E. (1989). Payment for assistive devices by the Veterans Administration. *Communication Outlook, 11,* 13–16.

Regenbogen, L. S., & Coscas, G. C. (1985). *Oculo-auditory syndromes*. New York: Masson Publishing.

Rehabilitation Engineering Research Center. (1996). *The guide to augmentative and alternative communication devices*. Wilmington, DE: E. I. du Pont Institute, University of Delaware.

Reichle, J. (1991). Defining the decision involved in designing and implementing augmentative and alternative communication systems. In J. Reichle, J. York, & J. Sigafoos (Eds.), *Implementing augmentative and alternative communication: Strategies for learners with severe disabilities* (pp. 39–60). Baltimore: Paul H. Brookes Publishing.

Reichle, J., & Brown, L. (1986). Teaching the use of a multipage direct selection communication board to an adult with autism. *Journal of the Association for Persons with Severe Handicaps, 11*, 68–73.

Reichle, J., & Karlan, G. (1985). The selection of an augmentative system in communication intervention: A critique of decision rules. *Journal of the Association for Persons with Severe Handicaps, 10*, 146–156.

Reichle, J., & Karlan, G. A. (1988). Selecting augmentative communication interventions: A critique of candidacy criteria and a proposed alternative. In R. L. Schiefelbusch & L. L. Lloyd (Eds.), *Language perspectives: Acquisition, retardation and intervention* (2nd ed., pp. 321–329). Austin, TX: Pro-Ed.

Reichle, J., & Sigafoos, J. (1991). Establishing spontaneity and generalization. In J. Reichle, J. York, & J. Sigafoos (Eds.), *Implementing augmentative and alternative communication: Strategies for learners with severe disabilities* (pp. 157–171). Baltimore: Paul H. Brookes Publishing.

Reichle, J. & Wacker, D. P. (1993). *Communicative alternatives to challenging behavior: Integrating functional assessment and intervention strategies*. Baltimore: Paul H. Brookes Publishing.

Reichle, J., Williams, W., & Ryan, S. (1981). Selecting signs for the formulation of an augmentative communicative modality. *Journal of the Association for the Severely Handicapped, 6*, 48–56.

Reichle, J., & Yoder, D. (1985). Communication board use in severely handicapped learners. *Language, Speech, and Hearing Services in Schools, 16*, 146–157.

Reichle, J., York, J., & Sigafoos, J. (1991). *Implementing augmentative and alternative communication: Strategies for learners with severe disabilities*. Baltimore: Paul H. Brookes Publishing.

Reimbursing Adaptive Technology. (1989). *NARIC Quarterly, 2*, 1, 7–10, 17.

Remington, B. (1991a). Behaviour analysis and intervention in mental handicap: The dialogue between research and application. In B. Remington (Ed.), *The challenge of severe mental handicap: A behaviour analytic approach* (pp. 1–22). Chichester, England: Wiley & Sons.

Remington, B. (1991b). Why use single subject methods in AAC? In J. Brodin & E. Björck-Akesson (Eds.), *Methodological issues in research in augmentative and alternative communication: Proceedings of the first international ISAAC research symposium in augmentative and alternative communication* (pp. 74–78). Stockholm: Swedish Handicap Institute.

Remington, B. (1994). Augmentative and alternative communication and behavior analysis: A productive partnership? *Augmentative and Alternative Communication, 10*, 3–13.

Repp, A. C., Felce, D., & Barton, L. E. (1988). Basing the treatment of stereotypic and self-injurious behavior on hypotheses of their causes. *Journal of Applied Behavior Analysis, 21*, 281–289.

RESNA. (1991). *RESNA technical assistance project: Assistive technology—A funding workbook*. Washington, DC: RESNA Press.

RESNA. (1992). *Proceedings of the national planners conference on assistive device service delivery* (pp. 159, 161). Washington, DC: RESNA.

RESNA. (1993). *Code of ethics*. Arlington, VA: RESNA.

RESNA Technical Assistance Project. (1992). *Assistive technology and the individualized education program*. Washington, DC: Author (Reprinted by Indiana Department of Education in conjunction with ATTAIN Project).

Reuss, V. (1991). Die Akzeptanz von BLISS in der Umwelt. In H. Becker, M. Gangkofer, & E. Schroeder (Eds.), *Kommunizieren mit BLISS: Sprechen ueber BLISS: Dokumente der ersten Bremer BLISS-Tagung (Communicating with Bliss: Speaking about Bliss. Documents of the first Bremer Bliss conference)* (pp. 42–56). Bremen, Germany: Selbstverlag des Paritaetischen Bildungswerks.

RE:view (1994). Decrease in corporate giving. *RE:view, 23*,13.

Rewcastle, M. B. (1991). Degenerative diseases of the central nervous system. In R. L. Davis & D. M. Robertson (Eds.), *Textbook of neuropathology* (pp. 905–961). Baltimore: Williams & Wilkins.

Rice, M., & Schiefelbusch, R. L. (1989). *The teachability of language*. Baltimore: Paul H. Brookes Publishing.

Rice, R. (1989). Federal legislation and assistive technology. *NICHCY News Digest, 13*, 4–5.

Rimland, B., & Edelson, S. M. (1994). The effects of auditory integration training on autism. *American Journal of Speech-Language Pathology, 3*(2), 16–24.

Rincover, A., & Devany, J. (1982). The application of sensory extinction procedures to self-injury. *Analysis and Intervention in Developmental Disabilities, 2*, 67–81.

Ripich, D. (1994). Functional communication with AD patients: A caregiver training program. *Alzheimer Disease and Associated Disorders, 8*, 95–109.

Ripley, S. (1989). Starting the funding process. *NICHCY News Digest, 13*, 14–17.

Robinson, G. C., Jan, J. E., & Kinnis, C. (1987). Congenital ocular blindness in children, 1945–1984. *American Journal of Diseases of Childhood, 141*, 1321–1324.

Robinson, L. & Owens, R. (1995). Clinical notes: Functional augmentative communication and positive behavior change. *Augmentative and Alternative Communication, 11*, 207–211.

Roe, F. H. (1948, February). *The evolution of my walkie-talkie*. Lecture at the Parents Association for Spastic Children's Aid, Chicago, Illinois.

Rogan, P., Hagner, D., & Murphy, S. (1993). Natural supports: Reconceptualizing job coach roles. *Journal of the Association for Persons with Severe Handicaps, 18,* 275–281.

Rohner, T. (1966). *Fonetic English spelling.* Evanston, IL: Fonetic English Spelling Associates.

Romski, M. A. (1989). Two decades of language research with great apes. *Asha, 31,* 81–82.

Romski, M. A., & Sevcik, R. (1988a). Augmentative and alternative communication systems: Considerations for individuals with severe intellectual disabilities. *Augmentative and Alternative Communication, 4,* 83–93.

Romski, M. A., & Sevcik, R. A. (1988b, November). *Speech output communication systems: Acquisition/use by youngsters with retardation.* Seminar presented at the Annual Convention of the American Speech-Language-Hearing Association, Boston.

Romski, M. A., & Sevcik, R. (1989). An analysis of visual-graphic symbol meanings for two nonspeaking adults with severe mental retardation. *Augmentative and Alternative Communication, 5,* 109–114.

Romski, M. A., & Sevcik, R. (1992). Augmented language development in children with severe mental retardation. In S. Warren & J. Reichle (Eds.), *Causes and effects in communication and language intervention* (pp. 131–156). Baltimore: Paul H. Brookes Publishing.

Romski, M. A., & Sevcik, R. (1993a). Language comprehension: Considerations for augmentative and alternative communication. *Augmentative and Alternative Communication, 9,* 281–285.

Romski, M. A., & Sevcik, R. A. (1993b). Language learning through augmented means: The process and its products (pp. 85–104). In A. P. Kaiser & D. B. Gray (Eds.), *Enhancing children's communication: Research foundations for intervention.* Baltimore: Paul H. Brookes Publishing.

Romski, M. A., & Sevcik, R. A. (1996). *Breaking the speech barrier.* Baltimore: Paul H. Brookes Publishing.

Romski, M. A., Sevcik, R., & Joyner, S. E. (1984). Nonspeech communication systems: Implications for language intervention with mildly retarded children. *Topics in Language Disorders, 5,* 66–81.

Romski, M. A., Sevcik, R., & Pate, J. (1988). Establishment of symbolic communication in persons with severe retardation. *Journal of Speech and Hearing Disorders, 53,* 94–107.

Romski, M. A., Sevcik, R., Pate, J., & Rumbaugh, D. (1985). Discrimination of lexigrams and traditional orthography by nonspeaking severely mentally retarded persons. *American Journal of Mental Deficiency, 90,* 185–189.

Romski, M. A., Sevcik, R., Robinson, B., & Bakeman, R. (1994). Adult-directed communication of youth with mental retardation using the System for Augmenting Language. *Journal of Speech and Hearing Research, 37,* 617–628.

Romski, M. A., Sevcik, R., & Rumbaugh, D. (1985). Retention of symbolic communication skills by severely mentally retarded persons. *American Journal of Mental Deficiency, 89,* 441–444.

Romski, M. A., White, R. A., Millen, C. E., & Rumbaugh, D. (1984). Effects of computer keyboard teaching on the symbolic communication of severely retarded persons: Five case studies. *Psychological Record, 34,* 39–54.

Rosado, L. R. (1994). Promoting partnerships with minority parents: A revolution in today's school restructuring efforts. *Journal of Educational Issues of Language Minority Students, 14,* 241–254.

Rosch, W. (1989). The evolution of the PC microprocessor. *PC Magazine, 8,* 96–97.

Rosenberg, S., & Beukelman, D. (1988). The participation model. In C. A. Coston (Ed.), *Proceedings of the national planners conference on assistive device service delivery* (pp. 159–161). Washington, DC: RESNA and the Association for the Advancement of Rehabilitation Technology.

Rosenthal, J. L. (1993). Special problems of people with diabetes and visual impairment. *Journal of Visual Impairment & Blindness, 87,* 331–333.

Ross, A. J. (1979). A study of the application of Blissymbols as a means of communication for a young brain damaged adult. *British Journal of Disorders of Communication, 14,* 103–109.

Rotholz, D. A., Berkowitz, S. F., & Burberry, J. (1989). Functionality of two modes of communication in the community by students with developmental disabilities: A comparison of signing and communication books. *Journal of the Association for Persons with Severe Handicaps, 14,* 227–233.

Rothstein, L. F. (1994). *Special education law.* New York: Longman Press.

Rousseau, J. J. (1762/1979). *Emile* (A. Bloom, Trans.). New York: Basic Books.

Rowland, C. (1990). Communication in the classroom for children with dual sensory impairments: Studies of teacher and child behavior. *Augmentative and Alternative Communication, 6,* 262–274.

Rowland, C., & Schweigert, P. (1989a). Tangible symbols: Symbolic communication for individuals with multisensory impairments. *Augmentative and Alternative Communication, 5,* 226–234.

Rowland, C., & Schweigert, P. (1989b). *Tangible symbol systems for individuals with multisensory impairments* (videotape and manual). Tucson, AZ: Communication Skill Builders.

Rowland, C., & Schweigert, P. (1990). *Tangible symbol systems: Symbolic communication for individuals with multisensory impairments.* Tucson, AZ: Communication Skill Builders.

Rowland, C., & Stremel-Campbell, K. (1987). Share and share alike: Conventional gestures to emergent language for learners with dual sensory impairments. In L. Goetz, D. Guess, & K. Stremel-Campbell (Eds.), *Innovative program design for individuals with dual sensory impairments (pp. 49–75). Baltimore: Paul H. Brookes Publishing.

Rubino, F., Hayhurst, A., Guejlman, J., Madison, W., & Plum, O. (1975). *Gestuno: International sign language of the deaf.* Carlisle Island, UK: The British Deaf Association.

Rumbaugh, D. M. (Ed.). (1977). *Language learning by a chimpanzee: The LANA Project.* New York: Academic Press.

Rumbaugh, D. M., Gill, T. V., & vonGlasserfield, E. C. (1973). A rejoinder to language in man, monkeys, and machine. *Science, 185,* 871–872.

Rusch, F. R. (Ed.). (1990). *Supported employment: Models, methods, and issues.* Sycamore, IL: Sycamore Publishing.

Rusk, H., Block, J., & Lowman, E. (1969). Rehabilitation of the brain injured patient: A report of 157 cases with long term follow-up of 118. In E. Walker, W. Caveness, & M. Critchley (Eds.), *The late effects of head injury.* Springfield, IL: Charles C. Thomas.

Russell, S. C., & Kaderavek, J. N. (1993). Alternative models for collaboration. *Language, Speech and Hearing Services in Schools, 24,* 76–78.

Rutter, M. (1978). Diagnosis and definition. In M. Rutter & E. Schopler (Eds.), *Autism: A reappraisal of concepts and treatment* (pp. 1–25). New York: Plenum Press.

Rygaard, K. (1990). *Can new technology enhance communicative competence for a person with Broca's aphasia?* (English Translation). Unpublished master's thesis, Copenhagen University, Denmark.

Sabin, L. A., & Donnellan, A. M. (1993). A qualitative study of the process of facilitated communication. *Journal of the Association for Persons with Severe Handicaps, 18,* 200–211.

Sacks, H., Goren, L. & Burke, L. (1991). Ophthalmologic screening of adults with mental retardation. *American Journal on Mental Retardation, 95,* 571–574.

Sacks, S., & Young, E. C. (1982). *Infant scale of communicative intent.* Philadelphia, PA: St. Christopher's Hospital for Children.

Salmon, S. J., & Goldstein, L. P. (1989). *The artificial larynx handbook.* New York: Grune & Stratton.

Salzberg, C. L., Lignugaris/Kraft, B., & McCuller, G. L. (1988). Reasons for job loss: A review of employment termination studies of mentally retarded workers. *Research in Developmental Disabilities, 9,* 153–170.

Samuels, S. J. (1967). Attentional processes in reading: The effects of pictures on the acquisition of reading responses. *Journal of Educational Psychology, 58,* 337–342.

San Francisco Unified School District. EHLR 507:416 (CA SEA, 1985).

Sanders, D. A. (1971). *Aural rehabilitation.* Englewood Cliffs, NJ: Prentice-Hall.

Sanders, D. A. (1976). A model for communication. In L. L. Lloyd (Ed.), *Communication assessment and intervention strategies* (pp. 1–32). Baltimore: University Park Press.

Sanders, D. A. (1982). *Aural rehabilitation* (2nd ed.). Englewood Cliffs, NJ: Prentice-Hall.

Sarno, M. (1969). *The functional communication profile.* New York: Institute of Rehabilitation Medicine.

Sarno, M., Buonaguro, A., & Levita, E. (1986). Characteristics of verbal impairment in closed head injury patients. *Archives of Physical Medicine and Rehabilitation, 67,* 400–405.

Sasanuma, S. (1986). Universal and language-specific symptomatology and treatment of aphasia. *Folia Phoniatrica, 38,* 121–175.

Saunders, R. J., & Solman, R. R. (1984). The effect of pictures on the acquisition of a small vocabulary of similar sight-words. *British Journal of Educational Psychology, 54,* 265–275.

Savage, R. D., Evans, L., & Savage, J. F. (1981). *Psychology and communication in deaf children.* Sydney: Grune & Stratton.

Saville-Troike, M. (1989). *The ethnography of communication: An introduction* (2nd ed.). Oxford, UK: Basil Blackwell.

Sawyer-Woods, L. (1987). Symbolic function in a severe nonverbal aphasic. *Aphasiology, 1,* 287–290.

Saya, M. (1979, November). *Adult aphasics and the Bliss symbol language.* Paper presented at the Annual Convention of the American Speech-Language-Hearing Association, Atlanta, GA.

Saylor, W., & Mix, B. J. (1975). *TARC assessment inventory for severely handicapped children.* Topeka, KS: Topeka Association for Retarded Citizens.

Scarborough, H. (1990, September). *Antecedents to reading disability: Preschool language development and literacy experiences of children from dyslexic families.* Presentation at the Boulder Rodin Conference, Boulder, CO.

Schaeffer, B., McDowell, P., Musil, A., & Kollinzas, G. (1976). Spontaneous verbal language for autistic children through signed speech. In *Research relating to children bulletin 37* (ERIC Clearinghouse for Early Childhood Education), pp. 98–99.

Scheerenberger, R. C. (1987). *A history of mental retardation: A quarter century of promise.* Baltimore: Paul H. Brookes Publishing.

Schepis, M. M., & Reid, D. H. (1995). The effects of a voice output communication aid on interactions between support personnel and an individual with multiple disabilities. *Journal of Applied Behavior Analysis, 28,* 73–77.

Schermer, G. (1990). *In search of a language: Influences from spoken Dutch on sign language of the Netherlands.* Delft, The Netherlands: Eburon.

Schermer, T., Fortgens, C., Harder, R., & de Nobel, E. (Eds.). (1991). *De Nederlandse Gebarentaal (Sign language of the Netherlands).* Amsterdam: Nederlandse Stichting voor het Dove en Slechthorende Kind (Dutch Foundation for the Deaf and Hearing Impaired Child).

Schlanger, P. H. (1976, November). *Training the adult aphasic to pantomime.* Paper presented at the 51st Annual Convention of the American Speech and Hearing Association, Chicago.

Schlinger, H. D. (1992). Theory in behavior analysis: An application to child development. *American Psychologist, 47,* 1396–1410.

Schlosser, R. W. (1993a, November). *Nomenclature and category levels in graphic AAC symbol sets and symbols.* Paper presented at the Annual Convention of the American Speech-Language-Hearing Association, San Antonio, TX.

Schlosser, R. W. (1993b, November). *Staff perspectives on the self-injurious behavior of a person with profound mental retardation.* Poster presented at the Annual Meeting of the Association for Persons with Severe Handicaps, Chicago.

Schlosser, R. W. (1995). Effectiveness of three teaching strategies on Blissymbol learning, retention, generalization, and use. (Doctoral dissertation, Purdue University, West Lafayette, IN, 1994). *Dissertation Abstracts International, 56,* (03) 892A.

Schlosser, R. W. (1997a). Nomenclature and category levels in graphic AAC symbols. Part I: Is a flower a flower a flower? *Augmentative and Alternative Communication, 13,* 4–13.

Schlosser, R. W. (1997b). Nomenclature of category levels in graphic AAC symbols. Part II: Role of similarity in categorization. *Augmentative and Alternative Communication, 13,* 14–19.

Schlosser, R. W., Belfiore, P. J., Blischak, D., Nigam, R., & Hetzroni, O. (1993, May). *Effectiveness and efficiency of voice output on symbol acquisition and maintenance.* Poster presented at the Annual Convention of the Association of Behavior Analysis, Chicago.

Schlosser, R. W., Belfiore, P. J., Nigam, R., Blischak, D., & Hetzroni, O. (1995). The effects of speech output technology in the learning of graphic symbols. *Journal of Applied Behavior Analysis, 28,* 537–549.

Schlosser, R. W., Blischak, D. M., Belfiore, P. J., Bartley, C., & Barnett, N. (in press). The effects of synthetic speech output and orthographic feedback in a student with autism: A preliminary study. *Journal of Autism and Developmental Disorders.*

Schlosser, R. W., & Goetze, H. (1991). Selbstverletzendes verhalten bei kindern und jugendlichen mit geistiger behinderung: Eine meta-analyse zur effektivität von interventionen. (Self-injurious behavior in children and adolescents with mental retardation: A meta-analysis of effectiveness of intervention). *Sonderpädagogik, 21,* 138–154.

Schlosser, R. W., & Goetze, H. (1992). Effectiveness and treatment validity of interventions addressing self-injurious behavior: From narrative reviews to meta-analyses. In T. E. Scruggs & M. A. Mastropieri (Eds.), *Advances in learning and behavioral disabilities* (Vol. 7, pp. 135–175). Greenwich, CT: JAI Press.

Schlosser, R. W., & Karlan, G. R. (1994). *Role of qualitative assessment and multimodality in functional communication training: A case study.* Unpublished manuscript, University of Oklahoma Health Sciences, Oklahoma City.

Schlosser, R. W., & Lloyd, L. L. (1993a, June). *An organizational framework to graphic AAC symbol research.* Paper presented at the Annual Conference of the American Association on Mental Retardation, Washington, DC.

Schlosser, R. W., & Lloyd, L. L. (1993b). Effects of initial element teaching in a storytelling context on Blissymbol acquisition and generalization. *Journal of Speech and Hearing Research, 36,* 979–995.

Schlosser, R. W., & Lloyd, L. L. (in press). Effects of paired-associated learning versus symbol explanations on Blissymbol comprehension and production. *Augmentative and Alternative Communication.*

Schlosser, R. W., Lloyd, L. L., & McNaughton, S. (1997). Graphic symbol selection in research and practice: Making the case for a goal driven process. In E. Bjorck-Akesson & P. Lindsay (Eds.), *Theoretical and methodological issues in augmentative and alternative communication: Proceedings of the fourth ISAAC research symposium, Vancouver, Canada, August 11–12, 1996.* Vasteras, Sweden: Malardalen University Press.

Schlosser, R. W., Lloyd, L. L., & Quist, R. (1991, November). *Effects of initial element teaching on Blissymbol learning and generalization.* Paper presented at the Annual Convention of the American Speech-Language-Hearing Association, Atlanta, GA.

Schmidt, M. J., Carrier, Jr., J. K., & Parsons, S. D. (1971, November). *Use of a nonspeech mode in teaching language.* Paper presented at the 46th Annual Convention of the American Speech and Hearing Association, Chicago.

Schoenberg, B. S. (1987). Environmental risk factors for Parkinson's disease: The epidemiologic evidence. *Canadian Journal of Neurological Sciences, 14,* 407–413.

Schonell, F. (1956). *Educating spastic children: The education and guidance of the cerebral palsied.* London: Oliver and Boyd.

Schow, R. L., & Nerbonne, M. A. (Eds.). (1989). *Introduction to aural rehabilitation.* Austin, TX: Pro-Ed.

Schrag, J. (1993). Policy letter. *Project ACTT: Funding technology for young children.* Macomb, IL: Western Illinois University.

Schuell, H. M. (1965). *The Minnesota test for differential diagnosis of aphasia.* Minneapolis, MN: University of Minnesota Press.

Schuler, A. L., Peck, C. A., Willard, C., & Theimer, K. (1989). Assessment of communicative means and functions through interview: Assessing the communicative abilities of individuals with limited language. *Seminars in Speech and Language, 10,* 51–62.

Schulte-Sasse, H. (1991). Lesen und BLISS: Frau S. lernt lesen (Reading and Bliss: Mrs. S. learns how to read). In H. Becker, M. Gangkofer, & E. Schroeder (Eds.), *Kommunizieren mit BLISS: Sprechen ueber BLISS: Dokumente der ersten Bremer BLISS-Tagung (Communicating with Bliss: Speaking about Bliss. Documents of the first Bremer Bliss conference)* (pp. 42–56). Bremen, Germany: Selbstverlag des Paritaetischen Bildungswerks.

Schure, A. (1961). *Basic transistor.* New York: J. F. Rider.

Schweigert, P. (1989). Use of microswitch technology to facilitate social contingency awareness as a basis for early communication skills. *Augmentative and Alternative Communication, 5,* 192–198.

Schweigert, P., & Rowland, C. (1992). Early communication and microtechnology: Instructional sequence and case studies of children with severe multiple disabilities. *Augmentative and Alternative Communication, 8,* 273–286.

Schweijda, P., & Vanderheiden, G. (1982). Adaptive firmware card for the Apple II. *Byte, 7*(9), 276–314.

Scouten, E. L. (1984). *Turning points in the education of deaf people.* Danville, IL: Interstate Printers & Publishers.

Section 504 Manual: A comprehensive manual for Indiana educators on Section 504 of the Rehabilitation Act of 1973 (Oct., 1992). Ch. 1, Summary of Section 504, p. 1.

Seidel, U., Chadwick, O., & Rutter, M. (1975). Psychological disorders in crippled children. A comparative study of children with and without brain damage. *Developmental Medicine and Child Neurology, 17,* 563–573.

Seligman, J. (1992). Horror story or big hoax: A new technique gives voice to abuse charges (facilitated communication for cognitively impaired). *Newsweek, 120*(12), 75–78.

Seligman-Wine, J. (1988). A Blissymbol bar mitzvah. *Communicating Together, 6,* 16–17.

Sellars, C. W., & Vegter, C. H. (1993). *Pediatric brain injury: A practical resource.* Tucson, AZ: Communication Skill Builders.

Sents, B., & Marks, H. (1988). Changes in preschool children's IQ scores as a function of positioning. *American Journal of Occupational Therapy, 43,* 685–687.

Sevcik, R., & Romski, M. A. (1984, November). *Group instruction: A viable communication approach to severely retarded persons.* Paper presented at the Annual Convention of the American Speech-Language-Hearing Association, San Francisco.

Sevcik, R., & Romski, M. A. (1986). Representational matching skills of persons with severe retardation. *Augmentative and Alternative Communication, 2,* 160–164.

Sevcik, R., Romski, M. A., & Wilkinson, K. M. (1991). Role of graphic symbols in the language acquisition process for persons with severe cognitive disabilities. *Augmentative and Alternative Communication, 7,* 161–170.

Seyfried, D. N, Hutchinson, J., & Smith, L. (1989). Language and speech of the hearing impaired. In R. Schow & M. Nerbonne (Eds.), *Introduction to aural rehabilitation* (pp. 181–239). Austin, TX: Pro-Ed.

Shalit, A., & Boonzaier, D. (1990). Macintosh™ based semantographic technique with adaptive-predictive algorithm for Blissymbolics communication. *Augmentative and Alternative Communication, 6,* 129. (Abstract)

Shane, H. C. (1986). Goals and uses. In S. Blackstone (Ed.), *Augmentative communication: An introduction* (pp. 29–48). Rockville, MD: American Speech-Language-Hearing Association.

Shane, H. C. (1993). F.C.: Facilitated or 'factitious' communication. *Communicating Together, 11*(2), 11–13.

Shane, H. C. (Ed.) (1994). *Facilitated communication: The clinical and social phenomenon.* San Diego, CA: Singular Publishing Group.

Shane, H. C., & Bashir, A. S. (1980). Election criteria for the adoption of an augmentative communication system: Preliminary considerations. *Journal of Speech and Hearing Disorders, 45,* 408–414.

Shane, H. C., & Kearns, K. (1994). An examination of the role of the facilitator in facilitated communication. *American Journal of Speech-Language Pathology, 3,* 48–54.

Shane, H. C., & Sauer, M. (1986). *Augmentative communication.* Austin, TX: Pro-Ed.

Shane, H. C., & Wilbur, R. (1989, November). *A conceptual framework for an AAC strategy based on sign language parameters.* Paper presented at the Annual Convention of the American Speech-Language-Hearing Association, St. Louis.

Shankweiler, D., & Crain, S. (1986). Language mechanisms and reading disorder: A modular approach. *Status Report on Speech Research* (pp. 86–87). New Haven, CT: Haskins Laboratories.

Shannon, C. E., & Weaver, W. W. (1949). *The mathematical theory of communication.* Urbana, IL: University of Illinois.

Shapiro, J. P. (1992). See me, hear me, touch me (facilitated communication for autistic people). *U.S. News & World Report, 113*(4), 63–64.

Shewan, C., & Blake, A. (1991). 1990 Omnibus survey: Augmentative and alternative communication. *Asha, 31,* 46.

Shipley, K. G., & McAfee, J. G. (1992). *Assessment in speech-language pathology: A resource manual.* San Diego, CA: Singular Publishing Group.

Shockley, W. (1950). *Electrons and holes in semiconductors with applications to transistor electronics.* New York: Van Nostrand.

Shodell, M. J., & Reiter, H. H. (1968). Self-mutilative behavior in verbal and nonverbal schizophrenic children. *Archives of General Psychiatry, 19,* 453–455.

Shumway-Cook, A., & Woollacott, M. (1993). Theoretical issues in assessing postural control. In I. J. Wilhelm (Ed.), *Physical therapy assessment in early infancy* (pp. 161–171). New York: Churchill Livingstone.

Sidman, M. (1971). Reading and auditory-visual equivalences. *Journal of Speech and Hearing Research, 14,* 5–13.

Sidman, M. (1986). Functional analysis of emergent verbal classes. In T. Thompson & M. D. Zeiler (Eds.), *Analysis and integration of behavioral units* (pp. 213–245). Hillsdale, NJ: Lawrence Erlbaum & Associates.

Sidman, M., & Cresson, O., Jr. (1973). Reading and cross-modal transfer of stimulus equivalences in severe retardation. *American Journal of Mental Deficiency, 77,* 515–523.

Sidman, M., & Tailby, W. (1982). Conditional discrimination versus matching-to-sample: An expansion of the testing paradigm. *Journal of the Experimental Analysis of Behavior, 37,* 5–22.

Siegel-Causey, E., & Guess, D. (1989). *Enhancing nonsymbolic communication interactions among learners with severe disabilities.* Baltimore: Paul H. Brookes Publishing.

Sienkiewicz-Mercer, R. (1995, June). *Acceptance: Key to the future*. Plenary session presented at the 119th Annual Meeting of the American Association on Mental Retardation, San Francisco.

Sienkiewicz-Mercer, R., & Kaplan, A. B. (1989). *I raise my eyes to say yes*. Hartford, CT: Whole Health Books.

Sigafoos, J., Doss, S., & Reichle, J. (1989). Developing mand and tact repertoires in persons with severe developmental disabilities using graphic symbols. *Research in Developmental Disabilities, 10*, 183–200.

Sigafoos, J., Mustonen, T., DePaepe, P., Reichle, J. & York, J. (1991). Defining the array of instructional prompts for teaching communication skills. In J. Reichle, J. York, & J. Sigafoos (Eds.), *Implementing augmentative and alternative communication: Strategies for learners with severe disabilities* (pp. 173–192). Baltimore: Paul H. Brookes Publishing.

Sigafoos, J., & York, J. (1991). Using ecological inventories to promote functional communication. In J. Reichle, J. York, & J. Sigafoos (Eds.), *Implementing augmentative and alternative communication: Strategies for learners with severe disabilities* (pp. 61–70). Baltimore: Paul H. Brookes Publishing.

Sigurdardottir, Z. G., Green, G., & Saunders, R. R. (1990). Equivalence classes generated by sequence training. *Journal of the Experimental Analysis of Behavior, 53*, 47–63.

Silliman, E. R. (1992). Three perspectives of facilitated communication: Unexpected literacy. Clever Hans, or enigma? *Topics in Language Disorders, 12*, 60–68.

Silva, P., Williams, S., & McGee, R. (1987). A longitudinal study of children with developmental language delay at age 3: Later intelligence, reading and behaviour problems. *Developmental Medicine and Child Neurology, 29*, 630–640.

Silverman, F. H. (1980). *Communication for the speechless*. Englewood Cliffs, NJ: Prentice Hall.

Silverman, F. H. (1989). *Communication for the speechless* (2nd ed.). Englewood Cliffs, NJ: Prentice Hall.

Silverman, F. H. (1994). Can AAC help persons with dementia? *Augmentative and Alternative Communication, 10*, 60.

Silverman, F. H. (1995). *Communication for the speechless* (3rd ed.). Boston, MA: Allyn & Bacon.

Silverman, H., McNaughton, S., & Kates, B. (1978). *Handbook of Blissymbolics*. Toronto: Blissymbolics Communication Institute.

Singh, N. N., Donatelli, L. S., Best, A., Williams, D. E., Barrera, F. J., Lenz, M. W., Landrum, T. J., Ellis, C. R., & Moe, T. L. (1993). Factor structure of the Motivation Assessment Scale. *Journal of Intellectual Disability Research, 37*, 65–74.

Singh, N. N., & Solman, R. T. (1990). A stimulus control analysis of the picture-word problem in children who are mentally retarded: The blocking effect. *Journal of Applied Behavior Analysis, 23*, 525–532.

Siple, P. (Ed.). (1978). *Understanding language through sign language research*. New York: Academic Press.

Siple, P., & Fischer, S. (Eds.). (1991). *Theoretical issues in sign language research. Vol. 2: Psychology*. Chicago: University of Chicago Press.

Skelly, M. (1979). *Amer-Ind gestural code based on universal American Indian hand talk*. New York: Elsevier.

Skelly, M., Schinsky, L., Smith, R., & Fust, R. (1974). American Indian sign (Amerind) as a facilitator of verbalization in the oral apraxic. *Journal of Speech and Hearing Disorders, 39*, 445–456.

Skinner, B. F. (1938). *The behavior of organisms*. New York: Appleton-Century-Crofts.

Skinner, B. F. (1957). *Verbal behavior*. New York: Appleton-Century-Crofts.

Skinner, B. F. (1969). *Contingencies of reinforcement: A theoretical analysis*. New York: Appleton-Century-Crofts.

Skinner, B. F. (1974). *About behaviorism*. New York: Knopf.

Skinner, B. F. (1989). The behavior of the listener. In S. C. Hayes (Ed.), *Rule-governed behavior: Cognition, contingencies, and instructional control* (pp. 85–96). New York: Plenum Press.

Sklar, M., & Bennett, D. (1956). Initial communication chart for aphasics. *Journal of the Association of Physical and Mental Rehabilitation, 10*, 43–53.

Smedley, T., & Plapinger, D. (1988). The nonfunctioning hearing aid: A case of double jeopardy. *The Volta Review, 90*, 77–84.

Smith, D. E. P., Miller, S., Stewart, M., Walter, T. L., & McConnell, J. V. (1988). Conductive hearing loss in autistic, learning-disabled, and normal children. *Journal of Autism and Developmental Disorders, 18*, 53–65.

Smith, F. (1982). *Understanding reading: A psycholinguistic analysis of reading and learning to read*. London: Holt, Rinehart and Winston.

Smith, M. M. (1989). Reading without speech: A study of children with cerebral palsy. *Irish Journal of Psychology, 10*, 601–614.

Smith, M. M. (1990). *School experiences of nonspeaking cerebral palsied children: Reading abilities and social interaction patterns*. Unpublished MSc thesis, Dublin University, Trinity College, Ireland.

Smith, M. M. (1991). Assessment of interaction patterns and AAC use: A case study. *Journal of Clinical Speech and Language Studies, 1*(1), 76–102.

Smith, M. M. (1992). Reading abilities of non-speaking students: Two case studies. *Augmentative and Alternative Communication, 8*, 57–66.

Smith, M. M. (1994, July). *Comprehension of graphic vs. verbal signs in two children with severe speech and physical impairments*. Presentation at 23rd International Congress of Applied Psychology, Madrid.

Smith-Lewis, M. (1994). Discontinuity in the development of aided augmentative and alternative communication systems. *Augmentative and Alternative Communication, 10*, 14–26.

Smith-Lewis, M., & Ford, A. (1987). A user's perspective on augmentative communication. *Augmentative and Alternative Communication, 3*, 12–17.

Snell, M. E., & Zirpoli, T. J. (1987). Intervention strategies. In M. E. Snell (Ed.), *Systematic instruction of persons with severe handicaps* (3rd ed., pp. 110–149). Columbus, OH: Charles E. Merrill.

Snidecor, J. C. (1962). *Speech rehabilitation of the laryngectomized.* Springfield, IL: Charles C. Thomas.

Snow, C. E., & Ferguson, C. A. (1977). *Talking to children: Language input and acquisition.* Cambridge, England: Cambridge University Press.

Snyder, L., & Downey D. (1991). The language-reading relationship in normal and reading-disabled children. *Journal of Speech and Hearing Research, 34,* 129–140.

Snyder-McLean, L. (1978, November). *Functional stimulus and response variables in sign training with retarded subjects.* Paper presented at the Annual Convention of the American Speech-Language-Hearing Association, San Francisco.

Snyder-McLean, L., McLean, J. F., & Etter, R. (1988). Clinical assessment of sensorimotor knowledge in nonverbal, severely retarded clients. *Topics in Language Disorders, 8*(4), 1–22.

Sobsey, D., & Wolf-Schein, E. G. (1991). Sensory impairments. In F. P. Orelove & D. Sobsey (Eds.), *Educating children with multiple disabilities: A transdisciplinary approach* (pp. 119–154). Baltimore: Paul H. Brookes Publishing.

Solomon, D. H. (1988). Geriatric assessment: Methods for clinical decision making. *Journal of the American Medical Association, 16,* 2450–2452.

Song, A. (1979). Acquisition and use of Blissymbols by severely mentally retarded adolescents. *Mental Retardation, 17,* 253–255.

Sonksen, P. M., Petrie, A., & Drew, K. J. (1991). Promotion of visual development of severely visually impaired babies. *Developmental Medicine and Child Neurology, 33,* 320–335.

Sosner, J., Wall, G. C., & Sznajder, J. (1993). Progressive supranuclear palsy: Clinical presentation and rehabilitation of two patients. *Archives of Physical Medicine and Rehabilitation, 74,* 537–539.

Soto, G. (1994, November). *Multicultural issues in AAC: Working with Hispanic clients.* A miniseminar at the Annual Convention of the American Speech-Language-Hearing Association, New Orleans.

Soto, G. (1995, March). *AAC intervention and maintenance with Hispanic and other culturally diverse clients.* Presentation at the Workshop on Multicultural Issues in Augmentative and Alternative Communication, Howard University, Washington, DC.

Soto, G., Belfiore, P. J., Schlosser, R. W., & Haynes, C. (1993). Teaching specific requests: A comparative analysis on skill acquisition and preference using two augmentative and alternative communication aids. *Education and Training in Mental Retardation, 28,* 169–178.

Spensley, S. (1989). Psychodynamically oriented psychotherapy in autism. In C. Gillberg (Ed.), *Diagnosis and treatment of autism* (pp. 237–250). New York: Plenum Press.

Sperber, D., & Wilson, D. (1986). *Relevance, communication and cognition.* Oxford, England: Blackwell.

Spiegel, B., Benjamin, B. J., & Spiegel, S. (1993). One method to increase spontaneous use of an assistive communication device: A case study. *Augmentative and Alternative Communication, 9,* 111–117.

Spradlin, J. E., Karlan, G. R., & Wetherby, B. (1976). Behavior analysis, behavior modification, and developmental disabilities. In L. L. Lloyd (Ed.), *Communication assessment and intervention strategies* (pp. 225–263). Baltimore: University Park Press.

Spragale, D., & Micucci, D. (1990). Signs of the week: A functional approach to manual sign training. *Augmentative and Alternative Communication, 6,* 29–37.

Stainback, S., & Stainback, W. (1985). *Integration of students with severe handicaps into regular schools.* Reston, VA: The Council for Exceptional Children.

Stainback, S., & Stainback, W. (Eds.). (1992). *Curriculum considerations in inclusive classrooms: Facilitating learning for all students.* Baltimore: Paul H. Brookes Publishing.

Stainback, S., & Stainback, W. (Eds.). (1996). *Inclusion: A guide for educators.* Baltimore: Paul H. Brookes Publishing.

Stanovich, K. (1986). Matthew effects in reading: Some consequences of individual differences in the acquisition of literacy. *Reading Research Quarterly, 21,* 360–407.

Steege, M. W., Wacker, D. P., Berg, W. K., Cigrand, K. K., & Cooper L. L. (1989). The use of behavioral assessment to prescribe and evaluate treatments for severely handicapped children. *Journal of Applied Behavior Analysis, 22,* 23–33.

Steege, M. W., Wacker, D. P., Cigrand, K. C., Berg, W. K., Novak, C. G., Reimers, T. M., Sasso, G. M., & DeRaad, A. (1990). Use of negative reinforcement in the treatment of self-injurious behavior. *Journal of Applied Behavior Analysis, 23,* 459–467.

Steele, R., Illes, J., Weinrich, M., & Lakin, F. (1985). Toward computer-aided visual communication for aphasia: Report of studies. In *Proceedings of the eighth annual RESNA conference.* Reston, VA: RESNA.

Steele, R., Weinrich, M., Wertz, R., Kleczewska, M, & Carlson, G. (1989). Computer-based visual communication in aphasia. *Neuropsychologia, 27,* 409–426.

Steelman, J. D. (1992, August). *Project TILLT: Technology, Interaction, Literacy Learning and Teaching.* Presentation at the Fifth Biennial Conference of the International Society for Augmentative and Alternative Communication, Philadelphia.

Steelman, J. D., Pierce, P. L., & Koppenhaver, D. A. (1993). The role of computers in promoting literacy in children with severe speech and physical impairments (SSPI). *Topics in Language Disorders, 13*(2), 76–88.

Sternberg, L., Ehren, B., Lefferts, L., & Eloranta, R. (1988). Assessing non-linguistic communication skills of students with severe or profound handicaps: Toward a research agenda. *Journal of Childhood Communication Disorders, 11*(2), 275–286.

Sternberg, M. L. (1980). *American Sign Language concise dictionary*. New York: Harper & Row.

Stevens, K. N., & House, A. S. (1955). Development of a quantitative description of vowel articulation. *Journal of the Acoustical Society of America, 27*, 484–493.

Stevens, K. N., & House, A. S. (1961). An acoustical theory of vowel production and some of its implications. *Journal of Speech and Hearing Research, 4*, 303–320.

Stevenson, J., & Richman, N. (1978). Behavior, language, and development in three-year-old children. *Journal of Autism and Childhood Schizophrenia, 8*, 299–313.

Stokoe, W. (1960). *Sign language structure: An outline of the visual communication system of the American deaf*. Washington, DC: Gallaudet College Press.

Stokoe, W. (1969). Sign language diglossia. *Studies in Linguistics, 21*, 27–41.

Stromer, R., & Mackay, H. A. (1993). Human sequential behavior, relations among stimuli, class formation, and derived sequences. *Psychological Record, 43*, 107–131.

Stuart, S., Vanderhoof, D., & Beukelman, D. (1993). Topic and vocabulary use patterns of elderly women. *Augmentative and Alternative Communication, 9*, 95–105.

Sudler, W. H., & Flexer, C. (1986). Low cost assistive listening device. *Language, Speech, and Hearing Services in Schools, 17*, 342–344.

Sue, D. (1981). *Counseling the culturally different: Theory and practice*. New York: John Wiley.

Sugishita, M., Iwata, M., Toyokura, Y., Yoshioka, M., & Yamada, R. (1978). Reading of ideograms and phonograms in Japanese patients after partial commissurotomy. *Neuropsychologia, 16*, 417–426.

Supalla, S. (1991). Manually coded English: The modality question in signed language development. In P. Siple & S. Fischer (Eds.), *Theoretical issues in sign language research. Vol. 2: Psychology* (pp. 85–109). Chicago: University of Chicago Press.

Suter, S. S. (1990). Foreword. In F. R. Rusch (Ed.), *Supported employment: Models, methods, and issues* (p. xiii). Sycamore, IL: Sycamore Publishing Company.

Sutton, V. (1981). *Sign writing for everyday use*. Newport Beach, CA: The Center for Movement Writing.

Swartz, S. (1984). Blissymbols go to India. *Communicating Together, 2*, 4–6.

Sweet, H. (1874, rev. 1888). *Handbook of phonetics*. Oxford, England: Clarendon Press.

Sweet, H. (1890). *A primer of phonetics*. Oxford, England: Clarendon Press.

Szempruch, J., & Jacobson, J. W. (1993). Evaluating facilitated communications of people with developmental disabilities. *Research in Developmental Disabilities, 14*, 253–264.

Tabe, N., & Jackson, M. (1989). Teaching sight word vocabulary to children with developmental disabilities. *Australia and New Zealand Journal of Developmental Disabilities, 15*, 27–39.

Talkington, L. W., Hall, S., & Altman, R. (1971). Communication deficits and aggression in the mentally retarded. *American Journal of Mental Deficiency, 76*, 235–237.

Tandan, R., & Bradley, B. (1985). Amyotrophic lateral sclerosis: Part 1. Clinical features, pathology, and ethical issues in management. *Annals of Neurology, 18*, 271–280.

Tardieu, C., Lespargot, A., Tabary, C., & Bret, M. D. (1988). For how long must the soleus muscle be stretched each day to prevent contracture? *Developmental Medicine and Child Neurology, 30*, 3–10.

Tavernier, G. G. F. (1993). The improvement of vision by vision stimulation and training: A review of the literature. *Journal of Visual Impairment & Blindness, 87*, 143–148.

Taylor, D., & Strickland, D. S. (1986). *Family storybook reading*. Portsmouth, NH: Heinemann Books.

Taylor, J. (1992). *Speech-language pathology: Services in the schools* (2nd ed.). Boston: Allyn & Bacon.

Taylor, O. L. (1986). *Nature of communication disorders in culturally and linguistically diverse populations*. San Diego, CA: College-Hill Press.

Taylor, O. L. (1989). Clinical practice as a social occasion. In L. Cole & V. R. Deal (Eds.), *Communication disorders in multicultural populations*. Rockville, MD: American Speech-Language-Hearing Association.

Taylor, O. L. (1994). Communication and communication disorders in a multicultural society. In F. D. Minifie (Ed.), *Introduction to communication sciences and disorders* (pp. 43–76). San Diego, CA: Singular Publishing Group.

Taylor, O. L., & Clarke, M. G. (1994). Culture and communication disorders: A theoretical framework. *Seminars in Speech and Language, 15*, 103–114.

Taylor, O. L., & Payne, K. T. (1983). Culturally valid testing: A proactive approach. *Topics in Language Disorders, 3*, 8–20.

Teale, W., & Sulzby, E. (1987). Literacy acquisition in early childhood: The roles of access and mediation in storybook telling. In D. A. Wagner (Ed.), *The future of literacy in a changing world* (pp. 111–130). New York: Pergamon Press.

Teale, W., & Sulzby, E. (1989). Emergent literacy: New perspectives on young children's reading and writing. In D. S. Strickland & L. M. Morrow (Eds.), *Emerging literacy: Young children learn to read and write* (pp. 1–15). Newark, DE: International Reading Association.

Terman, L. M., & Merrill, M. A. (1973). *Manual for the third revision (form L-M) of the Stanford-Binet intelligence scale*. Boston: Houghton-Mifflin.

Tervoort, B. T. (1984). Onderzoek naar een universele gebarentaal (Looking for a universal sign language). In R. Stes & R. Elen (Eds.), *Proceedings of the International Congress on Logopedics* (pp. 32–47). Antwerpen, Belgium: Katholieke Vlaamse Hogeschool.

Tervoort, B. T. (Ed.). (1986). *Signs of life: Proceedings of the second European congress on sign language research*. Amsterdam, The Netherlands: University of Amsterdam.

Test, D. W., Hinson, K. B., Solow, J., & Keul, P. (1993). Job satisfaction of persons in supported employment. *Education and Training in Mental Retardation, 28,* 38–46.

Thal, D. J., & Tobias, S. (1992). Communicative gestures in children with delayed onset of oral expressive vocabulary. *Journal of Speech and Hearing Research, 35,* 1281–1289.

Thompson, B., & Guess, D. (1989). Students who experience the most profound disabilities: Teacher perspectives. In F. Brown & D. H. Lehr (Eds.), *Persons with profound disabilities: Issues and practices* (pp. 3–41). Baltimore: Paul H. Brookes Publishing.

Thompson, L., Powers, G., & Houchard, B. (1992). The wage effects of supported employment. *Journal of the Association for Persons with Severe Handicaps, 17,* 87–94.

Thompson, T. (1993). A reign of error: Facilitated communication. *Vanderbilt University Kennedy Center News, 22,* 3–5.

Thousand, J. S., Villa, R. A., & Nevin, A. (Eds.). (1994). *Creativity and collaborative learning: A practical guide to empowering students and teachers.* Baltimore: Paul H. Brookes Publishing.

Thurman, S. K., & Widerstrom, A. H. (1990). *Infants and young children with special needs.* Baltimore: Paul H. Brookes Publishing.

Time-Life Books. (1985). *Understanding computers: Computer basics.* Alexandria, VA: Time-Life, Inc.

Timothy W. v. Rochester, New Hampshire School District. 875 F.2d 954 cert. den. 110 S. Ct. 519 (1st Cir., 1989).

Tomblin, J. B. (1994). Perspectives on diagnosis. In J. B. Tomblin, H. L. Morris, & D. C. Spriestersbach (Eds.), *Diagnosis in speech-language pathology.* San Diego, CA: Singular Publishing Group.

Tomkins, W. (1969). *Indian Sign Language.* New York: Dover Publications.

Tomoeda, C., & Bayles, K. (1990). The efficacy of speech-language pathology intervention: Dementia. *Seminars in Speech and Language, 11,* 311–319.

Touchette, P. E., MacDonald, R. F., & Langer, S. N. (1985). A scatter plot for identifying stimulus control of problem behavior. *Journal of Applied Behavior Analysis, 18,* 343–351.

Toulotte, J., Baudel-Cantgrit, B., & Trehou, G. (1990). Acceleration method using a dictionary access in a Blissymbolics communicator. *Augmentative and Alternative Communication, 6,* 122. (Abstract)

Trachtman, L. (1994). Tech Act reauthorization: Who wins? Who loses? (Editorial) *Assistive Technology, 6,* 1–2.

Trefler, E., Hobson, D. A., Taylor, S. J., Monahan, L. C., & Shaw, C. G. (1993). *Seating and mobility for persons with physical disabilities.* Tucson, AZ: Therapy Skill Builders.

Treviranus, J. (1994). Mastering alternative computer access: The role of understanding, trust, and automaticity. *Assistive Technology, 6,* 26–41.

Trief, E., Duckman, R., Morse, A. R., & Silberman, R. K. (1989). Retinopathy of prematurity. *Journal of Visual Impairment & Blindness, 83,* 500–504.

Trief, E., & Morse, A. R. (1988). Strabismus and amblyopia. *Journal of Visual Impairment & Blindness, 82,* 327–330.

Tronconi, A. (1990). Blissymbolics-based telecommunications. *Communication Outlook, 11,* 8–11.

Trunzo-Rahbar M. J. (1980). *Assessment of the Bliss symbol communication system in adult aphasics with severe oral and verbal apraxia.* Unpublished master's thesis, Wichita State University, Wichita, KS.

Tunmer, W. E., Herriman, M. L, & Nesdale, A. R. (1988). Metalinguistic abilities and beginning reading. *Reading Research Quarterly, 23,* 134–158.

Turnbull, H. R. (1993). *Free appropriate public education: The law and children with disabilities.* Denver, CO: Love Publishing.

Udwin, O., & Yule, W. (1990). Augmentative communication systems taught to cerebral palsy children—a longitudinal study. 1: The acquisition of signs and symbols and syntactic aspects of their use over time. *British Journal of Disorders of Communication, 25,* 295–309.

Ulatowska, H. K., Hayashi, M. M., Cannito, M. P. & Fleming, S. G. (1986). Disruption of reference in aging. *Brain and Language, 28,* 24–41.

United Nations. (1971). *Declaration of general and specific rights of the mentally retarded.* New York: Author.

Uslan, M. M. (1992). Barriers to acquiring assistive technology: Cost and lack of information. *Journal of Visual Impairment & Blindness, 86,* 402–407.

Uzgiris, I. C., & Hunt, J. M. (1975). *Assessment in infancy: Ordinal scales of psychological development.* Urbana, IL: University of Illinois Press.

Valentic, V. (1991). Successful integration from a student's perspective. *Communicating Together, 9*(2), 8–9.

van Balkom, H., & Welle Donker-Gimbrere, M. (1985). *Kiezen voor communicatie: van mensen met een motorische of meervoudige handicap (Choosing for communication: A handbook about the communication of motoric and multiple handicapped children).* Nijkerk, The Netherlands: Intro.

van Balkom, H., & Welle Donker-Gimbrere, M. (1994). *Kiezen voor communicatie: Een handboek voor mensen met een motorische of meervoudige handicap (Choosing for communication. A handbook for people with a motor or a multiple disability)* (2nd ed.). Nijkerk, The Netherlands: Intro.

Vanderheiden, G. C., & Harris-Vanderheiden, D. (1976). Communication techniques and aids for the nonverbal severely handicapped. In L. L. Lloyd (Ed.), *Communication assessment and intervention strategies* (pp. 607–652). Baltimore: University Park Press.

Vanderheiden, G. C., & Kelso, D. (1987). Comparative analysis of fixed-vocabulary communication acceleration techniques. *Augmentative and Alternative Communication, 3,* 196–206.

Vanderheiden, G. C., & Lloyd, L. L. (1986). Communication

systems and their components. In S. Blackstone (Ed.), *Augmentative communication: An introduction* (pp. 49–161). Rockville, MD: American Speech-Language-Hearing Association.

Vanderheiden, G. C., & Yoder, D. (1986). Overview. In S. Blackstone (Ed.), *Augmentative communication: An introduction* (pp. 1–28). Rockville, MD: American Speech-Language-Hearing Association.

Van Dijk, J. (1966). The first steps of the deaf-blind child towards language. *International Journal for the Education of the Blind, 15*, 112–114.

Van Dyke, D. C., Lang, D. J., Heide, F., van Duyne, S., & Soucek, M. J. (Eds.). (1990). *Clinical perspectives in the management of Down syndrome.* New York: Springer-Verlag.

van Hedel-van Grinsven, R. (1989). Communication and language development in a child with severe visual and auditory impairments: A case study and discussion of multiple modalities. *RE:view, 26*, 153–162.

van Oosterom, J., & Devereux, K. (1982). REBUS at Rees Thomas School. *Special Education: Forward Trends, 9*, 31–33.

van Oosterom, J., & Devereux, K. (1985). *Learning with rebuses.* Cambridgeshire, England: EARO, The Resource Centre.

Van Tatenhove, G. (1979, November). *Augmentative communication board development: A response training protocol.* Paper presented at the Annual Convention of the American Speech-Language-Hearing Association, Atlanta.

Van Tatenhove, G., Kovach, T., Privartsky, K. L., & Costello, J. (1993). Service delivery in augmentative and alternative communication: Expanding your resources. *Asha, 35*, 103–104.

Van Uden, A. (1983). *Diagnostic testing of deaf children: The syndrome of dyspraxia.* Lisse: Swets & Zeitlinger.

Varney, N. R. (1978). Linguistic correlates of pantomime recognition in aphasic patients. *Journal of Neurology, Neurosurgery and Psychiatry, 41*, 564–568.

Varney, N. R. (1982). Pantomime recognition defect in aphasia: Implications for the concept of asymbolia. *Brain and Language, 15*, 32–39.

Varney, N. R., & Benton, A. L. (1982). Qualitative aspects of pantomime recognition deficit in aphasia. *Brain and Cognition, 1*, 132–139.

Veale, T. K. (1994). Auditory integration training: The use of a new listening treatment within our profession. *American Journal of Speech-Language Pathology: A Journal of Clinical Practice, 3*(2), 12–15.

Venkatagiri, H. S. (1993). Efficiency of lexical prediction as a communication acceleration technique. *Augmentative and Alternative Communication, 9*, 161–167.

Venn, M. L., Wolery, M., Fleming, L. A., DeCesare, L. D., Morris, A., & Cuffs, M. S. (1993). Effects of teaching preschool peers to use the mand-model procedure during snack activities. *American Journal of Speech Language Pathology: A Journal of Clinical Practice, 3*, 38–46.

Vernon, M. (1972). Mind over mouth: A rationale for "total communication." *Volta Review, 74*, 529–540.

Vicker, B. (Ed.). (1974). *Nonoral communication system project 1964/1973.* Iowa City, IA: University of Iowa Campus Stores.

Viscardi, H. J., Jr., (1952). *A man's stature.* Middlebury, VT: Paul Eriksson.

Vision Research—A National Plan: 1983–1987. (1983). U.S. Department of Health and Human Services, NIH Publication No. 83-2472.

Visser, E. (1994). Barriers to employment. *Journal of Visual Impairment & Blindness, 88*, 177.

Volterra, V. (1990). Sign language acquisition and bilingualism. In S. Prillwitz & T. Vollhaber (Eds.), *Sign language research and application* (pp. 39–49). Hamburg, Germany: Signum Press.

von Glasserfeld, E. (1977). The Yerkish language and its automatic parser. In D. M. Rumbaugh (Ed.), *Language learning in a chimpanzee: The LANA Project.* New York: Academic Press.

von Tetzchner, S. (1985). Words and chips: Pragmatics and pidginization of computer-aided communication. *Child Language Teaching and Therapy, 1*, 298–305.

von Tetzchner, S., Grove, N., Loncke, F., Barnett, S., Woll, B., & Clibbens, J. (1996). Preliminaries to a comprehensive model of augmentative and alternative communication. In S. von Tetzchner & M. H. Jensen (Eds.), *European perspectives on augmentative and alternative communication* (pp. 19–36). London: Whurr.

von Tetzchner, S., & Martinsen, H. (1992). *Introduction to symbolic and augmentative communication.* San Diego, CA: Singular Publishing Group.

Wacker, D. P., Steege, M. W., Northrup, J., Sasso, G., Berg, W., Reimers, T., Cooper, L., Cigrand, K., & Donn, L. (1990). A component analysis of functional communication training across three topographies of severe behavior problems. *Journal of Applied Behavior Analysis, 23*, 417–429.

Wagner, P. A. (1994). Adaptations for administering the Peabody Picture Vocabulary Test-Revised to individuals with severe communication and motor dysfunctions. *Mental Retardation, 32*(2), 107–112.

Wagner, R., & Torgeson, J. (1987). The nature of phonological processing and its causal role in the acquisition of reading skills. *Psychological Bulletin, 101*, 192–212.

Walker, M. (1987, March). *The Makaton vocabulary: Uses and effectiveness.* Paper presented at the First International AFASIC Symposium, University of Reading, England.

Walker, M., Parsons, F., Cousins, S., Henderson, R., & Carpenter, B. (1985). *Symbols for Makaton.* Camberley, England: Makaton Vocabulary Development Project.

Wampler, D. (1971). *Linguistics of visual English.* Unpublished manuscript, Early Childhood Education Department, Aurally Handicapped Program, Santa Rosa City Schools, Santa Rosa, CA.

Wang, L., & Goodglass, H. (1992). Pantomime, praxis, and aphasia. *Brain and Language, 42*, 402–418.

Wanner, E., & Gleitman, L. R. (Eds.). (1982). *Language acquisition: The state of the art*. Cambridge, England: Cambridge University Press.

Wapner, W., & Gardner, H. (1981). Profiles of symbol-reading skills in organic patients. *Brain and Language, 12,* 303–312.

Ward, C. (1989). *Subsidy program for assistive devices*. Washington, DC: Rehabilitation Engineering Center.

Warren, S. F., & Rogers-Warren, A. K. (1985). Teaching functional language: An introduction. In S. F. Warren & A. K. Rogers-Warren (Eds.), *Teaching functional language* (pp. 3–23). Baltimore: University Park Press.

Warrick, A. (1984). Worldsign: A kinetic language. *Communicating Together, 2,* 17–19.

Washington State School for the Deaf. (1972). *An introduction to manual English*. Vancouver, WA: Author.

Wasson, C. (1994a). Multicultural demographics in AAC. *Special Interest Divisions: Augmentative and Alternative Communication (Division 12), 3*(3), 7.

Wasson, C. (1994b). Objective and subjective ratings of natural and synthetic speech passages by young adults without hearing impairment and older adults with and without hearing impairment. Unpublished manuscript, Purdue University, West Lafayette, IN.

Wasson, C., & Binnie, C. A. (1994, November). *Effects of synthetic speech on objective and subjective ratings by older adults with hearing impairment*. Paper presented at the Annual Convention of the American Speech-Language-Hearing Association, New Orleans.

Wasson, P., Tynan, T., & Gardiner, P. (1981). *Test adaptations for the handicapped*. San Antonio, TX: Education Service Center.

Watkins, L. T., Sprafkin, J. N., & Krolikowski, D. M. (1993). Using videotaped lessons to facilitate the development of manual signs skills in students with mental retardation. *Augmentative and Alternative Communication, 9,* 177–183.

Watkins, S. W., & Clark, T. C. (1991). A coactive sign system for children who are dual-sensory impaired. *American Annals of the Deaf, 136,* 321–324.

Watson, L. R., Layton, T. L., Pierce, P. L., & Abraham, L. M. (1994). Enhancing emerging literacy in a language preschool. *Language, Speech and Hearing Services in Schools, 25,* 136–145.

Watts, M., & Llewellyn-Jones, M. (1984a). *Teacher's handbook: Hands on*. Nottingham, England: Signit Project, Arnold Derrymount School.

Watts, M., & Llewellyn-Jones, M. (1984b). *User manual: Hands on*. Nottingham, England: Signit Project, Arnold Derrymount School.

Wayner, D. (1990). *Hearing aid handbook: Clinician's guide to client orientation*. Washington, DC: Gallaudet University Press.

Webster's new world dictionary of the American language. (1984). New York: Warner Books.

Webster's third international dictionary of the English language (Unabridged). (1976). Springfield, MA: G. & C. Merriam Company.

Wechsler, D. (1967). *Manual for the Wechsler preschool and primary scale of intelligence*. New York: The Psychological Corporation.

Wehman, P. (1993). *The ADA mandate for social change*. Baltimore: Paul H. Brookes Publishing.

Wehman, P., Wood, W., Everson, J. M., Goodwyn, R., & Conley, S. (1988). *Vocational education for multihandicapped youth with cerebral palsy*. Baltimore: Paul H. Brookes Publishing.

Weinrich, M. (1991). Computerized visual communication as an alternative communication system and therapeutic tool. *Journal of Neurolinguistics, 6,* 159–176.

Weinrich, M., McCall, D., Shoosmith, L., Thomas, K., Katzenberger, K., & Weber, C. (1993). Locative prepositional phrases in severe aphasia. *Brain and Language, 45,* 21–45.

Weinrich, M., McCall, D., Weber, C., Thomas, K., & Thornburg, L. (1995). Training on an iconic communication system for severe aphasia can improve natural language production. *Aphasiology, 9,* 343–364.

Weinrich, M., Steele, R., Carlson, G. S., Kleczewska, M., Wertz, R. T., & Baker, E. (1989). Processing of visual syntax by a globally aphasic patient. *Brain and Language, 36,* 391–405.

Weinrich, M., Steele, R., Kleczewska, M., Carlson, G. S., & Baker, E. (1987). Representation of verbs in a computerized visual communication system. In *Proceedings of the tenth annual RESNA conference*. Reston, VA: RESNA.

Weller, E. U., & Mahoney, G. (1983). A comparison of oral and total communication modalities on the language training of young mentally handicapped children. *Education and Training of the Mentally Retarded, 18,* 103–110.

Wells, G. (1986). *The meaning makers: Children learning language and using language to learn*. Portsmouth, NH: Heinemann Books.

Wendon, L. (1979). Exploring the scope of a picture code system for teaching reading and spelling. *Remedial Education, 7,* 33–42.

Wepman, J. M., & Jones, L. V. (1961). *The language modalities test for aphasia*. Chicago: Education Industry Service.

West, J. F., & Cannon, G. (1988). Essential collaborative consultation competencies for regular and special educators. *Journal of Learning Disabilities, 21,* 56–63.

West, J. F., & Idol, L. (1990). Collaborative consultation in the education of mildly handicapped and at-risk students. *Remedial and Special Education, 11,* 22–31.

Westby, C. E. (1990). Asking the right questions to the right people in the right ways. *Journal of Childhood Communication Disorders, 13,* 101–111.

Westminister School District. 21 IDELR 398 (CA SEA, 1994).

Wheeler, D. L., Jacobson, J. W., Paglieri, R. A., & Schwartz, A. A. (1993). An experimental assessment of facilitated communication. *Mental Retardation, 31,* 49–60.

Whitehouse, F. A. (1951). Teamwork: An approach to a higher professional level. *Exceptional Children, 18,* 75–82.

Whitley, K. (1985). Picture Communication Symbols (PCS): A review. *Aug-Communique, 3,* 3.

Wilbur, R., (1979). *American Sign Language and sign systems.* Baltimore: University Park Press.

Wilbur, R. (1987). *American Sign Language: Linguistic and applied dimensions* (2nd ed.). Boston: College-Hill.

Wilbur, R., & Jones, M. (1974). Some aspects of the bilingual/bimodal acquisition of sign language and English by three hearing children of deaf parents. In M. LaBally, R. Fox, & A. Bruck (Eds.), *Papers from the 10th regional meeting of the Chicago Linguistics Society.* Chicago: Chicago University Press.

Wilder, M. L. (1989). Effective use of technology with young children, *News Digest, 13,* 6–7.

Will, G. (1985). *James C. Hemphill lecture.* Paper presented at the Rehabilitation Institute of Chicago.

Williams, B. (1993). Kathy's story. *A.T. Quarterly, 4,* 7, 11.

Williams, B., Briggs, N., & Williams, R. (1979). Selecting, adapting, and understanding toys and recreation materials. In P. Weshman (Ed.), *Recreation programming for developmentally disabled persons* (pp. 15–36). Baltimore: University Park Press.

Williams, W. B., Stemach, G., Wolfe, S., & Stanger, C. (1993). *Lifespace access profile: Assistive technology planning for individuals with severe or multiple disabilities.* Sebastopol, CA: Lifespace Access.

Willows, D. M. (1991). Visual processes in learning disabilities. In B. Y. L. Wong (Ed.), *Learning about learning disabilities* (pp. 163–193). San Diego, CA: Academic Press.

Wills, K. (1981). Manual communication training for nonspeaking hearing children. *Journal of Pediatric Psychology, 6*(1), 15–27.

Wilson, K. D. (1980). Selection of a core lexicon for use with graphic communication systems. *Journal of Childhood Communication Disorders, 4,* 111–123.

Wilson, P. S. (1974, April). *Sign language as a means of communication for the mentally retarded.* Paper presented at the Eastern Psychological Association Conference.

Windsor, J., & Fristoe, M. (1991). Key word signing: Perceived and acoustic differences between signed and spoken narratives. *Journal of Speech and Hearing Research, 34,* 260–268.

Wing, L. (1989). The diagnosis of autism. In C. Gillberg (Ed.), *Diagnosis and treatment of autism* (pp. 5–32). New York: Plenum Press.

Wodlinger-Cohen, R. (1991). The manual representation of speech by deaf children, their mothers, and their teachers. In P. Siple & S. Fischer (Eds.), *Theoretical issues in sign language research. Vol. 2: Psychology* (pp. 149–169). Chicago: University of Chicago Press.

Wojcio, M., Gustason, G., & Zawolkow, E. (1983). *Music in motion.* Los Alamitos, CA: Modern Signs Press.

Wolery, M. (1989). Using direct observation in assessment. In D. B. Bailey & M. Wolery (Eds.) *Assessing infants and preschoolers with handicaps.* Columbus, OH: Merrill Publishing Co.

Wolfram, W. (1986). Language variation in the United States. In O. L. Taylor (Ed.), *Nature of communication disorders in culturally and linguistically diverse populations* (pp. 73–115). Austin, TX: Pro-Ed.

Woll, B. (1984). The comparative study of different sign languages. In F. Loncke, P. Boyes-Braem, & Y. Lebrun (Eds.), *Recent research on European sign languages* (pp. 79–91). Lisse: Swets & Zeitlinger.

Wood, C., Storr, J., & Reich, P. A. (Eds.). (1992). *Blissymbol reference guide.* Toronto, Canada: Blissymbolics Communication International.

Woodcock, R. W. (Ed.). (1965). *The rebus reading series.* Nashville, TN: George Peabody College, Institute on Mental Retardation and Intellectual Development.

Woodcock, R. W. (1968). *Rebuses as a medium in beginning reading instruction.* Nashville, TN: Institute on Mental Retardation and Intellectual Development.

Woodcock, R. W., Clark, C. R., & Davies, C. O. (1968). *Peabody rebus reading program.* Circle Pines, MN: American Guidance Service.

Woodcock, R. W., & Johnson, B. (1977). *Woodcock-Johnson psychoeducational battery.* Hingham, MA: Teaching Resources.

World Health Organization (1980). *International classification of impairments, disabilities, and handicaps.* Geneva, Switzerland: World Health Organization.

Worrall, N., & Singh, Y. (1983). Teaching TMR children to read using integrated picture cueing. *American Journal of Mental Deficiency, 8,* 422–429.

Wouts, W. (1987). Aka: Pourquoi? *Questions de Logopédie, 14,* 31–51.

Writer, J. (1984). A movement-based approach to the education of students who are sensory impaired/multihandicapped. In L. Goetz, D. Guess, & K. Stremel-Campbell (Eds.), *Innovative program designs for individuals with dual sensory impairments* (pp. 191–223). Baltimore: Paul H. Brookes Publishing.

Yaida, J., & Rubin, S. E. (1992). Job roles of assistive technology service providers in the United States. *Journal of Rehabilitation Research, 15,* 277–287.

Yamadori, A., Nagashima, T., & Tamaki, N. (1983). Ideogram writing in a disconnection syndrome. *Brain and Language, 19,* 346–356.

Yamadori, A., Osumi, Y., Ikeda, H., & Kanazawa, Y. (1980). Left unilateral agraphia and tactile anomia. *Archives of Neurology, 37,* 88–91.

Ylvisaker, M., & Urbanczyk, B. (1994). Assessment and treatment of speech, swallowing, and communication disorders following traumatic brain injury. In M. A. J. Finlayson & S. C. Garner (Eds.), *Brain injury rehabilitation: Clinical considerations* (pp. 157–187). Baltimore: Williams & Wilkins.

Yoder, D. E. (1980). Communication systems for non-speech children. *New Directions for Exceptional Children, 2,* 63–78.

York, J., Nietupski, J., & Hamre-Nietupski, S. (1985). A decision-making process for using microswitches. *Journal of the Association for Persons with Severe Handicaps, 10,* 214–223.

York, J., & Vandercook, T. (1990). Strategies for achieving an integrated education for middle school students with severe disabilities. *Remedial and Special Education, 11*, 6–16.

York, J., & Weimann, G. (1991). Accommodating severe physical disabilities. In J. Reichle, J. York, & J. Sigafoos (Eds.), *Implementing augmentative and alternative communication: Strategies for learners with severe disabilities* (pp. 239–256). Baltimore: Paul H. Brookes Publishing.

Yorkston, K. M. (1989). Early intervention in amyotrophic lateral sclerosis: A case presentation. *Augmentative and Alternative Communication, 5*, 67–70.

Yorkston, K. M., Beukelman, D., & Bell, K. (1988). *Clinical management of dysarthric speakers*. San Diego, CA: College-Hill Press.

Yorkston, K. M., Beukelman, D. R., Smith, K., & Tice, R. (1990). Extended communication samples of augmented communication II: Analysis of multiword sequences. *Journal of Speech and Hearing Disorders, 55*, 225–230.

Yorkston, K. M., Dowden, P., Honsinger, M., Marriner, N., & Smith, K. (1988). A comparison of standard and user vocabulary lists. *Augmentative and Alternative Communication, 4*, 189–210.

Yorkston, K. M., Honsinger, M. J., Dowden, P. A., & Marriner, N. (1989). Vocabulary selection: A case report. *Augmentative and Alternative Communication, 5*, 101–108.

Yorkston, K. M., & Karlan, G. R. (1986). Assessment procedures. In S. Blackstone (Ed.), *Augmentative communica-*tion: An introduction (pp. 163–196). Rockville, MD: American Speech-Language-Hearing Association.

Yorkston, K. M., Smith, K., & Beukelman, D. (1990). Extended communication samples of augmented communicators I: A comparison of individualized versus standard single word vocabularies. *Journal of Speech and Hearing Disorders, 55*, 217–224.

Young, C. V. (1986). Developmental disabilities. In J. Katz (Ed.), *Handbook of clinical audiology* (3rd ed., pp. 689–706). Baltimore: Williams & Wilkins.

Yovetich, W. S., & Paivio, A. (1980, August). Cognitive processing of Bliss-like symbols by normal populations: A report on four studies. *Proceedings of the European Association for Special Education*, Helsinki, Finland.

Zangari, C., Lloyd, L. L., & Vicker, B. (1994). Augmentative and alternative communication: An historic perspective. *Augmentative and Alternative Communication, 10*, 27–59.

Zantal-Weiner, K. (1994, June). *Emerging trends in technology for students with disabilities*. Paper presented at the Annual Conference of RESNA, Nashville, TN.

Zarcone, J. R., Rodgers, T. A., Iwata, B. A., Rourke, D. A., & Dorsey, M. F. (1991). Reliability analysis of the Motivation Assessment Scale: A failure to replicate. *Research in Developmental Disabilities, 12*, 349–360.

Zavalani, T. S. (1991). *Jet Era Glyphs: A pictographic communication system*. Panorama City, CA: Author.

Zimmerman, I. C., Steiner, V. S., & Pond, R. E. (1979). *Preschool language scale: Revised*. Columbus, OH: Merrill Publishing.

Author Index

Abraham, L. M., 430
Accardo, P. J., 299, 300
Acredolo, L., 312
Adamovich, B. B., 363
Adams, M. J., 421, 429, 436
Adams, M. R., 19, 90
Adamson, L. B., 75, 299, 300
Adler, S., 408
Ahlgren, I., 81, 82, 93
Aitchison, C., 267
Albano, M., 391
Albert, M. L., 359
Albin, R. W., 458
Albritton, E., 54, 222
Alcorn, S., 101
Alegria, J., 99
Alexander, G. C., 192
Alexander, P. K., 268, 271, 272, 273, 274
Alexander, R., 182, 284
Allaire, J. H., 254
Allen, D. A., 260, 264
Allen, G. D., 264, 477, 478
Allen, N., 412
Allen, P., 138
Allen, R. M., 186
Allport, A., 340, 341, 343, 348
Alpert, C. L., 249
Alpiner, J. G., 184, 254, 255, 256, 260
Altman, M., 349
Altman, R., 446
Alwell, M., 333, 445, 454
Amend, S., 73
American Speech-Language-Hearing
    Association (ASHA), 3, 384, 387
Anderson, E., 328
Anderson, N. B., 413
Anderson, R., 180, 420, 436
Anderson, S. R., 240
Ansel, B. M., 475
Anthony, D., 97
Apffel, J., 54
Aram, D. M., 446
Aristotle, 13
Arkell, C., 254
Arnason, B. G. W., 358
Aronson, A., 356
Arthur, G., 178
Arthur, M., 175
Arvidson, H. H., 1, 18, 127, 169, 199, 226,
    340, 474
Asher, P., 418
Atkinson, J., 272, 273, 274
Atwater, S. W., 284
Auerbach, S., 363
Ault, M. H., 460

Baer, D. M., 474
Bailey, B., 50–51, 273, 277–278, 324
Bailey, D. B., 169, 176, 185, 193, 194
Bailey, J. S., 458
Bailey, R. W., 117
Bakeman, R., 75
Baker, B., 66, 118, 210, 211, 442

Baker, C., 82, 93, 97
Baker, E., 340, 342, 344, 347, 348
Baker, L., 446
Baldwin, D. S., 401
Baldwin, V. L., 277
Balick, S., 236
Ball, E., 415
Bane, M. C., 272, 274
Bangs, T., 180
Bannatyne, A., 71
Barnes, H. D., 199
Barney, H. L., 474–475
Baroody, S. M., 187, 329, 330
Barresi, B., 340
Barron, R. W., 443
Barsch, R., 418
Barton, L. E., 460
Basil, C., 7
Bates, E., 446
Batshaw, M. L., 183, 267, 268, 269, 270,
    274, 299, 300
Batstone, S., 271, 272, 275, 276, 277
Battison, R., 99
Battle, D. E., 190, 408, 413
Baudel-Cantgrit, B., 59
Bauman, K. E., 460
Bauman, R. A., 473
Baumgart, D., 182, 303, 306, 320, 323
Bayles, K., 359
Bayley, N., 178
Beare, P. L., 337
Beatties, P. M., 401
Beaulac, D. A., 262
Bebian, R. A. A., 18
Beck, J., 332
Bedrosian, J. L., 187, 188
Beevers, R., 275
Begab, M. J., 20
Belfiore, P. J., 123, 336, 398, 399, 470, 478
Belkin, S. C., 284–285
Bell, K., 181, 357
Bellugi, U., 81, 85, 86, 90, 93, 218, 315,
    341, 353
Bender, R., 145
Benedict, H., 199–200
Benjamin, B. J., 436
Bennet, T. L., 257, 259
Bennett, D., 22, 236
Benson, H., 185
Bentler, R. A., 255
Bentley, D. W., 267
Benton, A. L., 354
Bergen, A. F., 281, 284, 285, 286, 287, 291,
    292
Berger, K., 199, 201, 203
Bergman, B., 81, 93
Bergman, J. S., 61
Berko, R. M., 27, 28, 29
Berkowitz, S. F., 55, 462
Berninger, V. W., 418, 425
Bernstein, M. E., 97–98
Berotti, D., 447
Berra, Y., 11

Berrigan, C., 330
Berry, T., 340, 347
Bersani, H. A., Jr., 78, 219, 224
Bertenthal, B. I., 285
Bertoni, B., 340, 343
Bess, F. H., 254, 257, 260, 261, 262
Beukelman, D. R., 10, 13, 14, 42, 46, 50, 51,
    56, 70, 71, 75, 116, 117, 118, 169, 170,
    172, 173, 174, 175, 181, 182, 185, 186,
    189, 191, 193, 194, 195, 199, 201, 205,
    206, 208, 209, 213, 226, 227, 228, 230,
    232, 236, 242, 278, 279, 306, 309, 310,
    315, 317, 320, 321, 335, 340, 350, 351,
    352, 356, 357, 358, 359, 362, 363, 364,
    365, 366, 410, 412, 422, 441, 442, 443,
    461, 475, 477
Bigge, J., 182, 266
Bihm, E. M., 458
Bijou, S. W., 460
Biklen, D., 330
Bilyeu, D., 201, 317
Binnie, C. A., 264
Biorn-Henriksen, T., 359
Birch, E. E., 272, 274
Bird, F., 448, 456, 458, 464
Bishop, D., 327, 419
Bishop, K., 436, 443
Bishop, V., 272, 273
Blachman, B. A., 414, 436, 439
Black, J., 331
Blackman, J. A., 254
Blackstone, S. W., 42, 129, 131, 169, 170,
    171, 175, 176, 185, 186, 187, 236, 430
Blake, A., 389
Blake, R., 262
Blau, A. F., 212, 431
Bligh, S. 387
Blischak, D. M., 38, 39, 40, 41, 42, 71, 104,
    109, 169, 191, 215, 233, 254, 276, 277,
    299, 315, 333, 414, 419, 436, 443, 447,
    470, 477, 478
Bliss, C., 22, 35, 58–59, 60
Block, J., 364
Blonsky, E. R., 357
Bloom, L., 179, 200, 201, 204–205, 206
Bloomberg, K., 54, 56, 58, 61
Blumbergs, P. C., 357
Blyden, A. E., 56
Boa, S., 232
Bodine, C., 181, 182
Boehme, R., 284
Boller, F., 357
Bolton, S. O., 180
Bonet, J. P., 80
Bonvillian, J., 18, 80, 315, 354
Boonzaier, D., 59
Boothe, R. G., 272
Boothroyd, A., 264
Borden, G. J., 148
Borel-Maisonny, S., 101, 104
Bornhoeft, D., 10
Bornstein, H., 67, 97, 316, 463
Borst, J. M., 474

SUBJECT INDEX

AAC. *See* Augmentative and alternative communication
AAC Feature Match Software, 231
AAC system, 41
  assessment of, 194–195, 478–479
AAC user, 38–39, 169
  assessment of, 175–191
  cultural background of, 215, 216, 406
  developing literacy in, 418–421
  experiential background of, 215
  preferences of, 224
  symbol selection and, 215, 216, 224
  variables involving, 215, 216
Abbreviation expansion, 117–118, 156, 161–162
Abstraction, level of, 77, 86–87
Abstract referent, 40–41
Academic and literacy abilities, assessment of, 184–185
Access, adapted, 162–163
AccessBliss™, 164
Accessibility, of symbols, 217
Access options, 132–135
Access Window™, 142
Accountability, 239–240
ACOLUG (Augmented Communicators On–Line Users' Group), 25
Acoustic symbols, 88
  electronically produced, 49, 77
  without linguistic characteristics, 88, 89
  pairing with graphic symbols, 470
Acquired disorders, 340–366
  Alzheimer's disease (AD), 359–362
  amyotrophic lateral sclerosis (ALS), 14, 19, 170, 236, 355–356
  aphasia, 19, 236, 340–355
  cervical spinal cord injury, 362–363
  multiple sclerosis, 14, 358–359
  Parkinson's disease, 14, 356–357
  progressive supranuclear palsy (PSP), 357–358
  traumatic brain injury (TBI), 2, 165, 235, 267, 363–366
ACS EvalPAC, 157, 158, 159
Acuity Card Procedure, 272
ADA. *See* Americans with Disabilities Act
ADAMLAB, 156, 157
Adapted access, 162–163
Adaptive Communication Systems, 71
Adaptive Firmware Card (AFC), 111, 142
Adobe™, 145
Adolescents, assessment of literacy in, 427–428
Adults
  assessment of literacy in, 427–428
  vocabularies of, 201–204
African Americans, 368, 406–407, 408
Age, and vocabulary selection, 205
Agglutinations, 78, 90
Aggression, 445, 446. *See also* Problem behavior

Aided communication, 1, 31, 34, 38, 44–46, 127, 278–279, 326–327
Aided language stimulation, 313–314
Aided symbols, 1, 31, 34, 38, 44–46, 48–79
  aided representations of manual signs and gestures, 49, 66–69
  alphabet-based, 49, 69–72
  arbitrary logographs and shapes, 49, 75–77
  characteristics of, 77–78
  communicative effectiveness of, 462
  electronically produced vibratory/acoustic, 49, 77
  encoding, 469–470
  existing repertoire of, 466
  intelligibility of, 461–462
  learnability of, 462
  object-based, 48–51
  partially picture-based symbols with linguistic characteristics, 49, 57–65
  phonemic- or phonic-based, 49, 72–75
  primarily picture-based symbols of dedicated VOCAs, 49, 65–66
  primarily picture-based symbols without linguistic characteristics, 49, 51–57
  problem behavior and, 461–468
  symbol selection and, 217, 221, 222–225
  unaided symbols vs., 217, 221, 222–225, 461–468
  See also specific types of symbols
Alexis B. v. Harwich Public Schools (1988), 377
Alphabet(s)
  manual, 80, 100
  phonetic, 73–74
Alphabet-based symbols
  aided symbols, 49, 69–72
  unaided symbols, 98–99, 101
Alphabet de Kinemes Assistes (AKA), 99, 101, 103
Alphabet encoding, 117
Alphabet glove, 278
Alphabetic/numeric arrangements, 131
Alphanumeric encoding, 118
AlphaTalker™, 120, 147, 148, 152, 157, 158, 159
ALS. *See* Amyotrophic lateral sclerosis
Altair 8800 computer, 138
Alzheimer's disease (AD), 359–362
Ambiguity, degree of, 46, 78
Amblyopia, 269
American Association on Mental Retardation (AAMR), 482
American Guidance Service (AGS), 53
American Indians, 408
American Manual Alphabet, 100
American Sign Language (ASL), 21, 37, 63, 81, 91
  conventionality of symbols in, 84
  defined, 41
  efficiency of, 221

  handshapes in, 92, 93
  symbols used in, 219
  See also Manual signs
American Speech-Language-Hearing Association (ASHA), 3, 15, 24–25, 173, 177, 192, 233, 254, 384, 481, 482, 483
  code of ethics of, 382, 384–385
  on facilitated communication, 330–331
Americans with Disabilities Act (ADA) of 1990 (PL 101–336), 15, 21, 369, 380, 400–401
Amer-Ind, 90
Amplification, of hearing, 261, 262, 263
Amyotrophic lateral sclerosis (ALS), 14, 19, 170, 236, 355–356
Analog recordings, 147
Animals, communication by, 19
Animated manual signs and gestures, 69
Anterior elements, in seating, 290, 291–292
Anterior superior iliac spines (ASIS), 288
Anterior visual pathway disorders, 270–271
Anticipatory behavior, preintentional, 302–303, 304
Aphasia, 19, 236, 340–355
  classification scheme used with, 350–353, 354
  communication characteristics of, 341
  defined, 340
  global, 341–355
  intervention with, 341, 348–355
  multiple profile of symbolic capacities in, 353–355
  severe, 341–355
Appeals, legal, 379
Apple® computers, 111–112, 138, 142, 143, 144
Apple Desktop Bus™ (ADP) port, 142
Apple+™, 140
AppleTalk®, 166
Apraxia, 181, 236, 355
Arbitrary logographs and shapes, 49, 75–77
Arbitrary symbols, 40, 49, 60, 75–77, 324–327
Arc, The. *See* The Arc
Arms, position in seating, 286, 292–293
Arousal problems, 283
Arthur Adaptation of the Leiter International Performance Scale, 178
Artificial larynx, 20, 34, 110, 111
Artificial sign systems, 81, 97
ASCII (American Standard Code Information Interchange), 142
ASHA. *See* American Speech-Language-Hearing Association
Asian Americans, 407, 408
ASL. *See* American Sign Language
Assertiveness, 470–472
Assessment, 169–198
  of AAC system, 194–195, 478–479
  of AAC user, 175–191
  of academic abilities, 184–185